Handbook of Autism

Handbook of Autism

Edited by Paul Hiddleston

hayle medical
New York

Hayle Medical,
750 Third Avenue, 9th Floor,
New York, NY 10017, USA

Visit us on the World Wide Web at:
www.haylemedical.com

ISBN: 978-1-63241-738-1

Printed in China.

Cataloging-in-Publication Data

Handbook of autism / edited by Paul Hiddleston.
p. cm.
Includes bibliographical references and index.
ISBN 978-1-63241-738-1
1. Autism. 2. Autism--Diagnosis. 3. Hyperlexia. 4. Autism spectrum disorders.
I. Hiddleston, Paul.
RC553.A88 H36 2019
616.858 82--dc23

Table of Contents

Preface IX

Chapter 1 **Video Game Playing Effects on Obesity in an Adolescent with Autism Spectrum Disorder** 1
Brandy E. Strahan and Jennifer H. Elder

Chapter 2 **Characteristics of Children who Lost the Diagnosis of Autism** 7
Nahit Motavalli Mukaddes, Mustafa Deniz Tutkunkardas, Oktay Sari, Aydan Aydin and Pınar Kozanoglu

Chapter 3 **Mental Health Services for Individuals with High Functioning Autism Spectrum Disorder** 17
Johanna K. Lake, Andrea Perry and Yona Lunsky

Chapter 4 **Dietary Intake and Plasma Levels of Choline and Betaine in Children with Autism Spectrum Disorders** 26
Joanna C. Hamlin, Margaret Pauly, Stepan Melnyk, Oleksandra Pavliv, William Starrett, Tina A. Crook and S. Jill James

Chapter 5 **Effectiveness of Methylcobalamin and Folinic Acid Treatment on Adaptive Behavior in Children with Autistic Disorder is Related to Glutathione Redox Status** 33
Richard E. Frye, Stepan Melnyk, George Fuchs, Tyra Reid, Stefanie Jernigan, Oleksandra Pavliv, Amanda Hubanks, David W. Gaylor, Laura Walters and S. Jill James

Chapter 6 **Gaze Behavior of Children with ASD toward Pictures of Facial Expressions** 42
Soichiro Matsuda, Yasuyo Minagawa and Junichi Yamamoto

Chapter 7 **The Michigan Autism Spectrum Questionnaire: A Rating Scale for High-Functioning Autism Spectrum Disorders** 50
M. Ghaziuddin and K.Welch

Chapter 8 ***Tsc2* Haploinsufficiency has Limited Effects on Fetal Brain Cytokine Levels during Gestational Immune Activation** 55
Dan Ehninger

Chapter 9 **The Effects of Rhythm and Robotic Interventions on the Imitation/Praxis, Interpersonal Synchrony and Motor Performance of Children with Autism Spectrum Disorder (ASD)** 62
Sudha M. Srinivasan, Maninderjit Kaur, Isabel K. Park, Timothy D. Gifford, Kerry L. Marsh and Anjana N. Bhat

Chapter 10 **Epigenetics and Autism** 80
Tafari Mbadiwe and Richard M. Millis

Chapter 11 **Back to Basic: Do Children with Autism Spontaneously Look at Screen Displaying a Face or an Object?** 89
Marie Guimard-Brunault, Nadia Hernandez, Laetitia Roché, Sylvie Roux, Catherine Barthélémy, Joëlle Martineau and Frédérique Bonnet-Brilhault

Chapter 12 **Parent Training Interventions for Toddlers with Autism Spectrum Disorder** 96
Audrée Jeanne Beaudoin, Guillaume Sébire, and Mélanie Couture

Chapter 13 **Early Intervention with a Parent-Delivered Massage Protocol Directed at Tactile Abnormalities Decreases Severity of Autism and Improves Child-to-Parent Interactions** 111
Louisa M. T. Silva, Mark Schalock, Kristen R. Gabrielsen, Sarojini S. Budden, Martha Buenrostro and Gretchen Horton

Chapter 14 **Computer Vision Tools for Low-Cost and Noninvasive Measurement of Autism-Related Behaviors in Infants** 127
Jordan Hashemi, Mariano Tepper, Thiago Vallin Spina, Amy Esler, Vassilios Morellas, Nikolaos Papanikolopoulos, Helen Egger, Geraldine Dawson and Guillermo Sapiro

Chapter 15 **Mild Dermatoglyphic Deviations in Adolescents with Autism Spectrum Disorders and Average Intellectual Abilities as Compared to Typically Developing Boys** 139
Esther I. de Bruin, John H. Graham, Anneke Louwerse and Anja C. Huizink

Chapter 16 **Longitudinal Study of Sensory Features in Children with Autism Spectrum Disorder** 145
Lucia Perez Repetto, Emmanuelle Jasmin, Eric Fombonne, Erika Gisel and Mélanie Couture

Chapter 17 **Autism Spectrum Disorder Screening Instruments for Very Young Children** 153
Patricia O. Towle and Patricia A. Patrick

Chapter 18 **Neuropsychological Characteristics of Children with Mixed Autism and ADHD** 182
Costanza Colombi and Mohammad Ghaziuddin

Chapter 19 **Social Skills Intervention Participation and Associated Improvements in Executive Function Performance** 187
Shawn E. Christ, Janine P. Stichter, Karen V. O'Connor, Kimberly Bodner, Amanda J. Moffitt and Melissa J. Herzog

Chapter 20 **What do Parents Think about Chromosomal Microarray Testing? A Qualitative Report from Parents of Children with Autism Spectrum Disorders** 200
Lei Xu, Linda Crane Mitchell, Alice R. Richman and Kaitlyn Clawson

Chapter 21 **Factor Structure, Internal Consistency and Screening Sensitivity of the GARS-2 in a Developmental Disabilities Sample** 209
Martin A. Volker, Elissa H. Dua, Christopher Lopata, Marcus L. Thomeer, Jennifer A. Toomey, Audrey M. Smerbeck, Jonathan D. Rodgers, Joshua R. Popkin, Andrew T. Nelson and Gloria K. Lee

Chapter 22 **Defining Autism: Variability in State Education Agency Definitions of and Evaluations for Autism Spectrum Disorders**.....221
Malinda L. Pennington, Douglas Cullinan and Louise B. Southern

Chapter 23 **Characteristics of Two-Year College Students on the Autism Spectrum and their Support Services Experiences**.....229
Anne M. Roux, Paul T. Shattuck, Jessica E. Rast, Julianna A. Rava, Amy D. Edwards, Xin Wei, Mary McCracken and Jennifer W. Yu

Chapter 24 **A Randomised Control Trial of the Impact of a Computer-based Activity Programme upon the Fitness of Children with Autism**.....239
Kathleen Dickinson and Maurice Place

Chapter 25 **Associations between Familial Rates of Psychiatric Disorders and De Novo Genetic Mutations in Autism**.....248
Kyleen Luhrs, Tracey Ward, Caitlin M. Hudac, Jennifer Gerdts, Holly A. F. Stessman, Evan E. Eichler and Raphael A. Bernier

Chapter 26 **Support Needs and Coping Strategies as Predictors of Stress Level among Mothers of Children with Autism Spectrum Disorder**.....256
Sheri R. Kiami and Shelley Goodgold

Chapter 27 **Experiences of Dental Care and Dental Anxiety in Adults with Autism Spectrum Disorder**.....266
My Blomqvist, Göran Dahllöf and Susanne Bejerot

Permissions

List of Contributors

Index

Preface

This book was inspired by the evolution of our times; to answer the curiosity of inquisitive minds. Many developments have occurred across the globe in the recent past which has transformed the progress in the field.

Autism is a developmental disorder. The main characteristics of this disorder are one's inability to socially interact in a proper manner, and one's restricted and repetitive behavior. Some common behavioral habits of autistic children include stereotyped behaviors, compulsive behaviors, ritualistic behaviors, staying stuck to restricted interests, and self-injury. Autism is a disease with a complex genetic basis. Such complexity arises due to the interaction among multiple genes, epigenetic factors and the environment, which influence gene expression. The diagnosis of autism is based on an examination of behavior. Autism Diagnostic Interview-Revised and Autism Diagnostic Observation Schedule are commonly used diagnostic tools. Increasing functional independence and better quality of care are the focus areas of autism management. Intensive and sustained special education programs, along with speech and behavioral therapies, help autistic individuals to achieve better social skills and communication skills. This book contains some path-breaking studies in autism. It includes some of the vital pieces of work being conducted across the world, on various topics related to autism. Those in search of information to further their knowledge will be greatly assisted by this book.

This book was developed from a mere concept to drafts to chapters and finally compiled together as a complete text to benefit the readers across all nations. To ensure the quality of the content we instilled two significant steps in our procedure. The first was to appoint an editorial team that would verify the data and statistics provided in the book and also select the most appropriate and valuable contributions from the plentiful contributions we received from authors worldwide. The next step was to appoint an expert of the topic as the Editor-in-Chief, who would head the project and finally make the necessary amendments and modifications to make the text reader-friendly. I was then commissioned to examine all the material to present the topics in the most comprehensible and productive format.

I would like to take this opportunity to thank all the contributing authors who were supportive enough to contribute their time and knowledge to this project. I also wish to convey my regards to my family who have been extremely supportive during the entire project.

Editor

1

Video Game Playing Effects on Obesity in an Adolescent with Autism Spectrum Disorder

Brandy E. Strahan[1] and Jennifer H. Elder[2]

[1] *University of West Florida, 11000 University Parkway, Building 37, Pensacola, FL 32514, USA*
[2] *University of Florida, College of Nursing, P.O. Box 100187, Gainesville, FL 32610-0187, USA*

Correspondence should be addressed to Brandy E. Strahan; bstrahan@uwf.edu

Academic Editor: Hansen Wang

Adolescent obesity has tripled in the past two decades, and adolescents with disabilities, specifically autism spectrum disorders (ASD), may be at greater risk for obesity due to the behavioral, physical, and psychosocial complications related to their disorder. This case study reports the effects of video game playing on an obese adolescent with ASD and illustrates the use of a multiple baseline single subject design. Over 12 weeks, the participant played inactive (6 weeks) and active video games (6 weeks) on the Wii console. Physiological data were evaluated weekly at home. Stress and anxiety were measured via the Stress Survey Schedule for Individuals with Autism and Other Pervasive Non-Developmental Disorders (SSS) and the Behavior Assessment System for Children Second Edition (BASC-2) pre- and postintervention. The Therapy Attitude Inventory (TAI) was used to determine parental perception of video game playing as a socially valid intervention to reduce stress and anxiety. Results demonstrated that active video game playing slowed and/or reduced weight and BMI with minimal changes to waist-to-hip ratios, triceps skinfolds, and stress and anxiety. This study demonstrates how alternative methods for physical activity may be used to improve health outcomes of overweight/obese adolescents with ASD and suggests directions for future research.

1. Introduction

Adolescent obesity has tripled over the past two decades across all race and ethnic groups, genders, and socioeconomic classes creating an epidemic and public health crisis [1]. Indeed adolescent obesity can contribute to serious health problems such as depression, diabetes mellitus, sleep apnea, and cardiovascular disease as well as social problems such as isolation, stigma, discrimination, and low self-esteem [2, 3]. Furthermore because nearly 70% of obese adolescents continue the trend into adulthood, [4, 5] consequences to their health are likely to be long term [6].

Children with developmental disabilities, such as those with autism spectrum disorders (ASD), may be particularly vulnerable to the development of obesity due to the behavioral, physical, and psychosocial complications related to their disorder [2, 7]. Indeed, children with ASD have a higher prevalence of obesity (30.4%) compared to children without ASD (23.6% [2]). Although numerous studies address obesity in typically developing adolescents, none address the problem among the ASD population.

ASD presents unique challenges for researchers and warrants novel interventions that can be tailored to meet the needs of individuals to address the challenge of obesity. Many caregivers of adolescents with ASD are often focused on problematic ASD features, with less concern for adverse health behaviors and weight [8], aberrant eating patterns and atypical physical activity [2], and/or excessive consumption of junk food [2, 9]. Although exercise has been shown to reduce stress and anxiety, which may be exhibited as tantrums in the ASD population, it may not be encouraged due to motor impairments, including poor motor skills, uneven developmental milestone acquisition, low muscle tone, and postural instability, frequently leading to decreased physical activity [2, 9]. Inactivity is not the only contributor to weight gain in children with ASD. Medications, such as Risperdal, often used to treat common features of ASD (such as self-injurious behavior, mood swings, and aggression towards others) have weight gain as a side effect [10]. Obesity is estimated to be 40% more likely in adolescents with ASD [2] than their typically developing peers and is rising at a rate that will outpace that of the general population [3].

Since nearly three-quarters of obese adolescents with ASD continue the obesity trend into adulthood, many develop comorbidities that are beyond the scope of previous interventions [5]. Additionally, young adults with ASD have a decrease in physical activity and become lethargic perpetuating the vicious cycle of caloric intake exceeding output. Indeed, one study of young adults with ASD found the mean sitting time in one day was 13 hours and that the lack of physical activity was due to disability; cost of equipment; lack of energy, leader, or partner, and athletic ability [5]. Clearly, there is a need to develop an intervention targeting the problem of obesity in adolescents with ASD.

One such creative approach is the use of electronic video games as an intervention to treat obesity in adolescents with ASD. Maddison et al. [11] conducted a randomized controlled trial with typically developing adolescents who were overweight or obese ($N = 322$) and were sedentary video gamers in order to evaluate the effects of physically active video games on participants' weight, body composition, physical activity, and fitness. Results revealed that the intervention group had a slight change in body mass index (BMI) from baseline ($p = .02$), a reduction in body fat ($p = .02$), and an increase in active video game play time ($p < .01$). In contrast, adolescents in the control group continued to gain weight playing inactive video games. These findings indicate that creative interventions have the potential to slow weight gain, an important component in reducing obesity.

Physical activity interventions represent an effective method to induce weight loss in adolescents with ASD. Active video gaming could have an effect on obesity in male adolescents with ASD since 41% of their free time is spent playing video games [12] and they may willingly adopt an active version of their favorite game or activity [11]. Thus, electronic video gaming provides an innovative alternative approach for treatment of obesity in adolescents with ASD that can be adapted to the individuals' preference of games and activities.

There are no studies to date that have examined the effects of video game playing on obese adolescents with ASD. Thus, the purpose of this case study was to determine the feasibility and effectiveness of active video game playing for an obese adolescent with ASD.

2. Method

The Institutional Review Board at University of Florida in Gainesville approved this work. The participant, "JD," was a Caucasian male adolescent with mild-to-moderate ASD, diagnosed at the age of 5, and was 15 years of age. JD's BMI classified him as obese, 28.7 kg/m^2, as defined by the CDC, and had other medical diagnoses such as Attention Deficit/Hyperactivity Disorder (ADHD) and Obsessive Compulsive Disorder (OCD). His daily medication regimen included Intuniv, 3 mg per day, Clonidine, 0.15 mg at night, Prozac, 20 mg per day, Trazadone, 75 mg at night, Clemastine, 0.67 mg in the morning and 4.02 mg at night, probiotics, and a multivitamin. He lived with his mother and a sibling and had weekend visitation with his father. JD was enrolled in public school and did not participate in any extracurricular activities. He typically stayed home and socialized with his family and a neighbor boy who is four years younger than JD. His diet consisted of two bowls of cereal or muffins for breakfast, pizza or sandwich with chips for lunch, and chicken nuggets, pasta, or pizza for dinner. Although his family offered healthier selections, he consistently chose these items.

2.1. Video Game Intervention. JD and his parents were told that they were participating in a video game playing intervention to learn more about exercise via active video game playing and weight in adolescents with ASD. JD and his mother were blinded to the study hypotheses and were told not to change any habitual physical activities or eating habits over the course of the study.

The active video game playing was completed using the Wii console and accessories needed. JD was given gaming options rated "E" for everyone for the Wii console. He chose an inactive and an active game. Baseline data were collected for four weeks prior to any gaming. JD's physiological data (height, weight, BMI, triceps skinfold, and waist-to-hip ratio) were collected during baseline and gaming weeks while gaming data (activity steps and playing time) were collected each week during interventional weeks of the study. JD also kept a daily food and activity log during all weeks of the study. After collection of baseline data, JD was instructed to play the chosen inactive video game for four or more days a week for a minimum of 30 minutes each day for a total of six weeks. Then, he played an active video game for four or more days a week for a minimum of 30 minutes each day for a total of six weeks.

2.2. Weight. JD was weighed at the same time of day using the same digital scale. Weight was obtained once a week during baseline and intervention phases in his home. JD wore similar clothing for weight assessment during the entire study.

2.3. Body Mass Index (BMI). Body mass index (BMI) was calculated using JD's height and weight as defined by the CDC [13] and obtained weekly during baseline and intervention phases. Height was measured in inches with JD standing flat footed with no shoes and his weight was measured in pounds. Height was then converted to meters and weight to kilograms (weight/height^2). Once the BMI was calculated, his weight status was determined using an age- and sex-specific percentile for children aged 2–19 years. Overweight was defined as "a BMI at or above the 85th percentile and lower than the 95th percentile for children of the same age and sex" and obese as "a BMI at or above the 95th percentile for children of the same age and sex" [13].

2.4. Waist-to-Hip Ratio. Waist-to-hip ratio was measured in inches using the same measuring tape and collected weekly during baseline and intervention phases. The ratio provides an indication of the overall health risk indicating low, moderate, or high risk for developing diseases such as cardiovascular disease or diabetes. Ratio norms are different for girls and boys, thus removing gender bias. Waist-to-hip ratio was obtained by measuring around the smallest part of the waist (just above the naval) and the widest part of the hips without pants or shorts but over underpants.

2.5. Triceps Skinfold. Anthropometric data, triceps skinfolds, were measured on the right arm using Harpenden calipers. Measurements were obtained weekly during baseline and intervention phases. Triceps skinfolds have been shown to more adequately correlate body fat percentages for children and adolescents while height and weight are better instruments for total body fat percentages [14].

2.6. Stress and Anxiety. Stress and anxiety were measured using the Stress Survey Schedule for Persons with Autism and Other Developmental Delays (SSS [15]) and Behavior Assessment System for Children-Second Edition (BASC-2 [16]) and completed by the same parent pre- and postintervention to assess stress and anxiety of JD. The SSS is a survey of 49 items rated on a Likert scale where 1 indicates none to mild and 5 indicates severe; the eight subscales range in reliability from 0.57 (the smallest subscale of social/environment interactions with three items) to 0.91. All subscales other than social/environment were above 0.75 for reliability, indicating that the SSS is a valid tool for assessing perceived stress in persons with autism [17]. Currently, the SSS is the only tool available to assess stress specifically in the target study population. Social validity was determined through Q-sort surveys among autism professionals, specifically the Autism Society of America's Panel of Professional Advisors, and results revealed that 94% of the stressors identified in the SSS are relevant to individuals with ASD [17]. The BASC-2 contains three forms (teacher, parent, and self) that can be used individually or in any combination. Due to the developmental issues associated with an autism diagnosis, this study included the parent form. It has 160 items and can be completed in 20–30 minutes. Results are reported in four categories, each with additional subcategories. The following are the categories and subcategories for the BASC-2 parent form: externalizing problems (hyperactivity, aggression, and conduct problems), internalizing problems (anxiety, depression, and somatization), behavioral symptoms index (atypicality, withdrawal, and attention problems), and adaptive skills (adaptability, activities of daily living, leadership, social skills, and functional communication). These results are reported as potential problem areas as clinically significant or at risk if the scores fall within a particular range. Reliability for the composite scores is 0.90, and test-retest reliability is 0.80. Validity was determined through parental, teacher, and psychologists' content as well as diagnostic criteria from the DSM-IV and DSM-IV-R [18] and has been used in previous studies of children with ASD [19, 20].

2.7. Therapy Attitude Inventory (TAI). Parental satisfaction with the video game playing intervention was measured by the Therapy Attitude Inventory (TAI [21]). The TAI is a 10-item questionnaire of parental satisfaction with the adolescent's behavior changes and type of treatment used. JD's parent was asked to rate each item on a 5-point scale where 1 indicates dissatisfaction or worsening of problems and 5 indicates maximum satisfaction. The scores are summed to yield a total score between 10 and 50. Cronbach's alpha has been reported at 0.91 [21]. The TAI was obtained at the conclusion of the intervention.

2.8. Procedure. JD and his mother provided assent and written informed consent, respectively. A pretreatment session lasted approximately one hour in which basic information, such as demographic and medical information, was collected. Following the pretreatment assessment, JD completed four baseline assessments for a level of experimental control to demonstrate change as a result of treatment. Each baseline session lasted approximately 30 minutes and consisted of weekly measurements of weight, BMI, waist-to-hip ratio, and triceps skinfolds. JD's mother also completed stress and anxiety surveys during the first session.

Following baseline sessions, JD was enrolled in treatment. The protocol involved 6 weeks of inactive video game playing for four days a week and a minimum of 30 minutes each day, followed by 6 weeks of active video game play for the same amount of time and days. Video games selected for the study were rated E (Everyone) by the Entertainment Software Rating Board and were considered suitable for ages of 6 years and older. Selection was based on current popularity, activity levels, and review of market ratings. During video game play, JD wore a Fitbit, a wireless tracker in a wristband that tracks steps taken, distance traveled, calories burned, and very active minutes, to ensure video game play as well as documenting video game play on their activity logs. The Fitbit was chosen for its convenience of wear, wrist only, and its proven reliability and validity of measuring step counts and energy expenditure in previous research [22–24]. Measurements of weight, BMI, waist-to-hip ratio, and triceps skinfold collected weekly during both inactive and active game playing phases (see Figure 1).

After completing all phases, JD's mother completed the stress and anxiety surveys as well as the TAI to determine social validity of the intervention and their perception of its effectiveness. Furthermore, feedback regarding barriers to performing the intervention and the feasibility of continuing a similar treatment to address obesity and health issues were discussed.

3. Results

JD had four baseline assessments that resulted in an increase in weight every week except the final baseline week, when there was a loss of 0.30 pounds (see Figure 2). Inactive video game playing, phase B, results demonstrate somewhat of a steady state in which his weight varied by 0.20 to 0.30 pounds in all but two weeks. JD's weight dropped by 2.20 pounds the second week and 2.30 pounds the fourth week of inactive video game playing. He increased in weight during the first two weeks of active video game playing by 1.70 pounds and 4.10 pounds; however, the remaining weeks of

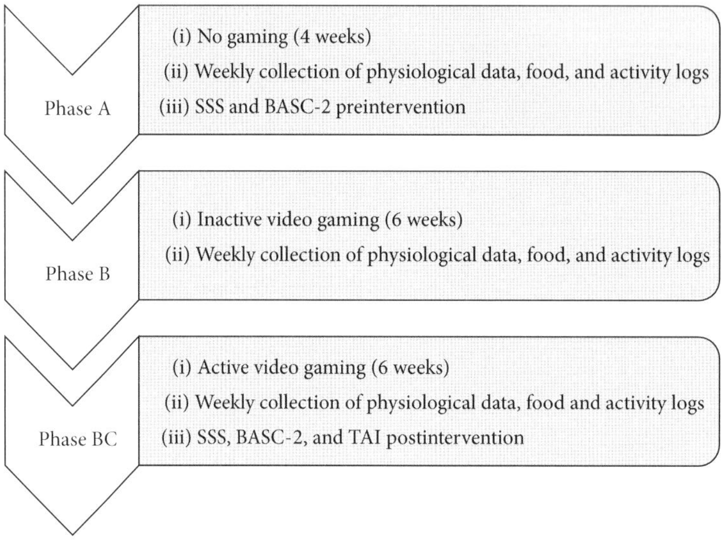

FIGURE 1: Procedure for baseline and interventional phases.

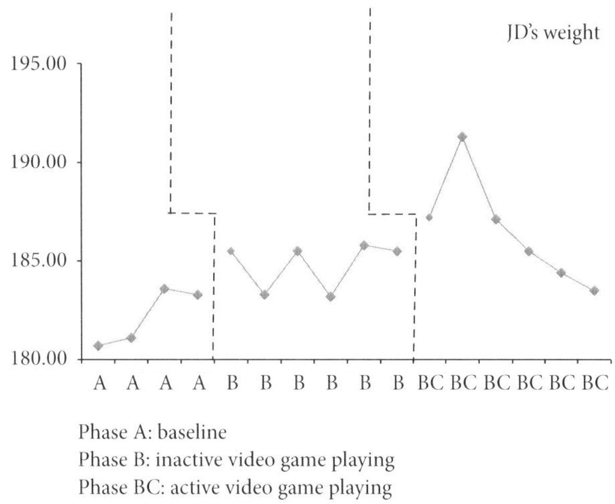

FIGURE 2: JD's weight across all phases.

this phase resulted in weight loss by 0.90 pounds to 4.20 pounds. The percent of weight change for JD from the final baseline assessment (phase A) to the end of inactive video game playing (phase B) was a 1.2% increase and for active video game playing (phase BC) was a 0.1% increase. BMI for JD remained in a stable state during baseline with a variation of only 0.01 kg/m^2 and in phase B a variation of only 0.30 to 0.40 kg/m^2 (see Figure 3). Active video game playing, phase BC, resulted in an increased BMI for the first two weeks and then a decrease for all remaining weeks. JD demonstrated minimal changes across all phases for waist-to-hip ratios with a range of 0.01 to 0.04 (see Figure 4). Similarly, triceps skinfold measurements were fairly consistent across all phases with a range of 0.20 to 0.40 mm (see Figure 5).

Preintervention results of stress and anxiety for JD demonstrated moderate-to-severe anxiety with the SSS instrument in the following categories: changes, unpleasant experiences, sensory/personal, food related, and rituals. Results for moderate anxiety were in the categories of anticipation, positive experiences, and social/environment. The preintervention results for the BASC-2 were noted to have clinically significant *T* scores in the following categories: externalizing problems (hyperactivity), internalizing problems (composite score, anxiety, and depression), behavioral symptoms index (composite score, atypicality, withdrawal, and attention problems), and adaptive skills (composite score, activities of daily living, leadership, and functional communication). The BASC-2 preintervention *T* scores that were classified as at-risk were externalizing problems (composite score) and adaptive skills (adaptability). Postintervention results for the SSS only had minimal changes that did not result in a difference in categorical classification. Postintervention BASC-2 results for JD did not result in any changes in *T* scores. The TAI results for JD revealed a score of 42 out of 50, demonstrating that the parents perceive active video game playing as an effective intervention in reducing stress and anxiety.

4. Discussion

JD had reductions in weight after the introduction of active video game playing; however, there was an overlap of data between phases. For example, JD's waist-to-hip ratios between finishing phase B and starting phase BC were the same measurement. Interestingly, JD gained weight after the introduction of the intervention designed to increase physical activity. As reported on weekly food logs and verbally by his mother, JD increased his food intake during the first few weeks of increased physical activity, which may account for the increase in weight gain. Furthermore, foods chosen to offset the caloric expenditure were the typical energy dense favorites: chicken nuggets, pizza, and hot dogs. An additional explanation for the weight gain after the introduction of the active video game may be an increase in muscle mass. However, after these first few weeks, JD continued to reduce

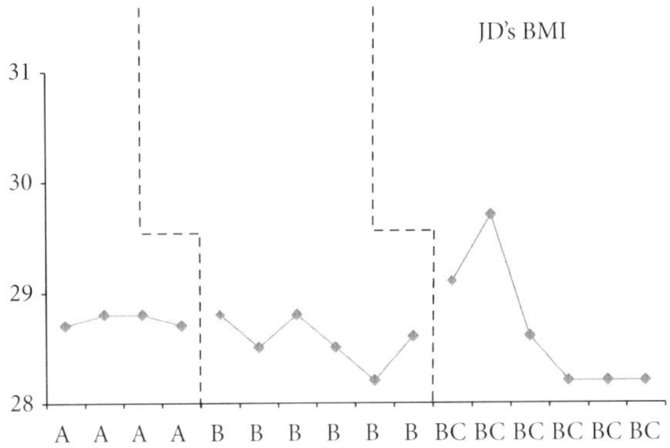

Phase A: baseline
Phase B: inactive video game playing
Phase BC: active video game playing

FIGURE 3: JD's BMI across all phases.

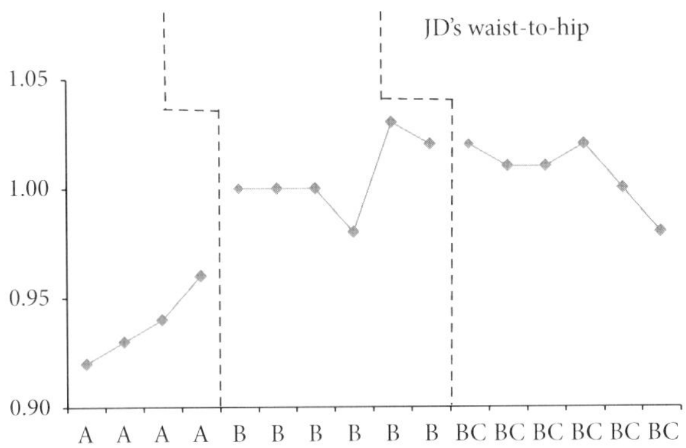

Phase A: baseline
Phase B: inactive video game playing
Phase BC: active video game playing

FIGURE 4: JD's waist-to-hip ratio across all phases.

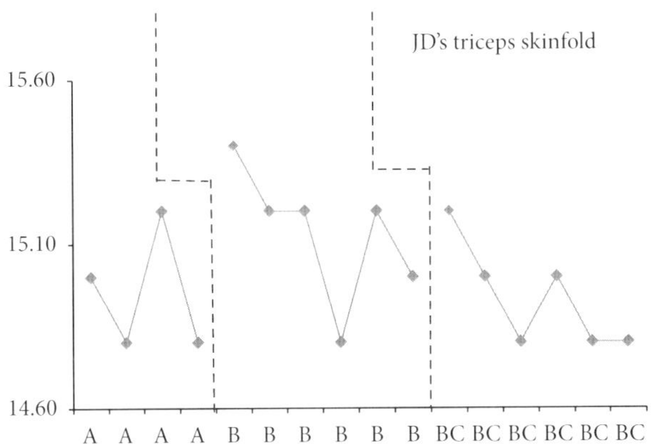

Phase A: baseline
Phase B: inactive video game playing
Phase BC: active video game playing

FIGURE 5: JD's triceps skinfolds across all phases.

his weight as well as BMI, even if minimally. Although JD's overall weight increased, the active video game playing slowed the progression of weight gain during phase BC. BMI also decreased due to changes in weight and height during the intervention. Similar to Maddison et al. [11], these results demonstrate that physically active video games may be a valid option to produce weight loss which could reduce the likelihood of serious health problems such as diabetes, cardiovascular disease, and sleep apnea as well as the financial strain of obesity. Along with improved health, the significance of reducing and/or slowing weight gain among overweight/obese adolescents with ASD is that parents can keep the focus on the problematic features of ASD rather than the weight. The waist-to-hip ratio demonstrated that JD was at moderate-to-high risk for the typical serious health problems associated with obesity. Although waist-to-hip ratio and triceps skinfolds did not have significant changes, the active video game playing slightly decreased those measurements over a six-week period of time which may slow the insidious progression of health problems associated with obesity.

Stress and anxiety results had minimal changes in pre- and postintervention phases demonstrating that physically active video game playing did not reduce stress or anxiety in all areas. Although these findings were counter to expectations, research has shown that approximately 40% of children under the age of 18 with a diagnosis of ASD also had at least one comorbid anxiety disorder [25]. Thus, stress and anxiety coexist within this population beyond the typical stressors and may not significantly improve with physical activity. Interestingly, his mother reported improved behavior with siblings and parental interactions, indicating added benefits of active video game playing and explaining parental satisfaction TAI scores.

Although the results from the case study are preliminary, there is a need for future research to address limitations and replicate findings. A clear limitation of this work is that it describes only a single participant and that these findings may not be generalizable. However, single subject design serves a distinct purpose in that it allows for exploration of individual patient characteristics on treatment outcomes and an opportunity to manipulate variables during intervention. Additionally, the present study results may have been influenced by expectations; that is, JD and his family were aware of active video game playing even though they were blinded to the hypotheses. This may have contributed to positive findings as JD and his mother may have consumed improved food choices and/or less food to produce weight loss. However, results obtained by multiple baseline design suggest that positive outcomes are less likely to explain treatment effects since changes were directly related to the intervention. The length of the intervention may be a limitation because the physiologic data of waist-to-hip ratio and triceps skinfold measurements may not demonstrate changes over short periods of time. Another possible limitation is that the stress and anxiety measures were based on parent report which has the potential for parental bias and may lack sufficient objectivity. Finally, JD demonstrated overlap of data between phases B and BC which may create difficulty in establishing a true functional relationship of variables. Therefore, study replication with extended baseline assessments and intervention phases is needed to determine if there is true cause and effect. Further research, including study replication and randomized controlled trials with larger samples of adolescents of both genders and varied ethnicities, is needed to determine if the treatment effects of active video game playing are robust and generalizable.

5. Conclusion

The case study report describes a protocol that can be replicated and provides preliminary evidence for the effectiveness of active video game playing with an overweight/obese adolescent with ASD. As noted previously, there are no studies yet published regarding the use of active video game playing in this population, a major gap in extant literature. Given the accumulating evidence for the effectiveness of physical activity in treating typically developing obese adolescents, it is critical that future research explores alternative solutions for physical activity among obese adolescents with ASD, for example, the active games used in this study.

References

[1] A. Y. Chen, S. E. Kim, A. J. Houtrow, and P. W. Newacheck, "Prevalence of obesity among children with chronic conditions," *Obesity*, vol. 18, no. 1, pp. 210–213, 2010.

[2] C. Curtin, S. E. Anderson, A. Must, and L. Bandini, "The prevalence of obesity in children with autism: a secondary data analysis using nationally representative data from the National Survey of Children's Health," *BMC Pediatrics*, vol. 10, article 11, 2010.

[3] M. J. Holcomb, L. A. Pufpaff, and D. E. Mcintosh, "Obesity rates in special populations of children and potential interventions," *Psychology in the Schools*, vol. 46, no. 8, pp. 797–804, 2009.

[4] E. Stice, H. Shaw, and C. N. Marti, "A meta-analytic review of obesity prevention programs for children and adolescents: the skinny on interventions that work," *Psychological Bulletin*, vol. 132, no. 5, pp. 667–691, 2006.

[5] L. C. Eaves and H. H. Ho, "Young adult outcome of autism spectrum disorders," *Journal of Autism and Developmental Disorders*, vol. 38, no. 4, pp. 739–747, 2008.

[6] M. D. Tsiros, N. Sinn, A. M. Coates, P. R. C. Howe, and J. D. Buckley, "Treatment of adolescent overweight and obesity," *European Journal of Pediatrics*, vol. 167, no. 1, pp. 9–16, 2007.

[7] H. Davies, J. Rennick, and A. Majnemer, "Transition from pediatric to adult health care for young adults with neurological disorders: parental perspectives," *Canadian Journal of Neuroscience Nursing*, vol. 33, no. 2, pp. 32–39, 2011.

[8] J. H. Rimmer, K. Yamaki, D. Lowry, E. Wang, and L. C. Vogel, "Obesity and obesity-related secondary conditions in adolescents with intellectual/developmental disabilities," *Journal of Intellectual Disability Research*, vol. 54, no. 9, pp. 787–794, 2010.

[9] N. Xiong, C. Ji, Y. Li, Z. He, H. Bo, and Y. Zhao, "The physical status of children with autism in China," *Research in Developmental Disabilities*, vol. 30, no. 1, pp. 70–76, 2009.

[10] B. E. Strahan and J. H. Elder, "Obesity in adolescents with autism spectrum disorders," *Research in Autism Spectrum Disorders*, vol. 7, no. 12, pp. 1497–1500, 2013.

[11] R. Maddison, L. Foley, C. N. Mhurchu et al., "Effects of active video games on body composition: a randomized controlled trial," *The American Journal of Clinical Nutrition*, vol. 94, no. 1, pp. 156–163, 2011.

[12] M. O. Mazurek, P. T. Shattuck, M. Wagner, and B. P. Cooper, "Prevalence and correlates of screen-based media use among youths with autism spectrum disorders," *Journal of Autism and Developmental Disorders*, vol. 42, no. 8, pp. 1757–1767, 2012.

[13] Centers for Disease Control and Prevention, Basics about childhood obesity, Centers for Disease Control and Prevention, http://www.cdc.gov/obesity/childhood/basics.html.

[14] A. F. Roche, R. M. Siervogel, W. C. Chumlea, and P. Webb, "Grading body fatness from limited anthropometric data," *The American Journal of Clinical Nutrition*, vol. 34, no. 12, pp. 2831–2838, 1981.

[15] J. Groden, A. Diller, M. Bausman, W. Velicer, G. Norman, and J. Cautela, "The development of a stress survey schedule for persons with autism and other developmental disabilities," *Journal of Autism and Developmental Disorders*, vol. 31, no. 2, pp. 207–217, 2001.

[16] C. Reynolds and R. Kamphaus, *Behavior Assessment System for Children*, Pearson, Bloomington, Minn, USA, 2nd edition, 2004.

[17] M. Goodwin, J. Groden, W. Velicer, and A. Diller, "Validating the stress survey schedule for persons with autism and other developmental disabilities," *Focus on Autism and Other Developmental Disabilities*, vol. 22, no. 3, pp. 183–189, 2007.

[18] Arkansas Department of Human Services website, https://ardhs.sharepointsite.net/default.aspx.

[19] M. A. Volker, C. Lopata, A. M. Smerbeck et al., "BASC-2 PRS profiles for students with high-functioning autism spectrum disorders," *Journal of Autism and Developmental Disorders*, vol. 40, no. 2, pp. 188–199, 2010.

[20] S. Mahan and J. L. Matson, "Children and adolescents with autism spectrum disorders compared to typically developing controls on the Behavioral Assessment System for Children, Second Edition (BASC-2)," *Research in Autism Spectrum Disorders*, vol. 5, no. 1, pp. 119–125, 2011.

[21] E. V. Brestan, J. R. Jacobs, A. D. Rayfield, and S. M. Eyberg, "A consumer satisfaction measure for parent-child treatments and its relation to measures of child behavior change," *Behavior Therapy*, vol. 30, no. 1, pp. 17–30, 1999.

[22] J. Takacs, C. L. Pollock, J. R. Guenther, M. Bahar, C. Napier, and M. A. Hunt, "Validation of the fitbit one activity monitor device during treadmill walking," *Journal of Science and Medicine in Sport*, vol. 17, no. 5, pp. 496–500, 2014.

[23] J. Adam Noah, D. K. Spierer, J. Gu, and S. Bronner, "Comparison of steps and energy expenditure assessment in adults of Fitbit Tracker and Ultra to the Actical and indirect calorimetry," *Journal of Medical Engineering and Technology*, vol. 37, no. 7, pp. 456–462, 2013.

2

Characteristics of Children Who Lost the Diagnosis of Autism: A Sample from Istanbul, Turkey

Nahit Motavalli Mukaddes,[1,2] Mustafa Deniz Tutkunkardas,[1] Oktay Sari,[3] Aydan Aydin,[3] and Pınar Kozanoglu[4]

[1] Child Psychiatry Department, Istanbul School of Medicine, Istanbul University, 34080 Istanbul, Turkey
[2] Istanbul Institute of Child & Adolescent Psychiatry, 34365 Istanbul, Turkey
[3] Department of Special Education, Marmara University, 34730 Istanbul, Turkey
[4] Private Education Center, 34140 Istanbul, Turkey

Correspondence should be addressed to Nahit Motavalli Mukaddes; nmotavalli@yahoo.com

Academic Editor: Bennett L. Leventhal

Aim. The aim of this study was to describe a group of children who lost a diagnosis of autism following participation in early educational programs. *Method.* This is a descriptive study reporting the characteristics of children (*n*: 39) who lost their diagnosis of autism and explaining the educational programs that these children followed. The data were collected by reviewing the participants' files and through examinations. *Results.* All of the children were placed at regular psychiatric follow-ups. The mean age at referral was 2.39±0.75 years, whereas the mean age at the time of optimal outcome reported was 5.11 ± 1.95 years. Two of the children were in early intensive behavioral intervention (EIBI), and the rest were in a comprehensive naturalistic behavioral program. The childhood autism rating scale (CARS) total scores at baseline and final were 32.75 ± 3.15 and 18.01 ± 1.76, respectively. The mean IQ of the group at final examination was 116.70 ± 18.88. *Conclusion.* It could be concluded that a group of children with an autism diagnosis could lose the diagnosis of autism upon early intervention. High IQ and the development of communicative and language skills at an early age could be the most powerful factors contributing to an optimal outcome.

1. Introduction

Autism spectrum disorders (ASD) are a group of disorders characterized by impairments in reciprocal social interaction, communication, restricted interests, and stereotypical behaviors [1].

Several studies on the consequences of ASD demonstrated unfavorable outcomes for the majority of individuals with a diagnosis of ASD. In an early longitudinal study, it was reported that 60% of subjects with ASD have a poor outcome and are severely handicapped, 35% have a "fair or good" adjustment, and only 1.5% were functioning normally [2]. Recent long-term studies on outcomes demonstrate unfavorable results for low-functioning individuals with autistic disorder (AD) [3, 4] and a favorable outcome in the majority of individuals with high-functioning autism (HFA) and Asperger's disorder (AS) [4, 5].

Over the last few decades, there has been an increase in the number of publications on the efficacy of different intervention programs. Improvements in the core symptoms of ASD, cognitive abilities, and adaptive functions have been reported in these studies [6–13]. Although these studies reported improvements in many aspects of autism, there are a limited number of studies that report "recovery" or optimal outcomes.

The first study in this field was performed by Lovaas [6], in which 47% of children with a diagnosis of autism who were in Applied Behavior Analysis (ABA) achieved the average IQ and could be placed in a regular educational situation without any specialized support [6]. Lovaas used the term "recovery" or "best outcome" to describe these children. Following this study, other investigations assessing the effectiveness of early behavioral approaches indicated that a substantial minority of children (ranging from 27% to 48%) perform within the average range in posttreatment assessments [14].

However, Mundy criticized Lovaas' approach, concluding that having average (or higher) IQ and attendance to a regular school program were not sufficient for "recovery." Many high-functioning children with a diagnosis of autism spectrum disorders may also possess an average or high IQ and be able to attend regular classrooms [15].

Among studies that assessed the effectiveness of different interventional approaches for autism's core symptoms, only some reported a "loss of diagnosis" or "optimal outcome." One of these studies was performed by Sallows and Graupner [8]. They compared the effectiveness of clinical and parent-directed behavioral intervention. After four years of treatment; they assessed outcomes, including cognitive, language, adaptive, social, and academic measures that were similar among groups. After combining groups, they reported that 48% (11 of 23) of all children showed "rapid learning." "Rapid learners" scored normally on IQ, language, adaptive functioning, and school placement tests. Additionally, 8 of the participants did not meet the criteria for an ASD according to the ADI-R [8]. According to Helt et al., these 8 individuals met the criteria for an optimal outcome [16]. The other important study in this field was performed by Fein et al. [17]. They reported eleven children with an earlier diagnosis of ASD who lost the diagnosis of ASD and developed attention deficit hyperactivity disorder (ADHD). Eight had received ABA treatment, and 3 had received intensive preschool classroom intervention. They reported that this group was at risk for significant attention problems as well as some subtle social difficulties and perseverative interests. Recently, Fein et al. published another comprehensive study assessing the functioning of 34 individuals with a previous history of autism. They compared the functioning of the optimal outcome (OO) group with individuals with high-functioning autism and a typical developing (TD) group. They reported that the OO and TD groups' mean scores did not differ regarding socialization, communication, face recognition, or most language subscales. They concluded that their result substantiates the possibility of an optimal outcome from ASD and demonstrates an overall level of functioning within normal limits for this group [18].

Another article in this field is a retrospective study reporting "recovery" from autism in thirty-eight individuals who received early intensive behavioral intervention [19].

In addition to studies that reported a loss of diagnosis of autism after intensive behavioral treatment, Zappella [20, 21] reported "reversible autism" in a group that had never been in behavioral treatment. First, he described a case series, all young males who showed autistic regression after age one. They all had motor and vocal tics. Autistic symptoms disappeared after naturalistic approaches and guidance; however, the children developed Tourette disorder [20]. In his later paper, Zappella described a heterogeneous group of children with a former diagnosis of pervasive developmental disorders (PDD) who lost their PDD diagnosis. Part of this group had concurrent tics and/or ADHD. Some had electroencephalographic (EEG) abnormalities comparable with Landau-Kleffner Syndrome (LKS). He stated that 7.3% of this group recovered spontaneously. It was also mentioned that none of the recovered individuals received ABA and that all underwent a more naturalistic treatment program [21].

Despite an increase in studies demonstrating an optimal outcome in autism, many professionals in this field have a skeptical approach to the idea of "loss of diagnosis" in ASD. Some believe that individuals with OO are initially misdiagnosed. However, evidence regarding similarities in the baseline between the optimal outcome group and persistent ASD in terms of social, communicative, and cognitive functions [22], as well as in head circumference as a biomarker of autism [23], supports the hypothesis of optimal outcome in autism. A recent comprehensive study reported no difference between an optimal outcome group and a typically developing group in socialization, communication, face recognition, or most language subscales; this clearly demonstrated the possibility of optimal outcomes in individuals with a history of autism [18].

As current evidence elucidates, there are only a limited number of studies that report and describe the characteristics of children who have lost a diagnosis of ASD. While some of these studies report optimal outcomes in groups that received intensive early intervention, only one study reported spontaneous recovery.

Therefore, the aim of this study was to describe the characteristics of subjects who lost the diagnosis of autism and to explain the interventional programs that they followed.

2. Methods and Material

This is a descriptive study to describe the characteristics of individuals who were previously diagnosed with ASD and who lost their diagnosis and achieved an optimal outcome.

2.1. Definition of "Recovery"/Optimal Outcome. To the best of our knowledge, the criteria that Helt et al. [16] defined are the only criteria that include either the loss of core symptoms of autism or the demonstration of an IQ in the normal range and normal adaptive functioning. Because our aim was to define a homogenous group that achieved a normal range of developmental trajectory in cognitive, social, and communicative areas, we did not include the group that lost the diagnosis of autism but met the criteria for language disorder and/or intellectual disability.

Our definition of optimal outcome was similar to that of Helt et al. [16]. We considered a case to have achieved an optimal outcome if he/she met the following criteria at baseline: (1) having a diagnosis of ASD at baseline based on DSM-IV criteria, (2) the presence of language delay (no words by 18 months and no word combinations by 24 months), and (3) total Childhood Autism Rating Scale (CARS) [24, 25] score over 25.5 based on scores reported by Chlebowski et al. [26], as well as these criteria at final assessment: (1) not meeting the criteria for any type of ASD based on DSM-IV, (2) not needing special education for the core symptoms of autism, (3) total score of CARS and Autism Behavior Checklist (ABC) [27, 28] in the nonautistic range, and (4) IQ in the nonretarded range (over 78).

2.2. Participants. Participants in our study were the regular patients of a psychiatry clinic, which is a referral center for developmental neuropsychiatric disorders. We included children who previously received a diagnosis of ASD and who did not meet the criteria for any ASD in the final examination. There were thirty-nine individuals (30 males and 9 females) with an age range of 18–54 months at referral. Thirty-eight met the full criteria for AD, and one met the criteria for pervasive developmental disorder-not otherwise specified (PDD-NOS) diagnosis at baseline according to DSM-IV-TR. Their age range at the time of final assessment was 3–10 years old.

2.3. Diagnosis and Follow-Up Procedure. The first assessment protocol was applied to all referrals with a probable diagnosis of ASD. The first assessment included an in-depth psychiatric examination of the child by taking detailed information from parents, watching home videos, and observation of the child's interaction with parents in a playroom. A diagnosis of ASD was made, based on DSM-IV-TR criteria, and the severity of autistic symptoms was measured using CARS. The Ankara Developmental Screening Inventory [29] was used to assess the social, self-help, communicative abilities and gross and fine motor skills of the child. A medical examination, including an auditory test, metabolic screening, and fragile X syndrome screening, was conducted.

The first diagnostic assessment of patients revealed that 39 individuals met the full criteria for AD and that 2 met the full criteria for PDD-NOS according to the DSM-IV-TR. Their CARS scores were between 26.5 and 43. The data of 2 children who had medical problems (auditory impairment and hypothyroidism) were excluded from the study. Therefore, we included 38 individuals with an initial diagnosis of autism and 1 with a diagnosis of PDD-NOS.

After receiving an ASD diagnosis, all children were referred to an education program.

Children were followed up psychiatrically every 3-4 months. In each follow-up visit, the examiner evaluated the child's social-communicative skills and behavioral patterns by watching home videos, observing the child in office, collecting information from parents, and reading written reports from senior educators. Each assessment aimed to evaluate ASD symptoms, such as social-communicative impairment, the severity and frequency of repetitive behaviors, self-help skills, and adaptive behaviors, as well as additional behavioral and medical problems. In addition to the progression of the child, the quality of the education program was also assessed based on information from parents' and educators' written reports. After every examination, a child psychiatrist shared their feedback with the senior educators and supervisors of the education program. Additionally, psychiatric follow-up helped parents to overcome their anxieties and concerns about their child's problems. During follow-up, when a child did not meet the criteria for any type of ASD according to the DSM-IV-TR, outcome measures were applied.

2.4. Measurements. (1) The Childhood Autism Rating Scale (CARS) is a behavioral rating scale used to assess the presence and severity of autism spectrum disorders [24]. It has been shown to have good sensitivity and specificity to distinguish ASD from non-ASD and other developmental disorders in children as young as 2 years of age [26]. A reliability and validity study of CARS was performed in Turkish [25]. CARS consists of 15 items that assess the severity of social-communicative impairments; therefore, CARS could be used for assessing and grading reductions in social-communicative impairments.

(2) The Autism Behavior Checklist (ABC) [27] consists of 57 behaviors that appear to be more commonly observed in autistic children than in children with other handicaps. The ABC was translated into Turkish, and reliability and validities studies were performed [28]. The total scores generated using the ABC ranged from 0 to 158. A total score of 67 or above was considered to indicate autism with "high probability." Parents were asked to fill out this scale during the final phase.

(3) The Ankara Developmental Screening Inventory (ADSI) [29] is a 154-item scale widely used in Turkey for the assessment of social, cognitive, and communicative abilities. The ADSI includes four subscales: the language-cognitive subscale, the fine motor subscale, the gross motor subscale, and the social interaction and self-care abilities subscales. In this study, educators utilized the scale during certain intervals (every 4–6 months) to evaluate the child's progression in these areas and to determine and tailor their educational program. Because it was not administered at a uniform point in time, it is not possible to report the result of the ADSI.

(4) IQ tests (the Stanford-Binet Intelligence Scale [30] or the Wechsler Intelligence Scale for Children-Revised (WISC-R) [31, 32]) were used to assess cognitive abilities.

2.5. Educational Program. The government of Turkey only funds 2 hours of the educational program for ASD per week in Turkey. The rehabilitation centers that provide this limited educational service usually do not have sufficient well-trained professionals who are familiar with ABA or other more effective behavioral treatments. There are a few institutes/schools that employ early intensive behavioral intervention (EIBI). The Turkish government does not provide funding for these programs, and a 20-hour per week program increases the financial burden on the family by €3,000 to €5,000 per month. There are also a few private centers that provide different modalities of educational programs (floor time, individualized social skills training, etc.) for children with ASD.

The patients in our clinic were primarily from upper-middle income families; thus, they had ample access to educational resources. Nevertheless, only 2 patients in this group were able to attend ABA programs with frequencies ranging from as low as 8 hours per week up to the recommended 20 hours per week.

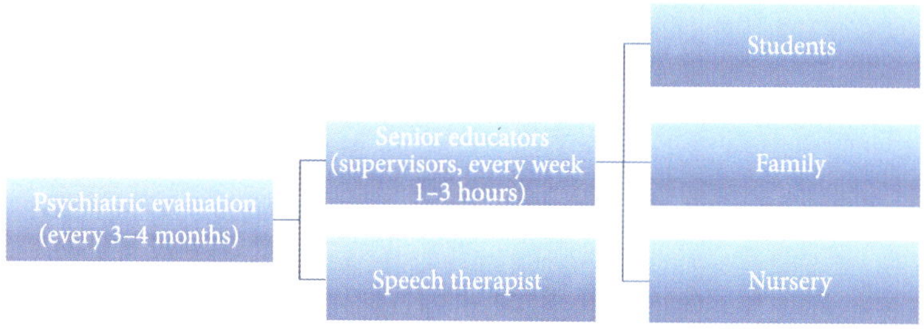

Figure 1: Providers of the educational program.

Thirty-seven individuals attended a comprehensive educational program, which is inspired by Pivotal Response Training (PRT) [33]. This program executes the principals of behavioral treatment and acquired abilities with a special focus on social-communicative development. It requires a more active collaboration with parents and other available family members. The program aims to enrich the environment and promote social responsiveness by working on eye contact, joint attention, imitative abilities, and pretend and make-believe plays. Other important goals include the prevention of interfering behaviors, practicing undeveloped skills, and the enhancement of verbal abilities.

Due to the scarcity of well-trained educators in this field, the senior educators who led the program could only see each patient for 1–3 sessions per week; however, these educators provided parents with intensive home programs and asked them to work with their children as much as they could. If parents struggled with the application of the home program, trained students were sent to their home to work with the child and to supervise the parents' interaction. These students were final-year students of special education programs. They had all observed their senior educators work with children with ASD for at least 6 months and had weekly supervision meetings with their senior educators.

As stated previously, this program required all available family members to be engaged; thus, they were encouraged to take responsibility for working with their child. We also encouraged healthy siblings and cousins to take part in the education program, at least as a "play partner."

Children who showed increased social responsiveness in individual education sessions and who showed progression in maintaining eye contact, joint attention, and imitative abilities were sent to the nursery to practice these abilities in a natural environment. The interval between intake and transfer to the nursery varied greatly between the children and ranged from 4 months to 19 months.

Although this education program works on enhancing verbal abilities, if a child failed to develop meaningful words by the age of 26–30 months, speech therapy was initiated.

In short, this is an individualized, comprehensive program that is widely applied across different settings and is in some respects similar to PRT.

A child psychiatrist who has 20 years of research and clinical background with ASD conducted the clinical diagnoses and follow-ups. A blind examiner, who is a child psychiatrist with 5 years of experience in the autism field, reviewed the records of all children at baseline and at the time of optimal outcome. Only individuals about whom both psychiatrists agreed regarding baseline diagnosis and optimal outcome were included in the study. The senior educators were educators with Ph.D. and M.S. degrees in special education and who had at least 10 years of experience in working with young children with ASD. These senior educators supervised the home program and the nursery program. They led this program in continuous consultation with child psychiatrists. See Figure 1 for the review of the providers of the educational program.

Because the behavioral interventions were not standardized or uniform, no treatment fidelity measures could be taken. However, parents were regularly consulted, and interventional progressions were periodically checked (every 4–6 months) using ADSI.

2.6. Statistical Analysis. All data were organized in Microsoft Excel 2010, and all statistical tests, excluding the correlation analysis, were conducted in Excel. Differences between means were calculated using a t-test. A P value <0.05 was regarded as statistically significant. For multiple comparisons for changes in each CARS item, a Bonferroni correction was conducted, and a P value < 0.0033 was considered statistically significant. Relationships between parametric values were assessed using the Pearson correlation coefficient in the Statistical Package for Social Sciences (SPSS) 16.0, SPSS Inc., Chicago, Illinois, USA.

3. Results

The mean age at referral was 2.39 ± 0.75 years (range: 1.5–4.5 years), which was also the age to start special education. The children started to talk with meaningful words at the age of 2.46 ± 0.92 years (range: 1.5–4.5 years) and used phrases at the age of 3.20 ± 0.91 years (range: 2–5 years). The mean age at optimal outcome was 5.11 ± 1.95 years. The mean number of psychiatric interviews from intake to the time of optimal outcome was 8.47 ± 3.89 sessions. Some patients are being followed up for other psychiatric problems after loss of ASD diagnosis. The education program of patients is summarized in Table 1.

The initial mean CARS score was 32.75 ± 3.15, and the CARS scores in the final evaluation decreased to 18.01 ± 1.76 ($P = 0.000$). The difference between the initial and final CARS scores was not related to the number of special

TABLE 1: Education program of the patients.

	Values
Years attending special education	2.00 ± 1.54 years
Psychiatric follow-up	3.10 ± 2.08 years
Special education hours per week	1.94 ± 1.61 hours
Number of home program providers	2.14 ± 1.41 persons
Number of patients attending mainstream education/nursery	31 patients (79.48%)
Age at starting mainstream education	3.00 ± 1.46 years
Number of patients attending speech therapy	15 patients (38.46%)

education sessions per week, age at the start special education, or the final IQ. See Table 2 for the changes in CARS items.

The final mean IQ score of the patients was 116.70 ± 18.88 (range: 80–148), and the final ABC score was 7.53 ± 7.83. The results of the outcome measures are summarized in Table 3.

The time from baseline to optimal outcome was 2.71 ± 1.67 years (range: 0.5–8 years).

Because some patients lost their diagnosis relatively quickly (8 patients required ≤1 year of intervention), a possible relationship between the time required to achieve optimal outcome and the number of weekly special education sessions, age at diagnosis, initial CARS score, IQ, and age of development of meaningful words and communicative phrases was examined. A negative relationship between the final IQ and the length of time between the initial diagnosis and optimal outcome was observed. That is, the higher the final IQ, the less the time required for achieving an optimal outcome. Additionally, a positive relationship was found between the age of language development and time to optimal outcome. There was no statistically significant relationship between the length of time to optimal outcome and the age at intake, CARS initial total score, or the number of weekly sessions. See Table 4 for details.

Of the 39 patients, 23 (58.9%) had an additional psychiatric disorder: 46.1% (18 patients) had ADHD, 23.07% (9 patients) had some type of anxiety disorder, and 7.69% (3 patients) had some type of tic disorder. Twenty-three patients (58.9%) were on medications with an average of 1.69 ± 0.82 medications per patient. Psychiatric comorbidity was assessed in psychiatric follow-up (every 3-4 months). The results presented here demonstrate the psychiatric comorbidities from initial intake until optimal outcome.

4. Discussion

This study documents the characteristics of children and the intervention programs that achieved an optimal outcome. The description and identification of factors that led to a favorable outcome in this group is a very important issue because it may shed light on the neurobiology of autism, provide information regarding the effectiveness of intervention programs, and also illuminate potential characteristics of children who may achieve an optimal outcome.

However, prior to discussing the characteristics of this group, it may be more pertinent to discuss diagnostic issues.

The first question that needs to be answered is whether the OO group was initially misdiagnosed. The early age at referral and therefore diagnosis at early age naturally raises a question regarding the probability of misdiagnosis. Psychiatric assessments of this group were performed in detail and were based on home videos, observations of child-parent interactions in play situations, and detailed developmental histories from parents. Additionally, we used instruments, such as CARS, that can distinguish between children with ASD and those with non-ASD. The psychiatric follow-up and assessment were repeated every 3-4 months. All psychiatric assessments and follow-ups were performed by a child psychiatrist with 20 years of experience in the field of autism. It is now agreed that clinical judgment by an experienced clinician is considered to be the "gold standard" for the diagnosis of autism in young children. Therefore, the probability of misdiagnosis is not likely.

The second question in this area is related to the diagnostic stability. The young age at referral also raises a question about the diagnostic stability. Some studies showed high rates of diagnostic stability (85%–89%) when autism was diagnosed at the age of 2 [34–36]; however, a study later showed lower diagnostic stability (63%) when autism was diagnosed at the age of 2 [37]. Another study reported that 18% of children with a diagnosis of ASD at age 2 lose the diagnosis of ASD by age 4. The group in that study was in an intervention program [23]. Our group was also in an intervention program and, despite the program, only 9 individuals moved off the autism spectrum prior to age 4, while 30 moved off after age 4. Taken together, it could be said that maturation may have contributed to improvements in social-communicative and cognitive areas [21]; however, we are not certain if the children in our group and other studies would have moved off the spectrum without any intervention. The important issue that we should consider here is the cohort effect. Increased awareness about autism among parents leads to patient referral at a younger age, with milder problems in social-communicative areas. It should be noted that children who are referred at an early age with major problems in one area of development often show deficits in several domains. Therefore, there is also the possibility of a different clinical manifestation later in life that may explain the developmental trajectory of some children who initially present with ASD.

The third point that needs to be clarified is the role of the inherent characteristics of the children, families, and intervention programs of this group. Although the mechanisms of improvement for any given child are not known, it could be assumed that the interaction of the child's own characteristics with an appropriate intervention program contributes to this favorable outcome.

We will discuss the inherent characteristics of children, families, and treatments in this group.

4.1. Age at Referral. Patients in this group were referred to us at an early age (mean age: 2.35 ± 0.75); 30 of 39 (76%) were referred at the age of 18–30 months. We assumed that the young age at intake could be one of the factors contributing to

Table 2: Changes in CARS items.

CARS item	Initial score mean	Initial score standard deviation	Final score mean	Final score standard deviation	P value
(1) Relating to people	2.40	0.37	1.14	0.23	<0.0001
(2) Imitation	2.45	0.46	1.06	0.20	<0.0001
(3) Emotional response	2.19	0.39	1.10	0.20	<0.0001
(4) Body use	2.26	0.54	1.06	0.17	<0.0001
(5) Object use	2.46	0.52	1.29	0.42	<0.0001
(6) Adaptation to change	2.03	0.54	1.27	0.36	<0.0001
(7) Visual response	2.27	0.44	1.14	0.23	<0.0001
(8) Listening response	2.41	0.32	1.18	0.27	<0.0001
(9) Taste, smell, and touch response	1.63	0.48	1.14	0.28	<0.0001
(10) Fear or nervousness	1.49	0.41	1.30	0.39	0.03*
(11) Verbal communication	2.69	0.42	1.25	0.30	<0.0001
(12) Nonverbal communication	2.41	0.36	1.14	0.23	<0.0001
(13) Activity level	1.73	0.59	1.91	0.79	0.13**
(14) Intellectual response	2.00	0.53	1.12	0.21	<0.0001
(15) General impressions	2.41	0.38	1.09	0.19	<0.0001

*Not significant after Bonferroni correction.
**Not significant.

Table 3: Results of the outcome measures.

	Values
Mean age at optimal outcome	5.11 ± 1.95 years
Time to optimal outcome (range)	2.71 ± 1.67 years (0.5–8 years)
Optimal outcome <4	9 patients (23.07%)
Optimal outcome ≥4	30 patients (76.9%)
Mean CARS score	18.01 ± 1.76
Mean ABC score	7.53 ± 7.83
Mean IQ score	116.70 ± 18.88

Table 4: Correlations of variables with length of time to optimal outcome.

	Time to recovery	
	Pearson correlation coefficient	P value
Final IQ	−0.491	0.009
Number of weekly special education sessions	0.173	NS
Age at diagnosis	0.179	NS
Use of first words (age)	0.607	0.027
Use of first phrases (age)	0.734	0.006
Initial CARS scores	0.274	NS

favorable outcome. Surprisingly, we did not find a statistically significant correlation between the age of intake and the length of time to achieve OO. Therefore, this study failed to show that an earlier age at intake leads to an earlier loss of diagnosis. Harris and Handleman [38] examined the predictive power of age and IQ at the time of admission to intensive behavioral treatment. They reported that a younger age and a higher IQ were predictive of placement in a regular education class [38]. Turner [35] examined the age 2 predictor of outcome at age 9 and reported that 70% of the children diagnosed prior to the age of 30 months had "more optimal" outcomes, while only 28% of children diagnosed older than 30 months achieved "more optimal" outcomes. The lack of a control group in our study limits our interpretation. Despite some controversy regarding the effect of early identification on outcome, it is accepted that an intervention, which is sufficiently early to coincide with the maximum neural plasticity, contributes to residual normality in various neurodevelopmental disorders [39].

4.2. Symptom Severity. Reviewing the scores of CARS items indicates the presence of mild to moderate impairment in all items at baseline. One important point is the statistically significant change from baseline to the time of optimal outcome in all autism-specific items. Thus, this group showed a great reduction in the core symptoms of autism from baseline to the time of optimal outcome. There were no statistically significant changes in only 2 items, which are not among the core symptoms of autism, namely, item number 10 (fear or nervousness) and number 13 (activity level).

According to the CARS total score, thirty-five of our patients (90%) were rated as having mild to moderate autism, and only 4 were rated as having severe autism. Therefore, it appears that mild to moderate autism was a common characteristic of the majority of our optimal outcome group. Our result is comparable with the results of Turner in which they showed that children who lost the diagnosis of autism at age 4 had a lower total CARS score at age 2 than a group that showed diagnostic stability [37]. Unfortunately, the lack of a control group in our study limits our interpretation of the effect of symptom severity on outcome. We examined the relationship between initial CARS scores and the length of time to optimal outcome. However, we did not observe a statistically significant relationship.

The influence of symptom severity on outcome is a controversial subject. While some studies claim that there are no significant effects of symptom severity on outcome [22], others mention that children with "milder social impairment" are more likely to show favorable outcomes [37]. In a recent study by Fein et al., the optimal outcome group had "milder autism" in childhood and "the milder presentation applied to social area but not communication and repetitive behaviors areas" [18]. Taken altogether, it could be suggested that individuals with milder symptoms are more likely to achieve optimal outcomes.

4.3. Early Communication and Language Development. Children in our group began to speak with meaningful words at the age of 2.47 ± 0.81 years and used phrases at the age of 3.15 ± 0.85 years. It was found that the time until optimal outcome was positively related to the first use of words (Pearson correlation coefficient: 0.607, $P = 0.027$) and first phrases (Pearson correlation coefficient: 0.734, $P = 0.006$). In other words, children who started to speak at a younger age more quickly achieved an optimal outcome. Improvements in verbal and communicative abilities are known as the most consistent prognostic factors [40]; thus, the age-appropriate acquisition of spoken language skills is an important factor leading to a favorable outcome. Naturally, children with verbal and communicative abilities have a greater chance to interact with other people—including peers—than nonverbal children. The presence of verbal abilities inevitably enhances social interaction and ultimately has a positive influence on outcome.

4.4. Intelligence Quotient (IQ). Although we could not test the initial IQ of the entire group, their final IQ scores point to their high intellectual potential. A total of 62.9% of the group had an IQ over 110, and the mean IQ of the group was 116.70± 18.8. Additionally, the relationship between IQ and the length of time from intake to loss of diagnosis showed a negative correlation. In other words, children with higher IQ scores achieved optimal outcomes more quickly than other children. This is consistent with previous studies that reported IQ as the strongest prognostic factor for outcomes of children with ASD [17, 18] due to expressive and receptive language skills [40]. Finally, other studies on optimal outcomes reported higher than average IQ in their OO group [17, 18]. Taking all factors into consideration, the hypothesis that higher IQ scores facilitate recovery appears to be plausible.

4.5. Absence of Medical Disorders. It is known that disorders affecting the central nervous system, such as epilepsy [41], have a negative influence on outcomes [42]. The absence of such disorders in this group appears to be another factor that influences outcomes.

4.6. Role of Intervention Program. The educational programs in which our patients participated were home-based educational interventions. Although we aimed to provide an intensive home program, our information about the intensity of the home program is limited to what parents reported to us (except for families that had home teachers). For that reason, we only considered the number of weekly in-office sessions that the patients had with education program supervisors.

The lack of a control group limits our interpretation of the effectiveness of the intervention program. Furthermore, assessing the relationship between the number of weekly sessions with educators and the length of time to optimal outcome failed to show a statistically significant difference. Finally, there was no statistically significant relationship between the number of special education sessions per week and the change in CARS score.

Previous studies reported OO in children who attended an ABA program [17, 19]. To the best of our knowledge, one study also reported recovery in which patients received only naturalistic, relation-based interventions [21]. In our group, only 2 individuals attended the ABA program, and the rest received home-based naturalistic behavioral interventions.

Our results may demonstrate the utility of developmentally appropriate, naturalistic behavioral programs in some toddlers with a diagnosis of ASD. However, intervention alone did not independently lead to a positive outcome. While intervention is highly important, it should be noted that the prognosis depends on the relationship between the child's characteristics and the intervention program.

4.7. Role of the Families. The parents of these children played an important role in each child's education. According to the clinical impressions of both the psychiatrists and educators, all parents in this group showed high motivation and great effort. However, it is important to remember that the majority of these families were comprised of well-educated parents from the upper-middle class. They showed excellent collaboration with all team members. In 9 of these families (23.07%), the loss of the diagnosis of ASD was relatively rapid (prior to the age of 4). However, the remaining families (30 patients, 76.9%) had to work diligently until their children were older (between the ages of 4 and 10).

One important point that affects the generalizability of the results of this study pertains to family characteristics. Because the majority of these parents were well-educated individuals with sufficient economic means, they provided a high quality assessment and intervention program for their children; they proficiently monitored and organized the program and had a very close collaboration with both the psychiatrist and educators.

In summary, reviewing the inherent characteristics of the children and their intervention program shows that a higher IQ and the development of communication and language skills at an earlier age are the most powerful factors contributing to a rapid recovery. Other factors, such as young age at identification and intervention, presence of mild to moderate symptoms, and the collaboration of families in the administration of education may have contributed to this favorable outcome. However, the lack of an appropriate control group limits our interpretation of these characteristics.

Another noteworthy point is the variability in the length of time from diagnosis to optimal outcome. The minimum time from intake to the loss of diagnosis was 6 months, while the maximum was 8 years. This indicates that OO is possible even in middle childhood. It is necessary to follow up with the individuals with ASD to determine if additional individuals lose the diagnosis as well as determining what happens to the children who move off the spectrum.

This study has some limitations, such as the lack of a diagnostic assessment with a structured interview form, such as the Autism Diagnostic Interview-Revised (ADI-R) [43] and the Autism Diagnostic Observation Schedule (ADOS) [44], due to the unavailability of these instruments in Turkish. Another limiting factor is that the information regarding the time and quality of the home-administered program was reported by the families and was not under our direct observation. The third factor that affects the generalizability of these results is the sample-specific characteristics of our group. This group is well educated, and the majority is from the upper-middle class, which has access to high quality health services. Additionally, the children had very high IQ scores, which again limits the generalizability of our results. Another limitation is that because this group was in a regular clinical follow-up, it was not possible to assess the children at uniform time points in terms of developmental periods, making it difficult to determine whether there were specific developmental factors that accounted for optimal outcomes at different time points. Finally, the lack of a control group limits our interpretation of the characteristics of children who can achieve an optimal outcome.

Nevertheless, this study has some strengths. One of the most important points is that it includes children who were followed by our study group; thus, the information given here is clinically based and prospective. All diagnostic and follow-up processes were completed by taking information from different and independent informants and by observing the child. Additionally, this study provides a follow-up intervention model for countries and settings with relatively limited resources for the treatment of ASD. Moreover, it provides information from a unique setting and culture, thus drawing attention to the need for new models of intervention to help families in low- and middle-income countries.

When interpreting the results of this study, it should be noted that it is not an effectiveness study; therefore, it would be difficult to predict the number of children who may benefit from the program. We have many children who are in similar programs (both ABA and naturalistic behavioral programs) and who remain in the ASD spectrum; we do not claim that this program represents a new gold standard in departing from the autism spectrum. Even so, we elucidated two main points; first, with early identification and an appropriate intervention program, an optimal outcome is possible for some children with ASD and, finally, in settings where there is a lack of community service for this group, motivating, teaching, and close collaboration with all available family members and schools may help to improve the clinical characteristics of this group and potentially even discard autism.

5. Conclusion

This study documented the data of children who lost a diagnosis of autism. It could be concluded that high IQ and the development of language at an early age are the most powerful factors contributing to optimal outcomes. Additionally, early identification and intervention, relatively mild symptoms, and, finally, a high motivation of parents in the administration of home programs are other common characteristics of this group.

It is important to mention that, in settings where there is a lack of resources for intervention programs, motivating and closely supervising family members could help to improve the social communicative abilities of this group.

References

[1] American Psychiatric Association, *Diagnostic and Statistical Manual of Mental Disorders*, American Psychiatric Association, Washington, DC, USA, 4th edition, 2000.

[2] M. Rutter, "Autistic children: infancy to adulthood," *Seminars in Psychiatry*, vol. 2, no. 4, pp. 435–450, 1970.

[3] E. Billstedt, C. Gillberg, and C. Gillberg, "Autism after adolescence: population-based 13- to 22-year follow-up study of 120 individuals with autism diagnosed in childhood," *Journal of Autism and Developmental Disorders*, vol. 35, no. 3, pp. 351–360, 2005.

[4] M. Cederlund, B. Hagberg, E. Billstedt, I. C. Gillberg, and C. Gillberg, "Asperger syndrome and autism: a comparative longitudinal follow-up study more than 5 years after original diagnosis," *Journal of Autism and Developmental Disorders*, vol. 38, no. 1, pp. 72–85, 2008.

[5] M. A. Farley, W. M. McMahon, E. Fombonne et al., "Twenty-year outcome for individuals with autism and average or near-average cognitive abilities," *Autism Research*, vol. 2, no. 2, pp. 109–118, 2009.

[6] O. I. Lovaas, "Behavioral treatment and normal educational and intellectual functioning in young autistic children," *Journal of Consulting and Clinical Psychology*, vol. 55, no. 1, pp. 3–9, 1987.

[7] J. S. Howard, C. R. Sparkman, H. G. Cohen, G. Green, and H. Stanislaw, "A comparison of intensive behavior analytic and eclectic treatments for young children with autism," *Research in Developmental Disabilities*, vol. 26, no. 4, pp. 359–383, 2005.

[8] G. O. Sallows and T. D. Graupner, "Intensive behavioral treatment for children with autism: four-year outcome and predictors," *The American Journal on Mental Retardation*, vol. 110, no. 6, pp. 417–438, 2005.

[9] C. Kasari, S. Freeman, and T. Paparella, "Joint attention and symbolic play in young children with autism: a randomized controlled intervention study," *Journal of Child Psychology and Psychiatry and Allied Disciplines*, vol. 47, no. 6, pp. 611–620, 2006.

[10] G. Dawson, S. Rogers, J. Munson et al., "Randomized, controlled trial of an intervention for toddlers with autism: the early start Denver model," *Pediatrics*, vol. 125, no. 1, pp. e17–e23, 2010.

[11] I. M. -Smith, R. L. Koegl, L. K. Koegl, D. A. Openden, K. L. Fossun, and S. E. Bryson, "Effectivness of a novel community-based early intervention model for children with autistic spectrum disorder," *The American Journal on Intellectual and Developmental Disabilities*, vol. 115, no. 6, pp. 504–523, 2010.

[12] L. Schreibman and A. C. Stahmer, "A randomized trial comparison of the effects of verbal and pictorial naturalistic communication startegies on spoken language for young children with autism," *Journal of Autism and Developmental Disorders*, 2013.

[13] S. J. Rogers and L. A. Vismara, "Evidence-based comprehensive treatments for early autism," *Journal of Clinical Child and Adolescent Psychology*, vol. 37, no. 1, pp. 8–38, 2008.

[14] T. Smith, "Applied behavior analysis and early intensive behavioral intervention," in *Autism Spectrum Disorders*, D. Amaral, G. Dawson, and D. Geschwind, Eds., Oxford University Press, New York, NY, USA, 2011.

[15] P. Mundy, "Normal versus High functioning status in children with autism," *The American Journal of Mental Retardation*, vol. 97, pp. 381–384, 1993.

[16] M. Helt, E. Kelley, M. Kinsbourne et al., "Can children with autism recover? If so, how?" *Neuropsychology Review*, vol. 18, no. 4, pp. 339–366, 2008.

[17] D. Fein, P. Dixon, J. Paul, and H. Levin, "Pervasive developmental disorder can evolve into ADHD: case illustrations," *Journal of Autism and Developmental Disorders*, vol. 35, no. 4, pp. 525–534, 2005.

[18] D. Fein, M. Barton, M. Eigsti et al., "Optimal outcome in individuals with a history of autism," *Journal of Child Psychology and Psychiatry*, vol. 54, no. 2, pp. 195–205, 2013.

[19] D. Granpeesheh, J. Tarbox, D. R. Dixon, E. Carr, and M. Herbert, "Retrospective analysis of clinical records in 38 cases of recovery from autism," *Annals of Clinical Psychiatry*, vol. 21, no. 4, pp. 195–204, 2009.

[20] M. Zappella, "Early-onset Tourette syndrome with reversible autistic behaviour: a dysmaturational disorder," *European Child and Adolescent Psychiatry*, vol. 11, no. 1, pp. 18–23, 2002.

[21] M. Zappella, "Autistic regression with and without EEG abnormalities followed by favourable outcome," *Brain and Development*, vol. 32, no. 9, pp. 739–745, 2010.

[22] S. Sutera, J. Pandey, E. L. Esser et al., "Predictors of optimal outcome in toddlers diagnosed with autism spectrum disorders," *Journal of Autism and Developmental Disorders*, vol. 37, no. 1, pp. 98–107, 2007.

[23] K. D. Mraz, J. Dixon, T. Dumont-Mathieu, and D. Fein, "Accelerated head and body growth in infants later diagnosed with autism spectrum disorders: a comparative study of optimal outcome children," *Journal of Child Neurology*, vol. 24, no. 7, pp. 833–845, 2009.

[24] E. Schopler, R. Reichler, and B. Renner, *The Childhood Autism Rating Scale*, Western Psychological Association, Los Angeles, Calif, USA, 1988.

[25] S. Incekas, B. Baykara, Y. Demiral, and S. Miral, "Cocukluk otizmini derecelendirme olcegi Turkce formunun gecerlilik ve guvenilirlik calismasi," in *19. Ulusal Cocuk ve Ergen Ruh Sagligi ve Hastaliklari Kongresi Ozet Kitabi*, Ulusal Cocuk ve Ergen Ruh Sagligi ve Hastaliklari Dernegi, Antakya, Turkey, 2009.

[26] C. Chlebowski, J. A. Green, M. L. Barton, and D. Fein, "Using the childhood autism rating scale to diagnose autism spectrum disorders," *Journal of Autism and Developmental Disorders*, vol. 40, no. 7, pp. 787–799, 2010.

[27] D. A. Krug, J. Arick, and P. Almond, "Behavior checklist for identifying severely handicapped individuals with high levels of autistic behavior," *Journal of Child Psychology and Psychiatry and Allied Disciplines*, vol. 21, no. 3, pp. 221–229, 1980.

[28] A. Gurkan and S. Sutcu, "Reliability and validity of Turkish translation of autism behavior checklist," in *Proceedings of the 2nd Istanbul Autism Symposium*, Istanbul, Turkey, 2004.

[29] I. Savasir, N. Sezgin, and N. Erol, *Ankara gelisim tarama envanteri el kitabi*, Turk Psikologlar Dernegi, Ankara, Turkey, 3rd edition, 2004.

[30] L. Terman and L. Merrill, *Stanford Binet Intelligence Scale Manual for the Third Revision, Form L-M*, Houghton Mifflin, Boston, Mass, USA, 1960.

[31] D. Wechsler, *Manual for the Wechsler Intelligence Scale for Children, Revised*, Psychological Corporation, New York, NY, USA, 1974.

[32] I. Savasir and N. Sahin, *Wechsler Cocuklar için Zeka Olcegi (WISC-R) El Kitabi*, Turk Psikologlar Dernegi, Ankara, Turkey, 1995.

[33] L. Shreibman and B. Ingersol, "Naturalistic Approaches to early behavioral intervention," in *Autism Spectrum Disorders*, D. Amaral, G. Dawson, and D. Geschwind, Eds., Oxford University Press, New York, NY, USA, 2011.

[34] T. Charman, E. Taylor, A. Drew, H. Cockerill, J. A. Brown, and G. Baird, "Outcome at 7 years of children diagnosed with autism at age 2: predictive validity of assessments conducted at 2 and 3 years of age and pattern of symptom change over time," *Journal of Child Psychology and Psychiatry and Allied Disciplines*, vol. 46, no. 5, pp. 500–513, 2005.

[35] L. M. Turner, W. L. Stone, S. L. Pozdol, and E. E. Coonrod, "Follow-up of children with autism spectrum disorders from age 2 to age 9," *Autism*, vol. 10, no. 3, pp. 243–265, 2006.

[36] C. Lord, S. Risi, P. S. DiLavore, C. Shulman, A. Thurm, and A. Pickles, "Autism from 2 to 9 years of age," *Archives of General Psychiatry*, vol. 63, no. 6, pp. 694–701, 2006.

[37] L. M. Turner and W. L. Stone, "Variability in outcome for children with an ASD diagnosis at age 2," *Journal of Child Psychology and Psychiatry and Allied Disciplines*, vol. 48, no. 8, pp. 793–802, 2007.

[38] S. L. Harris and J. S. Handleman, "Age and IQ at intake as predictors of placement for young children with autism: a four- to six-year follow-up," *Journal of Autism and Developmental Disorders*, vol. 30, no. 2, pp. 137–142, 2000.

[39] M. Thomas and A. Karmiloff-Smith, "Are developmental disorders like cases of adult brain damage? Implications from connectionist modelling," *Behavioral and Brain Sciences*, vol. 25, no. 6, pp. 727–750, 2002.

[40] R. Luyster, S. Qiu, K. Lopez, and C. Lord, "Predicting outcomes of children referred for autism using the MacArthur-Bates communicative development Inventory," *Journal of Speech, Language, and Hearing Research*, vol. 50, no. 3, pp. 667–681, 2007.

[41] M. Eriksson, J. Westerlund, A. Hedvall, P. Amark, C. Gillberg, and E. Fernell, "Medical conditions affect the outcome of early intervention in preschool children with autism spectrum disorders," *European Child and Adolescent Psychiatry*, vol. 22, no. 1, pp. 23–33, 2013.

[42] C. Darrou, R. Pry, E. Pernon, C. Michelon, C. Aussilloux, and A. Baghdadli, "Outcome of young children with autism: does the amount of intervention influence developmental trajectories?" *Autism*, vol. 14, no. 6, pp. 663–677, 2010.

[43] C. Lord, M. Rutter, and A. L. Couteur, "Autism diagnostic interview-revised: a revised version of a diagnostic interview for caregivers of individuals with possible pervasive developmental disorders," *Journal of Autism and Developmental Disorders*, vol. 24, no. 5, pp. 659–685, 1994.

[44] C. Lord, S. Risi, L. Lambrecht et al., "The autism diagnostic observation schedule-generic: a standard measure of social and communication deficits associated with the spectrum of autism," *Journal of Autism and Developmental Disorders*, vol. 30, no. 3, pp. 205–223, 2000.

3

Mental Health Services for Individuals with High Functioning Autism Spectrum Disorder

Johanna K. Lake,[1,2] Andrea Perry,[1] and Yona Lunsky[1,2]

[1] *Dual Diagnosis Service, Centre for Addiction and Mental Health, 501 Queen Street West, Toronto, ON, Canada M5V 2B4*
[2] *Department of Psychiatry, University of Toronto, 250 College Street, 8th Floor, Toronto, ON, Canada M5T 1R8*

Correspondence should be addressed to Johanna K. Lake; johanna.lake@camh.ca

Academic Editor: John A. Sweeney

Adolescents and adults with an autism spectrum disorder (ASD) who do not have an intellectual impairment or disability (ID), described here as individuals with high-functioning autism spectrum disorder (HFASD), represent a complex and underserved psychiatric population. While there is an emerging literature on the mental health needs of children with ASD with normal intelligence, we know less about these issues in adults. Of the few studies of adolescents and adults with HFASD completed to date, findings suggest that they face a multitude of cooccurring psychiatric (e.g., anxiety, depression), psychosocial, and functional issues, all of which occur in addition to their ASD symptomatology. Despite this, traditional mental health services and supports are falling short of meeting the needs of these adults. This review highlights the service needs and the corresponding gaps in care for this population. It also provides an overview of the literature on psychiatric risk factors, identifies areas requiring further study, and makes recommendations for how existing mental health services could include adults with HFASD.

1. Introduction

When it comes to supporting the needs of adolescents and adults with an autism spectrum disorder who do not have intellectual impairment or disability, described here as individuals with high-functioning autism spectrum disorder (HFASD), our mental health system is in crisis. We know that rates of mental health issues are high in this population; yet accessing services to address these symptoms remains difficult. Addressing the mental health and intervention needs of adolescents and adults with ASD is a recognized priority in Canada [1–3], the United States [4], and the United Kingdom [5–7], but most individuals with HFASD continue to encounter significant difficulties in social relationships, employment, and communication. These issues are further magnified in developing countries where there is an emerging literature on the diagnosis and treatment of ASD, but where the mental health needs of individuals with ASD often exceed available resources, and where limited training, policy, and mental health programs exist [8, 9].

The Centers for Disease Control and Prevention (CDC) in the United States estimate that 1 in 68 children have an autism spectrum disorder (ASD) and almost half (46%) function in the average or above average range of intellectual ability (IQ > 85) [10]. Previously defined as *Asperger syndrome* (AS) in the tenth revision of the International Statistical Classification of Diseases and Related Health Problems (ICD-10; [11]) and the fourth revised edition of the Diagnostic and Statistical Manual of Mental Disorders (DSM-IV-TR; [12]), individuals with HFASD are characterized by deficits in reciprocal social interaction and patterns of behaviour or interests in the absence of clinically significant delays in receptive language or cognitive development. In the DSM-5 [13], these individuals are now characterized as individuals with ASD who do not have an intellectual impairment. For the purpose of this review, we broadly refer to all individuals with AS or high-functioning autism as HFASD, even if some studies used different diagnostic terms. Although we know that children with ASD grow up to be adults with ASD, there are fewer mental health services available for adults with ASD, particularly for individuals without an ID. Despite improved recognition of individuals functioning at all levels across the spectrum, access to care for individuals with HFASD and research on this population has not kept pace with their needs.

As in the case with most developmental disorders, ASD symptomatology changes with age. While there is a significant body of literature on symptoms, service use, and interventions for children with ASD, there are fewer studies that have investigated these issues in adults [14, 15]. This is well articulated in the United Kingdom National Autistic Society document, "Ignored or ineligible? The reality for adults with autism spectrum disorders," where findings of 1200 adults with ASD demonstrated that many parents of these adults were confused about which statutory agency was responsible for their child's care and that the responsibility for funding and providing care and support often fell between agencies [16]. The issue of accessing mental health services is further complicated for adults with HFASD because community mental health agencies are not typically inclusive of individuals with ASD. The impact of this scenario is a lack of recognition among community mental health programs that this is a population needing their care for whom they are well equipped to support. Poor recognition occurs for a number of different reasons including restrictive intake criteria, misdiagnosis, limited knowledge or awareness of ASD, clinicians who lack confidence or exposure in caring for this population, and the notion that another service provider will provide this care.

Generally, individuals with HFASD have been unable to access developmental disability services because of the absence of significant cognitive impairments, leaving their needs to be addressed in community mental health settings. However, some adolescents and adults with HFASD, because of their ASD diagnosis, are excluded from community mental health services, leaving them grossly underserved. The purpose of this review, therefore, is to discuss some of the most common issues facing adolescents and adults with HFASD and to describe some of the interventions developed to support this population. In doing so, we also describe areas for future study, identify significant challenges and barriers to accessing mental health services, and highlight opportunities to address these barriers within existing community mental health systems and services. It is important to note that the interventions proposed in this review are services and supports which already form the foundation of many existing community mental health programs.

2. Mental Health Issues in HFASD

Comorbid psychiatric disorders are well documented in individuals with ASD across the lifespan [17–24]. Compared to studies of psychiatric comorbidity in individuals with ASD generally, research on cooccurring psychiatric disorders in adults and teens with HFASD, specifically, has been slower to progress. Most evidence comes from studies of youth (children and early adolescents), with fewer studies focusing on older adolescents and adults. Of these studies, findings suggest that a very high proportion of adults and teens with HFASD present with comorbid psychiatric disorders, particularly depression and anxiety [14, 17, 22, 25–29]. By contrast, studies of youth with HFASD tend to report higher rates of behavior and attention problems [27, 30, 31].

In a community and clinic-based study of adolescents with HFASD, results identified a prevalence rate of 74% for one or more comorbid psychiatric disorders, with 44% of individuals diagnosed with behavioural disorders and 44% diagnosed with anxiety disorders [27]. In another study, Ghaziuddin and Greden [32] identified that 65% of patients with HFASD also presented with symptoms of an additional psychiatric disorder. Children with HFASD were most likely to have a comorbid diagnosis of ADHD, while depression was the most common diagnosis in adolescents and adults. Similar findings were reported for rates of bipolar disorder in an outpatient clinic of 54 young adults with HFASD, where 36% of patients were diagnosed with a mood disorder [28]. More recently, in a study examining psychiatric comorbidity in young adults with AS, 70% had experienced at least one episode of major depression, 50% had suffered from recurrent depressive episodes, and 50% met criteria for an anxiety disorder [26]. Similar findings were reported in a study of adolescents with HFASD, where individuals with HFASD reported more psychiatric symptoms, particularly withdrawn, anxious/depressed, and social problems, compared to controls [25].

In summary, although research on adults and teens with HFASD is limited, studies to date suggest that the cooccurrence of psychiatric disorders in this population is remarkably high. Specifically, higher functioning adolescents and adults appear to be at heightened risk for developing depression and anxiety [33–35]. Despite these findings, several studies reported that comorbid psychiatric disorders and even the diagnosis of ASD itself often go unrecognized among adolescents and adults with HFASD seeking psychological or psychiatric care [28, 36]. This information is particularly noteworthy in the context of autism-related sociocommunicative deficits, which, when combined with psychiatric symptoms, can be quite debilitating in this population.

3. Long-Term Outcomes in HFASD

3.1. Challenges to Functional Autonomy and Quality of Life. A handful of longitudinal studies have demonstrated the many challenges youth with HFASD encounter once they become adults. Despite having intact cognitive skills, the large majority of adults and adolescents with HFASD continue to struggle with finding meaningful and gainful employment, as well as some degree of autonomy and independence in their lives [14]. For example, in a study examining outcomes of 19 men with HFASD, half had been educated in a special autism class, 5% had obtained independent employment, 16% worked in sheltered or voluntary jobs, and 11% were in full time education. In terms of housing, 50% of these adults lived in residential or supported accommodation, 40% with their parents, and 5% in a long-term facility for individuals with developmental delay [37]. Critically, only 10% of these high-functioning individuals lived independently.

Clearly, despite having normal intelligence, adults with HFASD present with significant delays in their adaptive skills. Most of these individuals continue to live at home with their parents and if employed obtain jobs in low level, poorly paid, sheltered or supported employment. It is hoped that in the future interventions will continue to improve for this population, with greater attention to social outcomes in school age youth and increased supports at the college level (e.g., mentorship programs). For example, findings of a recent case study of students with HFASD and their university coordinators demonstrated the benefits of explicit, organized routines and structures and of the importance of support systems (e.g., relatives) and services tailored to the individuals' needs [38].

3.2. Persistence of Social Challenges. Deficits in social functioning are a central feature of ASD regardless of level of intellectual functioning. Social skills deficits in this population do not remit with age and may in fact increase during adolescence and adulthood [39, 40]. Studies of children with HFASD demonstrate that despite having intact verbal skills, these individuals often fail to utilize language appropriately in social interactions, particularly in understanding nonliteral language, humor, and irony [41]. Individuals with HFASD may also be more acutely aware of the difficulties they encounter during social interactions compared to individuals with ASD with an ID and therefore appear to be at greater risk for developing depression, low self-esteem, and anxiety, when faced with peer rejection or bullying [42]. In a comparison study of adolescents and adults with HFASD and controls without ASD, individuals with HFASD reported significantly lower scores on measures of friendship [43]. Similarly, in another study, this time of 19 men with HFASD, only three reported close friendships and none had married [37]. Consistent findings were reported in several more recent studies of adolescents and adults with HFASD [44–46].

3.3. Challenges Accessing Services. Youth with ASD report significant difficulties accessing healthcare services, particularly comprehensive health services [47, 48]. Part of the reason for this difficulty stems from service providers feeling ill equipped to work with individuals with ASD, particularly individuals with comorbid mental health issues [1]. Challenges accessing services can often precipitate crises for individuals with ASD, leading families to be distrustful of healthcare services and service providers [49]. To date, no longitudinal research has examined whether these problems increase or decrease into adulthood.

In Ontario, as well as other parts of Canada and the world, the majority of services for adolescents and adults with ASD are designed for people with an intellectual disability [1]. Since these individuals do not meet criteria for an ID, adolescents and adults with HFASD have access to significantly fewer programs than adolescents and adults with other types of developmental disabilities. All of this occurs during a particularly difficult time of transition whereby social demands start to increase and educational and occupational structures are decreased [1, 50]. Not surprisingly then, a consistent theme for parents of individuals with HFASD is the fear that their child will fall through the cracks when transitioning from child to adult services [51]. Similar concerns have been voiced by the individuals with HFASD themselves, who describe how their needs are rarely recognized and the programs and services available are not designed for people with ASD in mind [52]. From the perspective of community mental health agencies, many services do not want to accept clients with ASD who have comorbid psychiatric or behaviour disorders because they do not feel equipped to manage their care.

While the majority of outcome studies showed improvement in ASD symptoms over time, most individuals with HFASD continue to encounter significant difficulties in social relationships, employment, and communication. Additionally, parents of these teens and adults report a number of challenges and concerns related to future independence and availability of appropriate services and supports.

4. Mental Health Interventions in HFASD

Outcome research on the effect of psychosocial and pharmacological interventions for people with HFASD has been relatively recent. A limited number of studies have investigated the efficacy of specific treatment approaches and, not surprisingly, no single methodology or intervention strategy has been identified as effective for all individuals with HFASD [53].

4.1. Pharmacological Interventions. While several studies document high rates of prescription medication use in children with ASD [54–58], very little is known about medication use in adolescence and adulthood. There is even less research on medication prevalence and pharmacological interventions for adults and teens with HFASD, despite high rates of psychiatric comorbidity in this population. In one of the only studies to examine these issues, Martin and colleagues [59] studied psychotropic drug use in a high-functioning (IQ > 70) sample of children, adolescents, and adults with autism, AS, and PDD-NOS. Across all diagnostic categories, 55% of participants reported taking psychotropic drugs, and 29% were taking 2 or more medications simultaneously. The most commonly prescribed medications were antidepressants (32%), followed by stimulants (20%) and neuroleptics (17%). Similar findings are described in a more recent study of psychotropic medication use in children with HFASD where 33% of the sample reported taking psychotropic drugs, with stimulant (25%), antidepressant (10%), and neuroleptic (6%) medications most commonly prescribed [60]. More general findings for studies of children, adolescents, and adults with ASD suggest that greater age, lower adaptive skills, lower social competence, higher levels of challenging behaviour, and living away from home are all associated with an increased likelihood of medication use [54, 55, 57, 58, 61, 62]. What these studies fail to describe in detail is the prescriber role and level of care received. Specifically, who is the prescriber and how well is medication monitored over time? The only study to look at medication profiles over time found that as adolescents with ASD aged, medications were only increased but never decreased [61]. Given high rates of psychotropic medication use observed in this population, combined with evidence of lack of psychiatric access, there remain significant concerns around prescribing and monitoring practices.

For studies evaluating the outcome of psychotropic medication use, it is important to ensure that validated, treatment-sensitive, rating scales, and side effects measures are utilized [63]. This is particularly pertinent for adults with HFASD, who can be quite sensitive to medication side effects and resistant in complying with medication regimens. It is also important to note that many medications have adverse or paradoxical side effects [63, 64] and that very few evidence-based approaches to psychopharmacologic management exist for this population [63, 65]. Training of future mental health clinicians must ensure that psychotropic prescription and monitoring for this population are included within curriculum alongside any other psychiatric disorder [33, 34].

4.2. Social Skills Interventions. A recent systematic review of research on behavioral interventions for young adults with HFASD identified 20 studies aimed at improving adaptive skills for this population [66]. Social interaction skills were most commonly targeted, followed by practical academic skills, vocational skills, and domestic skills. Improvements were noted in 19 of the 20 studies, and procedures involving visual cues, video modeling, self-reinforcement, contingencies, and corrective feedback showed greatest improvement. In another review of social skills training groups for youth with HFASD [67], most studies of social skills groups involving cognitive-behavioural or parent intervention components demonstrated success. Despite this, there are relatively few social skill interventions in place for individuals with HFASD. Several interventions have been developed with the aim of improving social appropriateness, social interest, and conversation skills, but results remain inconsistent [68–75]. Successful approaches have included those targeting social skill building, social skill training [42, 75–81], computer simulation [71, 82], and peer training [72]. The issue with these findings is a lack of consistent outcome measures, small sample sizes, and the limited number of programs studied, making comparisons between programs difficult and the significance of findings challenging to interpret. More rigorous, objective study of effective interventions and outcomes for this population is critical as individuals with HFASD transition into adulthood and the possibility of new vocational and residential environments.

4.3. Supported Employment. Very few vocational opportunities and supports exist for adults with ASD despite the fact that there are a number of well-informed, evidence-based vocational models (e.g., supported employment, job coach approaches [83–88]). Although adults with HFASD may be deemed more capable than individuals with ASD and an ID, organizational, sensory, and social deficits continue to impede successful and meaningful employment opportunities for this population.

Supported employment is a vocational rehabilitation system with demonstrated success in helping individuals with HFASD find and maintain employment [83, 84, 87]. For example, results of a two-year supported employment project for adults with HFASD reported significantly longer terms of employment and higher job levels and salaries, compared to individuals not in a supported program [89]. Additionally, in a more recent study involving an employment service for individuals with HFASD, results found that 68% of individuals involved with the service had found employment [85]. Some of the common features of successful supported employment programs include job matching, individualized, strengths-based job supports, communication supports, family supports, fostering self-determination and independence, autism awareness training, and strong relationships between employers, job coaches, and individuals with ASD [90, 91]. Obstacles to successful employment include completing job applications, acclimating to new job routines, communication, and navigating social interactions with coworkers and supervisors [91].

Findings suggest that supported employment systems may be beneficial for some individuals with ASD; however, barriers still exist from the perspective of employers. At the community level, employers must be engaged and incentivized to hire individuals with ASD through evidence that demonstrates the benefits of hiring individuals with autism to both employer and employee. This is particularly important in the context of knowledge that individuals who receive supported employment are hired faster, earn higher disposable incomes, and have lower individual allowances or disability support payments compared to individuals with disabilities who do not receive supported employment [92]. Given the existent foci of vocational rehabilitation within mental health services [93–97], inclusive of models like supportive employment, the request for similar models for individuals with HFASD suggests an opportunity for the mental health sector to take a leadership role in supporting the vocational needs of individuals with HFASD. Some of these efforts are already underway in the not-for-profit sector, such as the Specialist People Foundation (Specialisterne), but similar efforts are required in the mental health sector on a much broader scale. There is also a parallel need for more research on supported employment approaches and outcomes in this population as individuals with HFASD transition into adulthood.

4.4. Cognitive Behaviour Therapy (CBT) and Mindfulness-Based Therapy (MBT). The effectiveness of cognitive behaviour therapy (CBT) in addressing anxiety, anger, and social skills deficits in youth with HFASD is well documented in the literature [98–105]. There are fewer studies, however, which have examined the effectiveness of CBT in adults with HFASD. Although no large trials have been published on CBT and adults with HFASD, case study and case series reports suggest that CBT is a promising treatment for depression and anxiety in this population [49, 106, 107]. Results of a recent mindfulness-based therapy (MBT) randomized control trial suggest that this may also represent a promising treatment approach. Significant reductions in depression, anxiety, and rumination were observed in a sample of adults with HFASD who received MBT [108]. While further research is needed in this area, particularly large-scale studies which compare the effectiveness of CBT or MBT versus other treatment options (e.g., medication, counseling, etc.), it is important to note that many mental health clinicians already have the skills to effectively deliver these therapies. Another important next step is to look at what has been successfully employed in community mental health settings and adapting these effective, evidence-based psychiatric, employment, and academic interventions to include individuals with HFASD.

4.5. Supports for Families. Parents and other family members of individuals with ASD, because of the complexity of their mental health problems, as well as deficits in social and communicative functioning, frequently take on the role of coordinating the individual's healthcare well into adulthood [109]. It is not surprising then that caring for an individual with ASD is associated with high levels of caregiver burden [110, 111]. Despite this, there is a dearth of literature on interventions and supports for parents and siblings of individuals with ASD, particularly in adulthood. Of the few studies that have been conducted to date, results highlight the need to involve family in the individual's overall treatment plan and the need to support and address the mental health and parenting needs of those supporting and caring for individuals with ASD [112, 113]. Further research is needed to identify what supports are most effective for families of adolescents and adults with HFASD.

5. Conclusions

Adolescents and adults with HFASD represent a complex and underserved population. Of the studies completed to date, findings suggest that this subgroup of adolescents and adults faces a multitude of psychiatric and psychosocial issues, alongside significant challenges in accessing services. Social skills deficits for individuals with HFASD persist into adulthood, and adults appear to be at heightened risk for developing depression, low self-esteem, and anxiety. Despite this, very few studies have examined treatment patterns and interventions (pharmacological and psychosocial) for adolescents and adults with HFASD. Evidence is beginning to emerge for interventions targeting this population, including CBT, MBT, and SST, but further large-scale studies which compare the effectiveness of, for example, CBT or MBT versus other treatment options (e.g., medication, counseling, etc.) are required and the need for mental health clinicians trained to apply these techniques is now.

In developing interventions for these individuals, programs must consider what adolescents and adults want. For example, adolescents and adults with HFASD may be more interested in interventions targeting vocational opportunities than interventions targeting social skills. Individuals with HFASD and their family members must be viewed as valuable contributors and fully engaged in this process. Further, researchers must look at issues of service cost and efficiency when evaluating the impact of interventions [15].

The large majority of adults and adolescents with HFASD live at home with their families and, of those employed, most obtain jobs in low level, poorly paid, sheltered or supported employment. It is not surprising therefore that the parents of these teens and adults report a number of challenges and concerns related to future independence and availability of appropriate services and supports.

6. Recommendations

Together, findings point to a number of important practice recommendations. First, developmental disability agencies or agencies supporting individuals with ASD must partner with community mental health agencies to help train, mentor, and build capacity to care for this population across the lifespan. It is important to note that many clinicians working within community mental health agencies already have the skills to effectively deliver this care, but programs either preclude their ability to do so or they lack the confidence to work with this population. Second, there is a critical need for community mental health agencies to review their exclusion criteria to include persons with ASD. For example, agencies providing care for persons with mood or anxiety disorders should not exclude individuals on the basis of a diagnosis of ASD. Community mental health agencies have the resources and expertise in mental health, along with the programs to care for individuals with mental health issues (e.g., vocational programs, counseling, and therapies), but will need guidance from developmental disability agencies to successfully adapt these programs for adults with HFASD. Third, developmental disability agencies must reevaluate their inclusion criteria to include persons with HFASD, regardless of IQ, and across the lifespan. Organizations must work together, combining expertise in ASD from developmental disability agencies with knowledge and resources from community mental health agencies. Fourth, there is a need to study and identify programs and supports that are most effective in both school and community settings. To do this will require a full continuum of mental health services including counseling, vocational support, inpatient services, and outpatient services. It will also require a network of experienced clinicians and community partners. Many of these efforts are already underway in pediatric settings; however, these same efforts are required in adolescent and adult mental health services. Finally, there is a need to prepare and equip older youth with HFASD for the transition to adult services. A number of key recommendations and principles can be gleaned from the broader ID education/vocational literature [114] and from studies of individuals with ID transitioning from the pediatric to the adult medical system [115, 116], many of which could be tailored to persons with HFASD. For example, the use of meaningful transition tools (e.g., Transition Planning Inventory [117]; Good 2 Go Readiness Checklists https://www.sickkids.ca/Good2Go/What-we-do/Readiness-checklists/33789-G2G%20Transition%20Readiness%20Checklist%20for%20Patients%20-%20v.%20Nov%202010.pdf) and the importance of transition workers, protocols, and policies [118, 119] are required.

Acknowledgments

This work was supported by a fellowship award from the Centre for Addiction and Mental Health and the University of Toronto. The authors thank Susan Morris for her helpful input.

References

[1] Autism Ontario, "FORGOTTEN: Ontario Adults with Autism and Adults with Aspergers," 2008.

[2] Canadian Institutes of Health Research, *Report on the National Autism Research Symposium*, Policy Planning Plus, Ontario, Canada, 2007.

[3] Mental Health Commission of Canada, *Changing Directions, Changing Lives: The Mental Health Strategy for Canada*, Mental Health Commission of Canada, Calgary, Canada, 2012.

[4] National Institute of Mental Health, *Autism Spectrum Disorders (Pervasive Developmental Disorders)*, U.S. Government Printing Office, Bethesda , Md, USA, 2007.

[5] T. Charman and P. Clare, *Mapping Autism Research: Identifying UK Priorities for the Future*, The National Autistic Society, 2004.

[6] National Autistic Society, *Taking Responsibility: Good Practice Guidelines—Services for Adults with Asperger Syndrome*, Newnorth Print, London , UK, 2002.

[7] Royal College of Psychiatrists, "Psychiatric services for adolescents and adults with Asperger Syndrome and other autism spectrum disorders," Council Report CR 136, Royal College of Psychiatrists, London, UK, 2006.

[8] M. L. Belfer, "Child and adolescent mental disorders: the magnitude of the problem across the globe," *Journal of Child Psychology and Psychiatry and Allied Disciplines*, vol. 49, no. 3, pp. 226–236, 2008.

[9] A. Rahman, R. Harrington, M. Mubbashar, and R. Gater, "Annotation: developing child mental health services in developing countries," *Journal of Child Psychology and Psychiatry and Allied Disciplines*, vol. 41, no. 5, pp. 539–546, 2000.

[10] Autism and Developmental Disabilities Monitoring Network Surveillance Year 2010 Principal Investigators, "Prevalence of autism spectrum disorder among children aged 8 years—autism and developmental disabilities monitoring network, 11 sites, United States, 2010," *MMWR Surveillance Summaries*, vol. 63, no. 2, pp. 1–21, 2010.

[11] World Health Organization, *International Classification of Diseases, Tenth Revisions, Criteria for Research*, WHO, Geneva, Switzerland, 1992.

[12] American Psychiatric Association, *Diagnostic and Statistical Manual of Mental Disorders*, American Psychiatric Association, Washington, DC, USA, 4th edition, 2000.

[13] American Psychiatric Association, *Diagnostic and Statistical Manual of Mental Disorders*, American Psychiatric Association, Washington, DC, USA, 5th edition, 2013.

[14] P. Howlin and P. Moss, "Adults with autism spectrum disorders," *Canadian Journal of Psychiatry*, vol. 57, no. 5, pp. 275–283, 2012.

[15] P. T. Shattuck, A. M. Roux, L. E. Hudson, J. L. Taylor, M. J. Maenner, and J.-F. Trani, "Services for adults with an autism spectrum disorder," *Canadian Journal of Psychiatry*, vol. 57, no. 5, pp. 284–291, 2012.

[16] L. E. Barnard, V. Harvey, A. Prior, and D. Potter, *Ignored or Ineligible? The Reality for Adults with Autistic Spectrum Disorders*, National Autistic Society, London, UK, 2001.

[17] B. Hofvander, R. Delorme, P. Chaste et al., "Psychiatric and psychosocial problems in adults with normal-intelligence autism spectrum disorders," *BMC Psychiatry*, vol. 9, article 35, 2009.

[18] S. Mohiuddin, S. Bobak, D. Gih, and M. Ghaziuddin, "Autism spectrum disorders: comorbid psychopathology and treatment," in *International Handbook of Autism and Pervasive Developmental Disorders*, J. L. Matson and P. Sturmey, Eds., Autism and Child Psychopathology Series, pp. 463–478, Springer Science + Business Media, New York, NY, USA, 2011.

[19] D. S. Moseley, B. J. Tonge, A. V. Brereton, and S. L. Einfeld, "Psychiatric comorbidity in adolescents and young adults with autism," *Journal of Mental Health Research in Intellectual Disabilities*, vol. 4, no. 4, pp. 229–243, 2011.

[20] E. Simonoff, A. Pickles, T. Charman, S. Chandler, T. Loucas, and G. Baird, "Psychiatric disorders in children with autism spectrum disorders: prevalence, comorbidity, and associated factors in a population-derived sample," *Journal of the American Academy of Child and Adolescent Psychiatry*, vol. 47, no. 8, pp. 921–929, 2008.

[21] N. Skokauskas and L. Gallagher, "Mental health aspects of autistic spectrum disorders in children," *Journal of Intellectual Disability Research*, vol. 56, no. 3, pp. 248–257, 2012.

[22] M. Solomon, M. Miller, S. L. Taylor, S. P. Hinshaw, and C. S. Carter, "Autism symptoms and internalizing psychopathology in girls and boys with autism spectrum disorders," *Journal of Autism and Developmental Disorders*, vol. 42, no. 1, pp. 48–59, 2012.

[23] L. T. van Elst, M. Pick, M. Biscaldi, T. Fangmeier, and A. Riedel, "High-functioning autism spectrum disorder as a basic disorder in adult psychiatry and psychotherapy: Psychopathological presentation, clinical relevance and therapeutic concepts," *European Archives of Psychiatry and Clinical Neuroscience*, vol. 263, supplement 2, pp. 189–196, 2013.

[24] J. A. Worley and J. L. Matson, "Psychiatric symptoms in children diagnosed with an Autism spectrum disorder: an examination of gender differences," *Research in Autism Spectrum Disorders*, vol. 5, no. 3, pp. 1086–1091, 2011.

[25] T. Hurtig, S. Kuusikko, M.-L. Mattila et al., "Multi-informant reports of psychiatric symptoms among high-functioning adolescents with Asperger syndrome or autism," *Autism*, vol. 13, no. 6, pp. 583–598, 2009.

[26] T. Lugnegård, M. U. Hallerbäck, and C. Gillberg, "Psychiatric comorbidity in young adults with a clinical diagnosis of Asperger syndrome," *Research in Developmental Disabilities*, vol. 32, no. 5, pp. 1910–1917, 2011.

[27] M.-L. Mattila, T. Hurtig, H. Haapsamo et al., "Comorbid psychiatric disorders associated with asperger syndrome/high-functioning autism: a community- and clinic-based study," *Journal of Autism and Developmental Disorders*, vol. 40, no. 9, pp. 1080–1093, 2010.

[28] T. Munesue, Y. Ono, K. Mutoh, K. Shimoda, H. Nakatani, and M. Kikuchi, "High prevalence of bipolar disorder comorbidity in adolescents and young adults with high-functioning autism spectrum disorder: a preliminary study of 44 outpatients," *Journal of Affective Disorders*, vol. 111, no. 2-3, pp. 170–175, 2008.

[29] A. J. Russell, D. Mataix-Cols, M. Anson, and D. G. M. Murphy, "Obsessions and compulsions in Asperger syndrome and high-functioning autism," *The British Journal of Psychiatry*, vol. 186, pp. 525–528, 2005.

[30] H. Allik, J.-O. Larsson, and H. Smedje, "Health-related quality of life in parents of school-age children with Asperger syndrome

or high-functioning autism," *Health and Quality of Life Outcomes*, vol. 4, article 1, 2006.

[31] B. J. Tonge, A. V. Brereton, K. M. Gray, and S. L. Einfeld, "Behavioural and emotional disturbance in high-functioning autism and Asperger syndrome," *Autism*, vol. 3, no. 2, pp. 117–130, 1999.

[32] M. Ghaziuddin and J. Greden, "Depression in children with autism/pervasive developmental disorders: a case-control family history study," *Journal of Autism and Developmental Disorders*, vol. 28, no. 2, pp. 111–115, 1998.

[33] S. Bellini, "Social skills deficits and anxiety in high-functioning adolescents with autism spectrum disorders," *Focus on Autism and other Developmental Disorders*, vol. 19, pp. 78–86, 2004.

[34] M. Ghaziuddin, *Mental Health Aspects of Autism and Asperger Syndrome*, Jessica Kingsley Publishers, London, UK, 2005.

[35] N. M. Mukaddes, S. Hergner, and C. Tanidir, "Psychiatric disorders in individuals with high-functioning autism and Asperger's disorder: similarities and differences," *The World Journal of Biological Psychiatry*, vol. 11, no. 7-8, pp. 964–971, 2010.

[36] M. Raja and A. Azzoni, "Comorbidity of Asperger's syndrome and bipolar disorder," *Clinical Practice and Epidemiology in Mental Health*, vol. 4, article 26, 2008.

[37] P. Howlin, "Outcome in adult life for more able individuals with autism or Asperger syndrome," *Autism*, vol. 4, no. 1, pp. 63–83, 2000.

[38] A. S. Fleischer, "Support to students with Asperger syndrome in higher education—the perspectives of three relatives and three coordinators," *International Journal of Rehabilitation Research*, vol. 35, no. 1, pp. 54–61, 2012.

[39] M. D. Rutherford, S. Baron-Cohen, and S. Wheelwright, "Reading the mind in the voice: a study with normal adults and adults with Asperger syndrome and high functioning autism," *Journal of Autism and Developmental Disorders*, vol. 32, no. 3, pp. 189–194, 2002.

[40] D. Tantam, "The challenge of adolescents and adults with Asperger syndrome," *Child and Adolescent Psychiatric Clinics of North America*, vol. 12, no. 1, pp. 143–163, 2003.

[41] C. Kasari, E. Rotheram-Fuller, J. Locke, and A. Gulsrud, "Making the connection: randomized controlled trial of social skills at school for children with autism spectrum disorders," *Journal of Child Psychology and Psychiatry and Allied Disciplines*, vol. 53, no. 4, pp. 431–439, 2012.

[42] J. Tse, J. Strulovitch, V. Tagalakis, L. Meng, and E. Fombonne, "Social skills training for adolescents with Asperger syndrome and high-functioning autism," *Journal of Autism and Developmental Disorders*, vol. 37, no. 10, pp. 1960–1968, 2007.

[43] S. Baron-Cohen and S. Wheelwright, "The friendship questionnaire: an investigation of adults with Asperger syndrome or high-functioning autism, and normal sex differences," *Journal of Autism and Developmental Disorders*, vol. 33, no. 5, pp. 509–517, 2003.

[44] P. Howlin, S. Goode, J. Hutton, and M. Rutter, "Adult outcome for children with autism," *Journal of Child Psychology and Psychiatry and Allied Disciplines*, vol. 45, no. 2, pp. 212–229, 2004.

[45] P. Howlin, "The outcome in adult life for people with ASD," in *Autism and Pervasive Developmental Disorders*, F. Volkmar, Ed., Cambridge University Press, New York, NY, USA, 2nd edition, 2007.

[46] A. J. O. Whitehouse, K. Durkin, E. Jaquet, and K. Ziatas, "Friendship, loneliness and depression in adolescents with Asperger's Syndrome," *Journal of Adolescence*, vol. 32, no. 2, pp. 309–322, 2009.

[47] D. S. Mandell, C. M. Walrath, B. Manteuffel, G. Sgro, and J. Pinto-Martin, "Characteristics of children with autistic spectrum disorders served in comprehensive community-based mental health settings," *Journal of Autism and Developmental Disorders*, vol. 35, no. 3, pp. 313–321, 2005.

[48] S. C. Narendorf, P. T. Shattuck, and P. R. Sterzing, "Mental health service use among adolescents with an autism spectrum disorder," *Psychiatric Services*, vol. 62, no. 8, pp. 975–978, 2011.

[49] J. A. Weiss and Y. Lunsky, "Group cognitive behaviour therapy for adults with Asperger syndrome and anxiety or mood disorder: a case series," *Clinical Psychology and Psychotherapy*, vol. 17, no. 5, pp. 438–446, 2010.

[50] A. Ward and A. Russell, "Mental health services for adults with autism spectrum disorders," *Advances in Mental Health and Learning Disabilities*, vol. 1, pp. 23–28, 2007.

[51] J. Weiss, "The family study: parents share their experiences of caring for people with ASD in adolescence and adulthood," *Autism Matters*, vol. 5, pp. 6–8, 2008.

[52] T. Madar, "My use of mental health related services," *Advances in Mental Health and Learning Disabilities*, vol. 1, pp. 29–31, 2007.

[53] K. Toth and B. H. King, "Asperger's syndrome: diagnosis and treatment," *The American Journal of Psychiatry*, vol. 165, no. 8, pp. 958–963, 2008.

[54] D. L. Coury, E. Anagnostou, P. Manning-Courtney et al., "Use of psychotropic medication in children and adolescents with autism spectrum disorders," *Pediatrics*, vol. 130, no. 2, pp. S69–S76, 2012.

[55] R. E. Rosenberg, D. S. Mandell, J. E. Farmer, J. K. Law, A. R. Marvin, and P. A. Law, "Psychotropic medication use among children with autism spectrum disorders enrolled in a national registry, 2007-2008," *Journal of Autism and Developmental Disorders*, vol. 40, no. 3, pp. 342–351, 2010.

[56] D. S. Mandell, K. H. Morales, S. C. Marcus, A. C. Stahmer, J. Doshi, and D. E. Polsky, "Psychotropic medication use among medicaid-enrolled children with autism spectrum disorders," *Pediatrics*, vol. 121, no. 3, pp. e441–e448, 2008.

[57] D. Spencer, J. Marshall, B. Post et al., "Psychotropic medication use and polypharmacy in children with autism spectrum disorders," *Pediatrics*, vol. 132, pp. 833–840, 2013.

[58] A. Witwer and L. Lecavalier, "Treatment incidence and patterns in children and adolescents with autism spectrum disorders," *Journal of Child and Adolescent Psychopharmacology*, vol. 15, no. 4, pp. 671–681, 2005.

[59] A. Martin, L. Scahill, A. Klin, and F. R. Volkmar, "Higher-functioning pervasive developmental disorders: rates and patterns of psychotropic drug use," *Journal of the American Academy of Child and Adolescent Psychiatry*, vol. 38, no. 7, pp. 923–931, 1999.

[60] C. Lopata, J. A. Toomey, J. D. Fox, M. L. Thomeer, M. A. Volker, and G. K. Lee, "Prevalence and predictors of psychotropic use in children with high-functioning ASDs," *Autism Research and Treatment*, vol. 2013, Article ID 384527, 11 pages, 2013.

[61] A. J. Esbensen, J. S. Greenberg, M. M. Seltzer, and M. G. Aman, "A longitudinal investigation of psychotropic and non-psychotropic medication use among adolescents and adults with autism spectrum disorders," *Journal of Autism and Developmental Disorders*, vol. 39, no. 9, pp. 1339–1349, 2009.

[62] J. K. Lake, R. Balogh, and Y. Lunsky, "Polypharmacy profiles and predictors among adults with autism spectrum disorders,"

Research in Autism Spectrum Disorders, vol. 6, no. 3, pp. 1142–1149, 2012.

[63] S. M. Myers, "The status of pharmacotherapy for autism spectrum disorders," *Expert Opinion on Pharmacotherapy*, vol. 8, no. 11, pp. 1579–1603, 2007.

[64] E. Bradley and J. Lofchy, "Learning disability in the accident and emergency department," *Advances in Psychiatric Treatment*, vol. 11, no. 1, pp. 45–57, 2005.

[65] Z. Warren, M. L. McPheeters, N. Sathe, J. H. Foss-Feig, A. Glasser, and J. Veenstra-VanderWeele, "A systematic review of early intensive intervention for autism spectrum disorders," *Pediatrics*, vol. 127, no. 5, pp. e1303–e1311, 2011.

[66] A. Palmen, R. Didden, and R. Lang, "A systematic review of behavioral intervention research on adaptive skill building in high-functioning young adults with autism spectrum disorder," *Research in Autism Spectrum Disorders*, vol. 6, no. 2, pp. 602–617, 2012.

[67] M. C. Cappadocia and J. A. Weiss, "Review of social skills training groups for youth with Asperger Syndrome and high functioning autism," *Research in Autism Spectrum Disorders*, vol. 5, no. 1, pp. 70–78, 2011.

[68] C. Carter, L. Meckes, L. Pritchard, S. Swensen, P. P. Wittman, and B. Velde, "The friendship club: an after-school program for children with asperger syndrome," *Family and Community Health*, vol. 27, no. 2, pp. 143–150, 2004.

[69] P. Howlin and P. Yates, "The potential effectiveness of social skills groups for adults with autism," *Autism*, vol. 3, no. 3, pp. 299–307, 1999.

[70] A. Palmen, R. Didden, and M. Arts, "Improving question asking in high-functioning adolescents with autism spectrum disorders: effectiveness of small-group training," *Autism*, vol. 12, no. 1, pp. 83–98, 2008.

[71] S. Parsons, P. Mitchell, and A. Leonard, "The use and understanding of virtual environments by adolescents with autistic spectrum disorders," *Journal of Autism and Developmental Disorders*, vol. 34, no. 4, pp. 449–466, 2004.

[72] K. S. Thiemann and H. Goldstein, "Effects of peer training and written text cueing on social communication of school-age children with pervasive developmental disorder," *Journal of Speech, Language, and Hearing Research*, vol. 47, no. 1, pp. 126–144, 2004.

[73] C. Schmidt, J. P. Stichter, K. Lierheimer, S. McGhee, and K. V. O'Connor, "An initial investigation of the generalization of a school-based social competence intervention for youth with high-functioning autism," *Autism Research and Treatment*, vol. 2011, Article ID 589539, 11 pages, 2011.

[74] L. M. Turner-Brown, T. D. Perry, G. S. Dichter, J. W. Bodfish, and D. L. Penn, "Brief report: feasibility of social cognition and interaction training for adults with high functioning autism," *Journal of Autism and Developmental Disorders*, vol. 38, no. 9, pp. 1777–1784, 2008.

[75] B. J. Webb, S. P. Miller, T. B. Pierce, S. Strawser, and W. P. Jones, "Effects of social skill instruction for high functioning adolescents with autism spectrum disorders," *Focus on Autism and Other Developmental Disabilities*, vol. 19, no. 1, pp. 53–62, 2004.

[76] G. P. Barnhill, *Designing Social Skills Interventions for Students with Asperger Syndrome*, vol. 31, National Association of School Psychologists Communique, Bethesda, Md, USA, 2002.

[77] T. D. Barry, L. G. Klinger, J. M. Lee, N. Palardy, T. Gilmore, and S. D. Bodin, "Examining the effectiveness of an outpatient clinic-based social skills group for high-functioning children with autism," *Journal of Autism and Developmental Disorders*, vol. 33, no. 6, pp. 685–701, 2003.

[78] M. Konstantareas, "Social skills training in high functioning Autism and Asperger's disorder," *Hellenic Journal of Psychology*, vol. 3, no. 1, pp. 39–56, 2006.

[79] J. Rogers, "Interventions that facilitate socialization in children with autism," *Journal of Autism and Developmental Disorders*, vol. 30, no. 5, pp. 399–409, 2000.

[80] L. Sloman and J. Leef, "Child social interaction and parental self-efficacy: evaluating simultaneous groups for children with Asperger syndrome and their parents," in *Children, youth and adults with Asperger Syndrome*, K. P. Stoddart, Ed., Jessica Kingsley Publishers, London, UK, 2004.

[81] M. Solomon, B. L. Goodlin-Jones, and T. F. Anders, "A social adjustment enhancement intervention for high functioning autism, Asperger's syndrome, and pervasive developmental disorder NOS," *Journal of Autism and Developmental Disorders*, vol. 34, no. 6, pp. 649–668, 2004.

[82] P. Mitchell, S. Parsons, and A. Leonard, "Using virtual environments for teaching social understanding to 6 adolescents with autistic spectrum disorders," *Journal of Autism and Developmental Disorders*, vol. 37, no. 3, pp. 589–600, 2007.

[83] R. V. Burke, M. N. Andersen, S. L. Bowen, M. R. Howard, and K. D. Allen, "Evaluation of two instruction methods to increase employment options for young adults with autism spectrum disorders," *Research in Developmental Disabilities*, vol. 31, no. 6, pp. 1223–1233, 2010.

[84] D. García-Villamisar, P. Wehman, and M. D. Navarro, "Changes in the quality of autistic people's life that work in supported and sheltered employment. A 5-year follow-up study," *Journal of Vocational Rehabilitation*, vol. 17, no. 4, pp. 309–312, 2002.

[85] P. Howlin, J. Alcock, and C. Burkin, "An 8 year follow-up of a specialist supported employment service for high-ability adults with autism or Asperger syndrome," *Autism*, vol. 9, no. 5, pp. 533–549, 2005.

[86] L. Ling-Yi,, Y. Shu-Ning, and Y. Ya-Tsu, "A study of activities of daily living and employment in adults with autism spectrum disorders in Taiwan," *International Journal of Rehabilitation Research*, vol. 35, no. 2, pp. 109–115, 2012.

[87] L. Lawer, E. Brusilovskiy, M. S. Salzer, and D. S. Mandell, "Use of vocational rehabilitative services among adults with autism," *Journal of Autism and Developmental Disorders*, vol. 39, no. 3, pp. 487–494, 2009.

[88] K. Stoddart, L. Burke, and R. King, *Asperger Syndrome in Adulthood: A Comprehensive Guide for Clinicians*, W.W. Norton & Company, New York, NY, USA, 2012.

[89] L. Mawhood and P. Howlin, "The outcome of a supported employment scheme for high-functioning adults with autism or Asperger syndrome," *Autism*, vol. 3, no. 3, pp. 229–254, 1999.

[90] G. K. Lee and E. W. Carter, "Preparing transition-age students with high-functioning autism spectrum disorders for meaningful work," *Psychology in the Schools*, vol. 49, no. 10, pp. 988–1000, 2012.

[91] E. Müller, A. Schuler, B. A. Burton, and G. B. Yates, "Meeting the vocational support needs of individuals with Asperger Syndrome and other autism spectrum disabilities," *Journal of Vocational Rehabilitation*, vol. 18, no. 3, pp. 163–175, 2003.

[92] P. Germundsson, J. Gustafsson, M. Lind, and B. Danermark, "Disability and supported employment: impact on employment, income, and allowances," *International Journal of Rehabilitation Research*, vol. 35, no. 3, pp. 263–269, 2012.

[93] G. Bond, "Supported employment: evidence for an evidence-based practice," *Psychiatric Rehabilitation Journal*, vol. 27, no. 4, pp. 345–359, 2004.

[94] G. R. Bond, R. E. Drake, and D. R. Becker, "An update on randomized controlled trials of evidence-based supported employment," *Psychiatric Rehabilitation Journal*, vol. 31, no. 4, pp. 280–290, 2008.

[95] R. E. Drake and G. R. Bond, "IPS support employment: a 20-year update," *American Journal of Psychiatric Rehabilitation*, vol. 14, no. 3, pp. 155–164, 2011.

[96] R. E. Drake, H. H. Goldman, H. Stephen Leff et al., "Implementing evidence-based practices in routine mental health service settings," *Psychiatric Services*, vol. 52, no. 2, pp. 179–182, 2001.

[97] K. T. Mueser, R. E. Clark, M. Haines et al., "The Hartford study of supported employment for persons with severe mental illness," *Journal of Consulting and Clinical Psychology*, vol. 72, no. 3, pp. 479–490, 2004.

[98] A. Chalfant, R. Rapee, and L. Carroll, "Treating anxiety disorders in children with high functioning autism spectrum disorders: a controlled trial," *Journal of Autism and Developmental Disorders*, vol. 37, no. 10, pp. 1842–1857, 2007.

[99] A. Greig and T. MacKay, "Asperger's syndrome and cognitive behaviour therapy: new applications for educational psychologists," *Educational & Child Psychology*, vol. 22, pp. 4–15, 2005.

[100] J. A. Reaven, A. Blakeley-Smith, S. Nichols, M. Dasari, E. Flanigan, and S. Hepburn, "Cognitive-behavioral group treatment for anxiety symptoms in children with high-functioning autism spectrum disorders: a pilot study," *Focus on Autism and Other Developmental Disabilities*, vol. 24, no. 1, pp. 27–37, 2009.

[101] K. Sofronoff, T. Attwood, and S. Hinton, "A randomised controlled trial of a CBT intervention for anxiety in children with Asperger syndrome," *Journal of Child Psychology and Psychiatry and Allied Disciplines*, vol. 46, no. 11, pp. 1152–1160, 2005.

[102] K. M. Sze and J. J. Wood, "Cognitive behavioral treatment of comorbid anxiety disorders and social difficulties in children with high-functioning autism: a case report," *Journal of Contemporary Psychotherapy*, vol. 37, no. 3, pp. 133–143, 2007.

[103] K. M. Sze and J. J. Wood, "Enhancing CBT for the treatment of autism spectrum disorders and concurrent anxiety," *Behavioural and Cognitive Psychotherapy*, vol. 36, no. 4, pp. 403–409, 2008.

[104] S. W. White, A. M. Albano, C. R. Johnson et al., "Development of a cognitive-behavioral intervention program to treat anxiety and social deficits in teens with high-functioning autism," *Clinical Child and Family Psychology Review*, vol. 13, no. 1, pp. 77–90, 2010.

[105] J. J. Wood, A. Drahota, K. Sze, K. Har, A. Chiu, and D. A. Langer, "Cognitive behavioral therapy for anxiety in children with autism spectrum disorders: a randomized, controlled trial," *Journal of Child Psychology and Psychiatry and Allied Disciplines*, vol. 50, no. 3, pp. 224–234, 2009.

[106] L. Cardaciotto and J. D. Herbert, "Cognitive behavior therapy for social anxiety disorder in the context of Asperger's syndrome: a single-subject report," *Cognitive and Behavioral Practice*, vol. 11, no. 1, pp. 75–81, 2004.

[107] D. J. Hare, "The use of cognitive-behavioural therapy with people with Asperger syndrome—a case study," *Autism*, vol. 1, no. 2, pp. 215–225, 1997.

[108] A. A. Spek, N. C. van Ham, and I. Nyklíček, "Mindfulness-based therapy in adults with an autism spectrum disorder: a randomized controlled trial," *Research in Developmental Disabilities*, vol. 34, no. 1, pp. 246–253, 2013.

[109] P. S. Carbone, D. D. Behl, V. Azor, and N. A. Murphy, "The medical home for children with autism spectrum disorders: parent and pediatrician perspectives," *Journal of Autism and Developmental Disorders*, vol. 40, no. 3, pp. 317–324, 2010.

[110] T. Cadman, H. Eklund, D. Howley et al., "Caregiver burden as people with autism spectrum disorder and attention-deficit/hyperactivity disorder transition into adolescence and adulthood in the United Kingdom," *Journal of the American Academy of Child and Adolescent Psychiatry*, vol. 51, no. 9, pp. 879–888, 2012.

[111] S. R. Kring, J. S. Greenberg, and M. M. Seltzer, "Adolescents and adults with autism with and without co-morbid psychiatric disorders: differences in maternal well-being," *Journal of Mental Health Research in Intellectual Disabilities*, vol. 1, no. 2, pp. 53–74, 2008.

[112] N. N. Singh, G. E. Lancioni, A. S. W. Winton et al., "Mindful parenting decreases aggression, noncompliance, and self-injury in children with autism," *Journal of Emotional and Behavioral Disorders*, vol. 14, no. 3, pp. 169–177, 2006.

[113] K. P. Stoddart, "Adolescents with Asperger syndrome. Three case studies of individual and family therapy," *Autism*, vol. 3, no. 3, pp. 255–271, 1999.

[114] E. Carter, A. Trainor, Y. Sun, and L. Owens, "Assessing the transition-related strengths and needs of adolescents with high-incidence disabilities," *Exceptional Children*, vol. 76, no. 1, pp. 74–94, 2009.

[115] R. Burke, M. Spoerri, A. Price, A.-M. Cardosi, and P. Flanagan, "Survey of primary care pediatricians on the transition and transfer of adolescents to adult health care," *Clinical Pediatrics*, vol. 47, no. 4, pp. 347–354, 2008.

[116] N. G. Peter, C. M. Forke, K. R. Ginsburg, and D. F. Schwarz, "Transition from pediatric to adult care: internists' perspectives," *Pediatrics*, vol. 123, no. 2, pp. 417–423, 2009.

[117] G. M. Clark and J. R. Patton, *Transition Planning Inventory: Administration and Resource Guide*, PRO-ED, Austin, Tex, USA, 1997.

[118] S. P. Singh, "Transition of care from child to adult mental health services: the great divide," *Current Opinion in Psychiatry*, vol. 22, no. 4, pp. 386–390, 2009.

[119] S. P. Singh, M. Paul, T. Ford, T. Kramer, and T. Weaver, "Transitions of care from child and adolescent mental health services to adult mental health services (TRACK study): a study of protocols in Greater London," *BMC Health Services Research*, vol. 8, article 135, 2008.

4

Dietary Intake and Plasma Levels of Choline and Betaine in Children with Autism Spectrum Disorders

Joanna C. Hamlin,[1] Margaret Pauly,[2] Stepan Melnyk,[2] Oleksandra Pavliv,[2] William Starrett,[2] Tina A. Crook,[1] and S. Jill James[2,3]

[1] *Department of Dietetics and Nutrition, University of Arkansas for Medical Sciences, Little Rock, AR 72202, USA*
[2] *Department of Pediatrics, University of Arkansas for Medical Sciences, Little Rock, AR 72202, USA*
[3] *Department of Pediatrics, University of Arkansas for Medical Sciences, Arkansas Children's Hospital Research Institute, 13 Children's Way Slot 512-41B, Little Rock, AR 72202, USA*

Correspondence should be addressed to S. Jill James; jamesjill@uams.edu

Academic Editor: Geraldine Dawson

Abnormalities in folate-dependent one-carbon metabolism have been reported in many children with autism. Because inadequate choline and betaine can negatively affect folate metabolism and in turn downstream methylation and antioxidant capacity, we sought to determine whether dietary intake of choline and betaine in children with autism was adequate to meet nutritional needs based on national recommendations. Three-day food records were analyzed for 288 children with autism (ASDs) who participated in the national Autism Intervention Research Network for Physical Health (AIR-P) Study on Diet and Nutrition in children with autism. Plasma concentrations of choline and betaine were measured in a subgroup of 35 children with ASDs and 32 age-matched control children. The results indicated that 60–93% of children with ASDs were consuming less than the recommended Adequate Intake (AI) for choline. Strong positive correlations were found between dietary intake and plasma concentrations of choline and betaine in autistic children as well as lower plasma concentrations compared to the control group. We conclude that choline and betaine intake is inadequate in a significant subgroup of children with ASDs and is reflected in lower plasma levels. Inadequate intake of choline and betaine may contribute to the metabolic abnormalities observed in many children with autism and warrants attention in nutritional counseling.

1. Introduction

Autism is a complex, behaviorally-defined neurodevelopmental disorder characterized by significant impairments in social interaction, verbal and nonverbal communication, and by restrictive, repetitive, and stereotypic patterns of behavior. The Centers for Disease Control estimates that the current prevalence of autism spectrum disorders (ASD) in the United States is 1 in 110 children [1]. Nutritional screening and assessment of children with ASDs is an important clinical consideration for several reasons. First, these children often exhibit nutrition-related medical issues including gastrointestinal discomfort, bowel inflammation, diarrhea, constipation, and acid reflux [1]. Abnormal sensory processing can affect taste and texture perception leading to food avoidance and restricted food intake in many children with ASD. "Insistence on sameness" and compulsive repetitive behaviors reinforce rigid dietary preferences and lead to a limited food repertoire [2]. Finally, accumulating research indicates that nutrient metabolism and requirements may be altered in some children with ASDs compared to typically developing children [3–5]. Thus, children with ASDs have multiple risk factors that may increase the prevalence of nutrient deficiencies in this population.

Metabolic abnormalities reported in children with ASDs have primarily involved folate-dependent one-carbon metabolism. Paşca et al. reported hyperhomocysteinemia and abnormal methionine metabolite levels in children with AD and PDD-NOS [6]. They also noted an increased prevalence of the C677T MTHFR polymorphism in children with AD.

Polymorphisms in this pathway limit folate availability and increase the need for other interdependent metabolites including choline and betaine [7]. In addition, James et al. found that children with ASDs had significantly lower plasma concentrations of methionine, S-adenosylmethionine (SAM), cystathionine, cysteine, and total glutathione (GSH) and significantly higher concentrations of S-adenosylhomocysteine (SAH), adenosine, and oxidized glutathione (GSSG) when compared to age-matched control children [8–10]. These metabolic abnormalities can lead to compromised methylation (SAM/SAH) and antioxidant/detoxification capacity (GSH/GSSG). In one study, low plasma SAM/SAH was associated with DNA hypomethylation and low plasma GSH/GSSG was associated with biomarkers of protein oxidative damage (3-nitrotyrosine, 3-chlorotyrosine) and DNA oxidative damage (8-oxodeoxyguanine) [10]. Rose et al. found a similar decrease in GSH/GSSG and oxidative damage in postmortem brain samples from individuals with autism suggesting that oxidative stress and damage may be a systemic issue in some children with autism [11].

Choline, betaine, and folate are interchangeable sources of one-carbon units. As shown in Figure 1, the metabolism of choline intersects with folate-dependent one-carbon metabolism as an alternate pathway for methionine synthesis, especially when folate availability is limited. Choline is the precursor for betaine and methyl groups derived from betaine which are used for SAM-dependent methylation reactions including the synthesis of membrane phosphatidylcholine (PC). In this way, choline indirectly serves as a precursor for the synthesis of membrane phospholipids that are essential for normal membrane fluidity, signal transduction, membrane transport and integrity [12, 13]. Choline is also a precursor for the synthesis of acetylcholine (ACh), an important neurotransmitter in both the central and autonomic nervous systems. In the central nervous system, ACh is an important neuromodulator of sensory perceptions and inducer of REM sleep and is important for sustaining attention [14]. Finally, as a methyl donor for SAM synthesis, choline deficiency has been shown in animal models to contribute to global DNA hypomethylation and epigenetic abnormalities [15]. Low plasma SAM levels and DNA hypomethylation have also been shown to be present in children with autism [10].

Choline was recognized by the Institute of Medicine (IOM) as an essential nutrient in 1998 [16]. Good dietary sources of choline include eggs, liver, beef, chicken, fish, milk, cruciferous vegetables, beans, and peanuts, whereas betaine is primarily obtained from wheat bran, wheat germ, and spinach [9, 10]. Notably, betaine intake has been negatively associated with the Western diet high in meat, sugar, and fat [11]. Zeisel [17] observed the following symptoms when healthy individuals consumed a choline deficient diet: (1) hepatic steatosis, (2) muscle damage, (3) DNA damage, and (4) changes in lymphocyte gene expression. In addition, low plasma choline levels have been associated with increased anxiety [18].

Although choline and its metabolites are important contributors to normal folate-dependent one-carbon metabolism, dietary intake and plasma levels of these nutrients have not been investigated in the ASD population. Therefore, the purpose of the study was to determine whether age-specific dietary intake of these nutrients was within the adequate range by national standards and whether dietary intake was correlated with plasma levels in a subset of these children.

2. Subjects and Methods

2.1. Study Participants. Nutritional data on choline and betaine intake from food was obtained from 288 children with ASDs who participated in the Autism Intervention Research Network for Physical Health (AIR-P) Study on Diet and Nutrition in Children with Autism and they were recruited from four national sites including Pittsburg, Pennsylvania, Little Rock, Arkansas, Rochester, New York, and Denver, Colorado. A subgroup of 35 of the 288 ASD participants and 32 control participants whose parents consented to a blood draw participated in an ancillary study in which plasma choline metabolites were measured and compared between groups. Inclusion criteria for the ASD group included children 2–11 years of age with clinical diagnoses of an ASD based on the *Diagnostic and Statistical Manual IV* criteria and the Autism Diagnostic Observation Schedule (ADOS). Control participants were 3–10 years of age and had no medical history of behavioral or neurological abnormalities, as determined by parent report, and were control participants in an ongoing NICHD-sponsored study of children with autism (SJJ: R01HD051873). Control children were age and sex-matched to the case children for the plasma analysis and were limited to parents who agreed to have their child's blood drawn. The study protocols and informed consents were approved by the Institutional Review Boards at each site where data were collected.

2.2. Dietary Data. Three-day food records were collected from caregivers of the participants in the ASD group (n = 288). Trained personnel used a standardized method to instruct caregivers on recording all foods, beverages, and supplements consumed by the participants for three consecutive days, including one weekend day. Completed records were returned to each site for review and caregivers were contacted if information was missing or unclear. Records from each site were sent to Rochester, New York for analysis using the Nutrition Data System for Research (NDSR) software versions 2009 and 2010, developed by the Nutrition Coordinating Center (University of Minnesota, Minneapolis, MN). Individual food intake results were based on the mean intake from all three days of data collection.

2.3. Plasma Data. Plasma concentrations of choline and betaine were obtained from 67 participants (35 with ASD and 32 controls) whose parents consented to the blood draw. Participants were instructed to fast 12 hours prior to the blood draw. The maximum blood drawn was 25 mL per participant. The blood sample was obtained within two weeks of the completion of the 3-day food record. After samples were obtained and deidentified, they were sent to the Autism Treatment Network/Intellectual & Developmental

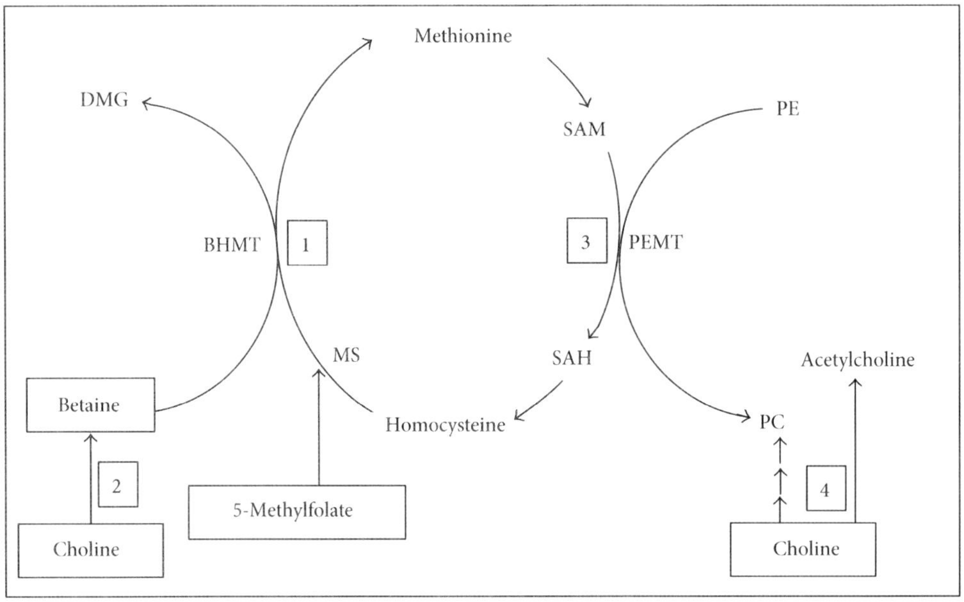

FIGURE 1: Interrelated and interdependent pathways of (1) folate- and betaine-dependent methionine resynthesis from homocysteine utilizing folate-dependent methionine synthase (MS) and betaine-dependent betaine:homocysteine methyltransferase (BHMT); (2) choline-dependent betaine synthesis; (3) phosphtidylethanoloamine methyltransferasse (PEMT) conversion of phosphatidylethanolamine (PE) to phosphatidylcholine (PC); and (4) choline-dependent synthesis of PC and acetylcholine.

Disabilities Research Center (ATN/IDDRC) Biorespository in Denver, Colorado for storage. A 250 uL aliquot was sent to the Autism Genomics Laboratory in Little Rock, Arkansas for analysis. Choline and betaine concentrations were measured using a Dionex High Performance Liquid Chromatography-Ultraviolet System coupled to an electrospray ionization (ESI) tandem mass spectrometer using Thermo-Finnagen LCQ. Samples of 30 μL were deprotenized with three volumes of acetonitrile and further analyzed using normal phase chromatography on silica gel column. It was equilibrated with a mixture of 15 mmol/L ammonium formate and acetonitrile in a ratio of 25 : 75 by volume. It was eluted with a linear gradient of increasing proportions of ammonium formate, as described in greater detail in Holm et al. [19].

2.4. Statistical Analysis. Statistical analyses were conducted using SPSS (version 21.0) and Excel software (Microsoft Office 2007; Microsoft Corp., Redmond, WA). Descriptive statistics were used to describe the study participants' demographic characteristics. Means, standard deviations, and ranges were used to describe the dietary intake of the ASD group. Pearson's product-moment correlation coefficients were used to test the relationships between dietary intake and plasma levels of choline and betaine in the ASD group. Student's t-tests were used to determine if differences existed in plasma concentrations between groups. Statistical significance was set at 0.0.

3. Results

3.1. Participant Characteristics. Among the 288 ASD participants, 86.1% were male, 25.7% (74) were in the 1–3-year-age category, 61.5% (177) were in the 4–8-year-age category, and 12.8% (37) were in the 9–11-year-age category. Greater than 90% of the participants were Caucasian. Within the subgroup of children evaluated for plasma and dietary intake of choline and betaine, 11 of the 35 children (32%) were 1–3 years old, 19 children (54%) were 4–8 years old, and 5 children (14%) were 8–11 years of age. Anthropometric data from the ASD subgroup (n = 35) and control group (n = 32) indicated that 27% of children in the ASD group were in the overweight and obese categories compared to 23% in the control group. Additionally, fewer children in the ASD group were classified as underweight compared to the control group (6% versus 10%, resp.).

3.2. Dietary Intake of Participants with ASD. Dietary intake data is based on three-day food records of the 288 ASD participants analyzed at the time of paper preparation. As shown in Table 1, choline intake was below the AI for more than 69% in all age categories. The proportion of children with intake below the AI increased progressively with age (range 69–93%). No dietary reference intake levels have been established for betaine; however, the average US adult betaine intake has been estimated to be ~5 mg/kg/day [20, 21]. The mean betaine intake in the children with autism was ~4.6 mg/kg/day across all age groups. However, the percent of children whose intake was less than 3.5 mg/Kg/day was 30% in the 1–3 yr age group, 23% in the 4–8 yr age group, and 18% in the 9–11 yr age group.

3.3. Relationships between Dietary Intake and Plasma Concentrations of Choline and Betaine in ASD Group. Relationships between dietary intake and plasma concentrations of choline

TABLE 1: Mean dietary intake of choline and betaine in children with ASD (n = 288).

Age	Choline intake (mg) (mean ± SE)	AI[a] for choline (mg)	Choline intake less than AI[a] (% children)	Betaine intake[b] (mg/kg) (mean ± SE)	Betaine intake less than 3.5 mg/kg (% children)
1–3 y (n = 72)	176 ± 10	200	68.7%	4.6 ± 0.18	30%
4–8 y (n = 178)	182 ± 5	250	84%	4.7 ± 0.47	23%
9–11 y (n = 38)	238 ± 14	375	93.2%	4.6 ± 0.20	18%

Note: [a]AI: adequate intake; [b]average adult betaine intake = ~5 mg/kg [14, 15].

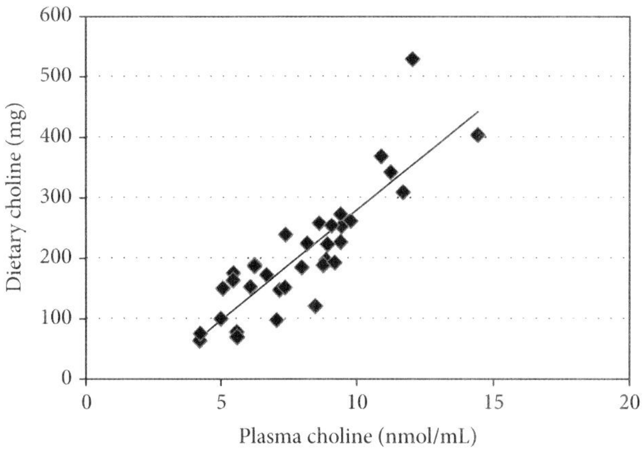

FIGURE 2: Correlation between dietary intake and plasma choline concentrations in children with ASD (n = 35). r = 0.86 and $P \leq 0.001$ using Pearson's product-moment correlation coefficient. ASD: autism spectrum disorder.

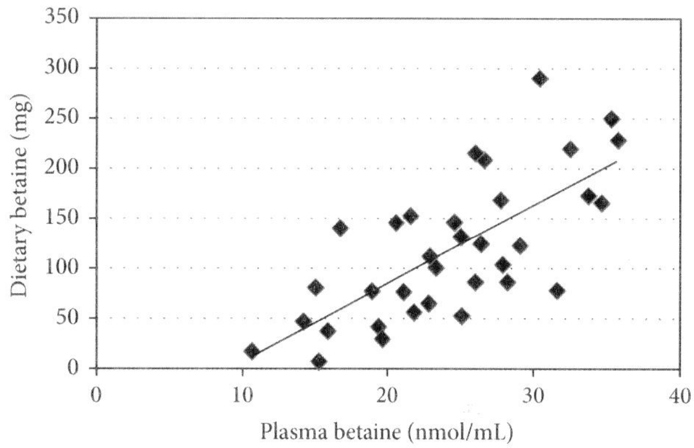

FIGURE 3: Correlation between dietary intake and plasma betaine concentrations in children with ASD (n = 35). r = 0.67 and $P \leq 0.001$ using Pearson's product-moment correlation coefficient. ASD: autism spectrum disorder.

and betaine in the ASD cohort (n = 35) were investigated using Pearson's product-moment correlation coefficients. There was a strong, positive correlation between dietary intake and plasma choline concentrations: r = 0.86, n = 35, and $P < 0.001$, with low intake associated with low plasma choline concentrations (Figure 2). Similarly, dietary intake and plasma betaine concentrations showed a strong, positive correlation: r = 0.67, n = 35, and $P < 0.001$, with low dietary intake associated with low plasma betaine concentrations (Figure 3).

3.4. Comparison of Plasma Metabolite Concentrations in ASD and Control Groups. A comparison of plasma concentrations of choline and betaine was made between the ASD cohort (n = 35) and the control group (n = 32) and is presented in Figure 4. Student's t-test demonstrated that participants in the ASD group had significantly lower plasma concentrations of choline and betaine compared to the control group ($P < 0.001$) as well as a significant decrease in the betaine : choline ratio.

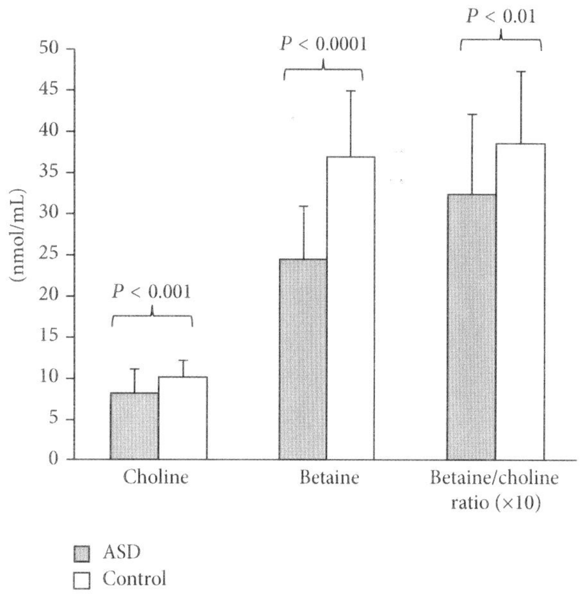

FIGURE 4: Plasma levels of choline, betaine, and the betaine/choline ratio in children with autism compared to age-matched controls.

4. Discussion

The results of the AIR-P study of diet and nutrition in children with autism demonstrate for the first time that the majority of children with ASDs between 3 and 11 years of age consume inadequate amounts of dietary choline. A strong correlation between choline and betaine dietary intake and plasma levels was observed in a subset of these children suggesting that the choline-betaine-homocysteine pathway for methionine synthesis may be compromised. The significant decrease in choline : betaine intake ratio presented in Figure 4 is consistent with this possibility. Research studies have shown that insufficient dietary folate increases requirement for choline and betaine-derived methyl groups and conversely, choline and betaine deficiency increases the requirement for folate-derived methyl groups [17]. Thus, dietary deficits in both pathways for methionine synthesis may be compromised in children with ASDs and additively contribute to the low methionine and SAM levels previously reported in these children [8–10]. Importantly, reduced synthesis of SAM, the major intracellular methyl donor, can lead to DNA hypomethylation and epigenetic abnormalities associated with abnormal gene expression, genomic imprinting, and genomic instability [22]. Significant decreases in plasma methioinine and SAM associated with DNA hypomethylation have been reported in children with ASDs relative to age-matched control children [10].

It is not known whether supplemental choline or betaine would increase methionine and SAM synthesis in children with autism. However, works by Atkinson et al. [23] and Innis et al. [24] support the positive effects of choline and betaine in other studies. Atkinson et al. conducted a randomized crossover study in healthy males ($n = 8$) that measured betaine and homocysteine concentrations after consuming meals or supplements containing choline or betaine. They found that betaine from meals and supplements acutely increased plasma betaine. Additionally, both betaine and choline helped alleviate the rise in homocysteine concentrations following a postmethionine load. Innis et al. found that a choline supplement in children with cystic fibrosis resulted in significant increased methionine, SAM, the SAM/SAH methylation ratio, and the GSH/GSSG redox ratio. Because the metabolic profile of children with ASDs is similar to that observed in children with cystic fibrosis, it is possible that choline supplementation may similarly improve methylation status in children with ASDs.

Consistent with low choline status, El-Ansary et al. [25] found that phosphatidylethanolamine, phosphatidylserine, and phosphatidylcholine were significantly lower in a group of Saudi Arabian children with ASDs ($n = 25$) compared to a control group ($n = 16$). They suggested that the lower levels of these phospholipids could be related to oxidative stress and inflammation. Similarly, James et al. found decreased plasma levels of cysteine, glutathione, and the ratio of reduced to oxidized glutathione (GSH/GSSG) in children with ASDs compared to a control group, indicating that some children with ASDs have reduced antioxidant capacity and evidence of oxidative stress [8]. Other researchers have reported higher homocysteine levels in children with ASDs [6] which is important to consider since choline and betaine have been shown to reduce these levels, especially when given in addition to methionine. In addition to inadequate intake of choline and betaine, the AIR-P study of diet and nutrition in children with autism reported that calcium, vitamin E, vitamin D, and fiber intake are also inadequate when compared to NHANES normative data [2].

A final consideration is the role of choline deficiency in brain development, memory, and anxiety. In rodent models, multiple studies have shown that choline deficiency and supplementation affect neurodevelopment. The offspring of choline-supplemented pregnant rodents have improved visuospatial and auditory memory and perform better in behavioral tests, whereas choline deficiency seems to have the opposite effect [26, 27]. Fewer studies have been done in humans, although the elderly and patients with Alzheimer's disease have reduced levels of free choline and phosphatidylcholine in the brain [28, 29]. A recent large population based study of 5,918 men and women participating in the Hordaland [18] Health Study, found that low plasma choline concentrations were significantly associated with higher anxiety levels. Behavioral alterations associated with low plasma choline levels in children with ASDs warrant further research consideration.

The present study had several possible limitations. First, it is possible that parents who consented to participate may have been more concerned about nutrition and feeding behaviors in their children such that their dietary patterns might be different from the general population of children with ASD. We were unable to make comparisons regarding the diets of the unaffected control children since food records were only collected for children with ASDs. Also, it is unclear if the differences observed in plasma concentrations between case and control groups are reflective of their dietary intake or abnormal metabolism or both. While the adequacy of choline intake was determined using the standard AI levels, a component of the dietary reference intakes that is intended for healthy individuals, it is uncertain if these standards can be applied to children with ASDs, especially since abnormalities in nutrient metabolism have been found in these children.

5. Conclusions

In summary, choline plays an essential role as a methyl-group donor in the synthesis of the membrane phospholipid components of cell membranes as well as in the synthesis of the neurotransmitter acetylcholine. The data in the AIR-P diet and nutrition study indicate that 69 to 93% of children with ASDs consumed diets that were inadequate in choline. Importantly, low choline and betaine intake were associated with low plasma levels of these nutrients suggesting that there could be functional consequences related to folate and phospholipid metabolism. Future research should consider whether these metabolic imbalances can be corrected with dietary counseling or supplement interventions and whether metabolic improvement is associated with improvement in some behavioral symptoms.

Abbreviations

ASDs:	Autism spectrum disorders
AIR-P:	Autism Intervention Research Network for Physical Health
NICHD:	National Institute of Child Health and Human Development
DMG:	Dimethylglycine
AI:	Adequate intake
AD:	Autistic disorder

PDD-NOS:	Pervasive developmental disorder not-otherwise specified
MTHFR:	Methylenetetrahydrofolate reductase
SAM:	S-adenosylmethionine
GSH:	Total glutathione
SAH:	S-adenosylhomocysteine
GSSG:	Oxidized glutathione
PC:	Phosphatidylcholine
ACh:	Acetylcholine
IOM:	Institute of Medicine
NDSR:	Nutrition Data System for Research
ATN/IDDRC:	Autism Treatment Network/Intellectual and Developmental Disabilities Research Center.

Authors' Contribution

The authors' responsibilities were as follows: Joanna C. Hamlin analyzed data, performed statistical analysis, and contributed to paper writing; Margaret Pauly is certified dietitian who collected dietary data; Stepan Melnyk is a laboratory director who developed metabolic assays; Oleksandra Pavliv conducted metabolic assays; William Starrett conducted metabolic assays; Tina A. Crook analyzed data, performed statistical analysis, and contributed to paper writing; S. Jill James (Principal Investigator) conducted the study, analyzed data, performed statistical analysis, interpreted the data, contributed to paper writing, and had primary responsibility for final content.

Acknowledgments

The authors would like to acknowledge the effort and participation of the mothers of children with autism without whom this study would not have been possible. This research was conducted as part of the Autism Speaks Autism Treatment Network. Further support came from cooperative agreement (UA3 MC 11054) from the U.S. Department of Health and Human Services, Health Resources and Services Administration, Maternal and Child Health Research Program, to the Massachusetts General Hospital. The views expressed in this paper do not necessarily reflect the views of Autism Speaks, Inc. It was also supported by HRSA: Autism Intervention for Physical Health (AIR-P); NICHD: R01HD051873 (SJJ); CTSI: Rochester University.

References

[1] T. Buie, D. B. Campbell, G. J. Fuchs 3rd et al., "Evaluation, diagnosis, and treatment of gastrointestinal disorders in individuals with ASDs: a consensus report," *Pediatrics*, vol. 125, supplement 1, pp. S1–18, 2010.

[2] S. L. Hyman, P. A. Stewart, B. Schmidt et al., "Nutrient intake from food in children with autism," *Pediatrics*, vol. 130, supplement 2, pp. S145–S153, 2012.

[3] D. A. Rossignol and R. E. Frye, "A review of research trends in physiological abnormalities in autism spectrum disorders: immune dysregulation, inflammation, oxidative stress, mitochondrial dysfunction and environmental toxicant exposures," *Molecular Psychiatry*, vol. 17, no. 4, pp. 389–401, 2012.

[4] R. E. Frye, L. C. Huffman, and G. R. Elliott, "Tetrahydrobiopterin as a novel therapeutic intervention for autism," *Neurotherapeutics*, vol. 7, no. 3, pp. 241–249, 2010.

[5] S. J. James, S. Melnyk, G. Fuchs et al., "Efficacy of methylcobalamin and folinic acid treatment on glutathione redox status in children with autism," *American Journal of Clinical Nutrition*, vol. 89, no. 1, pp. 425–430, 2009.

[6] S. P. Paşca, E. Dronca, T. Kaucsár et al., "One carbon metabolism disturbances and the C677T MTHFR gene polymorphism in children with autism spectrum disorders," *Journal of Cellular and Molecular Medicine*, vol. 13, no. 10, pp. 4229–4238, 2009.

[7] K.-A. Da Costa, O. G. Kozyreva, J. Song, J. A. Galanko, L. M. Fischer, and S. H. Zeisel, "Common genetic polymorphisms affect the human requirement for the nutrient choline," *The FASEB Journal*, vol. 20, no. 9, pp. 1336–1344, 2006.

[8] S. J. James, P. Cutler, S. Melnyk et al., "Metabolic biomarkers of increased oxidative stress and impaired methylation capacity in children with autism," *American Journal of Clinical Nutrition*, vol. 80, no. 6, pp. 1611–1617, 2004.

[9] S. J. James, S. Melnyk, S. Jernigan et al., "Metabolic endophenotype and related genotypes are associated with oxidative stress in children with autism," *American Journal of Medical Genetics B*, vol. 141, no. 8, pp. 947–956, 2006.

[10] S. Melnyk, G. J. Fuchs, E. Schulz et al., "Metabolic imbalance associated with methylation dysregulation and oxidative damage in children with autism," *Journal of Autism and Developmental Disorders*, vol. 42, no. 3, pp. 367–377, 2012.

[11] S. Rose, S. Melnyk, O. Pavliv et al., "Evidence of oxidative damage and inflammation associated with low glutathione redox status in the autism brain," *Translational Psychiatry*, vol. 2, article e134, 2012.

[12] D. E. Vance, "Physiological roles of phosphatidylethanolamine N-methyltransferase," *Biochimica et Biophysica Acta*, vol. 1831, no. 3, pp. 626–632, 2013.

[13] S. H. Zeisel, "Choline phospholipids: Signal transduction and carcinogenesis," *The FASEB Journal*, vol. 7, no. 6, pp. 551–557, 1993.

[14] F. Kimura, "Cholinergic modulation of cortical function: a hypothetical role in shifting the dynamics in cortical network," *Neuroscience Research*, vol. 38, no. 1, pp. 19–26, 2000.

[15] M. D. Niculescu, C. N. Craciunescu, and S. H. Zeisel, "Dietary choline deficiency alters global and gene-specific DNA methylation in the developing hippocampus of mouse fetal brains," *The FASEB Journal*, vol. 20, no. 1, pp. 43–49, 2006.

[16] L. M. Sanders and S. H. Zeisel, "Choline: dietary requirements and role in brain development," *Nutrition Today*, vol. 42, no. 4, pp. 181–186, 2007.

[17] S. H. Zeisel, "Choline: clinical nutrigenetic/nutrigenomic approaches for identification of functions and dietary requirements," *Journal of Nutrigenetics and Nutrigenomics*, vol. 3, no. 4-6, pp. 209–219, 2010.

[18] I. Bjelland, G. S. Tell, S. E. Vollset, S. Konstantinova, and P. M. Ueland, "Choline in anxiety and depression: The Hordaland

Health Study," *American Journal of Clinical Nutrition*, vol. 90, no. 4, pp. 1056–1060, 2009.

[19] P. I. Holm, P. M. Ueland, G. Kvalheim, and E. A. Lien, "Determination of choline, betaine, and dimethylglycine in plasma by a high-throughput method based on normal-phase chromatography-tandem mass spectrometry," *Clinical Chemistry*, vol. 49, no. 2, pp. 286–294, 2003.

[20] E. Cho, S. H. Zeisel, P. Jacques et al., "Dietary choline and betaine assessed by food-frequency questionnaire in relation to plasma total homocysteine concentration in the Framingham Offspring Study," *American Journal of Clinical Nutrition*, vol. 83, no. 4, pp. 905–911, 2006.

[21] A. Bidulescu, L. E. Chambless, A. M. Siega-Riz, S. H. Zeisel, and G. Heiss, "Usual choline and betaine dietary intake and incident coronary heart disease: The Atherosclerosis Risk in Communities (ARIC) Study," *BMC Cardiovascular Disorders*, vol. 7, article 20, 2007.

[22] M. A. Caudill, J. C. Wang, S. Melnyk et al., "Intracellular S-adenosylhomocysteine concentrations predict global DNA hypomethylation in tissues of methyl-deficient cystathionine β-synthase heterozygous mice," *Journal of Nutrition*, vol. 131, no. 11, pp. 2811–2818, 2001.

[23] W. Atkinson, J. Elmslie, M. Lever, S. T. Chambers, and P. M. George, "Dietary and supplementary betaine: acute effects on plasma betaine and homocysteine concentrations under standard and postmethionine load conditions in healthy male subjects," *American Journal of Clinical Nutrition*, vol. 87, no. 3, pp. 577–585, 2008.

[24] S. M. Innis, A. G. F. Davidson, S. Melynk, and S. J. James, "Choline-related supplements improve abnormal plasma methioninehomocysteine metabolites and glutathione status in children with cystic fibrosis," *American Journal of Clinical Nutrition*, vol. 85, no. 3, pp. 702–708, 2007.

[25] A. K. El-Ansary, A. G. Ben Bacha, and L. Y. Al- Ayahdi, "Impaired plasma phospholipids and relative amounts of essential polyunsaturated fatty acids in autistic patients from Saudi Arabia," *Lipids in Health and Disease*, vol. 10, article 63, 2011.

[26] S. H. Zeisel, "Choline: critical role during fetal development and dietary requirements in adults," *Annual Review of Nutrition*, vol. 26, pp. 229–250, 2006.

[27] S. H. Zeisel, "The fetal origins of memory: the role of dietary choline in optimal brain development," *Journal of Pediatrics*, vol. 149, supplement 5, pp. S131–S136, 2006.

[28] R. M. Nitsch, J. K. Blusztajn, A. G. Pittas, B. E. Slack, J. H. Growdon, and R. J. Wurtman, "Evidence for a membrane defect in Alzheimer disease brain," *Proceedings of the National Academy of Sciences of the United States of America*, vol. 89, no. 5, pp. 1671–1675, 1992.

[29] B. M. Cohen, P. F. Renshaw, A. L. Stoll, R. J. Wurtman, D. Yurgelun-Todd, and S. M. Babb, "Decreased brain choline uptake in older adults: an in vivo proton magnetic resonance spectroscopy study," *Journal of the American Medical Association*, vol. 274, no. 11, pp. 902–907, 1995.

5

Effectiveness of Methylcobalamin and Folinic Acid Treatment on Adaptive Behavior in Children with Autistic Disorder is Related to Glutathione Redox Status

Richard E. Frye,[1] Stepan Melnyk,[1] George Fuchs,[1] Tyra Reid,[1] Stefanie Jernigan,[1] Oleksandra Pavliv,[1] Amanda Hubanks,[1] David W. Gaylor,[2] Laura Walters,[1] and S. Jill James[1]

[1] *Department of Pediatrics, Arkansas Children's Hospital Research Institute, University of Arkansas for Medical Sciences, Little Rock, AR 72202, USA*
[2] *Department of Biostatistics, Arkansas Children's Hospital Research Institute, University of Arkansas for Medical Sciences, Little Rock, AR 72202, USA*

Correspondence should be addressed to Richard E. Frye; refrye@uams.edu

Academic Editor: Klaus-Peter Ossenkopp

Treatments targeting metabolic abnormalities in children with autism are limited. Previously we reported that a nutritional treatment significantly improved glutathione metabolism in children with autistic disorder. In this study we evaluated changes in adaptive behaviors in this cohort and determined whether such changes are related to changes in glutathione metabolism. Thirty-seven children diagnosed with autistic disorder and abnormal glutathione and methylation metabolism were treated with twice weekly 75 μg/Kg methylcobalamin and twice daily 400 μg folinic acid for 3 months in an open-label fashion. The Vineland Adaptive Behavior Scale (VABS) and glutathione redox metabolites were measured at baseline and at the end of the treatment period. Over the treatment period, all VABS subscales significantly improved with an average effect size of 0.59, and an average improvement in skills of 7.7 months. A greater improvement in glutathione redox status was associated with a greater improvement in expressive communication, personal and domestic daily living skills, and interpersonal, play-leisure, and coping social skills. Age, gender, and history of regression did not influence treatment response. The significant behavioral improvements observed and the relationship between these improvements to glutathione redox status suggest that nutritional interventions targeting redox metabolism may benefit some children with autism.

1. Introduction

Autism is a neurodevelopmental disorder characterized by significant impairment in reciprocal social interaction and communication as well as restricted interests and repetitive behaviors. An estimated 1 of 88 individuals in the United States is affected with an autism spectrum disorder (ASD) [1]. Although several genetic syndromes are associated with ASD, all of these genetic syndromes together only account for a minority of ASD cases [2]. Other areas of novel research have concentrated on systemic physiological abnormalities, such as mitochondrial dysfunction [3, 4], oxidative stress [5–7], and inflammation/immune dysregulation [8–10]. These novel areas of research have substantially grown over the last decade [11]. These emerging areas of research have provided a new understanding of the diverse mechanisms involved in ASD and have promoted the idea that the autism spectrum is composed of several subgroups or endophenotypes [12].

Several lines of evidence support the notion of an ASD endophenotype with abnormal redox and methylation metabolism. In two case-control studies we reported that redox and methylation metabolism in children diagnosed with autism was abnormal compared to that of unaffected control children [6, 13]. Briefly, the mean ratio of plasma S-adenosyl methionine (SAM) to S-adenosyl homocysteine (SAH), a reflection of cellular methylation capacity, was significantly reduced. Also, the mean concentration of free reduced glutathione (GSH), the major intracellular antioxidant and mechanism for detoxification, was also significantly decreased and the oxidized disulfide form of glutathione (GSSG) was significantly increased. This imbalance in reduced as compared to oxidized glutathione resulted in a 2-fold reduction in the GSH/GSSG redox ratio, an index known as the glutathione redox status. Several precursors for methylation and glutathione synthesis were also lower in the autistic children suggesting an insufficiency in the production of methylation and glutathione metabolites, at least in a subgroup of ASD children. In addition, we have also demonstrated that GSH is significantly reduced in the cytosol and isolated mitochondria from lymphoblastoid cell lines and fresh peripheral blood mononuclear cells derived from children with autistic disorder (AD) [14, 15].

The glutathione provides the essential intracellular reducing environment required for normal immune function, detoxification capacity, redox-sensitive enzyme activity, and membrane redox signaling [16–20]. Oxidative stress occurs when antioxidant defense mechanisms fail to counterbalance reactive oxygen species generated from endogenous oxidative metabolism or from prooxidant environmental exposures. The notion that abnormal glutathione metabolism is associated with oxidative cellular damage is consistent with studies from our laboratory which demonstrate an increase in oxidative damage to protein and DNA in peripheral blood mononuclear cells and postmortem brain derived from ASD individuals [15, 21]. Several recent reviews and research studies also lend support to the hypothesis that redox imbalance and oxidative stress may be a contributing factor to autism pathophysiology [6, 22].

These findings have particular clinical relevance since abnormalities in redox metabolism are potentially amenable to treatment. Glutathione is a tripeptide of cysteine, glycine, and glutamate that is synthesized *de novo* in all cells. Glutathione synthesis is tightly connected to methylation metabolism where it derives its cysteine precursor. As both methylation and glutathione metabolism have been shown to be abnormal in children with ASD and due to the fact that abnormal methylation metabolism will result in a depletion of the precursors needed for glutathione production, we previously conducted an open-label intervention trial where targeted metabolic cofactors for methylation and glutathione metabolism were provided. Specifically, in our previous study, we determine if glutathione redox status could be improved with a three-month intervention of subcutaneously injected methylcobalamin and oral folinic acid in children with AD and metabolic evidence of abnormal methylation and glutathione metabolism [23]. Although we measured adaptive behavior using the Vineland Adaptive Behavior Scale (VABS) during the trial, this behavioral data has not been previously reported. We now report the change in communication, daily living, and social skills domains of the VABS associated with the three-month intervention as well as investigate whether improvement in glutathione redox status was related to any change in VABS behavior scores.

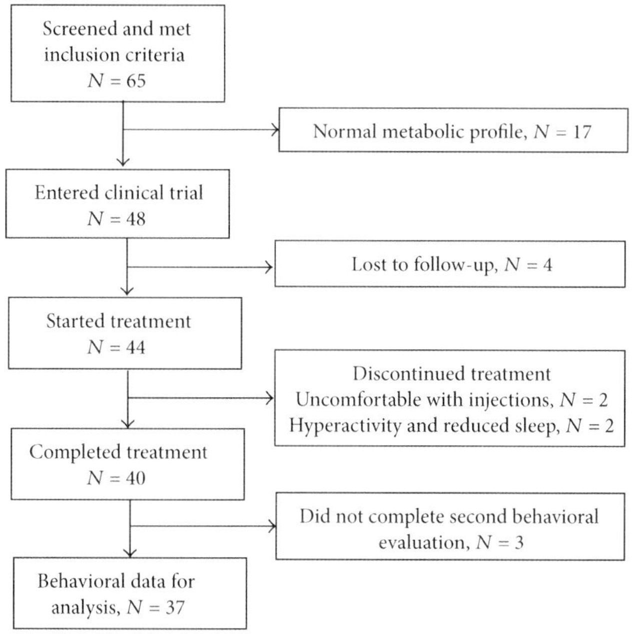

FIGURE 1: Flowchart of patients who met inclusion criteria for the study.

2. Methods and Materials

2.1. Participants. Forty-eight children with AD were enrolled in an open-label trial to test whether a three-month treatment of methylcobalamin (methyl B12) and folinic acid would improve glutathione synthesis as well as adaptive behavior. Inclusion criteria were a diagnosis of AD as defined by the *Diagnostic and Statistical Manual of Mental Disorders, Fourth Edition* (DSM-IV) criteria (299.0) and a Childhood Autism Rating Scales (CARS) score greater than 30. Exclusion criteria included Asperger's disorder, pervasive developmental disorder-not otherwise specified (PDD-NOS), genetic disorders, epilepsy, severe gastrointestinal symptoms, recent infections, and/or current use of high-dose vitamin or mineral supplements (i.e., above the recommend daily allowance). Metabolic and behavioral assessments were conducted at baseline and at the end of the 3-month intervention. A nurse contacted each family every two weeks to ensure compliance and monitor adverse effects.

Figure 1 provides a flowchart of the patients who met criteria for possible inclusion in the study. In order to determine if abnormal redox metabolism could be improved with the intervention, we selected children with abnormal glutathione redox status and methylation capacity for entry into the study. Normal glutathione redox status and methylation capacity were defined by measuring these same metabolites in typically developing control children. Sixty-five autistic children met the inclusion criteria and were initially screened for metabolic evidence of abnormal methylation capacity (SAM/SAH < 3.0) and glutathione redox metabolism (GSH/GSSG < 6.0). Of these, 48 (75%) children were found to have both abnormal methylation capacity and glutathione redox metabolism, thus meeting metabolic qualifications for inclusion. The remaining 17 (25%) were excluded because their baseline metabolic profile was within normal range. Four children dropped out during the study and another four children were lost to follow-up. Two children dropped out of the study because the parents were uncomfortable giving the methylcobalamin injections and 2 children dropped out because of hyperactivity and reduced sleep. For the four that were lost to follow-up, every attempt was made to contact the family but they either did not response to such requests or moved out of the area and could not return for follow-up. Of the 40 remaining children who completed the study, three of the parents did not complete the second behavioral evaluation, leaving 37 children who completed both the intervention and the behavioral evaluation. Characteristics of the children that completed the study are given in Table 1. Adverse effects were minimal with occasional reports of hyperactivity, as summarized in our previous study [23] and below. All parents signed informed consent approved by the Institutional Review Board at the University of Arkansas for Medical Sciences.

2.2. Intervention. Methylcobalamin was provided as a sterile injectable liquid from Hopewell Compounding Pharmacy (Hopewell, NJ). Tuberculin syringes fitted with a 1/4 inch 31 gauge needle were prefilled with 75 μg/Kg methylcobalamin and prepared individually based on each child's weight. A demonstration and instructions for the sterile subcutaneous injection of methylcobalamin in the fatty tissue of the buttocks were given to all parents. Parents were instructed to give methylcobalamin every third day for 3 months. Folinic acid (400 μg) obtained from Custom Compounding (Little Rock, AR) was administered orally twice each day as a powder mixed with a convenient food.

The subcutaneous injectable route of administration of methylcobalamin was selected based on preliminary observations that it resulted in improvement in speech and cognition [13] and the potential for support of methionine synthase activity under conditions of oxidative stress by substituting for the oxidized inactive form of coenzyme B12 [Cob (II)]. Folinic acid (5-formyltetrahydrofolate) was selected in light of the fact that it is absorbed as the reduced metabolite is rapidly polyglutamated and is more readily available for folate-dependent reactions than the synthetic vitamin form of folic acid. In our previous study, we demonstrated that this treatment significantly improved GSH and GSSG concentrations and glutathione redox status (i.e., the GSH/GSSG ratio) [23].

2.3. Glutathione Measurement. Fasting blood samples were collected into EDTA-Vacutainer tubes and immediately chilled on ice before centrifuging at 4000 ×g for 10 minutes at 4°C. To prevent metabolite interconversion, the ice-cold samples were centrifuged within 15 minutes of the blood collection and the plasma stored at −80°C until high-pressure liquid chromatography quantification within 2 weeks after receipt. Details of the methodology for high-pressure liquid chromatography with electrochemical detection and metabolite quantitation have been previously described [24, 25].

Table 1: Characteristics of the 37 participants with autistic disorder who completed the trial.

Gender (% male)	81%
Age (mean ± standard deviation)	5.1 ± 1.4 years
Regression (% regression)	35%
Childhood Autism Rating Scale score (mean ± standard deviation)	39.2 ± 7.8

2.4. Behavioral Evaluation. The VABS (1st Edition) is a validated parent interview that provides a numerical score for adaptive functioning in the domains of communication, socialization, and daily living skills which has been shown to have good reliability and validity [26]. Nine subscales represented these three domains, specifically receptive, expressive, and writing communication, personal, domestic, and community daily living skills, and interpersonal relations, play-leisure, and coping skills. Raw scores were used in the statistical analysis while age equivalent scores are used to illustrate the magnitude of the changes in behavioral development over the treatment period and domain scaled scores are provided as a comparison of the participant sample to the general population. Higher raw, age equivalent, and scaled scores represented better performance on these measures. The VABS was administered by a trained nurse at the baseline visit and again at the end of the treatment period.

2.5. Statistics. Mixed-effects regression models were conducted via SAS version 9.3 (Cary, NC) "glmmix" procedure [27]. Raw scores were used in the statistical analysis to represent the change in behavior over the intervention period. A similar approach was used in our recent study on the effect of sapropterin treatment in children with ASD [28]. Raw scores were used due to the fact that transformation of raw scores into scaled scores is not statistically valid to follow changes in adaptive behavior especially when examining the moderating effect of a biomarker on the change in behavior and especially when there is no reference control group. For example, many children with ASD have slow or stagnant development, so their development may not change over a typical three-month interval. With an intervention, their development may approach the rate of a typically developing child. However, a child whose development changes over the three-month period at a rate equal to that of a typically developing child would have a stable unchanging scaled score. Thus, in such a case, the scaled score would appear to reflect no developmental gains over the treatment period even though the child was making developmental gains. Since the null hypothesis is that there is no change over the treatment period, an unchanging scaled score would not be statistically significant even though it would indicate developmental progress.

The first statistical model included a linear effect of time on raw scores. A random intercept was used to account for each individual's symptom level. Two-tailed alpha of 0.05 was used in all analyses. In these initial models we tested whether age, gender, and/or a history of regression influenced

Table 2: Age equivalent scores from the Vineland Adaptive Behavior Scales at baseline before and after 3-month intervention with methylcobalamin and folinic acid. The change in age equivalent scores with 95% confidence interval (CI) is also given. The overall average of all subscales is also given in the last row of the table.

Vineland subscale	Baseline age equivalent (months) (mean ± SE)	Postintervention age equivalent (months) (mean ± SE)	Change in age equivalent (months) (mean; 95% CI)
Receptive language	23.1 ± 1.8	31.4 ± 3.4	8.3 (2.9, 13.7)
Expressive language	20.6 ± 1.9	27.5 ± 2.9	6.0 (3.3, 9.4)
Written language	40.5 ± 3.8	46.7 ± 4.0	6.2 (3.4, 9.0)
Personal skills	30.5 ± 2.3	40.5 ± 3.8	10.0 (3.8, 16.2)
Domestic skills	30.3 ± 4.1	39.3 ± 5.9	9.0 (−1.4, 19.4)
Community skills	32.9 ± 2.9	36.1 ± 3.8	2.0 (−3.0, 6.9)
Interpersonal skills	18.7 ± 2.7	24.1 ± 3.9	5.4 (0.0, 10.9)
Play/leisure skills	22.0 ± 4.5	34.0 ± 4.1	12.0 (4.1, 19.6)
Coping skills	25.8 ± 2.5	34.3 ± 4.0	11.5 (4.9, 18.0)
Overall skills	26.6 ± 2.3	34.3 ± 3.6	7.7 (3.4, 12.0)

the change in the outcome measure. To illustrate the relative strength of the effect we provide the Cohen's d effect size for each significant change in outcome variables. Next we determined whether baseline and/or change in glutathione redox status (i.e., the free reduced-to-oxidized glutathione ratio) moderated changes in the outcome variables. The glutathione redox status was investigated because it significantly changed with treatment in our previous study [23]. We did not investigate the moderating effect of other metabolites as multiple statistical tests would have increased our type I error rate. We conducted two sets of analyses; one examined the moderating effect of the overall glutathione redox status and another that examined the moderating effect of the change in glutathione redox status over the treatment period. The former analysis was conducted to determine whether glutathione redox status in general was related to VABS scores, while the latter analysis was conducted to determine if the change in glutathione status was related to the change in VABS scores over the treatment period. Age, gender, and/or regression factors were included in the analyses examining the moderating effect of glutathione if they were significant in the initial model.

3. Results

3.1. Behavior Change over the Intervention Period. The VABS was used to examine the impact of the intervention on measures of core behaviors associated with autism. The changes in VABS subscales with treatment were not influenced by gender, age, or history of regression, and neither gender nor history of regression was related to overall VABS subscale scores. Age was significantly related to overall raw scores for all subscales, except for interpersonal and coping skills.

Significant increases were found in all VABS subscale scores, including receptive ($F(1,36) = 11.90, P = 0.001; d = 0.59$), expressive ($F(1,36) = 32.80, P < 0.0001; d = 0.97$), and written ($F(1,36) = 11.07$, $P < 0.005$; $d = 0.56$) communication skills, personal ($F(1,36) = 14.69, P < 0.0005$; $d = 0.65$), domestic ($F(1,36) = 4.85, P < 0.05; d = 0.37$) and

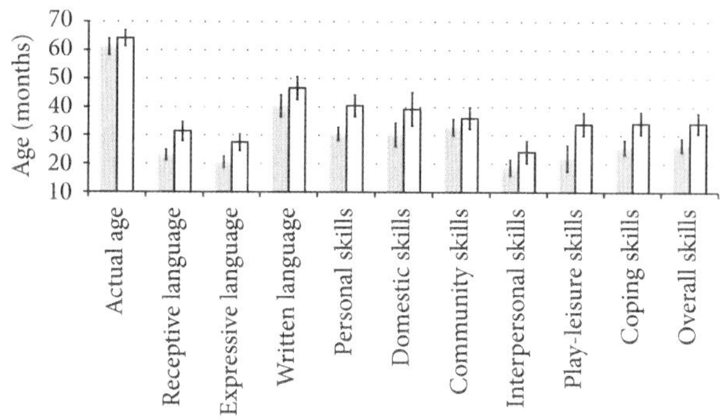

Figure 2: Histogram of actual age and age equivalents for the Vineland Adaptive Behavior Scale subscales. Error bars depict standard error.

community ($F(1,36) = 9.51, P < 0.005; d = 0.52$) daily living skills, and interpersonal ($F(1,36) = 6.45, P < 0.05; d = 0.43$), play-leisure ($F(1,36) = 12.36, P = 0.001; d = 0.59$), and coping ($F(1,36) = 15.68, P = 0.0005; d = 0.66$) social skills.

To illustrate the magnitude of the change in development with the intervention, Table 2 and Figure 2 present the average age equivalent for all subscales before and after the intervention. Table 2 also demonstrates the change in age equivalent with the intervention including confidence intervals. As evident from this table, many subscales, particularly those with larger effect sizes, demonstrate large gains with the three-month intervention. This is particularly true for the communication domain where skills improved between 6.0 and 8.3 months, on average, and in the social skills domain where skills improved between 5.4 and 12.0 months, on average, over a three-month period.

Baseline pretreatment scores of the individual domains and overall composite of the VABS (mean (SD): communication 65.4 (13.0); daily living skills 66.4 (13.4); social skills 67.3 (9.3); adaptive behavioral composite 66.1 (9.3)) were found to be within the range of previously published VABS scores for children with autistic disorder [15, 29]. Following intervention all individual domains and the overall

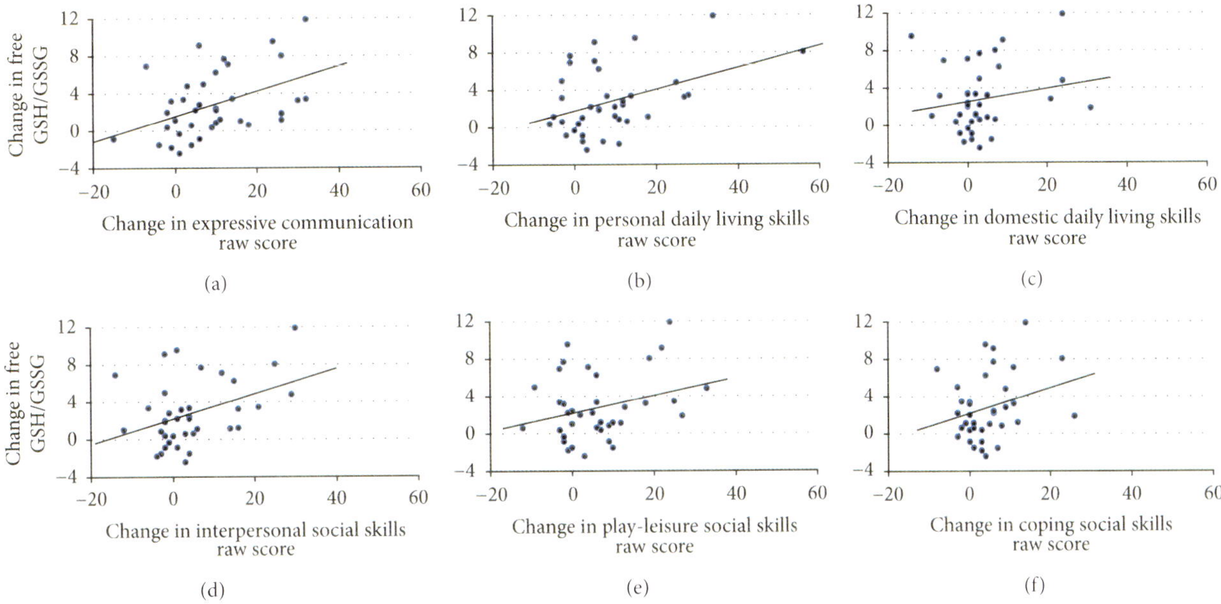

FIGURE 3: Significant relationships between the change in the glutathione redox status (reduced-to-oxidized glutathione ratio) and change in subscales of the Vineland Adaptive Behavior Scale (VABS) subscales. An improvement in glutathione redox status was associated with improvement in (a) expressive communication ($F(1,33) = 9.66, P < 0.01$), (b) personal daily living skills ($F(1,34) = 12.84, P = 0.001$), (c) domestic daily living skills ($F(1,34) = 4.69, P < 0.05$), (d) interpersonal social skills ($F(1,34) = 10.47, P < 0.005$), (e) play-leisure social skills ($F(1,34) = 8.16, P < 0.01$), and (f) coping social skills ($F(1.34) = 6.09, P < 0.05$). The moderating effect of glutathione redox status on the VABS subscale is provided in the graph as a representation of the relationship between the variables. Since the linear models examining the moderating effect of glutathione redox status on the VABS subscale takes into account age, simple correlation coefficients would not be accurate for inclusion in the graphs.

composite of the VABS markedly increased (Mean (SD): communication 72.1 (15.7); daily living skills 76.0 (18.0); social skills 75.6 (16.5); adaptive behavioral composite 73.8 (17.4)).

3.2. Relation between Behavior and Glutathione Redox Status. The overall glutathione redox status was not related to VABS subscales, indicating that overall development did not appear to be related to overall glutathione redox status. In order to determine whether changes in VABS subscales were related to changes in glutathione redox status, we examined whether the glutathione redox status moderated the change in the VABS subscales. We found that glutathione redox status moderated expressive communication ($F(1,33) = 9.66, P < 0.01$), personal ($F(1,34) = 12.84, P = 0.001$) and domestic ($F(1,34) = 4.69, P < 0.05$) daily living skills, and interpersonal ($F(1,34) = 10.47, P < 0.005$), play-leisure ($F(1,34) = 8.16, P < 0.01$), and coping ($F(1,34) = 6.09$, $P < 0.05$) social skills such that a greater increase in the glutathione redox status (i.e., greater improvement in glutathione) was associated with a greater improvement in VABS subscale scores (see Figure 3).

3.3. Adverse Effects. The adverse effect rates are outlined in Table 3. Out of the forty-four children that started the study and were not lost to follow-up, 72% reported no adverse effects of the treatment. For the four children that dropped out of the study two children (5%) dropped out because the parents were uncomfortable giving the methylcobalamin injections and 2 children (5%) dropped out because of hyperactivity and reduced sleep. Of the 4 families who reported hyperactivity but did not drop out of the study, the hyperactivity resolved with decreasing the folinic acid dose to 400 μg per day.

TABLE 3: Adverse effects reported of intervention with methylcobalamin and folinic acid. All 44 children who entered the study but were not lost to follow-up were included.

Adverse effect	% (*N*)
Hyperactivity	14% (6)
Reduced sleep	7% (3)
Discomfort with injections	5% (2)
Insomnia	2% (1)
Impulsivity	2% (1)
Irritability	2% (1)

4. Discussion

This intervention trial was undertaken to determine whether a nutritional intervention consisting of treatment with metabolic precursors for methionine and glutathione synthesis would improve autism symptoms in children with AD. Children meeting the inclusion criteria were initially screened for metabolic evidence of abnormal methylation capacity and glutathione redox status as an indication of potential benefit from the intervention. Our goal was to determine whether nutritional support with precursors for the abnormal metabolic pathways could result in improvement in ASD associated behavior as measured by the VABS. Overall, significant improvement was noted on all subscales of the VABS during the three-month intervention. In addition, improvement on several VABS subscales, including those related to communication and social skills, was related to the improvement in glutathione redox status. Overall, this study provides preliminary evidence that targeted nutritional support in children with AD who have metabolic abnormalities in glutathione and methylation pathways may be associated with improvements in certain behaviors associated with ASD, at least in a subset of AD children. In addition, a low rate of adverse effects with methylcobalamin and folinic acid treatment indicates that these supplements are safe and warrants further study as an intervention.

4.1. Behavioral Improvements with Intervention. A simple and safe nutritional intervention of methylcobalamin and folinic acid resulted in significant increases in VABS scores for all domains, including daily living, social, and communication skills, with an average effect size of 0.59, which is in the medium-to-large range. In fact, even the smallest effect size (domestic daily living skills, $d = 0.37$) was in the medium range and the largest effect size (expressive language skills, $d = 0.97$) was in the very large range. When considering changes in age equivalent skills over the treatment period, it was found that skills improved an average of 7.7 months over the three-month treatment period, with the lower end of the range being an average gain of 2.0 months for community daily living skills to the higher end of the range being an average gain of 12.0 months improvement for play-leisure skills. However, when we examine the overall change in scaled scores across the three-month treatment period, we find that, on average, the scaled score for the individual domains and the adaptive behavioral composite at the end of the treatment were still well below the average for typically developing children. In fact, these scaled scores were, on average, at the very lower end of normal range. Thus, although significantly improved, the behavior scores after treatment remained, on average, at the very low end of normal and for many children below the normal range. This suggests that further therapy may be required to promote continued improvement through continued nutritional treatment with metabolic precursors over a prolonged time period, the addition of intensive behavioral and educational therapy, or both.

4.2. The Relationship between Metabolic and Behavioral Changes. Change in glutathione redox status with treatment, but not baseline glutathione redox status prior to treatment, was found to be related to improvements in several VABS subscales, including all of the subscales in the social skills domain, two of three subscales in the daily living skills domain, and one of the subscales in the communication domain. Interestingly, many of the VABS subscales that were related to glutathione redox status were also subscales that demonstrated large effect sizes and larger age equivalent gains (e.g., personal daily living skills and play-leisure and coping social skills). This suggests that the marked changes in behaviors observed in these particular subscales were not simply due to a placebo-effect and may indeed be related to improvements in glutathione redox status over the three-month treatment period, although we will have to await double-blind placebo-controlled studies to validate these findings. The lack of a relationship between overall glutathione redox status and VABS scores most likely reflects the preselection of children with low glutathione redox status, thus decreasing the overall range in glutathione redox status.

In our previous study, we demonstrated that this open-label intervention significantly improved metabolites of glutathione metabolism, including total and free GSH and GSSG concentrations and the glutathione redox status (i.e., the GSH/GSSG ratio) [23]. However, despite this improvement, total and free GSH concentrations and the glutathione redox status remained significantly below those of age-matched control children. Additionally, methionine, SAM, and SAH concentrations did not significantly change with the intervention despite the fact that both methylcobalamin and folinic acid provide methyl groups for the methionine cycle. The fact that the treatment improved but did not normalize methionine, SAM and glutathione concentrations may reflect ongoing metabolic compensation for incompletely resolved oxidative stress. Thus, continued prooxidant conditions may promote glutathione synthesis as the metabolic priority at the expense of methionine transmethylation. Treatment with methylcobalamin and folinic acid appears to have rescued glutathione synthesis in this cohort of children, albeit incompletely, at the expense of transmethylation metabolism. Given the fact that some behavioral improvements were related to improvements in glutathione status, it is possible that longer-term treatment or treatments that include additional precursors or methylcobalamin and folinic acid at higher doses may result in additional behavioral improvements. For example, one recent open-label study demonstrated that high-dose folinic acid demonstrated potential efficacy in children with ASD [30] and another double-blind placebo controlled study demonstrated that N-acetylcysteine, a glutathione precursor, resulted in decreased irritability and improved social function [31]. However, neither of these aforementioned studies measured redox metabolism in order to determine whether the observed behavioral effects were related to changes in redox metabolism. Further studies will be needed to determine the optimal combination of precursors for the treatment of redox abnormalities in children with ASD.

4.3. The Use of Novel Interventions in Autism Spectrum Disorder. Our findings are consistent with smaller [31, 32] and larger [33] randomized control trials and large case series [30] demonstrating that nutritional interventions for children with ASD that target oxidative stress are associated with improvements in core ASD symptoms [30, 31], sleep and gastrointestinal symptoms [32], and hyperactivity, tantruming and parental impression of general functioning [33]. Besides the methylcobalamin and folinic acid treatment used in this study [23], the beneficial effect of nutritional treatments on redox metabolism in children with ASD has been documented in a randomized control trial [33] and a cross-sectional study [34]. Such studies suggest that glutathione metabolism can be improved by vitamin and mineral [33] and antioxidants, coenzyme Q10 and B vitamins supplementation [34], and sapropterin treatment [28]. Thus, although there is evidence for nutritional treatments improving redox metabolism and ASD symptoms and behaviors in children with ASD, there is no specific established treatment for correcting redox abnormalities in children with ASD and the evidence for efficacy of nutritional treatments which address oxidative stress on core and associated ASD behaviors is preliminary. Clearly more studies are needed to clarify the potential beneficial effect of nutritional treatments for children with ASD.

The nutritional treatment used in this study is considered, by some, as a complementary and alternative medicine (CAM) treatment [35]. However, CAM treatments refer to a much wider variety of treatments, including nonnutritional treatments such as acupuncture and homeopathy. The prevalence of CAM in children diagnosed with a ASD in western countries is estimated to be between 32% and 87% [35] which is believed to be much higher than CAM therapies used in typically developing children [36]. Children with ASD with a greater number of medical and behavioral problems receive more CAM treatments than those with fewer medical and behavioral problems [37]. Parents believe that most CAM-associated treatments are either helpful or without effect but not harmful [35]. The main reasons parents cite for choosing to use CAM for ASD are concerns about the safety and side effects of available medications for ASD and a need to be involved in decisions involving care of their child [38]. Because the majority of CAM therapies are based on anecdotal evidence, there is a clear need for clinical trials to evaluate the efficacy of these treatments [35]. In addition, it should be noted that for ASD, of all treatments considered CAM, nutritional treatments have the most evidence for effectiveness and efficacy. Thus, it may not be proper to consider nutritional treatments, which have been used in mainstream medicine for over a century, as equivalent to CAM treatments which have undergone much fewer investigations and have less support for their use.

4.4. Limitations. The reported improvement in behavior scores by parent report should be interpreted with caution in an open-label trial because of expectation bias [38]. In addition, without a control group it is difficult to know if, and to what extent, development would have changed without treatment. As this is a group with significant delays, it is unlikely that they would have demonstrated typical gains over the three-month period but it is possible they may have shown some developmental progress. However, it is reassuring that a significant number of improvements were moderated by improvements in glutathione metabolism, suggesting that changes in metabolism were indeed related to improvements in behavior.

This study prescreened and selected a subgroup of children with ASD that demonstrated abnormal glutathione redox status and methylation capacity as a means to increase sensitivity to treatment. The broad heterogeneity of clinical and behavioral symptoms in autistic children predicts that no single treatment will benefit every autistic child. Thus, the definition and characterization of subgroups of children who respond positively or negatively to intervention will be necessary to more sensitively identify those children who are most likely to benefit from a given treatment or medication.

4.5. Conclusions. This study demonstrates that a three-month treatment with methylcobalamin and folinic acid is associated with significant improvements in behavioral symptoms associated with ASD in a group of children with AD and metabolic markers of abnormal redox and methylation metabolism. Our previous study demonstrated that this treatment also improves metabolic markers of glutathione metabolism in these same children. This provides convergence of independent measures demonstrating the beneficial effect of this simple and safe nutritional intervention. Clearly this intervention requires further study in a double-blind placebo-controlled trial to eliminate the potential bias associated with an open-label study.

Authors' Contribution

Richard E. Frye was responsible for data analysis, interpretation, and writing of the paper. S. Jill James was the PI for this project and was responsible for the conduct of the study, interpretation of the data, and the writing of the paper. Stepan Melnyk is the laboratory director and provided HPLC expertise for metabolite analysis. George Fuchs and Tyra Reid provided clinical advice, assisted with the interpretation of data, and provided critical review of the paper. Oleksandra Pavliv provided technical assistance for the HPLC analysis. Amanda Hubanks was the study nurse who recruited patients and administered the Vineland behavior testing. David W. Gaylor provided statistical support for data analysis.

Acknowledgments

The authors gratefully acknowledge the support of the Arkansas families affected by autism whose participation made this study possible. They also thank the pediatricians and nurses at the University of Arkansas for Medical Sciences Dennis Developmental Center for patient referrals and Hopewell Compounding Pharmacy (Hopewell, NJ) for their generous donation of methylcobalamin for the study. This research was supported, in part, with funding from the National Institute of Child Health and Development (RO1 HD051873) to S. Jill James and by grants from the University of Arkansas for Medical Sciences Children's University Medical Group and the Arkansas Biosciences Institute (S. Jill James, Richard E. Frye).

References

[1] C. Rice, "Autism, Developmental Disabilities Monitoring Network Surveillance Year Principal I, Centers for Disease C, Prevention: prevalence of autism spectrum disorders—autism and developmental disabilities monitoring network, United States, 2006," *Morbidity and Mortality Weekly Report*, vol. 58, no. 10, pp. 1–20, 2009.

[2] G. B. Schaefer and N. J. Mendelsohn, "Clinical genetics evaluation in identifying the etiology of autism spectrum disorders," *Genetics in Medicine*, vol. 10, no. 4, pp. 301–305, 2008.

[3] R. E. Frye and D. A. Rossignol, "Mitochondrial dysfunction can connect the diverse medical symptoms associated with autism spectrum disorders," *Pediatric Research*, vol. 69, no. 5, pp. 41R–47R, 2011.

[4] D. A. Rossignol and R. E. Frye, "Mitochondrial dysfunction in autism spectrum disorders: a systematic review and meta-analysis," *Molecular Psychiatry*, vol. 17, no. 3, pp. 290–314, 2012.

[5] S. J. James, S. Melnyk, S. Jernigan, A. Hubanks, S. Rose, and D. W. Gaylor, "Abnormal transmethylation/transsulfuration metabolism and DNA hypomethylation among parents of children with autism," *Journal of Autism and Developmental Disorders*, vol. 38, no. 10, pp. 1966–1975, 2008.

[6] S. J. James, S. Melnyk, S. Jernigan et al., "Metabolic endophenotype and related genotypes are associated with oxidative stress in children with autism," *American Journal of Medical Genetics Part B*, vol. 141, no. 8, pp. 947–956, 2006.

[7] S. Melnyk, G. J. Fuchs, E. Schulz et al., "Metabolic imbalance associated with methylation dysregulation and oxidative damage in children with autism," *Journal of Autism and Developmental Disorders*, vol. 42, no. 3, pp. 367–377, 2012.

[8] P. Ashwood, B. A. Corbett, A. Kantor, H. Schulman, J. van de Water, and D. G. Amaral, "In search of cellular immunophenotypes in the blood of children with autism," *PLoS ONE*, vol. 6, no. 5, Article ID e19299, 2011.

[9] P. Ashwood, P. Krakowiak, I. Hertz-Picciotto, R. Hansen, I. N. Pessah, and J. Van de Water, "Associations of impaired behaviors with elevated plasma chemokines in autism spectrum disorders," *Journal of Neuroimmunology*, vol. 232, no. 1-2, pp. 196–199, 2011.

[10] P. Ashwood, P. Krakowiak, I. Hertz-Picciotto, R. Hansen, I. N. Pessah, and J. Van de Water, "Altered T cell responses in children with autism," *Brain, Behavior, and Immunity*, vol. 25, no. 5, pp. 840–849, 2011.

[11] D. A. Rossignol and R. E. Frye, "A review of research trends in physiological abnormalities in autism spectrum disorders: immune dysregulation, inflammation, oxidative stress, mitochondrial dysfunction and environmental toxicant exposures," *Molecular Psychiatry*, vol. 17, no. 4, pp. 389–401, 2012.

[12] E. Viding and S.-J. Blakemore, "Endophenotype approach to developmental psychopathology: implications for autism research," *Behavior Genetics*, vol. 37, no. 1, pp. 51–60, 2007.

[13] S. J. James, P. Cutler, S. Melnyk et al., "Metabolic biomarkers of increased oxidative stress and impaired methylation capacity in children with autism," *American Journal of Clinical Nutrition*, vol. 80, no. 6, pp. 1611–1617, 2004.

[14] S. J. James, S. Rose, S. Melnyk et al., "Cellular and mitochondrial glutathione redox imbalance in lymphoblastoid cells derived from children with autism," *FASEB Journal*, vol. 23, no. 8, pp. 2374–2383, 2009.

[15] S. Rose, S. Melnyk, T. A. Trusty et al., "Intracellular and extracellular redox status and free radical generation in primary immune cells from children with autism," *Autism Research and Treatment*, vol. 2012, Article ID 986519, 10 pages, 2012.

[16] W. Droge and R. Breitkreutz, "Glutathione and immune function," *Proceedings of the Nutrition Society*, vol. 59, no. 4, pp. 595–600, 2000.

[17] A. Pastore, G. Federici, E. Bertini, and F. Piemonte, "Analysis of glutathione: implication in redox and detoxification," *Clinica Chimica Acta*, vol. 333, no. 1-2, pp. 19–39, 2003.

[18] S. Biswas, A. S. Chida, and I. Rahman, "Redox modifications of protein-thiols: emerging roles in cell signaling," *Biochemical Pharmacology*, vol. 71, no. 5, pp. 551–564, 2006.

[19] F. Q. Schafer and G. R. Buettner, "Redox environment of the cell as viewed through the redox state of the glutathione disulfide/glutathione couple," *Free Radical Biology and Medicine*, vol. 30, no. 11, pp. 1191–1212, 2001.

[20] M. Reid and F. Jahoor, "Glutathione in disease," *Current Opinion in Clinical Nutrition and Metabolic Care*, vol. 4, no. 1, pp. 65–71, 2001.

[21] S. Rose, S. Melnyk, O. Pavliv et al., "Evidence of oxidative damage and inflammation associated with low glutathione redox status in the autism brain," *Translational Psychiatry*, vol. 2, article e134, 2012.

[22] A. Chauhan and V. Chauhan, "Oxidative stress in autism," *Pathophysiology*, vol. 13, no. 3, pp. 171–181, 2006.

[23] S. J. James, S. Melnyk, G. Fuchs et al., "Efficacy of methylcobalamin and folinic acid treatment on glutathione redox status in children with autism," *American Journal of Clinical Nutrition*, vol. 89, no. 1, pp. 425–430, 2009.

[24] S. Melnyk, M. Pogribna, I. Pogribny, R. J. Hine, and S. J. James, "A new HPLC method for the simultaneous determination of oxidized and reduced plasma aminothiols using coulometric electrochemical detection," *Journal of Nutritional Biochemistry*, vol. 10, no. 8, pp. 490–497, 1999.

[25] S. Melnyk, M. Pogribna, I. P. Pogribny, P. Yi, and S. J. James, "Measurement of plasma and intracellular S-adenosylmethionine and S-adenosylhomocysteine utilizing coulometric electrochemical detection: alterations with plasma homocysteine and pyridoxal 5′-phosphate concentrations," *Clinical Chemistry*, vol. 46, no. 2, pp. 265–272, 2000.

[26] S. Sparrow, D. Cicchetti, and D. Balla, *Vineland Adaptive Behavior Scales*, P. Assessment, Minneapolis, Minn, USA, 2nd edition, 2005.

[27] N. M. Laird and J. H. Ware, "Random-effects models for longitudinal data," *Biometrics*, vol. 38, no. 4, pp. 963–974, 1982.

[28] R. E. Frye, R. DeLatorre, H. B. Taylor et al., "Metabolic effects of sapropterin treatment in autism spectrum disorder: a preliminary study," *Translational Psychiatry*, vol. 3, article e237, 2013.

[29] S. M. Melnyk, K. F. More, and E. F. Miles, "Idiopathic radiation recall dermatitis developing nine months after cessation of Cisplatin therapy in treatment of squamous cell carcinoma of the tonsil," *Case Reports in Oncological Medicine*, vol. 2012, Article ID 271801, 3 pages, 2012.

[30] R. E. Frye, J. M. Sequeira, E. V. Quadros, S. J. James, and D. A. Rossignol, "Cerebral folate receptor autoantibodies in autism spectrum disorder," *Molecular Psychiatry*, vol. 18, no. 3, pp. 369–381, 2013.

[31] A. Y. Hardan, L. K. Fung, R. A. Libove et al., "A randomized controlled pilot trial of oral N-acetylcysteine in children with autism," *Biological Psychiatry*, vol. 71, no. 11, pp. 956–961, 2012.

[32] J. B. Adams and C. Holloway, "Pilot study of a moderate dose multivitamin/mineral supplement for children with autistic spectrum disorder," *Journal of Alternative and Complementary Medicine*, vol. 10, no. 6, pp. 1033–1039, 2004.

[33] J. B. Adams, T. Audhya, S. McDonough-Means et al., "Nutritional and metabolic status of children with autism vs. neurotypical children, and the association with autism severity," *Nutrition and Metabolism*, vol. 8, article 34, 2011.

[34] R. E. Frye, R. DeLatorre, and H. B. Taylor, "Redox metabolism abnormalities in autistic children associated with mitochondrial disease," *Translational Psychiatry*, 2013.

[35] N. Lofthouse, R. Hendren, E. Hurt, I. E. Arnold, and E. Butter, "A review of complementary and alternative treatments for autism spectrum disorders," *Autism Research and Treatment*, 2012.

[36] D. A. Rossignol, "Novel and emerging treatments for autism spectrum disorders: a systematic review," *Annals of Clinical Psychiatry*, vol. 21, no. 4, pp. 213–236, 2009.

[37] J. M. Perrin, D. L. Coury, S. L. Hyman, L. Cole, A. M. Reynolds, and T. Clemons, "Complementary and alternative medicine use in a large pediatric autism sample," *Pediatrics*, vol. 130, pp. S77–S82, 2012.

[38] S. L. Hyman and S. E. Levy, "Introduction: novel therapies in developmental disabilities—hope, reason, and evidence," *Mental Retardation and Developmental Disabilities Research Reviews*, vol. 11, no. 2, pp. 107–109, 2005.

6

Gaze Behavior of Children with ASD toward Pictures of Facial Expressions

Soichiro Matsuda,[1,2] Yasuyo Minagawa,[1,3] and Junichi Yamamoto[1,3]

[1]Department of Psychology, Keio University, 2-15-45 Mita, Minato-ku, Tokyo 108-0073, Japan
[2]Japan Society for the Promotion of Science, 5-3-1 Kojimachi, Chiyoda-ku, Tokyo 102-0083, Japan
[3]CREST, Japan Science and Technology Agency, 4-1-8 Honcho, Kawaguchi-shi, Saitama 332-0012, Japan

Correspondence should be addressed to Soichiro Matsuda; atom.opens.the.stargate@gmail.com

Academic Editor: Geraldine Dawson

Atypical gaze behavior in response to a face has been well documented in individuals with autism spectrum disorders (ASDs). Children with ASD appear to differ from typically developing (TD) children in gaze behavior for spoken and dynamic face stimuli but not for nonspeaking, static face stimuli. Furthermore, children with ASD and TD children show a difference in their gaze behavior for certain expressions. However, few studies have examined the relationship between autism severity and gaze behavior toward certain facial expressions. The present study replicated and extended previous studies by examining gaze behavior towards pictures of facial expressions. We presented ASD and TD children with pictures of surprised, happy, neutral, angry, and sad facial expressions. Autism severity was assessed using the Childhood Autism Rating Scale (CARS). The results showed that there was no group difference in gaze behavior when looking at pictures of facial expressions. Conversely, the children with ASD who had more severe autistic symptomatology had a tendency to gaze at angry facial expressions for a shorter duration in comparison to other facial expressions. These findings suggest that autism severity should be considered when examining atypical responses to certain facial expressions.

1. Introduction

Human faces provide important social cues, and the perception of facial expressions is fundamental to the development of social communication. Therefore, it is expected that individuals with autism spectrum disorders (ASDs), who are characterized by social communication difficulties, exhibit abnormalities in their perception of the face. Consistent with this view, several eye-tracking studies have shown atypical gaze behavior toward faces in individuals with ASD [1–3]. Certain other studies, however, have not found these abnormalities [4, 5]. Matsuda and Yamamoto [6–8] suggested that these mixed results were caused by the differing stimuli, ages, and/or autism severity of the participants.

When considering the face as a stimulus, we need to recognize that there are several variables which might affect gaze behavior [9, 10]. Gaze behavior toward the face differs because of variables such as speech (spoken or unspoken), movement (static or dynamic), or facial expression. However, in most previous investigations of gaze behavior toward faces in individuals with ASD, these variables have not been sufficiently examined.

It is possible that atypical gaze behavior toward a nonspeaking static facial expression in individuals with ASD could be related to age. Adults with ASD have exhibited shorter fixation durations on the eyes or longer fixation durations on the mouth than those with typical development [11–17]. However, studies of children or adolescents with ASD have not found such differences [18–20] and have indicated that children with ASD have the same gaze behavior as typically developing children for facial expressions.

In typical development, there is evidence that gaze behavior varies in response to different expressions. Infants and adults were found to look for a shorter duration at a feature area with fearful and angry facial expressions in comparison to neutral and sad expressions [21]. Adults looked longer at the mouth for happy expressions compared to sad, neutral, and fearful facial expressions [22] and longer at the feature area for fearful and angry expressions compared to happy, sad, and neutral expressions [23].

Recent eye-tracking studies in individuals with ASD have demonstrated that differences in gaze behavior in certain expressions were also observed in this population. van der Geest et al. [19] demonstrated that children with ASD looked longer at the mouth for surprised and happy expressions compared to angry and neutral expressions. Wagner et al. [20] also found that adolescents with ASD looked longer at the mouth for happy expressions compared to neutral and fearful facial expressions. In both studies, there was no significant difference between individuals with and without ASD for each of the facial expressions.

However, although previous research has suggested that autism severity is linked to fixation duration on the eyes or the mouth [2, 18, 24], no study has examined the relationship between autism severity and gaze behavior toward certain facial expressions. Some studies have reported that autism severity is negatively correlated with the percentage of correct responses in the naming of sad facial expressions [25], or fear facial expressions [26], which suggests that certain facial expressions may evoke a differential gaze behavior depending on autism severity.

In the current study, we presented children with ASD and typically developing children with pictures of surprised, happy, neutral, angry, and sad facial expressions. The participants' gaze behavior towards the facial expressions was assessed using an eye-tracking device. To investigate the role of autism severity in gaze behavior towards facial expressions, we examined the relationship degree between the total CARS scores (Childhood Autism Rating Scale) [27] and the proportion of total time spent looking at each facial expression.

2. Method

2.1. Participants. The participants included two groups of children: 18 with ASD and 11 typically developing (TD) children. Children in the ASD group had previously received a formal ASD diagnosis by an outside professional (one with Asperger's syndrome, 15 with autism, and two with Pervasive Developmental Disorders), according to the DSM-IV-TR criteria [28]. Children in the TD group were matched by their average age to the developmental age (DA) of those in the ASD group. Data analyses were conducted on a final sample of 15 boys with ASD (CA: $M = 7.5$, SD = 3.0, range: 3.6–13.7; DA: $M = 5.1$, SD = 2.0, range: 2.2–8.7) and 11 TD (CA: $M = 5.5$, SD = 1.8, range: 3.2–9.9; 3 female, 8 male) children. Three children with ASD were excluded from the analyses because they did not meet the CARS criteria for autism.

Developmental ages were derived using the Kyoto Scale of Psychological Development 2001 (KSPD) [29]. This assessment calculates the average scores of subitems for physical-motion, verbal-social, cognitive-adaptation, and total developmental age. The KSPD has been developed for typically developing infants and low-functioning children with ASD and other developmental disorders. In this study, the measure for the developmental age of the children was the total developmental age score in the KSPD.

Gold standard diagnostic measures, such as the Autism Diagnostic Interview–Revised [30, 31] and the Autism Diagnostic Observation Schedule [32], have not been officially translated and adopted to Japanese culture. Therefore, to confirm the diagnosis of ASD, we used the Japanese version of Childhood Autism Rating Scale [27]. A licensed psychologist and four therapists, who had at least five years' experience in the fields of behavior interventions, administered the CARS before the experiment. The mean autism severity of the children with ASD was 40.9 (SD = 6.5, range: 30.5–52.5). Autism severity was not associated with the CA ($r = 0.55$, $p = 0.035$, n.s. with Bonferroni correction) or DA ($r = -0.34$, $p = 0.217$).

The difference between the mean chronological age (CA) of each group approached significance; the participants in the ASD group were older than the participants in the TD group ($t(24) = 2.03$, $p = 0.054$). There were no significant differences between the mean DA in the ASD group and the CA in the TD group ($t(24) = -0.40$, $p = 0.693$).

2.2. Stimuli and Apparatus. The stimuli were color images of three female and two male Japanese actors' faces, each depicting a surprised, happy, neutral, angry, or sad expression. There were 25 images in total, with each image showing a single actor with one expression. All images were transformed with the Adobe Photoshop CS5 (Adobe, San Jose, CA) to control luminance, background colors, and face size. The emotions displayed in the images were selected from the list of six universal emotions identified by Ekman [33]: surprise, happiness, anger, sadness, fear, and disgust. In addition, a neutral expression was added. Emotions of fear and disgust were excluded from this study because Japanese participants in previous studies [34, 35] had had difficulty in identifying them. Prior to the study, a pilot study was conducted, in which 11 Japanese adults rated pictures of facial expressions. They were asked to rate the expressions on a 7-point Likert scale for each given emotion and the Affect Grid [36] for pleasure and arousal. The results of these ratings are presented in Table 1.

Participants sat in a chair facing the monitor in a testing room. With an approximately 75-cm viewing distance, the images (1024 × 731 px) measured approximately 24.0° and 17.3° of the vertical and horizontal visual angles, respectively. Eye-tracker calibration and stimulus presentation were controlled by Tobii Studio software (Tobii Technology).

Participant fixations were recorded using a Tobii X120 (Tobii Technology Japan, Ltd, Minato-ku Takanawa, Japan) at 60 Hz. Tobii has infrared light sources and cameras and uses corneal reflection techniques. Fixations were defined by an in-built automatic fixation detection algorithm that uses a sliding window average method (Tobii Fixation Filter). The velocity threshold was 35 pixel/window, and distance threshold was 35 pixels. The accuracy of this eye-tracker is approximately 0.5°. The eye-tracker was placed in front of a 27-inch monitor (1080 × 1920 px), which measured approximately 25.3° and 43.5° of the vertical and horizontal visual angles, respectively.

Table 1: Mean ratings for emotions, pleasure, and arousal for a stimuli based on a 7-point scale and an affect grid (9-point scale).

	7-point Likert scale				The Affect Grid (9-point)	
	Surprised	Happy	Angry	Sad	Pleasure	Arousal
Surprised	*5.6*	1.6	1.5	1.5	3.9	6.7
Happy	1.5	*5.3*	1.2	1.3	6.4	4.8
Neutral	1.5	1.7	2.0	2.3	3.6	3.6
Angry	1.6	1.2	*5.0*	3.1	1.3	5.4
Sad	1.7	1.2	2.2	*4.3*	1.9	3.3

Note. Ratings for predicted emotion are shown in italics.

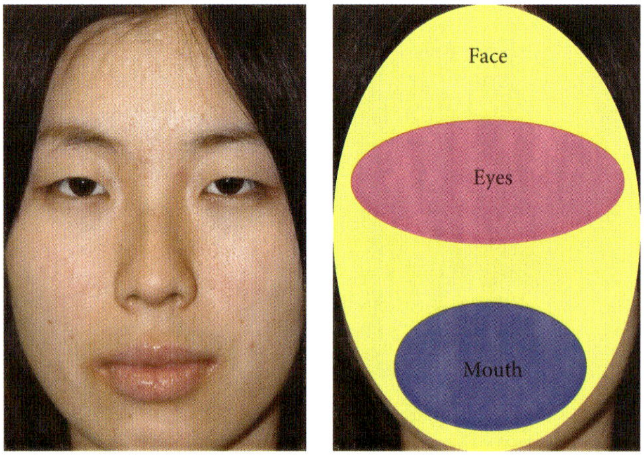

(a) (b)

Figure 1: Visual example of the (a) stimuli and (b) areas of interest (AOI). *Note.* This is printed with permission from the model.

2.3. Procedure. The experiment was conducted in a testing room at Keio University. The children were asked to sit in a chair in front of the monitor and instructed that they will be shown some pictures and movies on the monitor. Prior to testing, the gaze of each child was calibrated. We used a 5-point calibration procedure, in which a movie clip (i.e., a moving cat coupled with attractive sounds) was played sequentially at five locations on the screen. If all five points were calibrated successfully, the experimental phase began. The accuracy of the calibration was similar in the ASD and TD group. In this phase, all 25 images were shown for three seconds each, with an attention getter appearing before every five images. There was no interstimulus interval between five images. The attention getter was a 3-second movie clip (i.e., a moving star coupled with attractive sounds). The image order was pseudo-randomized.

2.4. Data Analysis

2.4.1. Areas of Interest (AOI). Three areas of interest (AOI) were manually defined: the face, eyes, and mouth. The face AOI covered the AOIs of both the eyes and the mouth, with the AOIs being equal for all images. The size of the AOIs was 78.1% of the image of the face AOI (24.0° and 17.2° of the vertical and horizontal visual angles), 19.1% for the image of the eyes AOI (15.5° and 6.1° of the vertical and horizontal visual angles), and 14.1% for the image of the mouth AOI (10.3° and 6.0° of the vertical and horizontal visual angles). An example of an image and AOIs are shown in Figure 1.

2.4.2. Statistical Analysis. All analyses were conducted using SPSS for windows, version 22. The first set of analyses examined the degree to which the children with ASD displayed different gaze behavior toward the facial expressions compared to the typically developing children. Repeated measures ANOVAs with the facial expression as the within-subject factor (surprised, happy, neutral, angry, and sad) and diagnosis as the between-subject factor (ASD, TD) were conducted for the dependent variables. We also examined the significant effects and interactions using post hoc t-tests with a Bonferroni correction. The dependent variables were based on the proportion of the fixation duration. The proportion of the total time spent looking at the face AOI (%Face) was standardized using the total duration of the stimulus display, and the proportion of the total time spent looking at the eyes AOI (%Eyes) and the mouth AOI (%Mouth) was standardized using the total time spent looking at the face AOI.

The second set of analyses explored the relationship degree between CA, DA, or autism severity (the total CARS scores) and the gaze behavior toward each expression using Pearson correlations. The gaze behavior toward each facial expression was calculated for each child by dividing

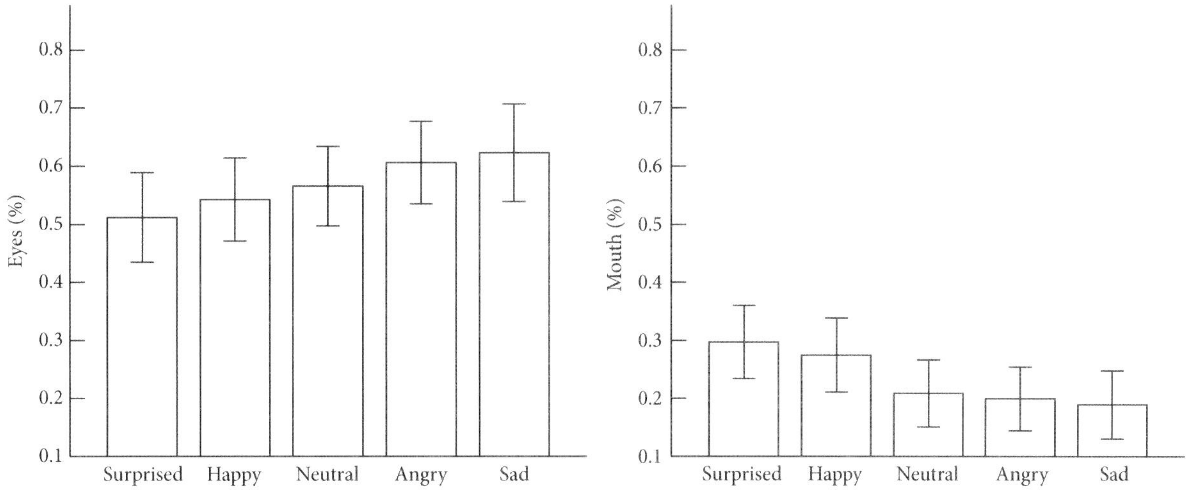

FIGURE 2: Mean proportion of total time spent looking at the eyes AOI and the mouth AOI for each facial expression category. The error bars indicate 95% confidence intervals.

the fixation duration on the face AOI for each expression (e.g., surprised) by the total fixation duration on the face AOI for all expressions (surprised, happy, neutral, angry, and sad).

3. Results

3.1. Total Time Spent Looking at the Face. The mean proportion of the total time spent looking at the face AOI was 65.1% (SD = 18.7) for children with ASD and 77.5% (SD = 20.0) for TDs. The diagnosis × facial expression ANOVA on % Face revealed no effects for diagnosis, $F(1, 24) = 2.49$, $p = 0.128$, $\eta p^2 = 0.09$, facial expression, $F(4, 96) = 1.05$, $p = 0.384$, $\eta p^2 = 0.04$, or diagnosis × facial expression interaction, $F(4, 96) = 0.31$, $p = 0.869$, $\eta p^2 = 0.01$.

3.2. Eyes and Mouth Ratios. Figure 2 shows the mean % Eyes and % Mouth for each facial expression category.

The diagnosis × facial expression ANOVA on % Eyes indicated a significant effect for facial expression, $F(4, 96) = 5.01$, $p = 0.001$, $\eta p^2 = 0.17$, but no effect for diagnosis, $F(1, 24) = 0.80$, $p = 0.380$, $\eta p^2 = 0.03$, or diagnosis × facial expression interaction, $F(4, 96) = 0.27$, $p = 0.895$, $\eta p^2 = 0.01$. Post hoc t-tests for the main facial expression effects revealed significantly shorter fixation durations on the eyes for the surprised expression compared to the sad expression, $t(25) = -3.61$, $p = 0.001$, and the angry expression, $t(25) = -3.31$, $p = 0.003$. Both groups tended to look for a shorter time at the eyes for the happy expression compared to the sad expression, $t(25) = -2.83$, $p = 0.009$ (n.s. with Bonferroni correction).

The diagnosis × facial expression ANOVA for % Mouth indicated a significant effect for facial expression, $F(4, 96) = 8.54$, $p < 0.001$, $\eta p^2 = 0.26$, but no effect for diagnosis, $F(1, 24) = 0.57$, $p = 0.457$, $\eta p^2 = 0.02$, or diagnosis × facial expression interaction, $F(4, 96) = 0.38$, $p = 0.823$, $\eta p^2 = 0.02$. Post hoc t-tests for the main facial expression effects revealed significantly longer fixation durations on the mouth for the surprised expression compared to the sad, $t(25) = 4.47$, $p < 0.001$, angry, $t(25) = 4.57$, $p < 0.001$, and the neutral, $t(25) = 3.27$, $p = 0.003$, expressions. In addition, both groups looked longer at the mouth for the happy expression compared to the sad, $t(25) = 3.57$, $p = 0.001$, angry, $t(25) = 3.05$, $p = 0.005$, and neutral, $t(25) = 2.60$, $p = 0.015$ (n.s. with Bonferroni correction), expressions.

3.3. Associations between CA, DA, and Fixation Durations for Each Facial Expression in ASD. CA was not associated with the proportion of total time spent looking at the surprised ($r = 0.29$, $p = 0.104$); happy ($r = -0.10$, $p = 0.735$); neutral ($r = 0.02$, $p = 0.959$); angry ($r = -0.38$, $p = 0.167$); or sad ($r = -0.15$, $p = 0.603$) expressions. DA was also not associated with the proportion of total time spent looking at the surprised ($r = -0.10$, $p = 0.735$); happy ($r = 0.12$, $p = 0.957$); neutral ($r = 0.10$, $p = 0.717$); angry ($r = 0.20$, $p = 0.466$); or sad ($r = -0.18$, $p = 0.518$) expressions.

3.4. Associations between Autism Severity and Fixation Durations for Each Facial Expression in ASD. Finally, we examined the correlation between autism severity and the proportion of total time spent looking at each facial expression. Autism severity was not associated with the proportion of total time spent looking at the surprised ($r = 0.23$, $p = 0.420$), happy ($r = 0.23$, $p = 0.418$), neutral ($r = 0.17$, $p = 0.172$), or sad ($r = 0.19$, $p = 0.491$) expressions. On the other hand, there was a significant negative correlation between autism severity and the proportion of total time spent looking at the angry expression, $r = -0.77$, $p = 0.001$ (Figure 3).

4. Discussion

In the current study, we examined gaze behavior in children with ASD and TD toward pictures of facial expressions.

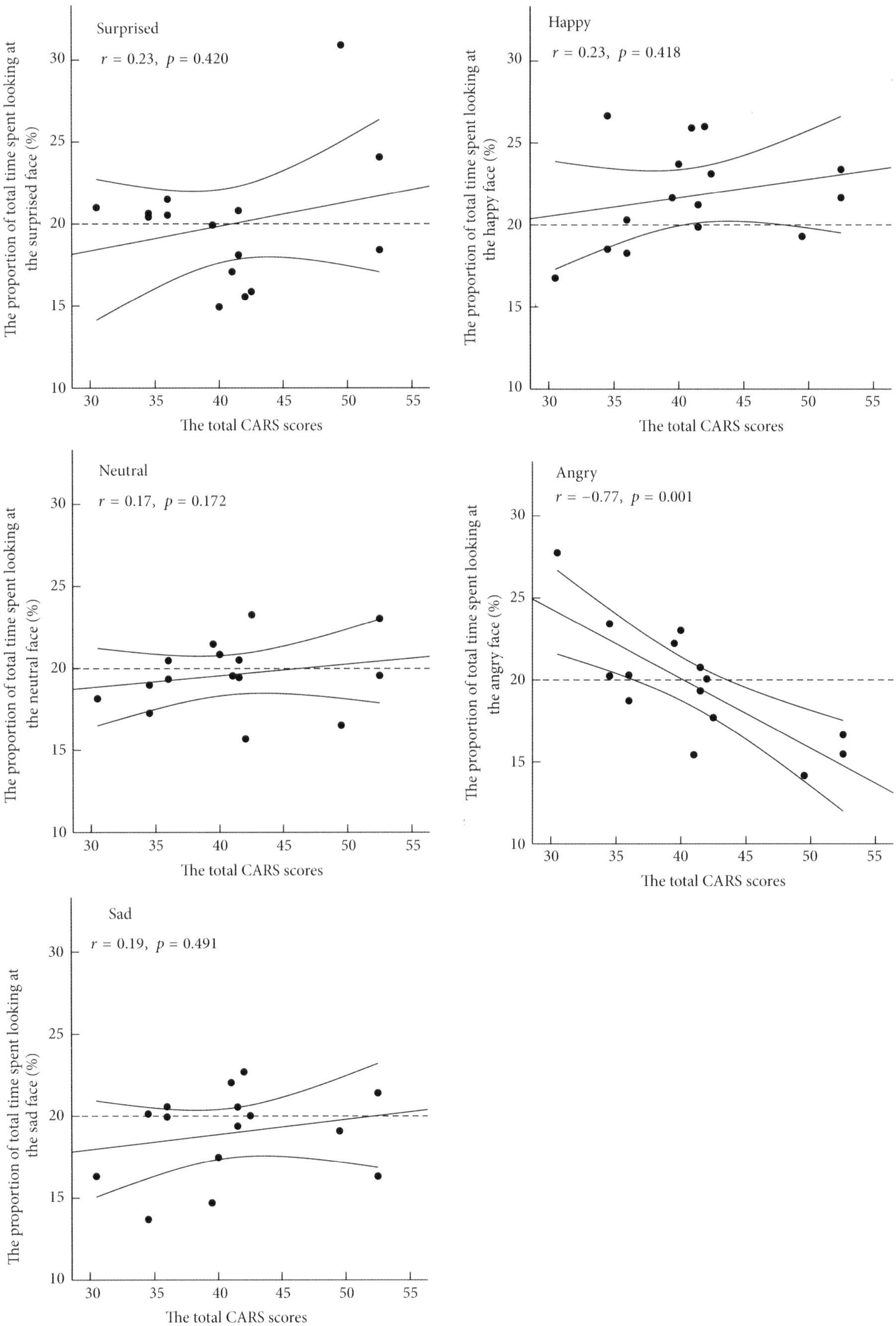

FIGURE 3: Correlation of the total CARS scores and the proportion of total time spent looking at each facial expression in ASD group.

Overall, we found no group differences in gaze behavior toward the pictures of facial expressions. Further, the results of total time spent looking at the face and the proportion of time spent looking at the eyes and the mouth regions revealed no differences between children with ASD and TD. In both groups, the eyes of the angry and sad facial expressions were fixated on longer than the eyes of the surprised, and the mouth of the surprised and happy facial expressions was fixated on longer than the mouth of the angry and sad facial expressions. CA and DA were not associated with the proportion of total time spent looking at all facial expressions. While autism severity was not found to be associated with the proportion of total time spent looking at the surprised, happy, neutral, or sad facial expressions, it was found to be associated with a lower proportion of total time spent looking at the angry facial expression.

Our study demonstrated that there was no difference in gaze behavior between children with ASD and TD toward nonspeaking static facial expressions. This result is in accordance with recent eye-tracking studies of children and adolescents with ASD [18–20]. Although other eye-tracking studies on children or adolescents with ASD have found differences between ASD and TD [1, 3], one implication of this finding is that the presence of speech (spoken) and movement (dynamic) might be responsible for such differences.

It has regularly been reported that typically developing children show a specific fixation pattern when looking at certain facial expressions [21–23]. Several studies using visual search tasks have also demonstrated that mouth region had importance for surprised and happy expression, while eye region played important role for angry and sad expressions [37, 38]. The present study indicates that children with ASD have the same gaze behavior toward each facial expression. This result is in line with previous studies, which suggests that certain facial expressions do not cause atypical gaze behavior in children with ASD [19, 20].

Even though there were no group differences in gaze behavior toward certain facial expressions, the proportion of total time spent looking at the angry facial expression was found to be associated with autism severity. This result suggests that children with ASD who have a more severe autistic symptomatology tend to look for a shorter duration on angry facial expressions in comparison to other facial expressions. Children with ASD show atypical responses to angry faces on a visual search task [39], although adults with ASD show a similar response to those with a typical development [40, 41]. It is possible that both the autism severity and the participant ages may affect the atypical response to an angry facial expression.

There were several limitations to the study. First, we need to be cautious about interpreting lack of significant results between groups due to small sample size. Studies including more participants are needed. Second, the two groups differed slightly in CA. Future studies should include a CA matched control group to confirm that CA is not an important factor for lack of significant difference between two groups. Third, we used CARS to determine both eligibility and severity in this study. Further studies will be required to use other diagnostic measures in order that eligibility and severity are separately determined. Also, the ASD and TD groups were not matched on participant's gender.

Despite limitations, to our knowledge, this study is the first to demonstrate relationships between autism severity and gaze behaviors toward facial expressions. While previous studies examine the association between autism severity and fixation duration on the eyes or the mouth [2, 18, 24], our findings showed that angry expressions evoke a differential gaze behavior depending on autism severity. The current study contributes to a growing body of evidence that the demographic factor, including autism severity, affects the results of eye-tracking studies.

5. Conclusion

The present data suggested that there is no difference between children with ASD and TD when looking at a picture of a facial expression. Both groups showed differences in gaze behavior for certain expressions. That is, both groups looked longer at the eyes for the angry and sad facial expressions compared to the happy and surprised facial expressions. Furthermore, the results suggested that an atypical response to an angry facial expression might be because of autism severity.

Acknowledgments

This research was supported by the CREST research project on Social Imaging, JST. Soichiro Matsuda was supported by a fellowship from the Japan Society for the Promotion of Science.

References

[1] W. Jones, K. Carr, and A. Klin, "Absence of preferential looking to the eyes of approaching adults predicts level of social disability in 2-year-old toddlers with autism spectrum disorder," *Archives of General Psychiatry*, vol. 65, no. 8, pp. 946–954, 2008.

[2] A. Klin, W. Jones, R. Schultz, F. Volkmar, and D. Cohen, "Visual fixation patterns during viewing of naturalistic social situations as predictors of social competence in individuals with autism," *Archives of General Psychiatry*, vol. 59, no. 9, pp. 809–816, 2002.

[3] K. Rice, J. M. Moriuchi, W. Jones, and A. Klin, "Parsing heterogeneity in autism spectrum disorders: visual scanning of dynamic social scenes in school-aged children," *Journal of the American Academy of Child & Adolescent Psychiatry*, vol. 51, no. 3, pp. 238–248, 2012.

[4] J. Fischer, K. Koldewyn, Y. V. Jiang, and N. Kanwisher, "Unimpaired attentional disengagement and social orienting in children with autism," *Clinical Psychological Science*, vol. 2, no. 2, pp. 214–223, 2014.

[5] J. C. McPartland, S. J. Webb, B. Keehn, and G. Dawson, "Patterns of visual attention to faces and objects in autism spectrum

disorder," *Journal of Autism and Developmental Disorders*, vol. 41, no. 2, pp. 148–157, 2011.

[6] S. Matsuda and J. Yamamoto, "Intervention for increasing the comprehension of affective prosody in children with autism spectrum disorders," *Research in Autism Spectrum Disorders*, vol. 7, no. 8, pp. 938–946, 2013.

[7] S. Matsuda and J. Yamamoto, "Computer-based intervention for inferring facial expressions from the socio-emotional context in two children with autism spectrum disorders," *Research in Autism Spectrum Disorders*, vol. 8, no. 8, pp. 944–950, 2014.

[8] S. Matsuda and J. Yamamoto, "Intramodal and cross-modal matching of emotional expression in young children with autism spectrum disorders," *Research in Autism Spectrum Disorders*, vol. 10, pp. 109–115, 2015.

[9] J. V. Haxby, E. A. Hoffman, and M. I. Gobbini, "The distributed human neural system for face perception," *Trends in Cognitive Sciences*, vol. 4, no. 6, pp. 223–233, 2000.

[10] L. L. Speer, A. E. Cook, W. M. McMahon, and E. Clark, "Face processing in children with autism," *Autism*, vol. 11, no. 3, pp. 265–277, 2007.

[11] B. Corden, R. Chilvers, and D. Skuse, "Avoidance of emotionally arousing stimuli predicts social-perceptual impairment in Asperger's syndrome," *Neuropsychologia*, vol. 46, no. 1, pp. 137–147, 2008.

[12] N. Hernandez, A. Metzger, R. Magné et al., "Exploration of core features of a human face by healthy and autistic adults analyzed by visual scanning," *Neuropsychologia*, vol. 47, no. 4, pp. 1004–1012, 2009.

[13] D. Neumann, M. L. Spezio, J. Piven, and R. Adolphs, "Looking you in the mouth: abnormal gaze in autism resulting from impaired top-down modulation of visual attention," *Social Cognitive and Affective Neuroscience*, vol. 1, no. 3, pp. 194–202, 2006.

[14] K. A. Pelphrey, N. J. Sasson, J. S. Reznick, G. Paul, B. D. Goldman, and J. Piven, "Visual scanning of faces in autism," *Journal of Autism and Developmental Disorders*, vol. 32, no. 4, pp. 249–261, 2002.

[15] M. D. Rutherford and A. M. Towns, "Scan path differences and similarities during emotion perception in those with and without autism spectrum disorders," *Journal of Autism and Developmental Disorders*, vol. 38, no. 7, pp. 1371–1381, 2008.

[16] M. L. Spezio, R. Adolphs, R. S. E. Hurley, and J. Piven, "Analysis of face gaze in autism using 'bubbles'," *Neuropsychologia*, vol. 45, no. 1, pp. 144–151, 2007.

[17] M. L. Spezio, R. Adolphs, R. S. E. Hurley, and J. Piven, "Abnormal use of facial information in high-functioning autism," *Journal of Autism and Developmental Disorders*, vol. 37, no. 5, pp. 929–939, 2007.

[18] T. C. J. de Wit, T. Falck-Ytter, and C. von Hofsten, "Young children with autism spectrum disorder look differently at positive versus negative emotional faces," *Research in Autism Spectrum Disorders*, vol. 2, no. 4, pp. 651–659, 2008.

[19] J. N. van der Geest, C. Kemner, M. N. Verbaten, and H. van Engeland, "Gaze behavior of children with pervasive developmental disorder toward human faces: a fixation time study," *Journal of Child Psychology and Psychiatry and Allied Disciplines*, vol. 43, no. 5, pp. 669–678, 2002.

[20] J. B. Wagner, S. B. Hirsch, V. K. Vogel-Farley, E. Redcay, and C. A. Nelson, "Eye-tracking, autonomic, and electrophysiological correlates of emotional face processing in adolescents with autism spectrum disorder," *Journal of Autism and Developmental Disorders*, vol. 43, no. 1, pp. 188–199, 2013.

[21] S. Hunnius, T. C. J. de Wit, S. Vrins, and C. von Hofsten, "Facing threat: infants' and adults' visual scanning of faces with neutral, happy, sad, angry, and fearful emotional expressions," *Cognition and Emotion*, vol. 25, no. 2, pp. 193–205, 2011.

[22] H. Eisenbarth and G. W. Alpers, "Happy mouth and sad eyes: scanning emotional facial expressions," *Emotion*, vol. 11, no. 4, pp. 860–865, 2011.

[23] M. J. Green, L. M. Williams, and D. Davidson, "In the face of danger: specific viewing strategies for facial expressions of threat?" *Cognition and Emotion*, vol. 17, no. 5, pp. 779–786, 2003.

[24] T. Falck-Ytter, E. Fernell, C. Gillberg, and C. von Hofsten, "Face scanning distinguishes social from communication impairments in Autism," *Developmental Science*, vol. 13, no. 6, pp. 864–875, 2010.

[25] G. L. Wallace, L. K. Case, M. B. Harms, J. A. Silvers, L. Kenworthy, and A. Martin, "Diminished sensitivity to sad facial expressions in high functioning autism spectrum disorders is associated with symptomatology and adaptive functioning," *Journal of Autism and Developmental Disorders*, vol. 41, no. 11, pp. 1475–1486, 2011.

[26] K. Humphreys, N. Minshew, G. L. Leonard, and M. Behrmann, "A fine-grained analysis of facial expression processing in high-functioning adults with autism," *Neuropsychologia*, vol. 45, no. 4, pp. 685–695, 2007.

[27] E. Schopler, R. J. Reichler, and B. R. Renner, *The Childhood Autism Rating Scales (CARS)*, Western Psychological Services, Los Angeles, Calif, USA, 1988.

[28] American Psychiatric Association, *Diagnostic and Statistical Manual of Mental Disorders*, American Psychiatric Association, Washington, DC, USA, 4th edition, 2000.

[29] M. Ikuzawa, Y. Matsushita, and A. Nakase, Eds., *Kyoto Scale of Psychological Development 2001*, Kyoto International Social Welfare Exchange Centre, Kyoto, Japan, 2002, (Japanese).

[30] A. le Couteur, M. Rutter, C. Lord et al., "Autism diagnostic interview: a standardized investigator-based instrument," *Journal of Autism and Developmental Disorders*, vol. 19, no. 3, pp. 363–387, 1989.

[31] C. Lord, M. Rutter, and A. Le Couteur, "Autism diagnostic interview–revised: a revised version of a diagnostic interview for caregivers of individuals with possible pervasive developmental disorders," *Journal of Autism and Developmental Disorders*, vol. 24, no. 5, pp. 659–685, 1994.

[32] C. Lord, S. Risi, L. Lambrecht et al., "The autism diagnostic observation schedule-generic: a standard measure of social and communication deficits associated with the spectrum of autism," *Journal of Autism and Developmental Disorders*, vol. 30, no. 3, pp. 205–223, 2000.

[33] P. Ekman, "An argument for basic emotions," *Cognition & Emotion*, vol. 6, no. 3, pp. 169–200, 1992.

[34] P. Ekman, W. V. Friesen, M. O'Sullivan et al., "Universals and cultural differences in the judgments of facial expressions of emotion," *Journal of Personality and Social Psychology*, vol. 53, no. 4, pp. 712–717, 1987.

[35] J. A. Russell, N. Suzuki, and N. Ishida, "Canadian, Greek, and Japanese freely produced emotion labels for facial expressions," *Motivation and Emotion*, vol. 17, no. 4, pp. 337–351, 1993.

[36] J. A. Russell, A. Weiss, and G. A. Mendelsohn, "Affect grid: a single-item scale of pleasure and arousal," *Journal of Personality and Social Psychology*, vol. 57, no. 3, pp. 493–502, 1989.

[37] M. G. Calvo and L. Nummenmaa, "Detection of emotional faces: salient physical features guide effective visual search,"

Journal of Experimental Psychology: General, vol. 137, no. 3, pp. 471–494, 2008.

[38] A. J. Calder, A. W. Young, J. Keane, and M. Dean, "Configural information in facial expression perception," *Journal of Experimental Psychology: Human Perception and Performance*, vol. 26, no. 2, pp. 527–551, 2000.

[39] T. Isomura, H. Ito, S. Ogawa, and N. Masataka, "Absence of predispositional attentional sensitivity to angry faces in children with autism spectrum disorders," *Scientific Reports*, vol. 4, article 7525, 2014.

[40] C. Ashwin, S. Wheelwright, and S. Baron-Cohen, "Finding a face in the crowd: testing the anger superiority effect in Asperger Syndrome," *Brain and Cognition*, vol. 61, no. 1, pp. 78–95, 2006.

[41] K. M. Krysko and M. D. Rutherford, "A threat-detection advantage in those with autism spectrum disorders," *Brain and Cognition*, vol. 69, no. 3, pp. 472–480, 2009.

7

The Michigan Autism Spectrum Questionnaire: A Rating Scale for High-Functioning Autism Spectrum Disorders

M. Ghaziuddin[1] **and K. Welch**[2]

[1] *Department of Psychiatry, University of Michigan Medical Center, Plymouth Road, Ann Arbor, MI 48109-0277, USA*
[2] *Center for Statistical Consultation and Research (CSCAR), University of Michigan Medical Center, Plymouth Road, Ann Arbor, MI 48109-0277, USA*

Correspondence should be addressed to M. Ghaziuddin; mghaziud@umich.edu

Academic Editor: Herbert Roeyers

Although the DSM-5 has recently created a single category of autism spectrum disorder (ASD), delineation of its putative subtypes remains clinically useful. For this process, screening instruments should ideally be brief, simple, and easily available. The aim of this study is to describe the validity of one such instrument. We administered the Michigan Autism Spectrum Questionnaire (MASQ), a 10-item questionnaire, to 42 patients with ASD (age range 6–13 years, mean 9.7 years, SD 2.5, one female) and 18 patients with other psychiatric disorders (age range 6–17 years, mean 11.7 years, SD 3.8, 6 females). Responses to each item were scored from 0 to 4 yielding a total score of 30. Patients with intellectual disability were excluded. As a group, patients with ASD scored higher than those with other psychiatric disorders (Chi-square test with 1 df = 16.019, $P < 0.0001$). Within the ASD group, a linear discriminant analysis found that the best cut-off points were 22 or above for Asperger syndrome, 14 to 21 for autism/PDDNOS, and less than 14 for those with other psychiatric disorders. We propose that the MASQ can be used as a brief measure to screen high-functioning ASD from other psychiatric disorders and to identify its possible subtypes.

1. Introduction

Autism is a developmental disorder characterized by a distinct pattern of social and communication impairment with rigid ritualistic interests first described by Kanner [1]. It is sometimes divided into high- and low-functioning types depending on the level of intelligence of the affected individual. Almost 40 years after its initial description, it was introduced as infantile autism in the DSM-III [2]. Subsequently, the DSM-III-R [3] introduced the concept of Pervasive Developmental Disorders (PDD) to describe a group of conditions marked by similar deficits of socialization, communication, and imagination, consisting of the main category of autistic disorder and a residual entity of Pervasive Developmental Disorder Not Otherwise Specified (PDDNOS). Reflecting the increasing interest in Asperger Disorder (or Asperger syndrome) [4], the DSM-IV [5] added it to the group of PDD along with Rett's Disorder and Disintegrative Disorder and retained PDDNOS. However, the recently published DSM-5 has combined autistic disorder, Asperger syndrome, and PDDNOS into a single category of autism spectrum disorder (ASD) and eliminated Rett's and Disintegrative Disorders [6]. The decision to merge the three disorders was apparently taken because they could not be easily distinguished from each other. However, differentiating Asperger syndrome from autism has clinical utility, and delineating the subtypes of the autism spectrum has treatment implications [7, 8]. For example, children with Asperger syndrome may respond better to different kinds of communication skills training than those with autism. Likewise, certain kinds of behaviors and symptoms may be more common in some individuals with high-functioning autism and Asperger syndrome than in those with low-functioning autism [9]. Although several rating scales exist for the assessment of autism spectrum disorders, their diagnosis remains expensive and time consuming, especially in those who are high functioning and who suffer from comorbid psychiatric conditions. In this preliminary study, we describe the use of a brief rating scale to screen for the presence of high-functioning autism spectrum disorders in psychiatric settings.

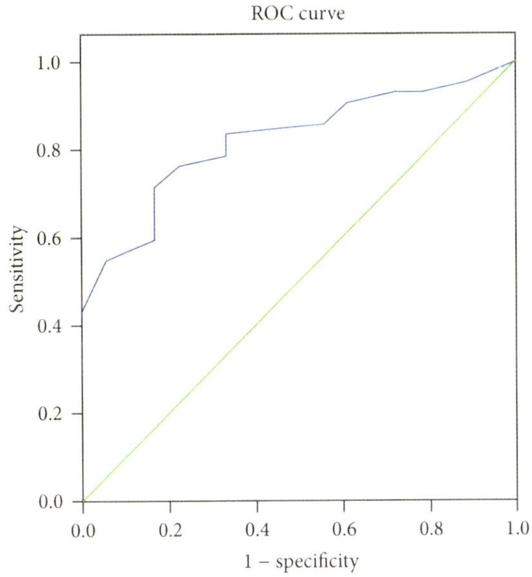

FIGURE 1: Diagonal segments are produced by ties. Roc Curve for AS, Aut./PDDNOS versus mixed subjects.

2. Method

2.1. Participants. The study was conducted at the University of Michigan Child Psychiatry Clinic in Ann Arbor, USA. The sample consisted of forty-two participants with autism spectrum disorders (age range 6–13 years, mean 9.78 years, SD 2.5, one female). Of these, 15 had Asperger syndrome (AS), 5 had autistic disorder (autism), and 22 had PDDNOS based on the DSM IV-TR criteria [5]. Because of the low numbers of patients with autism and because one purpose was to determine if the scale can identify patients with Asperger syndrome, the autism/PDDNOS groups were merged into a single category. Eighteen participants with other psychiatric disorders (mixed group, age range 6–17 years, mean 11.7 years, SD 3.8, 6 females) formed the comparison group. Comorbid psychiatric disorders in the autistic group were ADHD only ($n = 19$), Mood/Anxiety Disorder only (4), ADHD plus Mood/Anxiety Disorder (5), and Specific Language Impairment (SLI) (1). Eight subjects did not have any comorbid disorder. Psychiatric disorders in the mixed group consisted of ADHD only ($n = 7$), ADHD/Conduct Disorder ($n = 2$), Mood/Anxiety Disorder only ($n = 5$), ADHD plus Mood/Anxiety Disorder ($n = 3$), and SLI plus ADHD ($n = 2$). In all, 9 patients had more than one diagnosis. Since the focus of the study was on high-functioning individuals, participants with a full scale IQ below 70 were excluded. In the absence of an IQ, the level of functioning was estimated on clinical grounds.

2.2. Materials. For the diagnosis of ASD, each subject was administered an assessment battery consisting of a brief neuropsychological examination; a speech and language assessment; and a detailed psychiatric interview. In addition, caregivers completed the Child Behavior Checklist [10]; the Conner's Parent Rating Scale-Revised Long Form [11]; the Autism Behavior Checklist [12]; and the Social and Communication Questionnaire [13]. All available records were also examined. The Michigan Autism Spectrum Questionnaire (MASQ) was designed on the basis of the clinical characteristics of high-functioning autism and Asperger syndrome described in the literature. The purpose was to construct a scale that would be brief and easy to administer and incorporate questions targeting behaviors suggestive of Asperger syndrome. The aim was to focus on two main areas: quality of social interactions and form/content of communication. For example, questions 2 to 5 were intended to capture the pedantic style of communication said to be typical of this condition [14]. Question 8 attempted to describe the "active but odd" style of social interaction said to be common in Asperger syndrome as opposed to the "aloof and passive" manner typical of high-functioning autism [15]. Question 9 reflected the clinical impression that persons with AS tend to speak fluently by three years of age and sometimes even earlier, while question 10 referred to the fact that in many cases, features of AS become more apparent as the child grows older, usually by 7-8 years of age. Each question had four responses ranging from 0 to 4, yielding a total score of 30. Approval to perform the study was obtained from the Institutional Review Board (IRB).

Data Analysis. Data were analyzed to answer two questions. First, can the MASQ differentiate between autism spectrum disorders and other psychiatric disorders? Second, can the MASQ differentiate between Asperger syndrome and other autistic spectrum disorders?

To determine if the MASQ can differentiate between ASD and other psychiatric disorders, a binary logistic model on the total MASQ score was used. This model was found to be significant (Likelihood Ratio Chi-square test with 1 df = 16.019, $P < 0.0001$; the Nagelkerke R-square was 0.332, and the Area Under Curve was 0.821). A discriminant analysis showed that the total score correctly classified 73.3% of the entire group, 85.7% of the ASD group, and 44.4% of the mixed group as shown in Figure 1.

Table 1: MASQ scores of the three groups.

	Asperger syndrome	Autism/PDDNOS	Mixed group
Number	15	27	18
Male : female	15 : 0	26 : 1	12 : 6
Mean age (SD)	9.26 (2.5)	10.07 (2.5)	11.72 (3.8)
Mean MASQ (SD)	21.86 (4.3)	16.96 (4.5)	12.88 (3.9)

Table 2: Classification of the sample by the MASQ.

Observed	Predicted			
	AS	Aut/PD NOS	Mixed	Percent correct
AS	10	4	1	66.7%
Aut./PDDNOS	3	19	5	70.4%
Mixed	0	10	8	44.4%
Overall percentage	21.7%	55.0%	23.3%	61.7%

Overall, 61.7% of patients were correctly classified (66.7% of AS patients, 70.4% of Aut./PDD patients, and 44.4% of mixed patients).

To find out if the MASQ can differentiate between the various subtypes of ASD, the sample was divided into three groups: 15 with Asperger syndrome, 22 with autism/PDDNOS, and 18 with other psychiatric disorders. Using a multinomial logistic regression, the MASQ scores of the three groups were compared. The overall model was again found to be significant (Likelihood Ratio Chi-square with 2 df = 28.579, $P < 0.001$; Nagelkerke R-square was 0.430). Thus, the total score could distinguish between AS and autism/PDDNOS (Wald Chi-square = 8.116, 1 df, $P = 0.0004$) and also between AS and other psychiatric disorders (Wald Chi-square = 15.338, 1 df, $P < 0.0001$).

To ascertain the best cut-off points from the total score that could discriminate between the three groups, we used a linear discriminant analysis. The cut-off points were 22 or above for Asperger syndrome, 14 to 21 for autism/PDDNOS, and less than 14 for the mixed group. Using a discriminant function analysis, 66.7% of patients were correctly classified overall, and 66.7% were correctly classified in each diagnostic group. The leave-one-out cross-validation classification also correctly classified 66.7% of the patients as shown in Table 2.

3. Results

Participants with ASD scored higher than those with other psychiatric disorders as shown in Table 1. Within the ASD group, those with Asperger syndrome scored higher than those with autism and PDDNOS.

4. Discussion

These findings suggest that the MASQ can screen patients with high-functioning autism spectrum disorders from other psychiatric conditions and to identify patients with possible Asperger syndrome. In this clinic sample, patients with ASD scored higher than those with other psychiatric disorders, and, within the ASD group, those with Asperger syndrome scored the highest. Thus, the highest total scores (>22) predicted Asperger syndrome, the intermediate scores (14 through 21) predicted autism/PDDNOS, and the lowest scores (<14) predicted other psychiatric disorders. Thirteen out of 15 participants (86.7%) with Asperger syndrome scored 20 or higher. On the other hand, the autism/PDDNOS group had a wider range of scores, with 10/27 (26%) scoring 20 or higher and 6/27 (22%) scoring less than 14. One of the 18 participants in the mixed group (5.6%) scored 20, while 12/18 (66.7%) scored less than 14. The fact that 86% of the AS group scored higher than 20 while that autism/PDDNOS group had a much wider spread suggests that in this sample subjects with AS were more homogeneous than those with autism/PDDNOS. This also suggests that within the group of high-functioning autistic spectrum disorders, a subgroup of individuals may be identified based on the *quality* of social interaction and the *style* of communication rather than on the presence/absence of language delay, which is dependent on parental recall. If the central feature of Asperger syndrome is the history of language delay, it cannot be reliably differentiated from high-functioning autism. If, however, the disorder is conceptualized primarily on the *quality* of social deficits, the presence of a *distinct manner of communication*, and the occurrence of focused excessive interests, it may be possible to diagnose a distinct group of affected individuals. As opposed to most rating scales of Asperger syndrome, which rest on the premise that it is a mild form of high-functioning autism, this scale attempts to incorporate the clinical variables of AS that may define its qualitative differences from other types of autism spectrum disorders. While rating scales and structured interviews are not diagnostic on their own and only serve to collect data in a systematic and comprehensive manner, these results suggest that within the ASD spectrum, the scores may index different subtypes. However, before generalizing the findings of the study, it is important to discuss some of its limitations. First, the sample consisted of a relatively small number of participants, mostly males, underscoring the need to replicate the findings in a large group, with adequate numbers of patients with autism, Asperger syndrome, and PDDNOS. Also, the average age of the ASD group was about 10 years. As the symptoms of those with Asperger syndrome and higher functioning autism tend to become more apparent with age, the scale may prove to be equally useful in older adolescents and young adults. Second, as the sample was drawn from an outpatient psychiatric clinic, it will be important to replicate the findings in community samples.

In summary, this pilot study describes the use of a brief rating scale to distinguish between high-functioning autism spectrum disorders (autism and Asperger syndrome) and other psychiatric disorders. The highest total scores (>22) predicted Asperger syndrome while the intermediate scores (14 through 21) predicted autism/PDDNOS. In a psychiatric clinic setting, the MASQ can be used as a simple screening tool to identify children with suspected autism and Asperger syndrome. Future studies should examine its utility in both clinic and community samples.

Appendix

Michigan Autism Spectrum Questionnaire (MASQ)

Circle the Appropriate Answer for Each Question.

(1) Is he/she able to have a back and forth conversation with you?

Not at all	Just a little	Pretty much	Very much
0	1	2	3

(2) Does he/she have special interests or hobbies that seem to be excessive compared to those of other people of the same age? (Examples: interest in astronomy; roads and bridges; Japanese culture, etc.)

Not at all	Just a little	Pretty much	Very much
0	1	2	3

(3) Does he/she have a tendency to talk excessively on certain topics? (Examples: speaks like a "Little Professor," pays no attention to the needs of the listener; appears to go on talking even when not necessary, etc.)

Not at all	Just a little	Pretty much	Very much
0	1	2	3

(4) Does he/she offer excessive details about certain topics while speaking? (Examples: gives precise information about animals beginning with the Letter B; offers details about the classification of dinosaurs, etc.)

Not at all	Just a little	Pretty much	Very much
0	1	2	3

(5) Does he/she have an odd manner of speaking? (Examples: uses uncommon or high-flown words; speaks in a formal manner; has an odd intonation, etc.)

Not at all	Just a little	Pretty much	Very much
0	1	2	3

(6) Does he/she make an attempt to interact with others in an inappropriate manner? (Examples: on meeting a person, asks intrusive details about his/her marriage or salary; keeps staring at a stranger just to be "friendly with," appears over formal and stilted when not expected to do so, etc.)

Not at all	Just a little	Pretty much	Very much
0	1	2	3

(7) Does he/she appear intelligent yet, lacking in common sense?

Not at all	Just a little	Pretty much	Very much
0	1	2	3

(8) Does he/she appear to be physically clumsy? (Examples: bumps into objects; breaks things without realizing it, etc.)

Not at all	Just a little	Pretty much	Very much
0	1	2	3

(9) Did he/she speak at the normal age when growing up? (Example: by 3-4 years of age was able to speak in simple three word sentences, such as, "Give me milk")

Not at all	Just a little	Pretty much	Very much
0	1	2	3

(10) When did you first suspect that something was different or unusual with your child's behavior?

Before 3 years of age	Between 3 and 4 years	Between 4 and 5 years	After 5 years of age
0	1	2	3

Total Score. . . .

References

[1] L. Kanner, "Autistic disturbances of affective contact," *Nervous Child*, vol. 2, pp. 217–250, 1943.

[2] American Psychiatric Association, *Diagnostic and Statistical Manual of Mental Disorders*, Washington, DC, USA, 3rd edition, 1980.

[3] American Psychiatric Association, *Diagnostic and Statistical Manual of Mental Disorders*, revised, Washington, DC, USA, 3rd edition, 1987.

[4] H. Asperger, "Die "Autistischen Psychopathen" im Kindesalter," *Archiv für Psychiatrie und Nervenkrankheiten*, vol. 117, no. 1, pp. 76–136, 1944.

[5] American Psychiatric Association, *Diagnostic and Statistical Manual of Mental Disorders*, text revision, Washington, DC, USA, 4th edition, 2000.

[6] American Psychiatric Association, *Diagnostic and Statistical Manual of Mental Disorders*, Washington, DC, USA, 5th edition, 2013.

[7] M. Ghaziuddin, "Asperger disorder in the DSM-V: sacrificing utility for validity," *Journal of the American Academy of Child and Adolescent Psychiatry*, vol. 50, no. 2, pp. 192–193, 2011.

[8] M. R. Woodbury-Smith and F. R. Volkmar, "Asperger syndrome," *European Child and Adolescent Psychiatry*, vol. 18, no. 1, pp. 2–11, 2009.

[9] L. Bartak and M. Rutter, "Differences between mentally retarded and normally intelligent autistic children," *Journal of Autism and Childhood Schizophrenia*, vol. 6, no. 2, pp. 109–120, 1976.

[10] T. M. Achenbach, *Integrative Guide for the 1991 CBCL 4–18, YSR and TRF Profiles*, University of Vermont, Department of Psychiatry, Burlington, Vt, USA, 1991.

[11] K. C. Conners, *Conner's Rating Scales-Revised (CRS-R)*, Pearson Education, 2009.

[12] D. A. Krug, J. Arick, and P. Almond, "Behavior checklist for identifying severely handicapped individuals with high levels of autistic behavior," *Journal of Child Psychology and Psychiatry and Allied Disciplines*, vol. 21, no. 3, pp. 221–229, 1980.

[13] M. Rutter, A. Bailey, S. K. Berument, C. Lord, and A. Pickles, *Social Communication Questionnaire (SCQ) Lifetime Version*, Western Psychological Services, Los Angeles, Calif, USA, 2003.

[14] M. Ghaziuddin and L. Gerstein, "Pedantic speaking style differentiates Asperger syndrome from high-functioning autism," *Journal of Autism and Developmental Disorders*, vol. 26, no. 6, pp. 585–595, 1996.

[15] M. Ghaziuddin, "Defining the behavioral phenotype of Asperger syndrome," *Journal of Autism and Developmental Disorders*, vol. 38, no. 1, pp. 138–142, 2008.

8

Tsc2 Haploinsufficiency Has Limited Effects on Fetal Brain Cytokine Levels during Gestational Immune Activation

Dan Ehninger

German Center for Neurodegenerative Diseases (DZNE), Ludwig-Erhard-Allee 2, 53175 Bonn, Germany

Correspondence should be addressed to Dan Ehninger; dan.ehninger@dzne.de

Academic Editor: Geraldine Dawson

Dysregulated TSC/mTOR signaling may play a pathogenetic role in forms of syndromic autism, such as autism associated with tuberous sclerosis, a genetic disorder caused by heterozygous *TSC1* or *TSC2* mutations. Environmental risk factors, such as gestational viral infections, may, in some cases, also contribute to the pathogenesis of autism and related neuropsychiatric disorders. We have recently found that a heterozygous *Tsc2* mutation and the poly I:C model of maternal immune activation (MIA) interactively perturb fetal development and adult social behavior in mice, suggesting that these factors converge on shared pathways. TSC/mTOR signaling plays an important role in the modulation of immune responses, raising the possibility that the damage caused by MIA was greater in $Tsc2^{+/-}$ than in wildtype fetuses because of an exacerbated immune response in the mutants. Here, cytokine antibody arrays were employed to measure relative cytokine abundances in the fetal brain and the placenta during MIA. Cytokines were induced by gestational poly I:C but there was no obvious modulatory effect of *Tsc2* haploinsufficiency. The data indicate that cytokine exposure during MIA is comparable in *Tsc2* haploinsufficient and wildtype control fetuses, suggesting that downstream molecular and cellular processes may account for the interactive effects of *Tsc2* haploinsufficiency and MIA.

1. Introduction

Dysregulated mTOR signaling and altered protein synthesis are emerging as common themes in the biology of autism [1–3]. In brief, heterozygous mutations in the *TSC1* or *TSC2* gene cause tuberous sclerosis, a multisystem disorder, which is associated with autism in 20–60% of cases [4–6]. Additionally, mutations in the genes encoding for the upstream regulators PTEN and NF1, as well as in the downstream effector eIF4E, have been linked to autism [7–9]. Moreover, fragile X syndrome, another single gene disorder, in which the regulation of mRNA translation is perturbed [1], is associated with autism [11]. These data collectively highlight the mTOR pathway and protein synthesis as one important theme in the pathogenesis of autism-related disorders.

In addition to genetic factors, environmental risk factors may also contribute to the pathogenesis of autism spectrum disorders. At least some prenatal viral infections elevate the risk for neuropsychiatric disorders (such as autism spectrum disorders and schizophrenia) in the offspring [10, 12–16]. Moreover, there is a growing literature suggesting the presence of inflammatory or immunological changes in the brains of at least a subset of individuals affected by autism [17–21], suggesting that immune activation/inflammatory processes may play a role (primary and/or secondary) in the pathogenesis of some cases of autism.

Prenatal viral infections have been modeled in mice by injection of poly I:C [19], a synthetic double-stranded RNA that elicits an immune response via activation of toll-like receptor 3. Gestational poly I:C injections in mice and rats elicit behavioral, neurochemical, and structural abnormalities in the developing offspring [19, 22, 23], which is consistent with the notion that maternal immune activation during gestational periods can alter proper neurodevelopment and, hence, results in behavioral consequences in the offspring generation.

Heterozygous *Tsc2* mutations and the poly I:C paradigm of maternal immune activation (MIA) showed significant interactive effects in mice, indicating a cooperative influence on gestational survival and postnatal behavioral traits [24]: fewer $Tsc2^{+/-}$ pups than wildtype (WT) pups were born to poly I:C injected dams, while the number of $Tsc2^{+/-}$

pups and WT pups born to vehicle-injected mothers did not differ. Moreover, grown-up mice exposed to both gestational poly I:C and *Tsc2* haploinsufficiency showed deficient social exploratory behavior, while this was not the case in the animals exposed to one of these factors alone.

Gestational immune activation may disrupt normal brain development at least in part because of crosstalk between cytokines and the developing CNS [19, 22, 25–27]. TSC/mTOR signaling regulates immunological and inflammatory processes [28, 29] and, accordingly, it is possible that an exacerbated immune response in the *Tsc*2 mutant fetus accounts for the more severe consequences of gestational poly I:C in the $Tsc2^{+/-}$ background. To address this possibility, $Tsc2^{+/-}$ fetuses and WT control fetuses were gestationally exposed to poly I:C or saline and cytokine responses were measured in the placenta, as well as the fetal $Tsc2^{+/-}$ and WT control brain.

2. Materials and Methods

2.1. Mice. Mice were generated as previously described [24]. In brief, in order to generate $Tsc2^{+/-}$ and WT offspring gestationally exposed to either poly I:C or saline, $Tsc2^{+/-}$ male breeders (on a C57BL6/Ncrl genetic background) were mated with C57BL6/J wildtype females. After overnight mating, female breeders with a vaginal plug were designated as E0, single-housed, and left undisturbed, except for weekly cage change. At E12.5, pregnant females received a single intraperitoneal injection of 20 mg/kg poly I:C (Sigma) or vehicle (see below). Poly I:C is supplied as potassium salt and poly I:C constitutes 10% of the total weight of the salt. The dosage was based on the actual weight of poly I:C itself. Poly I:C was dissolved in 0.9% sterile saline and a volume of 10 μL/g was injected. Local and federal regulations regarding animal welfare were followed.

2.2. Tissue Extraction. Two hours or 6.5 hours after poly I:C, pregnant females were anaesthetized with isoflurane and were decapitated. The uterus was extracted and briefly washed in ice-cold phosphate-buffered saline. Subsequently, fetal brains and placentas were isolated in fresh ice-cold phosphate-buffered saline under a dissection microscope. Tissue was flash frozen and stored at −80°C until processed for cytokine antibody arrays.

2.3. Cytokine Antibody Arrays. Cytokine antibody arrays (RayBio Mouse Cytokine Antibody Array 3 and RayBio Mouse Cytokine Antibody Array 2) were used according to the manufacturer's instructions. In brief, tissue was lysed in the cell lysis buffer provided after addition of proteinase inhibitors (Sigma, P8340), homogenized, and centrifuged at 5000 g for 10 min (4°C) and the supernatant was isolated. Protein concentrations were established with BCA assays. Next, the volume containing 125 μg protein was taken from each sample and pooled by group (WT/saline, WT/poly I:C, $Tsc2^{+/-}$/saline, and $Tsc2^{+/-}$/poly I:C; materials of 4 animals from 4 different litters were pooled per group for each experiment; at the 6.5 h time point, only fetal brain from the following groups was analyzed: WT/saline, WT/poly I:C, and $Tsc2^{+/-}$/poly I:C). Pooled lysates were then diluted at least 10-fold in 1x blocking buffer to a total volume of 2.5 mL. After a blocking step, array membranes were incubated in pooled lysates at 4°C overnight. Next, membranes were washed 3 times in 2 mL wash buffer I for 5 min each followed by washing steps in wash buffer II (2 × 5 min; room temperature). Array membranes were then incubated in biotin-conjugated antibody solutions for 2 h at room temperature followed by washing steps in wash buffer I (3 × 5 min) and II (2 × 5 min). Next, membranes were incubated in HRP-conjugated streptavidin (1 : 1000) at room temperature for 2 h. After washing (wash buffer I, 3 × 5 min; wash buffer II, 2 × 5 min), array membranes were incubated in ECL-plus and imaged on a Typhoon 9400 scanner. Image analyses were performed in ImageQuant 5.2. Array membranes contained a total of 62 or 32 different cytokine antibody probes (RayBio Mouse Cytokine Antibody Array 3 and RayBio Mouse Cytokine Antibody Array 2, resp.), in addition to positive controls and negative controls. Fluorescent intensities were measured for cytokine probes and positive and negative controls. After subtraction of background, data for cytokine probes were normalized to the average fluorescence intensity of the positive controls. All data are expressed as percentage of the corresponding value of the WT/saline group and are based on duplicate measurements for each cytokine probe (shown as mean +/− SEM).

2.4. Statistics. In order to compare relative cytokine abundances across genotypes and treatment groups, multifactorial ANOVAs were performed (with genotype and/or treatment as between-subjects factor and/or cytokine as within-subjects factor) as described in the main text.

3. Results

To evaluate if fetal *Tsc2* haploinsufficiency modifies gestational cytokine responses during a maternal immune activation paradigm [22], pregnant C57BL6/J female mice were subjected to a single poly I:C injection (20 mg/kg, i.p.) or saline control at E12.5. Fetal brains and placental tissue were extracted 2 h or 6.5 h after the injection and the relative cytokine abundance in these tissues was assessed using cytokine antibody arrays.

In placental tissue (6.5 h after poly I:C), poly I:C caused a robust increase of several cytokines, including the proinflammatory cytokine IL-6 (Figure 1). An overall comparison of cytokine profiles by three-way ANOVA with genotype and treatment as between-subjects factors and cytokine as within-subjects factor yielded a significant main effect of poly I:C treatment ($P = 0.0003$). Additional analyses on the level of individual cytokines (using two-way ANOVAs with genotype and treatment as between-subjects factors) showed clear increases of G-CSF, IL-6, IL12 p40/p70, KC, MCP-1, MIP-2, and RANTES in the placental samples of poly I:C treated animals (Figure 1). Poly I:C-induced placental cytokine levels were similar in $Tsc2^{+/-}$ and WT samples (Figure 1).

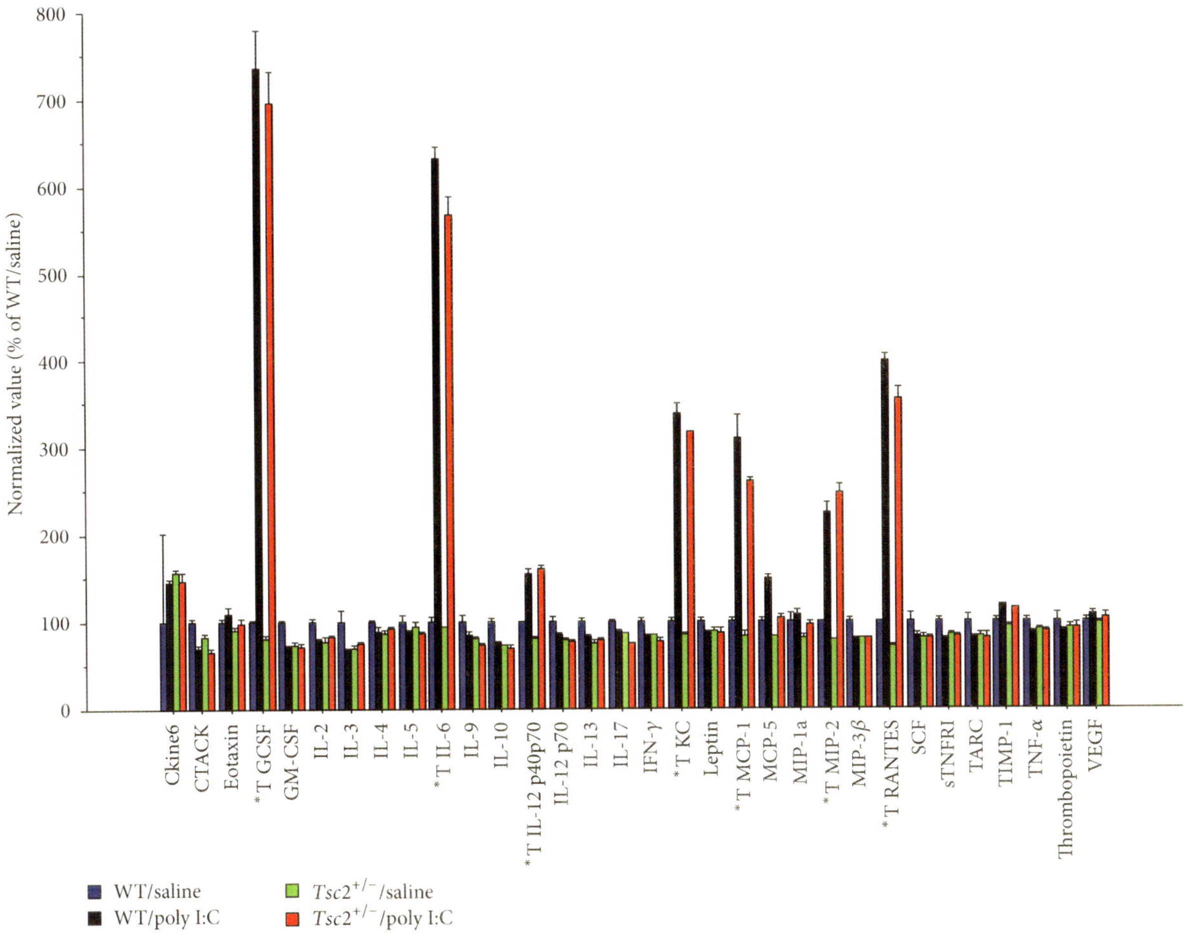

FIGURE 1: The graph shows relative cytokine abundances in placental tissue lysates at 6.5 h after poly I:C injection as measured by cytokine antibody array. *T denotes individual cytokines with main effect of treatment at $P < 0.01$ and a fold change > 1.5. Plotted are means +/− SEM.

Poly I:C effects on cytokines in fetal whole brain extracts were more moderate than those seen in the placenta: At 2 h after poly I:C, the levels of several cytokines appeared to be decreased in the treated group compared to saline controls (Figures 2(a) and 2(b)). An overall comparison of cytokine profiles (by three-way ANOVA with genotype and treatment as between-subjects factors and cytokine as within-subjects factor) showed a nonsignificant trend towards an effect of poly I:C ($P = 0.09$), while there was no effect of genotype ($P = 0.34$) and no genotype x treatment interaction ($P = 0.95$). Exploratory statistical analyses focusing on individual cytokines (using two-way ANOVAs with genotype and treatment as between-subjects factors) revealed a number of molecules with significantly altered abundances in the poly I:C groups (Figures 2(a) and 2(b)), such as Fas ligand, fractalkine, IL-3, IL-4, IL-5, lymphotactin, MCP-5, M-CSF, MIG, MIP-1alpha, TARC, TECK, TNF-alpha, and VCAM-1. These analyses, however, showed few effects of *Tsc2* haploinsufficiency on fetal cytokine levels (Figures 2(a) and 2(b)).

At 6.5 h after poly I:C, cytokines appeared to be, overall, modestly elevated in poly I:C fetal brains relative to controls, although this finding did not reach statistical significance (Figures 3(a) and 3(b); two-way ANOVA, WT/saline versus poly I:C, treatment as between-subjects factor and cytokine as within-subjects factor: effect of treatment, $P = 0.09$). *Tsc2* haploinsufficiency did not seem to modulate the cytokine response induced by gestational poly I:C in any obvious way (Figures 3(a) and 3(b); two-way ANOVA, WT/poly I:C versus $Tsc2^{+/-}$/poly I:C, genotype as between-subjects factor and cytokine as within-subjects factor: effect of genotype, $P = 0.89$; measure x genotype interaction, $P = 0.34$).

Taken together, these provisional data indicate that alterations in fetal brain cytokine abundance during MIA are less pronounced than placental changes and they suggest that cytokine responses during MIA are not substantially influenced by a heterozygous *Tsc2* mutation.

4. Discussion

In a previous study, we have found an interactive influence of *Tsc2* haploinsufficiency and gestational poly I:C on fetal development and adult behavioral traits in mice [24]: fewer $Tsc2^{+/-}$ than WT pups were born to poly I:C-injected

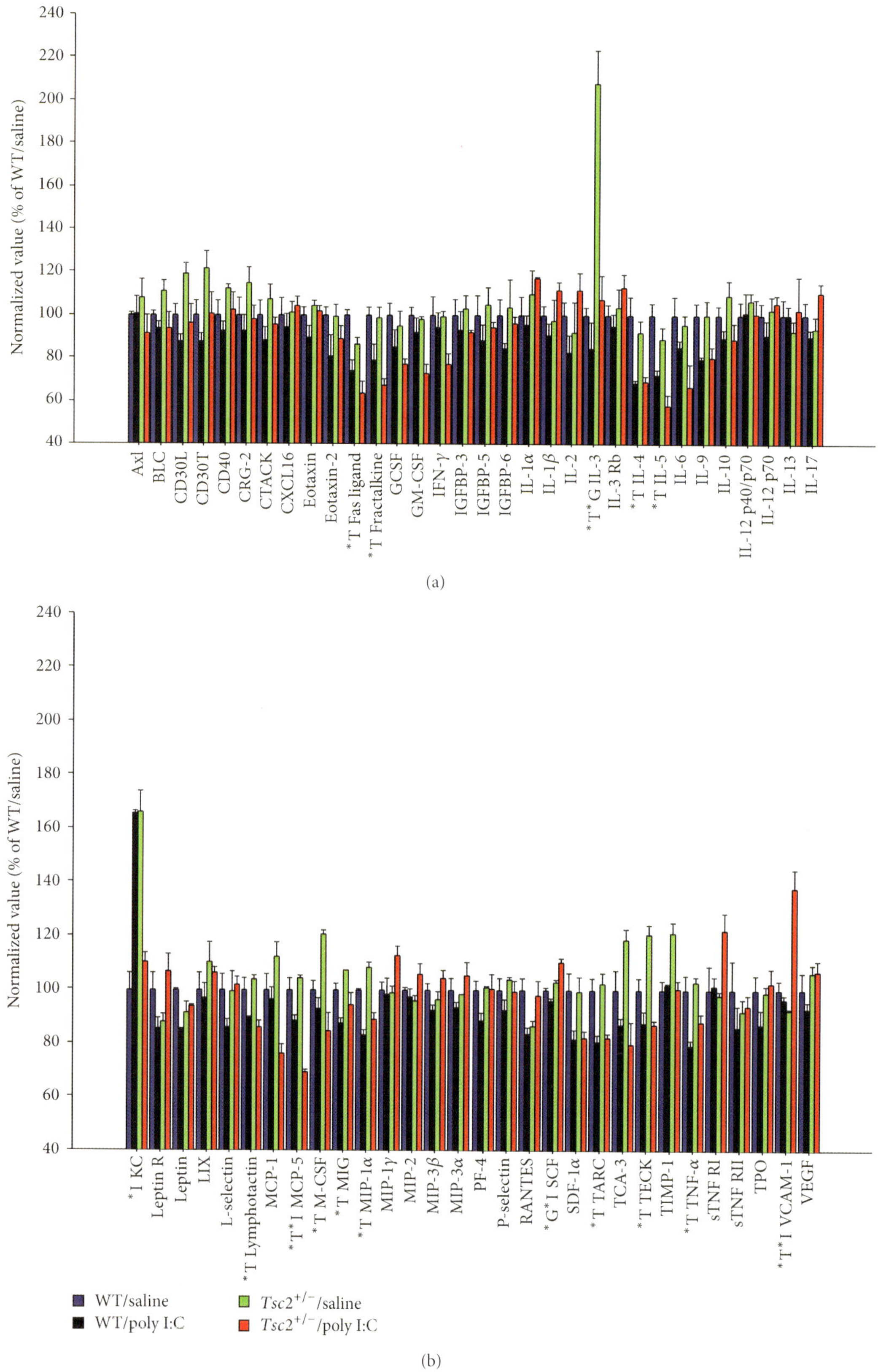

FIGURE 2: (a) and (b) The figure shows relative cytokine abundances as measured by cytokine antibody arrays in fetal brain at 2 h after gestational poly I:C. Individual cytokines with a main effect of treatment (*T; $P < 0.01$), genotype (*G; $P < 0.01$), or a genotype x treatment interaction (*I; $P < 0.01$) are highlighted. Shown are means +/− SEM.

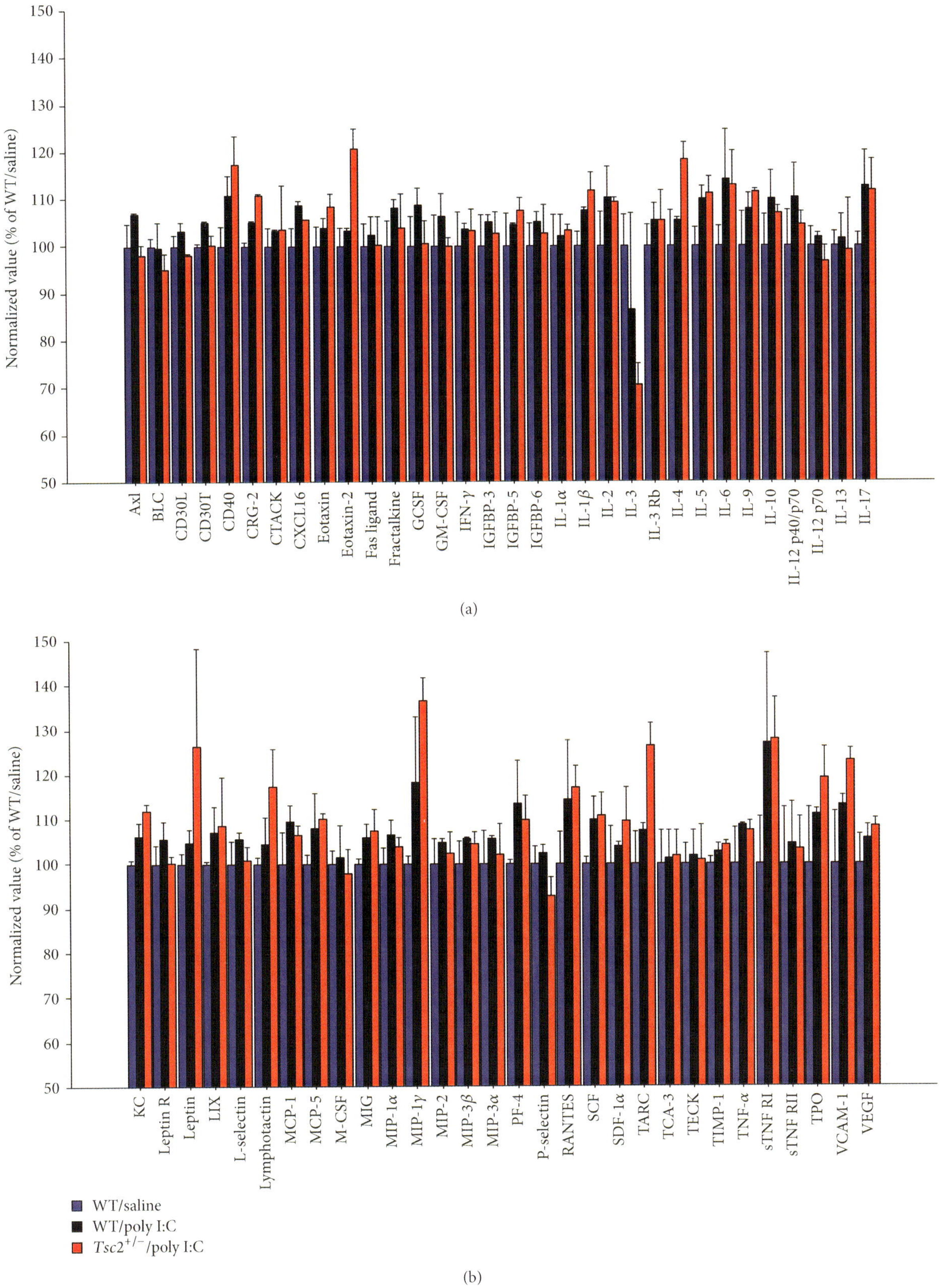

Figure 3: (a) and (b) This graph shows relative cytokine abundances as measured by cytokine antibody arrays in fetal brain at 6.5 h after gestational poly I:C. Shown are means +/− SEM.

mothers, while the genotype ratio was balanced in vehicle-treated mothers, which suggested, together with the presence of fetal resorption, that gestational poly I:C triggered the preferential elimination of $Tsc2^{+/-}$ fetuses *in utero*. Surviving poly I:C-exposed $Tsc2^{+/-}$ animals, but not $Tsc2^{+/-}$/saline and WT/poly I:C mice, showed abnormal social approach behavior when tested in adulthood [24]. Collectively, these data indicated that poly I:C-related gestational immune activation and *Tsc2* haploinsufficiency interact to perturb fetal development.

Gestational immune activation may, at least to some extent, interfere with normal fetal development because of adverse effects of cytokines on the developing organism [19, 22, 25–27]. TSC-related cell signaling regulates immunological and inflammatory processes [28, 29] and, therefore, it is conceivable that an exacerbated immune response in the $Tsc2^{+/-}$ fetal brain to gestational poly I:C contributes to the interactive effects of *Tsc2* haploinsufficiency and maternal immune activation.

The present analysis of poly I:C-triggered cytokine responses suggests that $Tsc2^{+/-}$ and WT fetal brains are exposed to qualitatively and quantitatively similar cytokine responses upon midgestational poly I:C administration. Cytokine antibody arrays revealed a pronounced increase in the abundance of specific cytokines in the placenta at 6.5 h after poly I:C, representing evidence for the mounted maternal immune activation triggered by poly I:C. Poly I:C caused a complex alteration in cytokine levels in the fetal brain that comprised an initial phase of decreased cytokine abundance (at 2 h after poly I:C) and a subsequent phase of modestly elevated tissue cytokine levels (at 6.5 h after poly I:C), which is consistent with prior data that show that the fetal brain cytokine response during maternal immune activation is a complex function of various parameters, such as time after poly I:C injection and gestational age [30]. Cytokine levels were similar in fetal $Tsc2^{+/-}$ and WT brains, suggesting that genotype-dependent differences in cytokine exposure are unlikely to account for the interactive effects of *Tsc2* haploinsufficiency and gestational immune activation [24].

As TSC/mTOR signaling not only regulates immune responses, but also is a downstream signaling mediator of many cytokines and other factors induced by poly I:C, it remains to be explored if altered TSC-related cell signaling downstream of cytokines/other poly I:C-induced factors contributes to the genotype-dependent effects of poly I:C [24]. In addition, it is also possible that the disruptive effects of *Tsc2* haploinsufficiency and gestational immune activation converge on certain developmental processes ongoing at the time of poly I:C injection (E12.5). For instance, both gestational poly I:C and TSC gene mutations interfere with and disrupt neurogenesis, neuroblast migration, and proper cortical layering [31–33], which are important features of the developing CNS at E12.5. Accordingly, gestational immune activation and *Tsc2* haploinsufficiency may display synergistic effects on these processes and interactively lead to the phenotypic precipitation of otherwise subthreshold neurobiological changes.

5. Conclusion

The present study revealed a similar cytokine induction profile in *Tsc2* mutant and WT control brains in the context of a midgestational immune activation paradigm. These findings indicate that an exacerbated cytokine response in *Tsc2* mutants is unlikely to account for the interactive effects of *Tsc2* haploinsufficiency and maternal immune activation identified in a previous study [24]. Future experiments will address if *Tsc2* haploinsufficiency and gestational immune activation may possibly interact by converging on cytokine-induced cell signaling and/or by jointly disrupting midgestational neurodevelopmental processes, such as neurogenesis and/or cell migration.

References

[1] B. D. Auerbach, E. K. Osterweil, and M. F. Bear, "Mutations causing syndromic autism define an axis of synaptic pathophysiology," *Nature*, vol. 480, no. 7375, pp. 63–68, 2011.

[2] D. Ehninger and A. J. Silva, "Rapamycin for treating Tuberous sclerosis and Autism spectrum disorders," *Trends in Molecular Medicine*, vol. 17, no. 2, pp. 78–87, 2011.

[3] R. J. Kelleher III and M. F. Bear, "The autistic neuron: troubled translation?" *Cell*, vol. 135, no. 3, pp. 401–406, 2008.

[4] E. Fombonne, "Epidemiological surveys of autism and other pervasive developmental disorders: an update," *Journal of Autism and Developmental Disorders*, vol. 33, no. 4, pp. 365–382, 2003.

[5] S. L. Smalley, "Autism and tuberous sclerosis," *Journal of Autism and Developmental Disorders*, vol. 28, no. 5, pp. 407–414, 1998.

[6] S. L. Smalley, P. E. Tanguay, M. Smith, and G. Gutierrez, "Autism and tuberous sclerosis," *Journal of Autism and Developmental Disorders*, vol. 22, no. 3, pp. 339–355, 1992.

[7] M. G. Butler, M. J. Dazouki, X. Zhou et al., "Subset of individuals with autism spectrum disorders and extreme macrocephaly associated with germline PTEN tumour suppressor gene mutations," *Journal of Medical Genetics*, vol. 42, no. 4, pp. 318–321, 2005.

[8] M. Neves-Pereira, B. Müller, D. Massie et al., "Deregulation of EIF4E: a novel mechanism for autism," *Journal of Medical Genetics*, vol. 46, no. 11, pp. 759–765, 2009.

[9] P. G. Williams and J. H. Hersh, "Brief report: the association of neurofibromatosis type 1 and autism," *Journal of Autism and Developmental Disorders*, vol. 28, no. 6, pp. 567–571, 1998.

[10] H. Ó. Atladóttir, P. Thorsen, L. Østergaard et al., "Maternal infection requiring hospitalization during pregnancy and autism spectrum disorders," *Journal of Autism and Developmental Disorders*, vol. 40, no. 12, pp. 1423–1430, 2010.

[11] R. J. Hagerman, A. W. Jackson III, A. Levitas, B. Rimland, and M. Braden, "An analysis of autism in fifty males with the fragile X syndrome," *American Journal of Medical Genetics*, vol. 23, no. 1-2, pp. 359–374, 1986.

[12] S. Chess, "Autism in children with congenital rubella," *Journal of Autism and Childhood Schizophrenia*, vol. 1, no. 1, pp. 33–47, 1971.

[13] S. Chess, "Follow up report on autism in congenital rubella," *Journal of Autism and Childhood Schizophrenia*, vol. 7, no. 1, pp. 69–81, 1977.

[14] S. Chess, P. Fernandez, and S. Korn, "Behavioral consequences of congenital rubella," *Journal of Pediatrics*, vol. 93, no. 4, pp. 699–703, 1978.

[15] T. L. Sweeten, D. J. Posey, and C. J. McDougle, "Brief report: autistic disorder in three children with cytomegalovirus infection," *Journal of Autism and Developmental Disorders*, vol. 34, no. 5, pp. 583–586, 2004.

[16] Y. Yamashita, C. Fujimoto, E. Nakajima, T. Isagai, and T. Matsuishi, "Possible association between congenital cytomegalovirus infection and autistic disorder," *Journal of Autism and Developmental Disorders*, vol. 33, no. 4, pp. 455–459, 2003.

[17] K. Garbett, P. J. Ebert, A. Mitchell et al., "Immune transcriptome alterations in the temporal cortex of subjects with autism," *Neurobiology of Disease*, vol. 30, no. 3, pp. 303–311, 2008.

[18] J. T. Morgan, G. Chana, C. A. Pardo et al., "Microglial activation and increased microglial density observed in the dorsolateral prefrontal cortex in autism," *Biological Psychiatry*, vol. 68, no. 4, pp. 368–376, 2010.

[19] P. H. Patterson, "Immune involvement in Schizophrenia and Autism: etiology, pathology and animal models," *Behavioural Brain Research*, vol. 204, no. 2, pp. 313–321, 2009.

[20] D. L. Vargas, C. Nascimbene, C. Krishnan, A. W. Zimmerman, and C. A. Pardo, "Neuroglial activation and neuroinflammation in the brain of patients with autism," *Annals of Neurology*, vol. 57, no. 1, pp. 67–81, 2005.

[21] I. Voineagu, X. Wang, P. Johnston et al., "Transcriptomic analysis of autistic brain reveals convergent molecular pathology," *Nature*, vol. 474, no. 7351, pp. 380–384, 2011.

[22] S. E. P. Smith, J. Li, K. Garbett, K. Mirnics, and P. H. Patterson, "Maternal immune activation alters fetal brain development through interleukin-6," *Journal of Neuroscience*, vol. 27, no. 40, pp. 10695–10702, 2007.

[23] L. Zuckerman and I. Weiner, "Post-pubertal emergence of disrupted latent inhibition following prenatal immune activation," *Psychopharmacology*, vol. 169, no. 3-4, pp. 308–313, 2003.

[24] D. Ehninger, Y. Sano, P. J. De Vries et al., "Gestational immune activation and Tsc2 haploinsufficiency cooperate to disrupt fetal survival and may perturb social behavior in adult mice," *Molecular Psychiatry*, vol. 17, no. 1, pp. 62–70, 2012.

[25] B. E. Deverman and P. H. Patterson, "Cytokines and CNS development," *Neuron*, vol. 64, no. 1, pp. 61–78, 2009.

[26] H. Nawa, M. Takahashi, and P. H. Patterson, "Cytokine and growth factor involvement in schizophrenia—support for the developmental model," *Molecular Psychiatry*, vol. 5, no. 6, pp. 594–603, 2000.

[27] L. Shi, N. Tu, and P. H. Patterson, "Maternal influenza infection is likely to alter fetal brain development indirectly: the virus is not detected in the fetus," *International Journal of Developmental Neuroscience*, vol. 23, no. 2-3, pp. 299–305, 2005.

[28] W. Cao, S. Manicassamy, H. Tang et al., "Toll-like receptor-mediated induction of type I interferon in plasmacytoid dendritic cells requires the rapamycin-sensitive PI(3)K-mTOR-p70S6K pathway," *Nature Immunology*, vol. 9, no. 10, pp. 1157–1164, 2008.

[29] R. Colina, M. Costa-Mattioli, R. J. O. Dowling et al., "Translational control of the innate immune response through IRF-7," *Nature*, vol. 452, no. 7185, pp. 323–328, 2008.

[30] U. Meyer, M. Nyffeler, A. Engler et al., "The time of prenatal immune challenge determines the specificity of inflammation-mediated brain and behavioral pathology," *Journal of Neuroscience*, vol. 26, no. 18, pp. 4752–4762, 2006.

[31] J. de Miranda, K. Yaddanapudi, M. Hornig, G. Villar, R. Serge, and W. I. Lipkin, "Induction of toll-like receptor 3-mediated immunity during gestation inhibits cortical neurogenesis and causes behavioral disturbances," *mBio*, vol. 1, no. 4, Article ID e00176-10, 2010.

[32] L. Magri, M. Cominelli, M. Cambiaghi et al., "Timing of mTOR activation affects tuberous sclerosis complex neuropathology in mouse models," *Disease Models & Mechanisms*, vol. 6, pp. 1185–1197, 2013.

[33] H. Soumiya, H. Fukumitsu, and S. Furukawa, "Prenatal immune challenge compromises the normal course of neurogenesis during development of the mouse cerebral cortex," *Journal of Neuroscience Research*, vol. 89, no. 10, pp. 1575–1585, 2011.

9

The Effects of Rhythm and Robotic Interventions on the Imitation/Praxis, Interpersonal Synchrony, and Motor Performance of Children with Autism Spectrum Disorder (ASD)

Sudha M. Srinivasan,[1] Maninderjit Kaur,[1] Isabel K. Park,[2] Timothy D. Gifford,[3] Kerry L. Marsh,[3] and Anjana N. Bhat[1,2,3,4]

[1] *Department of Physical Therapy, Biomechanics and Movement Sciences, University of Delaware, Newark, DE 19713, USA*
[2] *Physical Therapy Program, Department of Kinesiology, University of Connecticut, Storrs, CT 06269, USA*
[3] *Center for Health, Intervention, and Prevention, Department of Psychology, University of Connecticut, Storrs, CT 06269, USA*
[4] *Behavioral Neuroscience Program, Department of Psychology, University of Delaware, Newark, DE 19713, USA*

Correspondence should be addressed to Anjana N. Bhat; abhat@udel.edu

Academic Editor: Klaus-Peter Ossenkopp

We assessed the effects of three interventions, rhythm, robotic, and standard-of-care, on the imitation/praxis, interpersonal synchrony, and overall motor performance of 36 children with Autism Spectrum Disorder (ASD) between 5 and 12 years of age. Children were matched on age, level of functioning, and services received, prior to random assignment to one of the three groups. Training was provided for 8 weeks with 4 sessions provided each week. We assessed generalized changes in motor skills from the pretest to the posttest using a standardized test of motor performance, the Bruininks-Oseretsky Test of Motor Proficiency, 2nd edition (BOT-2). We also assessed training-specific changes in imitation/praxis and interpersonal synchrony during an early and a late session. Consistent with the training activities practiced, the rhythm and robot groups improved on the body coordination composite of the BOT-2, whereas the comparison group improved on the fine manual control composite of the BOT-2. All three groups demonstrated improvements in imitation/praxis. The rhythm and robot groups also showed improved interpersonal synchrony performance from the early to the late session. Overall, socially embedded movement-based contexts are valuable in promoting imitation/praxis, interpersonal synchrony, and motor performance and should be included within the standard-of-care treatment for children with ASD.

1. Introduction

Children with Autism Spectrum Disorder (ASD) have persistent impairments in social communication skills including impaired initiation of social interactions, poor sharing of interests with social partners, impairments in verbal and nonverbal communication skills as well as repetitive and restricted interests including repetitive actions on objects, circumscribed interests, and stereotyped speech [1–4]. In addition, between 50 and 100% of individuals with ASD have motor difficulties including incoordination during gross and fine motor activities, poor balance skills, and clumsy gait patterns [5–10]. They also demonstrate impairments in motor imitation, praxis, and interpersonal synchrony [11–15]. Motor impairments in infancy and early childhood have implications for future social, cognitive, and communication development in autism [16]. For example, impairments in basic gross motor skills such as running, jumping, and hopping as well as poor interpersonal synchrony can limit children's play with peers and restrict their opportunities to build social connections and friendships [5, 16]. Similarly, poor manual motor skills such as pointing, requesting, and reaching have implications for nonverbal modes of communication such as use of gestures and engaging in joint attention bids [17]. Poor imitation and praxis skills will limit children's opportunities to learn and refine complex motor skills such as bicycling, playing soccer, and so forth through observation of others' actions [5, 9, 18–20]. Overall, there is substantial evidence supporting the far-reaching cascading effects of motor difficulties on the core impairments in autism. Not surprisingly, motor skills of children with ASD at age 2 were predictive of optimal outcomes at age 4 [21]. Given this unequivocal evidence on the impact of motor skills in ASD, there is a need for intensive research dedicated towards understanding and remediating the motor impairments in children with ASD.

Impairments in gross and fine motor performance as well as interpersonal synchrony are evident from an early age in individuals with ASD [14, 22–26]. In terms of gross motor performance, children have significant impairments in postural control [27–30], gait patterns [6, 31, 32], and bilateral coordination skills [14, 26]. Similarly, children with ASD have impaired fine motor skills involving object control and manual dexterity [33–36], visuomotor integration [9], and handwriting [37–39]. A recent meta-analysis based on 51 studies comparing children with ASD and typically developing (TD) controls demonstrated a large effect size of 1.2 for motor issues in gait, postural control, motor coordination, upper limb control, and motor planning in ASD [10]. Moreover, overall motor performance is associated with the severity of diagnostic symptoms [8, 40], level of adaptive functioning [41], and level of social withdrawal [29] in autism. Children with ASD also have difficulties in interpersonal synchrony [14]. Interpersonal synchrony involves coordinating one's actions with those of social partners and it requires appropriate social attention, imitation, and turn taking skills [13, 26, 42–47]. For example, during a rocking chair task that examined spontaneous interpersonal synchrony between the parent and their child, children with autism showed significantly less in-phase rocking coordination compared to TD children [14]. Overall, given the pervasive nature of motor impairments, it is critical that goals related to motor performance and interpersonal synchrony be brought to the forefront during planning and implementation of interventions for children with ASD.

Difficulties in imitation have been documented in toddlers and young children with ASD [11, 48, 49] and are thought to continue into adulthood [11, 12, 50, 51]. Poor imitation skills may be associated with the core social communication, affective, and cognitive impairments in ASD [52, 53]. Two different types of imitative actions have been described in the literature. Based on object use, there are transitive actions or actions on objects (e.g., hammering a nail) and intransitive actions or actions without objects (e.g., clapping hands). Based on purpose, there are meaningful actions (e.g., actions that convey communicative intent such as waving "bye") and nonmeaningful actions (e.g., noncommunicative actions such as placing hand on chest) [54, 55]. Young children with ASD had lower imitation scores compared to TD children and children with developmental delays, with greater difficulties in imitation of intransitive compared to transitive actions [49]. Similarly, children had greater impairments in imitation of meaningless versus meaningful actions and imitation impairments were associated with children's overall motor ability levels [56]. Deficits in imitation have also been hypothesized to be part of a more generalized impairment in praxis [57, 58]. Praxis is the ability to plan and execute a series of actions/gestures following imitation, on verbal command, and during tool use [57, 58]. High-functioning children with ASD had impairments in production of gestures on imitation, on verbal command, and during tool use compared to TD children, suggestive of a broader impairment in praxis [58]. Taken together, imitation and praxis impairments are associated with language and play skills as well as levels of symptom severity in children with ASD [40, 49, 59–61]. In spite of considerable evidence on motor impairments, there is little previous research supporting the use of movement-based interventions in ASD. However, recently, there has been growing emphasis on the need for early interventions with a focus on active play and enriched movement experiences to promote multisystem development in ASD [5, 18].

Contemporary interventions that target imitation skills include naturalistic and developmental clinician/caregiver-mediated interventions [62, 63], peer-mediated interventions [64, 65], and video-modeling interventions [66]. Naturalistic and developmental interventions aim to teach imitation within naturalistic, developmentally appropriate social interactions [62, 63]. A 10-week randomized controlled trial using clinician-delivered Reciprocal Imitation Training (RIT) techniques such as contingent imitation, linguistic mapping, modeling, prompting, and contingent natural reinforcement led to improvements in imitation skills in the treatment group but not in the control group that received treatment as usual [67]. In contrast, peer-mediated training involves adults prompting children with ASD to imitate the behaviors of their TD peers; such training led to improvements in imitation of actions on objects as well as generalization of learned skills to novel actions within novel environments [64]. Lastly, motivating approaches such as video modeling, where children with ASD are asked to watch a video clip of the target behavior and then imitate the modeled behavior, have led to better learning of skills such as toy play, brushing, and greeting compared to live modeling techniques [66]. Although several contemporary autism interventions target social imitation, there is currently a lack of evidence on interventions targeting gross/fine motor performance and interpersonal synchrony. In the current study, we explored the effects of two 8-week novel, movement-based rhythm and robotic interventions on the overall motor performance, imitation/praxis, and interpersonal synchrony skills of children with ASD.

Recently, novel intervention approaches such as rhythm and robotic therapies have been used to promote social communication skills in children with ASD [68–70]. Children with autism have a predisposition for musical stimuli, find musical experiences very enjoyable, and have intact musical perception in spite of significant impairments in language skills [68, 71, 72]. Therefore, rhythm-based contexts have been used to enhance verbal and nonverbal communication as well as behavioral skills in ASD [68, 69, 73, 74]. For example, a meta-analysis based on 10 studies and 165 individuals with

ASD showed improvements in primary core symptoms of autism including social interaction, verbal communication, initiation of behavior, and social-emotional reciprocity as well as secondary outcomes including social adaptation skills and quality of parent-child relationships [73]. Despite considerable evidence on positive effects of rhythmic interventions on core social communication symptoms, interestingly, few studies have used such contexts to facilitate motor skills in children with ASD [75, 76]. For example, a musical social routine focusing on reciprocal imitation between the child and the experimenter led to improved spontaneous word and action imitation in 3 out of 4 children with ASD, with carry-over effects observed in 2 children [75]. In contrast to the limited literature in autism, there is considerable evidence that rhythmic accompaniment using music can promote gross and fine motor skills in TD children [77–81]. A 10-week music and movement program in preschoolers led to greater improvements in locomotor skills assessed on the standardized, Test of Gross Motor Development (TGMD), compared to a control group that engaged in free play [79]. Overall, music-based contexts seem to be a promising tool to facilitate motor skills in children with ASD [74]. In the current study, we systematically examined the effects of a prolonged rhythm intervention on the motor skills of children with ASD using a randomized controlled trial (RCT) design.

Robotic interactions are highly motivating environments for children with ASD due to the simple, predictable, and nonintimidating nature of robots compared to humans [82, 83]. Children can use robots as a "social crutch" to practice turn taking, language, and joint attention skills; it is hypothesized that they would eventually transfer learned skills to interactions with humans [70, 82, 84]. Robot-child interactions have also been used to encourage imitation skills within structured as well as free play environments [83, 85–90]. For example, following 7 weeks of structured training, low-functioning children paired with a robot mediator demonstrated greater shared attention and imitation of facial expressions of the robot compared to children paired with the human mediator [85]. In spite of these promising results, none of the aforementioned studies systematically assessed changes in imitation or praxis performance following training. Furthermore, studies did not use standardized tests to assess changes in overall motor performance following robotic interactions. Our own previous work suggests objective improvements in imitation/praxis and bilateral coordination following a 4-week robot-adult-child intervention protocol using a 7-inch humanoid robot, Isobot (Tony, Inc.) in 15 TD children and 1 child with autism [91–93]. In the present study, we address limitations in the current literature by extending our work to a larger sample of children with ASD and systematically examining the effects of a prolonged robotic intervention using a humanoid robot, Nao, on training-specific measures of imitation/praxis and interpersonal synchrony assessed within the training context, as well as overall motor performance assessed on a standardized test outside the training context.

Taken together, in spite of the growing recognition of motor impairments in ASD, there is currently little evidence on comprehensive intervention programs that target gross and fine motor performance in autism. Moreover, evidence on novel rhythm and robotic therapies is anecdotal and limited in its application due to small sample sizes, limited training durations, lack of use of standardized assessments, and detailed coding schemes, as well as lack of methodological rigor and experimental controls. The current RCT aimed to address these gaps by comparing the effects of prolonged 8-week rhythm and robotic interventions to those of a standard-of-care comparison intervention on the motor skills of children with ASD. Note that we are currently reporting effects of these interventions on the social communication and behavioral skills through other publications. All three groups engaged in imitation-based activities within group contexts. The movement groups engaged in whole-body gross motor and fine motor imitation games to the beat of music whereas the comparison group engaged in sedentary tabletop fine motor imitation activities. We assessed changes in generalized motor performance from pretest to posttest using a standardized test of motor performance, namely, the Bruininks-Oseretsky Test of Motor Proficiency, 2nd edition (BOT-2) [93]. We also assessed changes in training-specific measures of imitation/praxis and interpersonal synchrony from an early to a late training session. We hypothesized that consistent with the training demands, the movement groups would show improvements in gross motor performance (balance and bilateral coordination subtests), whereas the comparison group would demonstrate improvements in fine motor performance (fine motor precision and fine motor integration subtests) on the BOT-2. Due to the strong focus on imitation-based games in all groups, we hypothesized that all groups would demonstrate improvements in training-specific measures of imitation/praxis. Given the nature of the training activities, we assessed interpersonal synchrony only in the rhythm and robot groups and hypothesized that both groups would demonstrate improvements in synchrony with training.

2. Method

2.1. Participants. We recruited 36 children (32 M and 4 F, 20 Caucasian, 6 African American, 4 Asian, 3 Hispanic, and 3 of mixed ethnicity) between 5 and 12 years of age (M (SD) = 7.63 (2.24)) (see Table 1(a) for demographic details) (see Figure 1 for enrollment and allocation details). Children were recruited through fliers posted online and onsite in local schools, services, and self/parent advocacy groups. The Social Communication Questionnaire (SCQ) [94] was used as a screener prior to enrollment. Eligibility was confirmed using the gold standard diagnostic assessment, the Autism Diagnostic Observation Schedule, 2nd edition (ADOS-2) [95], and clinician judgment during a clinical psychology evaluation. Children with significant behavioral impairments or severe receptive language impairments that limited comprehension of 2-step simple instructions were excluded (see Figure 1). All children were enrolled following written parental consent as approved by the Institutional Review Board at the University of Connecticut. All participating families belonged to the upper-middle to upper

TABLE 1: (a) Demographic characteristics of children in the rhythm, robot, and comparison groups. (b) Baseline motor performance, adaptive behavior, and autism severity of children in rhythm, robot, and comparison groups.

(a)

Participant characteristics	Rhythm group M (SD)	Robot group M (SD)	Comparison group M (SD)	F or χ^2 value	p value
Age	7.88 (2.56)	7.52 (2.22)	7.36 (2.02)	0.44	0.65
Gender	10 M, 2 F	11 M, 1 F	11 M, 1 F	0.56	0.76
Socioeconomic status	47.33 (10.86)	47.75 (8.75)	52.46 (10.37)	0.97	0.39

(b)

Participant characteristics	Rhythm group M (SD) and range	Robot group M (SD) and range	Comparison Group M (SD) and Range	F value	p value
Adaptive behavior composite on the VABS	71.45 (11.75) 35 to 94	67.91 (15.01) 41 to 88	75.92 (18.43) 39 to 100	0.80	p values > 0.5
Percentage of children with scores lower than 1 SD below the mean	81.82	90.91	66.67		
Total motor scores on the MABC-2 checklist	30.92 (16.40) 7 to 62	37.5 (13.06) 3 to 50	30.5 (14.50) 8 to 50	1.45	p values > 0.3
Percentage of children below age-based cut-off scores	75	83.33	66.67		
ADOS-2 comparison score	8.5 (1.24) 6 to 10	7.92 (1.78) 5 to 10	8.42 (1.72) 5 to 10	0.46	p values > 0.3

Note. On the VABS, higher scores indicate better functioning; on the MABC-2 caregiver checklist, higher scores indicate poor motor performance; on the ADOS-2, and higher comparison scores indicate high autism severity.

class in terms of their socioeconomic status (M (SD) = 49.18 (10.03)) [96] (see Table 1(a)).

Following enrollment, children were matched on age (4-5, 6-7, 8-9, and 10–12 years), level of functioning, and amount of prior services and then randomly assigned to one of three groups, rhythm, robot, or comparison using the random number generator in MS Excel (see Table 1(a)). We assessed autism severity using the comparison scores on the ADOS-2. The comparison score is a continuous metric ranging from 1 to 10 that describes the severity of a child's autism symptoms compared to children with ASD of similar age and language levels [95]. Low comparison scores are indicative of minimal to no evidence of autism symptoms whereas high scores are indicative of severe autism symptoms. All participating children showed moderate to severe symptoms of ASD and there were no group differences in terms of levels of autism severity (p values > 0.3, see Table 1(b)). We assessed children's level of adaptive functioning using the Vineland Adaptive Behavior Scales (VABS) parent questionnaire [97] (see Table 1(b)). Overall, 82% of our participants had significant delays (>1 SD below the mean) on the Adaptive Behavior Composite; specifically, 70% children had communication delays, 80% had delays in daily living skills, and 82% had delays on the socialization domain with no group differences (p values > 0.5). We used the caregiver checklist of the Movement Assessment Battery for Children, 2nd edition (MABC-2), to assess motor competence of children between 5 and 12 years of age on a variety of fine and gross motor activities [98] (see Table 1(b)). Overall, 75% of children in the study had MABC scores below the 15th percentile on the MABC-2 checklist with no group differences (p values > 0.3).

2.2. Study Characteristics. Our pilot randomized controlled trial lasted for 10 weeks with the pretest and posttest sessions conducted during the first and last weeks of the study, respectively. The training sessions were provided during the intermediate 8 weeks of the study. Children in all three groups, rhythm, robotic, and comparison, were provided a total of 32 sessions (16 expert and 16 parent sessions). Children were provided 2 expert sessions per week with each session lasting for around 45 minutes. In addition, we provided caregivers with detailed instruction manuals, session supplies, and in-person training to practice similar activities during 2 additional home sessions each week. Out of the 32 sessions, all families completed more than 50% of the sessions (Rhythm: M (SD) = 73.18 (19.74), Robot: M (SD) = 76.82 (16.72), Comparison: M (SD) = 80.21 (15.27), p values > 0.05).

2.3. Training Protocol. In all three groups, children engaged in training activities within a triadic context involving the child, an expert trainer, and an adult model (see Figures 2(a), 2(b), and 2(c)). The expert trainer was the instructor and guided the child through the activities of the session. In the robot group, the robot was the instructor and the human trainer controlled the robot using a laptop. The adult model served as a buddy and a visual model for the child and provided hand-on-hand assistance, if needed, during the session. The rhythm and robot groups engaged in socially embedded whole-body movement games (see Figures 2(a) and 2(b)), whereas the comparison group engaged in tabletop activities promoting fine motor, social communication, and academic skills within a group setting (see Figure 2(c)).

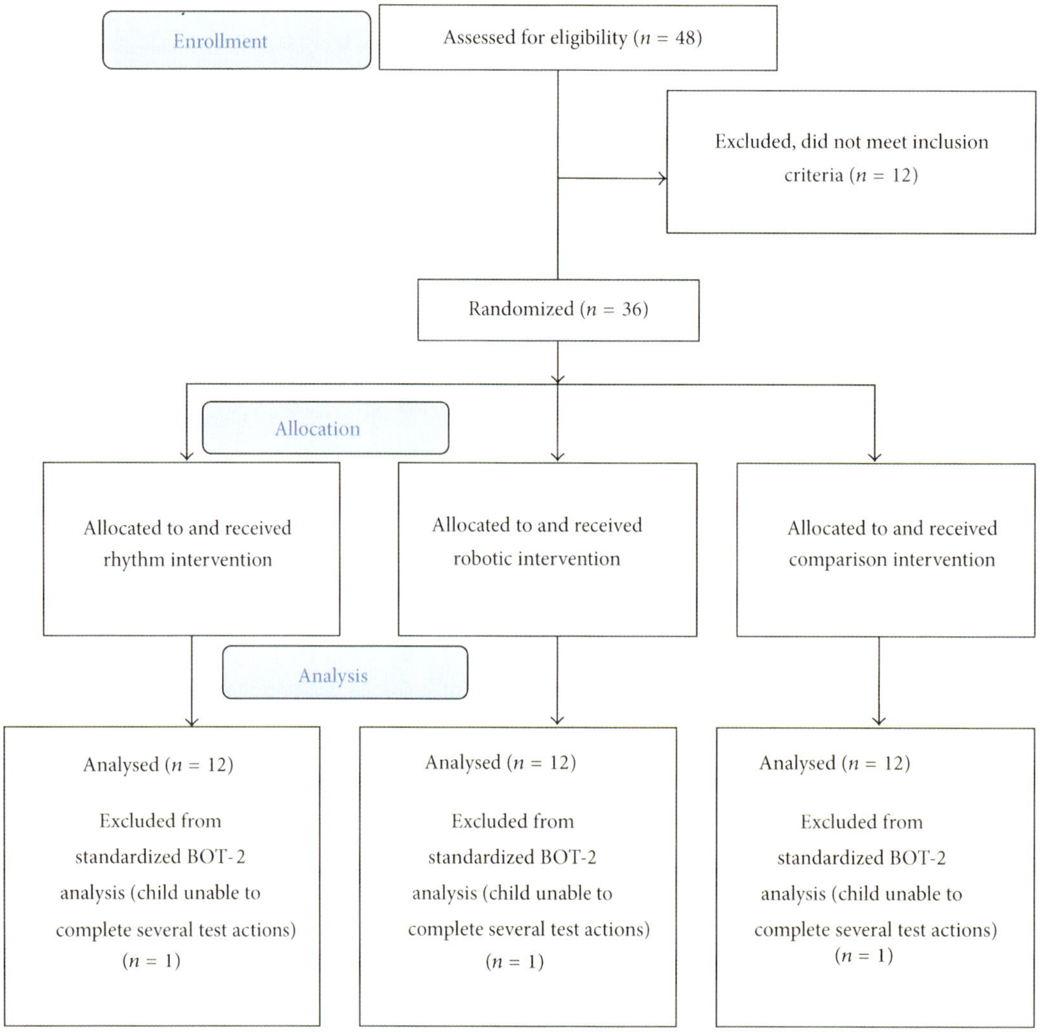

FIGURE 1: CONSORT flow diagram.

The comparison group was structured to mimic the types of activities that children with autism typically receive in special education settings. In all three groups, we promoted social communication skills such as eye contact, turn taking, greeting/farewell, responding to questions, commenting, asking for help, and use of gestures. In addition, the rhythm and robot groups promoted gross motor skills including balance, bilateral coordination, imitation, interpersonal synchrony, and manual dexterity during joint action games, whereas the comparison group promoted fine motor skills such as symmetrical and asymmetrical grips and pinches, coloring, drawing, cutting, and gluing. All training sessions were videotaped for further behavioral coding.

In all groups, we used training principles derived from current mainstream autism interventions including Applied Behavioral Analysis (ABA) [99], Teaching and Education of Autistic and Related Communication Handicapped Children (TEACCH) [100], and Picture Exchange Communication System (PECS) [101]. For example, we used strategies such as repetition, graded prompting, ensuring structure and consistency in the environment and the individuals involved in the training, and the use of pictures to facilitate transitions. All trainers involved in the study were pediatric physical therapists or physical therapy/kinesiology graduate students who received intensive training from the last author, a music educator, and ABA experts prior to the training sessions. Similarly, all models involved in the study were undergraduate students experienced in working with children with special needs and they received significant training from the last author prior to participation. To assess treatment fidelity, a naïve coder randomly chose and coded one early (sessions 1–5), mid (sessions 6–11), and late (sessions 12–16) session for each child using a comprehensive checklist developed to assess trainer and model behaviors (see Table 4). The coder evaluated (1) accurate completion of critical components of training activities (maximum score = 74 points), (2) trainer and model behaviors including instructions, prompts, and trainer/model affect (scored on a scale of 1 to 5 with 1 indicating poor quality and 5 indicating highest quality), and (3) child's compliance (scored on a scale of 1 to 5 with 1 indicating poor interest and 5 indicating maximum interest). Overall, across groups, training activities were completed

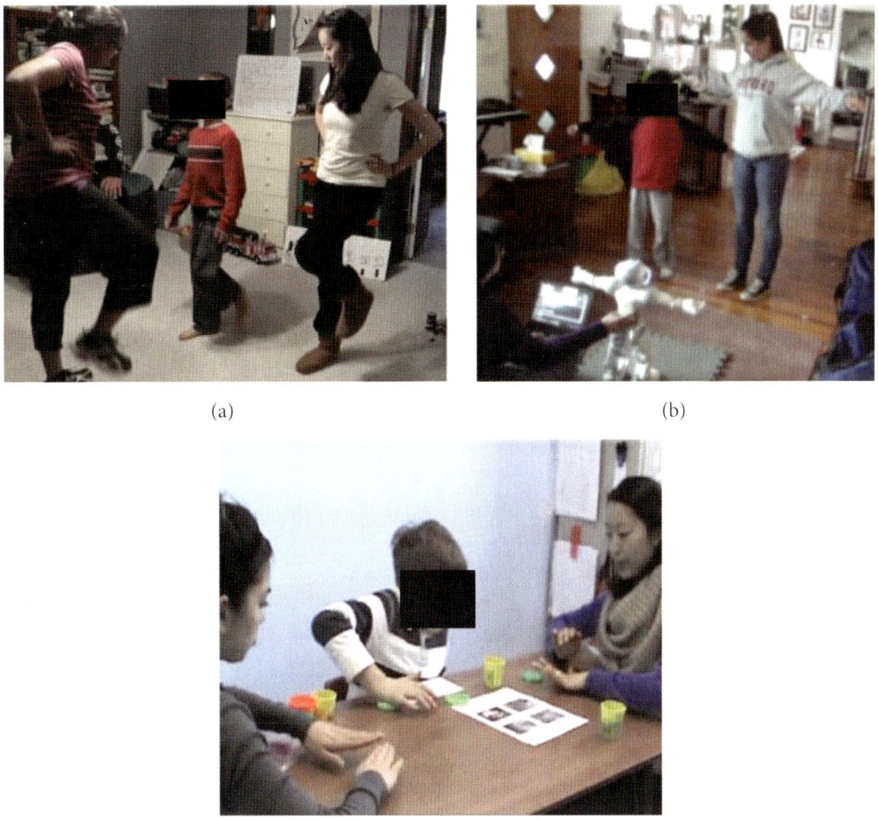

(a) (b) (c)

Figure 2: (a) Experimental set-up for a rhythm group training session. (b) Experimental set-up for a robot group training session. (c) Experimental set-up for a comparison group training session.

accurately across sessions (Rhythm: 92.16% (8.32), Robot: 90.73% (17.7), Comparison: 91.51% (5.67)), trainers and models demonstrated greater than optimal adherence to the training protocol (Rhythm: 4.68 (0.39), Robot: 4.36 (0.34), Comparison: 4.65 (0.27)), and children showed moderate to high levels of compliance with training (Rhythm: 3.27 (1.14), Robot: 2.67 (0.79), Comparison: 3.95 (0.81)). Next, we describe training activities in each group.

In the rhythm group, children engaged in simple and complex whole-body discrete imitation and interpersonal synchrony-based rhythmic joint action games set to music with the expert trainer and the adult model. Specifically, children engaged in the following movement-based games: action songs that involved finger play, beat keeping routines involving synchronous whole body movements with the adults, improvisational music making that involved synchronous playing of musical instruments, and moving games involving synchronous, locomotor actions such as skipping and jumping (see Table 5).

In the robot group, children engaged with a 23-inch humanoid robot, Nao, and a mobile robot, Rovio, during a variety of dual and multilimb imitation and synchrony-based games. Children practiced the following movement-based activities in each session: warm-up game involving body stretches, action game involving upper and lower body synchrony games, drumming game involving practice of simple and complex drumming patterns, and walking game involving tracing letters and shapes on the floor while following the Rovio robot (see Table 5).

In the comparison group, children engaged in several tabletop activities that promoted academic and fine motor skills. Children engaged in reading developmentally appropriate books, building games that involved making creations using supplies such as Play-Doh, Duplos/Legos, and Zoob (Infinitoy), and art-craft activities involving drawing, cutting, coloring, gluing, and pasting to build theme-based creations. We encouraged fine motor skills including symmetrical and asymmetrical hand movements such as rolling, pressing, pulling apart, pushing together, and different types of grips and pinches, as children engaged in imitation games involving building supplies (see Table 5).

2.4. Testing Protocol. We assessed generalized changes in gross and fine motor performance using the standardized test, Bruininks-Oseretsky Test of Motor Proficiency, 2nd edition (BOT-2) [93]. In addition, we assessed training-specific changes in imitation/praxis and interpersonal synchrony by coding custom-developed test activities in the early and late part of the intervention.

2.4.1. Standardized Test of Motor Performance. The BOT-2 is a reliable and valid assessment of gross and fine motor performance for individuals between 4 and 21 years of age [93]. We assessed changes in motor performance using the fine motor precision (FMP), fine motor integration (FMI), bilateral coordination (BC), and balance (BA) subtests of the BOT-2. The FMP subtest consists of 7 activities that assess precise hand and finger control, the FMI subtest includes 8 items that assess the ability to reproduce drawings of geometric shapes, the BC subtest consists of 8 items that assess the ability to sequentially and simultaneously synchronize upper and lower limbs, and the BA subtest consists of 9 items that evaluate postural control skills during standing and walking. We used the standard scores on the body coordination composite and fine manual control composite to assess for training-related changes in motor performance. The body coordination composite is based on the on the BC and BA subtests and the fine manual control composite is based on the FMP and FMI subtests of the BOT-2. A novel tester blinded to the grouping of the child conducted the BOT-2 assessment during the pretest and posttest sessions. The first and the third author coded the entire dataset after establishing inter- and intrarater reliability of greater than 85% using 20% of the dataset. The dependent variable was the standard scores on the body coordination and fine manual control composites of the BOT-2 in the pretest and posttest sessions.

2.4.2. Training-Specific Test of Imitation/Praxis. We developed a set of test actions that were representative of the training activities practiced in each group and administered these activities during an early and late training session. Imitation was assessed during the action song and xylophone games in the rhythm group, during the action and drumming games in the robot group, and during building games using Play-Doh, Duplo/Lego blocks, and Zoob (Infinitoy) pieces in the comparison group (see Table 2 for details). Using video data from the training session, we coded imitation accuracy of children during test actions by assessing errors in spatial and temporal aspects of movement execution relative to actions of the trainer. This coding scheme was developed using the error classification reported in the praxis literature [102] (see Table 3 for details). A score of 0 indicated no error and a score of 1 indicated an error within the specific error category. We also recorded the types of prompts, visual, verbal, or manual hand-on-hand assistance, that children required to complete the actions. The total imitation error score was calculated as the sum of error scores on all individual error categories during the test actions. A single coder coded the entire dataset after establishing inter- and intrarater reliability of over 90% using 20% of the dataset. Our dependent variable was the percent total imitation error during test actions administered in the early and late training sessions in each group.

2.4.3. Training-Specific Test of Interpersonal Synchrony. We assessed changes in interpersonal synchrony between children and their adult partners in the rhythm and robot groups during an early and late training session. Interpersonal synchrony was assessed during the beat keeping, music making, and moving game activities in the rhythm group and during the action, drumming, and walking game activities in the robot group (see Table 2 for details). The comparison group was excluded from this analysis, since they did not engage in whole-body rhythmic actions promoting interpersonal synchrony. In the rhythm and robot groups, we assessed for the percent duration of time that children were in-synchrony (movements synchronized in time and spatially in the same or opposite direction as the adult), out-of-synchrony (movements not synchronized in time and space with the adult), and in assisted-synchrony (manual assistance provided to synchronize movements with the adult) relative to the adult. A single coder coded all the data using Openshapa video coding software after establishing inter- and intrarater reliability of >84% using 20% of the dataset.

2.5. Statistical Analysis. We checked our data for assumptions of normality and homogeneity of variances. The data from the standardized BOT-2 test satisfied all assumptions of parametric statistics. We used repeated measures ANCOVA with composite type (body coordination and fine manual control) and test session (pretest and posttest) as within-subjects factors and group as the between-subjects factor. In addition, to control for the effect of autism severity on motor performance, we added the ADOS-2 comparison scores as a covariate in the analysis. Data from our training-specific measure of imitation/praxis and interpersonal synchrony were not normally distributed. Hence, we conducted a square root transformation and used transformed data in our analyses. Moreover, since the tests employed to assess imitation/praxis and synchrony were different in the three groups, we conducted separate analyses for each group. We used dependent t-tests to assess changes in imitation/praxis from the early to the late session within each group. For assessing changes in interpersonal synchrony, we conducted separate repeated measures ANOVAs for the rhythm and robot groups with session (early, late) and synchrony type (in-synchrony, out-of-synchrony, assisted-synchrony) as the within-subjects factors. For the ANOVAs, in case of main and interaction effects involving the same factor, we assessed the interaction effects only. In case of violations of the assumption of sphericity, Greenhouse Geisser corrections were applied. Post hoc testing was done using dependent t-tests. We report effect sizes using partial eta-squared (η_p^2) and standardized mean difference (SMD) [103] values. Statistical significance was set at $p \leq 0.05$.

3. Results

3.1. Standardized Test of Motor Performance. For this analysis, we excluded 3 out of the 36 children since they were low functioning and could not perform a majority of the test actions of the BOT-2, in both the pretest and posttest sessions. The final analysis was therefore based on 11 children per group. The repeated measures ANCOVA indicated significant interaction effect of test session x composite type x group ($F(2, 29) = 3.44$, $p = 0.05$, $\eta_p^2 = 0.19$). We report post hoc analysis of the significant interaction as between-group differences and within-group changes.

TABLE 2: Training-specific measures of imitation/praxis and interpersonal synchrony.

Rhythm group		Robot group		Comparison group	
Test of imitation/praxis					
Action song	(i) Finger play (ii) Whole body discrete movements	Action game	Whole body discrete movements	Play-doh game	(i) Roll (ii) Flatten (iii) Pinch Play-Doh
Xylophone game	(i) Unilateral (ii) Bilateral symmetrical (iii) Bilateral alternating (iv) Crossover patterns	Drumming game	(i) Unilateral (ii) Bilateral symmetrical (iii) Bilateral alternating sequences	Duplos/Lego blocks and Zoob pieces	(i) Push (ii) Pull blocks/pieces
Test of interpersonal synchrony					
Beat keeping	(i) Rhythmic symmetrical (ii) Alternating arm actions	Action game	Rhythmic asymmetrical arm and leg actions	Not applicable	
Music making	(i) Rhythmic unilateral (ii) Bilateral symmetrical (iii) Bilateral alternating drum sequences	Drumming game	(i) Rhythmic unilateral (ii) Bilateral asymmetrical drum sequences		
Moving game	(i) Jumping (ii) Stomping (iii) March and clap (iv) Skipping	Walking game	Walking synchronously with the model to follow mobile robot		

Note. The comparison group did not engage in interpersonal synchrony activities; hence, no training-specific synchrony tests are reported for this group.

TABLE 3: Coding scheme to assess imitation/praxis errors.

Imitation errors	Definitions
Spatial	Incorrect positioning and orientation of joints involved
Body part	Use of incorrect body parts
Movement modulation	Movements are either insufficient or exaggerated in terms of effort and range of motion compared to the trainer
Movement precision	Incorrect sequence of movements within a pattern including omission of steps or addition of extra steps
Pace	Movements slower or faster than the trainer
Symmetry/reciprocity	Two sides of the body are used incorrectly or immaturely to perform test actions
Mirroring	Child failed to mirror actions of the trainer

TABLE 4: A checklist to assess fidelity of the training sessions.

Checklist criteria	Exemplar behaviors assessed
Eye contact	Trainer and model elicit eye contact from child during social interactions
Ready response	Trainer asks child if he/she is ready before each activity
Use of PECS board	Trainer takes child through the activities of the day using the PECS board
Session theme	Trainer explains the theme of the session to the child Example: "Today's theme is turn taking. When I move you watch, and when I stop it is your turn to move"
Activity introduction using PECS	Trainer introduces activity using picture boards Example: "Let's get ready for music making" while pointing at the picture for "music making"
Help with setup	Trainer and model ask child to help with setup for each activity. Example: "Can you pass that blue Lego block to me. . ."
Presentation of activity	At the beginning of each activity, trainer gives simple instructions for the activity Example: "Now, we will copy the robot"
Activity-specific bids	Appropriate bids to promote motor and social communication skills during each activity were provided Example: For building activity, "Let's roll the Play-Doh into a ball. Roll with me"
Trials	Trainer asks child to repeat each activity twice
Spontaneous exploration	Trainer and model provide children with opportunities for free play and spontaneous exploration Example: "It is free music time. You can play the drums in any way you want"
Social praise	Trainer and model provide verbal and gestural praise to child as required
Help with cleanup	Trainer and model ask child to help with cleanup of supplies after completion of each activity
Activity completion	After each activity, trainer asks child to move down the picture for the activity on the PECS board
General characteristics in the session	The overall session is evaluated for the following characteristics: number of activities completed, environmental arrangement (supplies in close proximity but out of the sight of the child to avoid distractions), and incremental prompts (visual, verbal, gestural, and lastly manual prompts/assistance provided if child is unable to perform the activity)
Trainer and model behaviors	The trainer's and model's behaviors are evaluated for the following criteria on a scale of 1 to 5: (i) appropriateness of instructions, prompts, and reinforcement, (ii) voice and affect modulation, (iii) appropriateness of movements
Child interest	Child's interest and compliance during session assessed on a scale of 1 to 5.

3.1.1. Between-Group Differences. At baseline, the comparison group had significantly greater scores on the fine manual control composite than the rhythm group (Rhythm: M (SD) = 33.5 (5.02), Comparison: M (SD) = 41.44 (8.72), $p = 0.02$). Based on the pretest session, there were no other baseline differences between groups on the body coordination and fine manual control composite standard scores. In the posttest session, after controlling for baseline levels of autism severity, the comparison group had significantly higher scores on the fine manual control composite compared to the robot and rhythm groups (Rhythm: M (SD) = 34.38 (4.36), Robot: M (SD) = 34.13 (8.72), Comparison: M (SD) = 44.52 (10.82), p values < 0.02) (see Figure 3(b)).

3.1.2. Within-Group Changes. In the *rhythm group*, after controlling for baseline levels of autism severity, children

TABLE 5: An exemplar rhythm, robot, and comparison group training session.

Activity	Rhythm group	Robot group	Comparison group
1	Hello song (i) Child asked to sing to trainer and model (ii) Song: hello everybody, yes indeed	Introduction Child asked to greet the trainer, model, and robot	Introduction Child asked to greet the trainer and model
2	Action song (i) Child asked to sing and engage in finger play (ii) Song: open shut them	Warm-up game Child asked to copy whole-body stretching moves of the Nao robot	Book reading Child reads age-appropriate book while taking turns with trainer and model
3	Beat keeping (i) Child asked to copy trainer during rhythmic arm and leg actions (ii) Song: stop, go, go, go	Action game (i) Child asked to engage in upper and lower body synchrony games with Nao robot and model (ii) Theme: start and stop game	Building (i) Child builds creations using Play-Doh, Lego, and so forth (ii) Theme: make a Lego car
4	Music making (i) Child asked to play instruments like drums, xylophones, cymbals, tambourines, and so forth (ii) Song: jingle jingle jingle jive	Drumming game (i) Child asked to practice simple and complex drum patterns with Nao robot and model (ii) Theme: start and stop game	Arts and crafts (i) Child makes creations by drawing, coloring, cutting, and so forth (ii) Theme: make a vegetable basket
5	Moving game (i) Child asked to copy trainer during gross motor actions like skipping, hopping, jumping, and so forth (ii) Song: on the bridge of Newtown	Walking (i) Child asked to follow Rovio robot with the model to trace letters and shapes on the floor (ii) Theme: tracing letter "L"	Cleanup Child asked to clean up all supplies used for the session
6	Farewell song (i) Child asked to sing to trainer and model (ii) Song: it was good to see you	Farewell Child asked to bid goodbye to the trainer, model, and robot	Farewell Child asked to bid goodbye to trainer and model

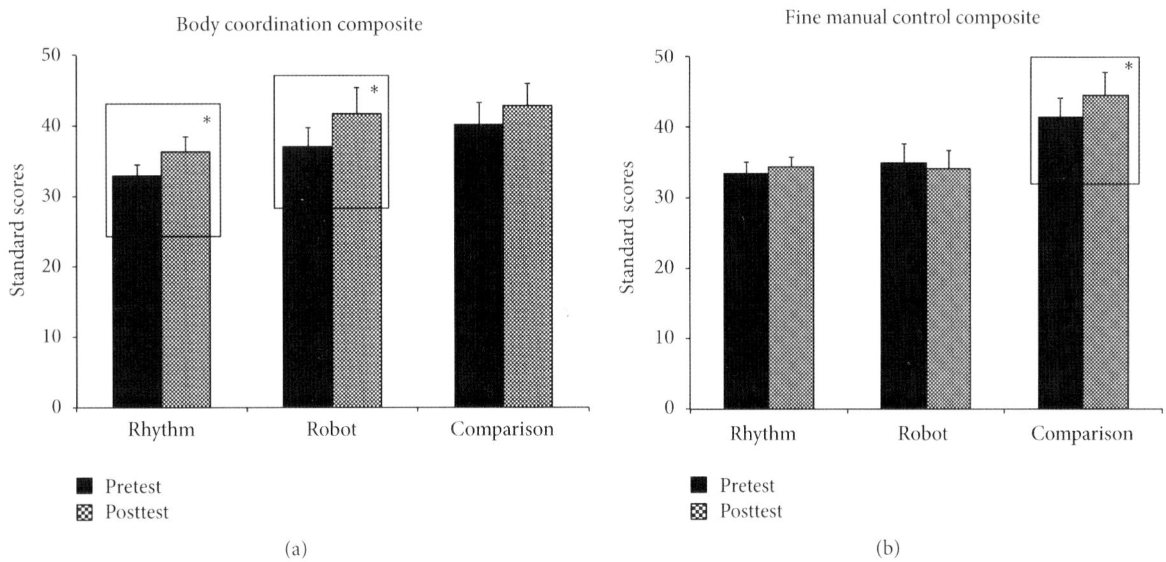

FIGURE 3: (a) Training-related changes on the body coordination composite of BOT-2. Error bars represent standard errors. (b) Training-related changes on the fine manual control composite of BOT-2. Error bars represent standard errors. $^{*}p \leq 0.05$.

improved their scores on the body coordination composite in the posttest compared to the pretest (Pretest: M (SD) = 32.91 (5.34), Posttest: M (SD) = 36.36 (6.90), $p = 0.01$, SMD = 0.60) (see Figure 3(a)). Specifically, 9 out of 11 children followed the group trends. Similarly, in the *robot group*, children significantly improved their performance on the body coordination composite in the posttest compared to the pretest, while controlling for the effects of autism severity (Pretest: M (SD) = 37 (9.15), Posttest: M (SD) = 41.73 (12.02), $p = 0.02$, SMD = 0.48) (see Figure 3(a)).

Specifically, 8 out of 11 children followed the group trends. Children in the rhythm and robot groups did not demonstrate any improvements in fine motor performance (see Figure 3(b)). In the *comparison group*, after controlling for baseline autism severity levels, children significantly increased their scores on the fine manual control composite of the BOT-2 from the pretest to the posttest session (Pretest: M (SD) = 41.44 (8.72), Posttest: M (SD) = 44.52 (10.83), $p = 0.05$, SMD = 0.33) (see Figure 2(b)). Individual data show that 9 out of 11 children followed the group trends. This group did not show any improvements on the body coordination composite of the BOT-2 (see Figure 3(a)).

3.2. Training-Specific Test of Imitation/Praxis. In the *rhythm group*, children demonstrated a significant reduction in imitation error scores from the early to the late session (Early: M (SD) = 35.55 (26.85), Late: M (SD) = 16.72 (18.21), $t(23) = 6.16$, $p < 0.001$, SMD = −0.65) (see Figure 4). Individual data show that all 12 children in the group demonstrated improvements in imitation performance. In the *robot group*, children significantly improved imitation performance from the early to the late session (Early: M (SD) = 27.91 (21.66), Late: M (SD) = 22.60 (17.59), $t(23) = 2.96$, $p = 0.007$, SMD = −0.23) (see Figure 4), with 10 out of the 12 children following the group trends. Along the same lines, the *comparison group* also demonstrated significant improvements in imitation performance from the early to the late session, with 9 out of 12 children following the group trend (Early: M (SD) = 24.85 (20.69), Late: M (SD) = 9.38 (8.91), $t(23) = 4.77$, $p < 0.001$, SMD = −0.70) (see Figure 4).

3.3. Training-Specific Test of Interpersonal Synchrony. The repeated measures ANOVA in the rhythm group revealed main effects of session ($F(1,35) = 4.57$, $p = 0.04$, $\eta_p^2 = 0.12$) and synchrony type ($F(1.263, 44.21) = 51.98$, $p < 0.001$, $\eta_p^2 = 0.60$) as well as a significant session x synchrony type interaction ($F(2,70) = 3.99$, $p = 0.023$, $\eta_p^2 = 0.10$). Post hoc analysis of the session x synchrony type interaction showed that the rhythm group increased amount of time spent in-synchrony with the adult from the early to the late session (Early: M (SD) = 45.59 (29.45), Late: M (SD) = 52.91 (30.57), $p = 0.02$, SMD = 0.23) (see Figure 5). Individual data show that 10 out of the 12 children followed the group trends.

The repeated measures ANOVA in the robot group showed a significant main effect of synchrony type ($F(1.35, 47.22) = 15.66$, $p < 0.001$, $\eta_p^2 = 0.31$) and a significant session x synchrony type interaction ($F(2,70) = 3.78$, $p = 0.028$, $\eta_p^2 = 0.10$). Post hoc analysis of the session x synchrony type interaction indicated that the robot group increased the amount of time spent in-synchrony with the adult from the early to the late session (Early: M (SD) = 37.88 (28.55), Late: M (SD) = 46.99 (30.28), $p = 0.04$, SMD = 0.30), with 10 out of the 12 children following the group trends.

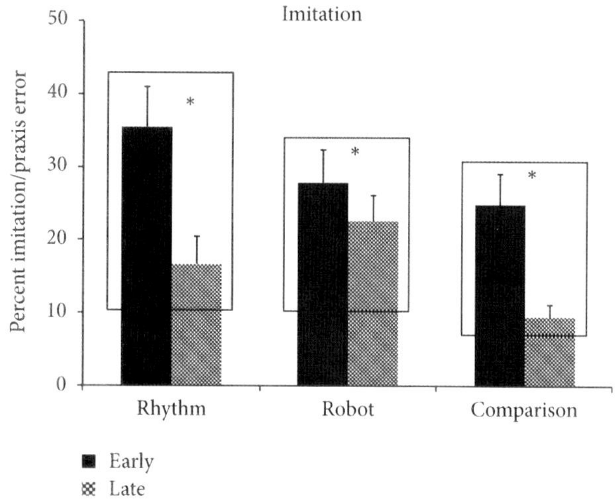

FIGURE 4: Training-related changes in percent imitation error in the rhythm, robot, and comparison groups. Error bars represent standard errors. $^*p \le 0.05$.

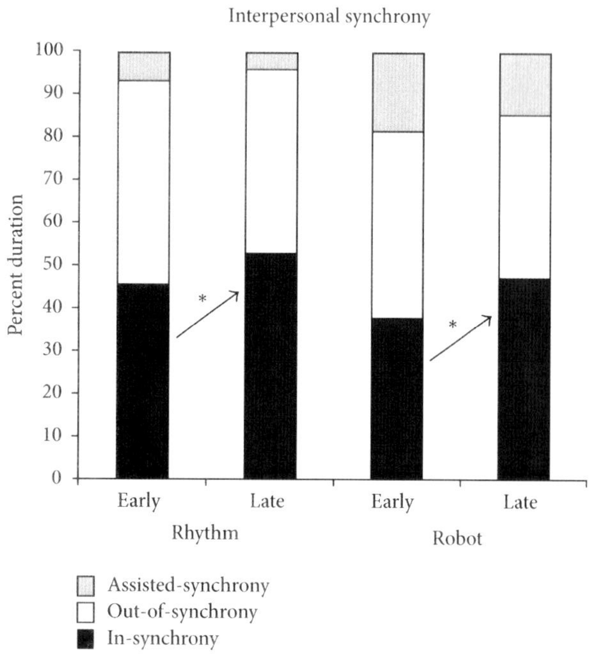

FIGURE 5: Training-related changes in interpersonal synchrony in the rhythm and robot groups. Error bars represent standard errors. $^*p < 0.05$.

4. Discussion

We examined the effects of rhythm and robotic interventions compared to a stationary comparison intervention on the gross and fine motor performance, imitation/praxis, and interpersonal synchrony skills of children with ASD. After controlling for the level of autism severity, the rhythm and robot groups demonstrated improvements in gross motor performance (i.e., body coordination composite) as measured on the BOT-2 from the pretest to the posttest session with no similar improvements on the fine manual control composite (see Figures 3(a) and 3(b)). Children in both groups also reduced their imitation/praxis errors and improved their interpersonal synchrony skills from the early to the late session (see Figures 4 and 5). Consistent with the type of training provided, the comparison group demonstrated an improvement on the fine manual control composite of the BOT-2 from the pretest to the posttest after controlling for level of autism severity, with no significant changes in gross motor performance (see Figures 3(a) and 3(b)). Moreover, children also significantly reduced their imitation errors from the early to the late session (see Figure 4). In the subsequent sections, we discuss possible reasons for our findings and also highlight the implications of our study results.

4.1. Changes in Motor Skills within the Standardized and Training-Specific Tests: Rhythm Group. The rhythm group demonstrated an improvement of medium effect size on the body coordination composite of the BOT-2 and the training-specific test of imitation/praxis as well as a small improvement on the training-specific test of interpersonal synchrony. Our findings fit with the limited existing literature on the use of music therapy in children with ASD and the broader music education literature on the effects of music-based experiences on motor skills of TD children [75, 80, 81, 104, 105]. For example, within the context of one-on-one reciprocal musical imitation games involving music-making, singing, and dancing between children with autism and an adult therapist, 3 out of 4 children demonstrated an increase in spontaneous imitation of actions and words of the therapist [75]. In TD children, music has frequently been used as an accompaniment in physical education programs to improve balance and bilateral coordination skills [77, 79, 106, 107]. For example, a developmentally appropriate music and movement program led to greater improvements in jumping and dynamic balance skills of preschool children compared to a control group that engaged in physical education activities that were not based on music [78]. Similarly, following a music- and movement-based program, TD children improved dual and multilimb coordination skills during galloping, leaping, jumping, and skipping actions compared to a control group [107]. Along the same lines, prolonged musical training also led to improvement in accuracy on a motor sequencing task compared to a control group that did not receive musical instruction [80]. In terms of interpersonal synchrony, even 2.5–4.5 year old TD children were able to synchronize more accurately with their adult human partner compared to a machine during a joint drumming task [108]. Moreover, joint music making experiences such as singing or dancing foster prosocial cooperative/synchronous behaviors in 4-year old TD children [109]. Along these lines, the training activities in the rhythm group involved group-based symmetrical and asymmetrical movements of hands and legs such as jumping, galloping, hopping, and so forth to the beat of music. Across training weeks, children may have improved their visuomotor and bilateral coordination as well as balance skills, their ability to plan and execute multistep sequences, the speed and timing of their motor responses, and their ability to synchronize with social partners; this in turn could have led to improvements on standardized and training-specific measures of motor performance.

4.2. Changes in Motor Skills within the Standardized and Training-Specific Tests: Robot Group. The robot group also demonstrated small improvements in motor performance on the standardized and training-specific tests following training. Our previous proof-of-concept study on 14 TD children and 1 child with autism suggested improvements in children's ability to coordinate actions with social partners following 4 weeks of imitation-based training using the 7-inch humanoid robot, Isobot (Tony, Inc.) [92]. In the current study, we were able to replicate our previous work and further extend it to a larger sample of children with ASD. Our findings are also similar to the few other studies within the robotics literature that have used robots to facilitate motor skills in children with ASD [85–87, 110–112]. For example, children with ASD were faster at imitating a reach-to-grasp action following observation of a robotic versus a human model performing the task, whereas the reverse trend was observed in TD children [110]. Similarly, repeated short bouts of interactions with a humanoid doll robot, Robota, over 101 days led to a trend for improved imitation of simple actions of the robot in children with ASD [86]. In a different study, during repeated unconstrained interactions with a child-sized humanoid robot, KASPAR, a minimally expressive teenager with autism learned to imitate the actions of the robot as a part of turn taking games played with the therapist and another child [89]. Although the results of the above studies are encouraging, none of the aforementioned studies assessed motor performance using standardized tests or detailed coding schemes to evaluate changes in spatial and temporal aspects of movement execution following intervention. Our findings add to the current body of knowledge by systematically assessing motor performance using training-specific and standardized measures. Over training weeks, children may have improved their perception of the anthropomorphic characteristics of the robot, their balance, motor imitation, and multilimb coordination skills, as well as their social monitoring abilities; this could have contributed to the improvements in imitation/praxis, interpersonal synchrony, and overall gross motor performance seen in this group.

4.3. Changes in Motor Skills within the Standardized and Training-Specific Tests: Comparison Group. The comparison group demonstrated an improvement of small effect size on the fine motor subtests of the BOT-2 as well as an improvement of medium effect size on the training-specific test of imitation following the intervention. Our standard-of-care comparison group was designed to mimic the kind of fine motor activities that children with ASD receive during school-based therapies [113]. These services typically address fine motor problems including handwriting skills (illegible writing, inability to stay on the line, letter reversals, etc.), desk skills (using scissors, folding, cutting, rolling Play-Doh, manipulating small objects, etc.), and organization skills (keeping materials in order, completing homework, remembering sequence of tasks, etc.) [114–116]. In line with the types of object manipulation, manual, and desk skills practiced during training sessions, the comparison group demonstrated improvements in fine motor skills. Our findings also fit with existing literature in children with fine motor problems that reports improvements in fine motor and visuomotor skills following prolonged interventions [115, 117]. For example, an 8-month intervention targeting fine motor problems in 44 preschool children led to improvements in standardized tests assessing in-hand manipulation, eye-hand coordination, fine motor skills, visuomotor skills, and functional performance, with the amount of improvement associated with the intensity of training [115]. Similarly, at one-year follow-up following training to address fine motor, visuomotor, and gross motor skills, children with developmental disabilities showed improvements in visuomotor skills as assessed on standardized tests [117]. Overall, it was encouraging to see improvements in fine motor skills both within and outside the training context following a relatively short-term 8-week intervention program.

5. Clinical Implications

We assessed the effects of rhythm, robotic, and standard-of-care comparison interventions on the gross and fine motor performance, imitation/praxis, and interpersonal synchrony skills of children with ASD between 5 and 12 years of age. Consistent with the training demands, the movement groups demonstrated improvements in balance, bilateral coordination, gross motor imitation, and interpersonal synchrony skills on standardized and training-specific tests following the 8-week intervention. Similarly, the comparison group demonstrated improvements in fine motor skills on the standardized BOT-2 test and the training-specific test of imitation. Given the association between motor impairments and core symptoms in ASD [8, 40, 118], it would be critical to include both gross and fine motor goals in the treatment plan of children with ASD. Our data show that socially embedded movement-based contexts such as rhythm and robotic therapies that focus on imitation, bilateral coordination, balance, and synchrony skills are enjoyable for children and can be used to promote gross motor skills in this population. In fact, other data from this study show that movement-based contexts can also promote social communication skills such as social monitoring and verbal communication that are considered core impairments in autism. Therefore, in addition to the existing emphasis on remediating fine motor issues in children with ASD within predominantly sedentary contexts, socially embedded creative movement ideas involving rhythm, dance, and active play must also be introduced in the standard-of-care treatments for children with ASD.

We assessed the effects of interventions on training-specific as well as standardized tests of motor performance. The standardized test involved novel actions that were administered by a novel unfamiliar tester outside the training context during the pretest and posttest sessions. In contrast, the training-specific tests involved activities similar to the training activities and were administered by the familiar trainer within the training context during an early and late session. Improvements in the training-specific tests could therefore be attributed to some extent to familiarity effects. In contrast, improvements in the standardized test are indicative of carryover of skills learned during training sessions to novel contexts. It was encouraging to see that there were training-related improvements in both standardized and training-specific tests in all three groups. Clinicians using similar movement-based games for children with ASD should aim to assess training-related changes in motor skills both within and outside the training context and should further evaluate sustenance of treatment effects at follow-up visits.

In the present study, although both rhythm and robot groups demonstrated improvements in motor skills, we observed several limitations in the robotic technology. First, the robot had a limited movement repertoire and could not train children for complex actions such as running, jumping, galloping, hopping, skipping, or even walking at different speeds. Secondly, the robot's movements were slower, less varied, and less precise than those of a human. Lastly, the robot could not train fine motor skills such as cutting, coloring, and drawing. Therefore, although our results look promising, at this point, we recommend that robots be used as adjunct therapies for children with ASD. Future efforts must be directed towards designing training activities that are engaging and functionally meaningful for children with autism, as well as developing contingent, semiautonomous robots that can adapt to the needs of the children.

6. Limitations

In spite of the promising results, our study is limited in many ways including a small sample size, limited intervention duration, limited generalization to activities of daily living, and lack of long-term follow-up. Our study was a preliminary study with a relatively small sample size of 36 children with 12 children per group. Further, there was some group variability in our sample due to the nature of the ASD diagnosis. In terms of behavioral coding, the coders of the training-specific measures were not blinded to the grouping of the child. The limited training duration of 8 weeks may have contributed to the small-to-moderate size improvements on the standardized and training-specific measures as well as the lack of significant between-group differences on the standardized BOT-2 test. Overall, in spite of the encouraging nature of our results, we recommend that they be interpreted with caution until future studies can replicate these results using larger sample sizes and extensive training protocols.

7. Conclusions

We assessed the effects of novel rhythm and robotic interventions compared to a standard-of-care comparison intervention on the gross and fine motor performance, imitation/praxis, and interpersonal synchrony skills of children with ASD. To the best of our knowledge, this is the first study to systematically assess the effects of rhythm and robotic interventions on motor skills of children using standardized motor tests and custom-developed coding schemes to evaluate imitation/praxis and interpersonal synchrony. Consistent with the training demands of the contexts, the movement groups demonstrated improvements in gross motor performance, whereas the comparison group demonstrated improvements in fine motor performance on the standardized BOT-2 test. All groups demonstrated improvements on the training-specific test of imitation and both the rhythm and robot groups improved their interpersonal synchrony performance following training. Overall, given the perceptuo-motor impairments in ASD, we argue for the inclusion of goals promoting gross and fine motor proficiency within the treatment plan of children with ASD. Our data showed that embodied, whole-body movement-based activities such as rhythm and robotic therapies are valuable contexts to promote motor skills in children with ASD.

Disclosure

This work was completed when Dr. Kerry L. Marsh was serving at the National Science Foundation.

Disclaimer

The views expressed here are solely of the authors and do not necessarily represent views of the National Science Foundation or the funding agencies, National Institutes of Health or Autism Speaks.

Acknowledgments

The authors would like to thank the children and families who participated in this study. They thank Christian Wanamaker for his help with the programming of the Nao robot. They thank Dr. Linda Neelly for her support in developing the rhythm intervention protocol. They thank the undergraduate students who contributed to this project through data collection, data processing, and behavioral coding, Sara Balakrishnan, Margaret Reiss, Dominica Gilewska, Christina O'Hara, Chaitali Korgaonkar, Lyly Tran, Kathleen Lynch, Carolyn Susca, Sean Walsh, Debbie Lee, Cassondra Hunter, Tracy Sooklall, Caitlyn Metsack, Jenna Shaw, and Joanna Sajdlowska. They thank Dr. Marianne Barton, Director of the Psychological Services Clinic at the University of Connecticut, and clinical psychology doctoral students, Dasal Jashar and Lauren Haisley for their support in conducting ADOS testing. Last but not the least, they thank Dr. Deborah Bubela for her assistance with the testing and training administration for a subset of the participating children. The authors thank the National Institute of Mental Health for the R21MH089441 and R33MH089441 awards, Autism Speaks for the pilot treatment award #8137, and the UConn Foundation for their large grant awarded to the last author, Dr. Anjana N. Bhat.

References

[1] American Psychiatric Association, Ed., *Diagnostic and Statistical Manual of Mental Disorders*, American Psychiatric Association, Arlington, Va, USA, 2013.

[2] G. Dawson, K. Toth, R. Abbott et al., "Early social attention impairments in autism: social orienting, joint attention, and attention to distress," *Developmental Psychology*, vol. 40, no. 2, pp. 271–283, 2004.

[3] H. Tager-Flusberg, R. Paul, and C. Lord, "Language and communication in autism," in *Handbook of Autism and Pervasive Developmental Disorders*, vol. 1, pp. 335–364, Wiley, 2005.

[4] S. R. Leekam, M. R. Prior, and M. Uljarevic, "Restricted and repetitive behaviors in autism spectrum disorders: a review of research in the last decade," *Psychological Bulletin*, vol. 137, no. 4, pp. 562–593, 2011.

[5] A. N. Bhat, R. J. Landa, and J. C. Galloway, "Current perspectives on motor functioning in infants, children, and adults with autism spectrum disorders," *Physical Therapy*, vol. 91, no. 7, pp. 1116–1129, 2011.

[6] M. Hallett, M. K. Lebiedowska, S. L. Thomas, S. J. Stanhope, M. B. Denckla, and J. Rumsey, "Locomotion of autistic adults," *Archives of Neurology*, vol. 50, no. 12, pp. 1304–1308, 1993.

[7] D. Green, T. Charman, A. Pickles et al., "Impairment in movement skills of children with autistic spectrum disorders," *Developmental Medicine & Child Neurology*, vol. 51, no. 4, pp. 311–316, 2009.

[8] C. L. Hilton, Y. Zhang, M. R. Whilte, C. L. Klohr, and J. Constantino, "Motor impairment in sibling pairs concordant and discordant for autism spectrum disorders," *Autism*, vol. 16, no. 4, pp. 430–441, 2012.

[9] B. Provost, S. Heimerl, and B. R. Lopez, "Levels of gross and fine motor development in young children with autism spectrum disorder," *Physical and Occupational Therapy in Pediatrics*, vol. 27, no. 3, pp. 21–36, 2007.

[10] K. A. Fournier, C. J. Hass, S. K. Naik, N. Lodha, and J. H. Cauraugh, "Motor coordination in autism spectrum disorders: a synthesis and meta-analysis," *Journal of Autism and Developmental Disorders*, vol. 40, no. 10, pp. 1227–1240, 2010.

[11] S. J. Rogers, L. Bennetto, R. McEvoy, and B. F. Pennington, "Imitation and pantomime in high-functioning adolescents with autism spectrum disorders," *Child Development*, vol. 67, no. 5, pp. 2060–2073, 1996.

[12] R. P. Hobson and A. Lee, "Imitation and identification in autism," *Journal of Child Psychology and Psychiatry*, vol. 40, no. 4, pp. 649–659, 1999.

[13] G. Vivanti, D. Trembath, and C. Dissanayake, "Mechanisms of imitation impairment in autism spectrum disorder," *Journal of Abnormal Child Psychology*, vol. 42, no. 8, pp. 1395–1405, 2014.

[14] K. L. Marsh, R. W. Isenhower, M. J. Richardson et al., "Autism and social disconnection in interpersonal rocking," *Frontiers in Integrative Neuroscience*, vol. 7, 2013.

[15] L. R. Dowell, E. M. Mahone, and S. H. Mostofsky, "Associations of postural knowledge and basic motor skill with dyspraxia in autism: implication for abnormalities in distributed connectivity and motor learning," *Neuropsychology*, vol. 23, no. 5, pp. 563–570, 2009.

[16] M. R. Leary and D. A. Hill, "Moving on: autism and movement disturbance," *Mental Retardation*, vol. 34, no. 1, pp. 39–53, 1996.

[17] M. A. Gernsbacher, J. L. Stevenson, S. Khandakar, and H. H. Goldsmith, "Why does joint attention look atypical in autism?" *Child Development Perspectives*, vol. 2, no. 1, pp. 38–45, 2008.

[18] M. Lloyd, M. MacDonald, and C. Lord, "Motor skills of toddlers with autism spectrum disorders," *Autism*, vol. 17, no. 2, pp. 133–146, 2013.

[19] C.-Y. Pan, C.-L. Tsai, and C.-H. Chu, "Fundamental movement skills in children diagnosed with autism spectrum disorders and attention deficit hyperactivity disorder," *Journal of Autism and Developmental Disorders*, vol. 39, no. 12, pp. 1694–1705, 2009.

[20] E. M. Jansiewicz, M. C. Goldberg, C. J. Newschaffer, M. B. Denckla, R. Landa, and S. H. Mostofsky, "Motor signs distinguish children with high functioning autism and Asperger's syndrome from controls," *Journal of Autism and Developmental Disorders*, vol. 36, no. 5, pp. 613–621, 2006.

[21] S. Sutera, J. Pandey, E. L. Esser et al., "Predictors of optimal outcome in toddlers diagnosed with autism spectrum disorders," *Journal of Autism and Developmental Disorders*, vol. 37, no. 1, pp. 98–107, 2007.

[22] R. Landa and E. Garrett-Mayer, "Development in infants with autism spectrum disorders: a prospective study," *Journal of Child Psychology and Psychiatry*, vol. 47, no. 6, pp. 629–638, 2006.

[23] J. E. Flanagan, R. Landa, A. Bhat, and M. Bauman, "Head lag in infants at risk for autism: a preliminary study," *The American Journal of Occupational Therapy*, vol. 66, no. 5, pp. 577–585, 2012.

[24] S. Ozonoff, S. Macari, G. S. Young, S. Goldring, M. Thompson, and S. J. Rogers, "Atypical object exploration at 12 months of age is associated with autism in a prospective sample," *Autism*, vol. 12, no. 5, pp. 457–472, 2008.

[25] G. Esposito, P. Venuti, S. Maestro, and F. Muratori, "An exploration of symmetry in early autism spectrum disorders: analysis of lying," *Brain and Development*, vol. 31, no. 2, pp. 131–138, 2009.

[26] R. W. Isenhower, K. L. Marsh, M. J. Richardson, M. Helt, R. C. Schmidt, and D. Fein, "Rhythmic bimanual coordination is impaired in young children with autism spectrum disorder," *Research in Autism Spectrum Disorders*, vol. 6, no. 1, pp. 25–31, 2012.

[27] J. L. Adrien, P. Lenoir, J. Martineau et al., "Blind ratings of early symptoms of autism based upon family home movies," *Journal of the American Academy of Child & Adolescent Psychiatry*, vol. 32, no. 3, pp. 617–626, 1993.

[28] P. Teitelbaum, O. Teitelbaum, J. Nye, J. Fryman, and R. G. Maurer, "Movement analysis in infancy may be useful for early diagnosis of autism," *Proceedings of the National Academy of Sciences of the United States of America*, vol. 95, no. 23, pp. 13982–13987, 1998.

[29] C. M. Freitag, C. Kleser, M. Schneider, and A. von Gontard, "Quantitative assessment of neuromotor function in adolescents with high functioning autism and Asperger syndrome," *Journal of Autism and Developmental Disorders*, vol. 37, no. 5, pp. 948–959, 2007.

[30] N. J. Minshew, K. Sung, B. L. Jones, and J. M. Furman, "Underdevelopment of the postural control system in autism," *Neurology*, vol. 63, no. 11, pp. 2056–2061, 2004.

[31] N. J. Rinehart, M. A. Bellgrove, B. J. Tonge, A. V. Brereton, D. Howells-Rankin, and J. L. Bradshaw, "An examination of movement kinematics in young people with high-functioning autism and Asperger's disorder: further evidence for a motor planning deficit," *Journal of Autism and Developmental Disorders*, vol. 36, no. 6, pp. 757–767, 2006.

[32] J. A. Vilensky, A. R. Damasio, and R. G. Maurer, "Gait disturbances in patients with autistic behavior: a preliminary study," *Archives of Neurology*, vol. 38, no. 10, pp. 646–649, 1981.

[33] S. L. Berkeley, L. L. Zittel, L. V. Pitney, and S. E. Nichols, "Locomotor and object control skills of children diagnosed with autism," *Adapted Physical Activity Quarterly*, vol. 18, no. 4, pp. 405–416, 2001.

[34] D. Green, G. Baird, A. L. Barnett, L. Henderson, J. Huber, and S. E. Henderson, "The severity and nature of motor impairment in Asperger's syndrome: a comparison with specific developmental disorder of motor function," *Journal of Child Psychology and Psychiatry and Allied Disciplines*, vol. 43, no. 5, pp. 655–668, 2002.

[35] M. Miyahara, M. Tsujii, M. Hori, K. Nakanishi, H. Kageyama, and T. Sugiyama, "Brief report: motor incoordination in children with Asperger syndrome and learning disabilities," *Journal of Autism and Developmental Disorders*, vol. 27, no. 5, pp. 595–603, 1997.

[36] L.-A. R. Sacrey, T. Germani, S. E. Bryson, and L. Zwaigenbaum, "Reaching and grasping in autism spectrum disorder: a review of recent literature," *Frontiers in Neurology*, vol. 5, article 6, 2014.

[37] A. Kushki, T. Chau, and E. Anagnostou, "Handwriting difficulties in children with autism spectrum disorders: a scoping review," *Journal of Autism and Developmental Disorders*, vol. 41, no. 12, pp. 1706–1716, 2011.

[38] C. T. Fuentes, S. H. Mostofsky, and A. J. Bastian, "Children with autism show specific handwriting impairments," *Neurology*, vol. 73, no. 19, pp. 1532–1537, 2009.

[39] S. Dickerson Mayes and S. L. Calhoun, "Ability profiles in children with autism: influence of age and IQ," *Autism*, vol. 7, no. 1, pp. 65–80, 2003.

[40] M. A. Dziuk, J. C. G. Larson, A. Apostu, E. M. Mahone, M. B. Denckla, and S. H. Mostofsky, "Dyspraxia in autism: association with motor, social, and communicative deficits," *Developmental Medicine & Child Neurology*, vol. 49, no. 10, pp. 734–739, 2007.

[41] S. Kopp, E. Beckung, and C. Gillberg, "Developmental coordination disorder and other motor control problems in girls with autism spectrum disorder and/or attention-deficit/hyperactivity disorder," *Research in Developmental Disabilities*, vol. 31, no. 2, pp. 350–361, 2010.

[42] A. Kleinspehn-Ammerlahn, M. Riediger, F. Schmiedek, T. von Oertzen, S.-C. Li, and U. Lindenberger, "Dyadic drumming across the lifespan reveals a zone of proximal development in children," *Developmental Psychology*, vol. 47, no. 3, pp. 632–644, 2011.

[43] C. Colombi, K. Liebal, M. Tomasello, G. Young, F. Warneken, and S. J. Rogers, "Examining correlates of cooperation in autism: imitation, joint attention, and understanding intentions," *Autism*, vol. 13, no. 2, pp. 143–163, 2009.

[44] K. L. Marsh, M. J. Richardson, and R. C. Schmidt, "Social connection through joint action and interpersonal coordination," *Topics in Cognitive Science*, vol. 1, no. 2, pp. 320–339, 2009.

[45] P. Fitzpatrick, R. Diorio, M. J. Richardson, and R. C. Schmidt, "Dynamical methods for evaluating the time-dependent unfolding of social coordination in children with autism," *Frontiers in Integrative Neuroscience*, vol. 7, article 21, 2013.

[46] A. McDuffie, L. Turner, W. Stone, P. Yoder, M. Wolery, and T. Ulman, "Developmental correlates of different types of motor

imitation in young children with autism spectrum disorders," *Journal of Autism and Developmental Disorders*, vol. 37, no. 3, pp. 401–412, 2007.

[47] N. I. Berger and B. Ingersoll, "An exploration of imitation recognition in young children with autism spectrum disorders," *Autism Research*, vol. 6, no. 5, pp. 411–416, 2013.

[48] T. Charman, J. Swettenham, S. Baron-Cohen, A. Cox, G. Baird, and A. Drew, "Infants with autism: an investigation of empathy, pretend play, joint attention, and imitation," *Developmental Psychology*, vol. 33, no. 5, pp. 781–789, 1997.

[49] W. L. Stone, O. Y. Ousley, and C. D. Littleford, "Motor imitation in young children with autism: what's the object?" *Journal of Abnormal Child Psychology*, vol. 25, no. 6, pp. 475–485, 1997.

[50] R. Bernier, G. Dawson, S. Webb, and M. Murias, "EEG mu rhythm and imitation impairments in individuals with autism spectrum disorder," *Brain and Cognition*, vol. 64, no. 3, pp. 228–237, 2007.

[51] S. Avikainen, A. Wohlschläger, S. Liuhanen, R. Hänninen, and R. Hari, "Impaired mirror-image imitation in Asperger and high-functioning autistic subjects," *Current Biology*, vol. 13, no. 4, pp. 339–341, 2003.

[52] A. N. Meltzoff and A. Gopnik, "The role of imitation in understanding persons and developing a theory of mind," in *Understanding Other Minds: Perspectives from Autism*, pp. 335–366, Oxford University Press, Oxford, UK, 1993.

[53] S. J. Rogers and B. F. Pennington, "A theoretical approach to the deficits in infantile autism," *Development and Psychopathology*, vol. 3, no. 2, pp. 137–162, 1991.

[54] I. M. Smith and S. E. Bryson, "Imitation and action in autism: a critical review," *Psychological Bulletin*, vol. 116, no. 2, pp. 259–273, 1994.

[55] J. H. G. Williams, A. Whiten, and T. Singh, "A systematic review of action imitation in autistic spectrum disorder," *Journal of Autism and Developmental Disorders*, vol. 34, no. 3, pp. 285–299, 2004.

[56] M. Vanvuchelen, H. Roeyers, and W. De Weerdt, "Nature of motor imitation problems in school-aged boys with autism: a motor or a cognitive problem?" *Autism*, vol. 11, no. 3, pp. 225–240, 2007.

[57] D. Dewey, M. Cantell, and S. G. Crawford, "Motor and gestural performance in children with autism spectrum disorders, developmental coordination disorder, and/or attention deficit hyperactivity disorder," *Journal of the International Neuropsychological Society*, vol. 13, no. 2, pp. 246–256, 2007.

[58] S. H. Mostofsky, P. Dubey, V. K. Jerath, E. M. Jansiewicz, M. C. Goldberg, and M. B. Denckla, "Developmental dyspraxia is not limited to imitation in children with autism spectrum disorders," *Journal of the International Neuropsychological Society*, vol. 12, no. 3, pp. 314–326, 2006.

[59] B. Ingersoll and K. Meyer, "Examination of correlates of different imitative functions in young children with autism spectrum disorders," *Research in Autism Spectrum Disorders*, vol. 5, no. 3, pp. 1078–1085, 2011.

[60] K. Toth, J. Munson, A. N. Meltzoff, and G. Dawson, "Early predictors of communication development in young children with autism spectrum disorder: joint attention, imitation, and toy play," *Journal of Autism and Developmental Disorders*, vol. 36, no. 8, pp. 993–1005, 2006.

[61] D. A. Zachor, T. Ilanit, and E. B. Itzchak, "Autism severity and motor abilities correlates of imitation situations in children with autism spectrum disorders," *Research in Autism Spectrum Disorders*, vol. 4, no. 3, pp. 438–443, 2010.

[62] B. Ingersoll and L. Schreibman, "Teaching reciprocal imitation skills to young children with autism using a naturalistic behavioral approach: effects on language, pretend play, and joint attention," *Journal of Autism and Developmental Disorders*, vol. 36, no. 4, pp. 487–505, 2006.

[63] R. J. Landa, K. C. Holman, A. H. O'Neill, and E. A. Stuart, "Intervention targeting development of socially synchronous engagement in toddlers with autism spectrum disorder: a randomized controlled trial," *Journal of Child Psychology and Psychiatry*, vol. 52, no. 1, pp. 13–21, 2011.

[64] E. G. Carr and M. Darcy, "Setting generality of peer modeling in children with autism," *Journal of Autism and Developmental Disorders*, vol. 20, no. 1, pp. 45–59, 1990.

[65] A. N. Garfinkle and I. S. Schwartz, "Peer imitation: increasing social interactions in children with autism and other developmental disabilities in inclusive preschool classrooms," *Topics in Early Childhood Special Education*, vol. 22, no. 1, pp. 26–38, 2002.

[66] M. H. Charlop-Christy, L. Le, and K. A. Freeman, "A comparison of video modeling with in vivo modeling for teaching children with autism," *Journal of Autism and Developmental Disorders*, vol. 30, no. 6, pp. 537–552, 2000.

[67] B. Ingersoll, "Brief report: pilot randomized controlled trial of reciprocal imitation training for teaching elicited and spontaneous imitation to children with autism," *Journal of Autism and Developmental Disorders*, vol. 40, no. 9, pp. 1154–1160, 2010.

[68] K. Simpson and D. Keen, "Music interventions for children with autism: narrative review of the literature," *Journal of Autism and Developmental Disorders*, vol. 41, no. 11, pp. 1507–1514, 2011.

[69] J. Whipple, "Music in intervention for children and adolescents with autism: a meta-analysis," *Journal of Music Therapy*, vol. 41, no. 2, pp. 90–106, 2004.

[70] J. J. Diehl, L. M. Schmitt, M. Villano, and C. R. Crowell, "The clinical use of robots for individuals with Autism Spectrum Disorders: a critical review," *Research in Autism Spectrum Disorders*, vol. 6, no. 1, pp. 249–262, 2012.

[71] P. Heaton, B. Hermelin, and L. Pring, "Can children with autistic spectrum disorders perceive affect in music? An experimental investigation," *Psychological Medicine*, vol. 29, no. 6, pp. 1405–1410, 1999.

[72] A. Bonnel, L. Mottron, I. Peretz, M. Trudel, E. Gallun, and A.-M. Bonnel, "Enhanced pitch sensitivity in individuals with autism: a signal detection analysis," *Journal of Cognitive Neuroscience*, vol. 15, no. 2, pp. 226–235, 2003.

[73] M. Geretsegger, C. Elefant, K. A. Mössler, and C. Gold, "Music therapy for people with autism spectrum disorder," *Cochrane Database of Systematic Reviews*, no. 6, Article ID CD004381, pp. 1–23, 2014.

[74] S. M. Srinivasan and A. N. Bhat, "A review of 'music and movement' therapies for children with autism: embodied interventions for multisystem development," *Frontiers in Integrative Neuroscience*, vol. 7, article 22, 2013.

[75] C. E. Stephens, "Spontaneous imitation by children with autism during a repetitive musical play routine," *Autism*, vol. 12, no. 6, pp. 645–671, 2008.

[76] E. M. Buday, "The effects of signed and spoken words taught with music on sign and speech imitation by children with autism," *Journal of Music Therapy*, vol. 32, no. 3, pp. 189–202, 1995.

[77] E. Deli, I. Bakle, and E. Zachopoulou, "Implementing intervention movement programs for kindergarten children," *Journal of Early Childhood Research*, vol. 4, no. 1, pp. 5–18, 2006.

[78] E. Zachopoulou, A. Tsapakidou, and V. Derri, "The effects of a developmentally appropriate music and movement program on motor performance," *Early Childhood Research Quarterly*, vol. 19, no. 4, pp. 631–642, 2004.

[79] V. Derri, A. Tsapakidou, E. Zachopoulou, and E. Kioumourtzoglou, "Effect of a music and movement programme on development of locomotor skills by children 4 to 6 years of age," *European Journal of Physical Education*, vol. 6, no. 1, pp. 16–25, 2001.

[80] M. Forgeard, E. Winner, A. Norton, and G. Schlaug, "Practicing a musical instrument in childhood is associated with enhanced verbal ability and nonverbal reasoning," *PLoS ONE*, vol. 3, no. 10, Article ID e3566, 2008.

[81] E. Costa-Giomi, "Does music instruction improve fine motor abilities?" *Annals of the New York Academy of Sciences*, vol. 1060, pp. 262–264, 2005.

[82] B. B. Scassellati, "How social robots will help us to diagnose, treat, and understand autism," in *Robotics Research: Results of the 12th International Symposium ISRR*, vol. 28 of *Springer Tracts in Advanced Robotics*, pp. 552–563, Springer, Berlin, Germany, 2007.

[83] B. Robins, K. Dautenhahn, R. Te Boekhorst, and A. Billard, "Robotic assistants in therapy and education of children with autism: can a small humanoid robot help encourage social interaction skills?" *Universal Access in the Information Society*, vol. 4, no. 2, pp. 105–120, 2005.

[84] A. Tapus, M. J. Mataric, and B. Scassellati, "Socially assistive robotics [Grand Challenges of Robotics]," *IEEE Robotics & Automation Magazine*, vol. 14, no. 1, pp. 35–42, 2007.

[85] A. Duquette, F. Michaud, and H. Mercier, "Exploring the use of a mobile robot as an imitation agent with children with low-functioning autism," *Autonomous Robots*, vol. 24, no. 2, pp. 147–157, 2008.

[86] B. Robins, K. Dautenhahn, R. te Boekhorst, and A. Billard, "Effects of repeated exposure to a humanoid robot on children with autism," in *Universal Access and Assistive Technology*, Springer, Cambrige, UK, 2004.

[87] I. Fujimoto, T. Matsumoto, P. R. De Silva, M. Kobayashi, and M. Higashi, "Mimicking and evaluating human motion to improve the imitation skill of children with autism through a robot," *International Journal of Social Robotics*, vol. 3, no. 4, pp. 349–357, 2011.

[88] H. Kozima, C. Nakagawa, and Y. Yasuda, "Children-robot interaction: a pilot study in autism therapy," *Progress in Brain Research*, vol. 164, pp. 385–400, 2007.

[89] B. Robins, K. Dautenhahn, and P. Dickerson, "From isolation to communication: a case study evaluation of robot assisted play for children with autism with a minimally expressive humanoid robot," in *Proceedings of the 2nd International Conferences on Advances in Computer-Human Interactions (ACHI '09)*, pp. 205–211, IEEE, Cancún, Mexico, February 2009.

[90] B. Scassellati, H. Admoni, and M. Matarić, "Robots for use in autism research," *Annual Review of Biomedical Engineering*, vol. 14, no. 1, pp. 275–294, 2012.

[91] S. M. Srinivasan, K. A. Lynch, D. J. Bubela, T. D. Gifford, and A. N. Bhat, "Effect of interactions between a child and a robot on the imitation and praxis performance of typically devloping children and a child with autism: a preliminary study," *Perceptual and Motor Skills*, vol. 116, no. 3, pp. 885–904, 2013.

[92] M. Kaur, T. Gifford, K. L. Marsh, and A. Bhat, "Effect of robot-child interactions on bilateral coordination skills of typically developing children and a child with autism spectrum disorder: a preliminary study," *Journal of Motor Learning and Development*, vol. 1, no. 2, pp. 31–37, 2013.

[93] R. Bruininks and B. Bruininks, *Bruininks-Oseretsky Test of Motor Proficiency Second Edition (BOT2)*, AGS Publishing, Circle Pines, Minn, USA, 2005.

[94] M. Rutter, A. Bailey, and C. Lord, *The Social Communication Questionnaire: Manual*, Western Psychological Services, 2003.

[95] C. Lord, M. Rutter, P. C. DiLavore, S. Risi, K. Gotham, and S. L. Bishop, *Autism Diagnostic Observation Schedule, Second Edition (ADOS-2) Manual (Part 1): Modules 1–4*, Western Psychological Services, Torrance, Calif, USA, 2012.

[96] A. Hollingshead, *Four Factor Index of Social Status*, Yale University, New Haven, Conn, USA, 1975.

[97] S. S. Sparrow, D. V. Cicchetti, and D. A. Balla, *The Vineland Adaptive Behavior Scales*, Springer, 2005.

[98] S. E. Henderson, D. A. Sugden, and A. L. Barnett, *Movement Assessment Battery for Children-2: Movement ABC-2: Examiner's Manual*, Pearson, 2007.

[99] O. I. Lovaas, "Behavioral treatment and normal educational and intellectual functioning in young autistic children," *Journal of Consulting and Clinical Psychology*, vol. 55, no. 1, pp. 3–9, 1987.

[100] G. B. Mesibov, V. Shea, and E. Schopler, *The TEACCH Approach to Autism Spectrum Disorders*, Springer, New York, NY, USA, 2004.

[101] A. Bondy and A. Frost, "Communication strategies for visual learners," in *Teaching Individuals with Developmental Delays: Basic Intervention Techniques*, O. I. Lovaas, Ed., pp. 291–304, PRO-ED, Austin, Tex, USA, 2003.

[102] D. Dewey, "Error analysis of limb and orofacial praxis in children with developmental motor deficits," *Brain and Cognition*, vol. 23, no. 2, pp. 203–221, 1993.

[103] L. V. Hedges, "Distribution theory for Glass's estimator of effect size and related estimators," *Journal of Educational and Behavioral Statistics*, vol. 6, no. 2, pp. 107–128, 1981.

[104] E. Costa-Giomi, "Effects of three years of piano instruction on children's academic achievement, school performance and self-esteem," *Psychology of Music*, vol. 32, no. 2, pp. 139–152, 2004.

[105] I. Hurwitz, P. H. Wolff, B. D. Bortnick, and K. Kokas, "Nonmusicol effects of the Kodaly music curriculum in primary grade children," *Journal of Learning Disabilities*, vol. 8, no. 3, pp. 167–174, 1975.

[106] J. Brown, C. Sherrill, and B. Gench, "Effects of an integrated physical education/music program in changing early childhood perceptual-motor performance," *Perceptual and Motor Skills*, vol. 53, no. 1, pp. 151–154, 1981.

[107] B. Ulrich and D. Ulrich, "The role of balancing ability in performance of fundamental motor skills in 3-, 4-, 5-year-old children," *Motor Development: Current Selected Research*, vol. 1, pp. 87–97, 1985.

[108] S. Kirschner and M. Tomasello, "Joint drumming: social context facilitates synchronization in preschool children," *Journal of Experimental Child Psychology*, vol. 102, no. 3, pp. 299–314, 2009.

[109] S. Kirschner and M. Tomasello, "Joint music making promotes prosocial behavior in 4-year-old children," *Evolution and Human Behavior*, vol. 31, no. 5, pp. 354–364, 2010.

[110] A. C. Pierno, M. Mari, D. Lusher, and U. Castiello, "Robotic movement elicits visuomotor priming in children with autism," *Neuropsychologia*, vol. 46, no. 2, pp. 448–454, 2008.

[111] D. Hanson, D. Mazzei, C. Garver et al., "Realistic humanlike robots for treatment of ASD, social training, and research;

shown to appeal to youths with ASD, cause physiological arousal, and increase human-to-human social engagement," in *Proceedings of the 5th ACM International Conference on Pervasive Technologies Related to Assistive Environments (PETRA '12)*, Heraklion, Greece, June 2012.

[112] G. Pioggia, R. Igliozzi, M. L. Sica et al., "Exploring emotional and imitational android-based interactions in autistic spectrum disorders," *Journal of Cyber Therapy & Rehabilitation*, vol. 1, no. 1, pp. 49–61, 2008.

[113] J. Case-Smith and H. Miller, "Occupational therapy with children with pervasive developmental disorders," *American Journal of Occupational Therapy*, vol. 53, no. 5, pp. 506–513, 1999.

[114] D. Reid, T. Chiu, G. Sinclair, S. Wehrmann, and Z. Naseer, "Outcomes of an occupational therapy school-based consultation service for students with fine motor difficulties," *Canadian Journal of Occupational Therapy*, vol. 73, no. 4, pp. 215–224, 2006.

[115] J. Case-Smith, "Effectiveness of school-based occupational therapy intervention on handwriting," *American Journal of Occupational Therapy*, vol. 56, no. 1, pp. 17–25, 2002.

[116] K. McHale and S. A. Cermak, "Fine motor activities in elementary school: preliminary findings and provisional implications for children with fine motor problems," *American Journal of Occupational Therapy*, vol. 46, no. 10, pp. 898–903, 1992.

[117] H. L. Dankert, P. L. Davies, and W. J. Gavin, "Occupational therapy effects on visual-motor skills in preschool children," *American Journal of Occupational Therapy*, vol. 57, no. 5, pp. 542–549, 2003.

[118] C. Hilton, L. Wente, P. LaVesser, M. Ito, C. Reed, and G. Herzberg, "Relationship between motor skill impairment and severity in children with Asperger syndrome," *Research in Autism Spectrum Disorders*, vol. 1, no. 4, pp. 339–349, 2007.

10

Epigenetics and Autism

Tafari Mbadiwe and Richard M. Millis

Department of Physiology & Biophysics, The Howard University College of Medicine, Washington, DC 20059, USA

Correspondence should be addressed to Richard M. Millis; rickmillis@aol.com

Academic Editor: Jean-Louis Adrien

This review identifies mechanisms for altering DNA-histone interactions of cell chromatin to upregulate or downregulate gene expression that could serve as epigenetic targets for therapeutic interventions in autism. DNA methyltransferases (DNMTs) can phosphorylate histone H3 at T6. Aided by protein kinase Cβ1, the DNMT lysine-specific demethylase-1 prevents demethylation of H3 at K4. During androgen-receptor-(AR-) dependent gene activation, this sequence may produce AR-dependent gene overactivation which may partly explain the male predominance of autism. AR-dependent gene overactivation in conjunction with a DNMT mechanism for methylating oxytocin receptors could produce high arousal inputs to the amygdala resulting in aberrant socialization, a prime characteristic of autism. Dysregulation of histone methyltransferases and histone deacetylases (HDACs) associated with low activity of methyl CpG binding protein-2 at cytosine-guanine sites in genes may reduce the capacity for condensing chromatin and silencing genes in frontal cortex, a site characterized by decreased cortical interconnectivity in autistic subjects. HDAC1 inhibition can overactivate mRNA transcription, a putative mechanism for the increased number of cerebral cortical columns and local frontal cortex hyperactivity in autistic individuals. These epigenetic mechanisms underlying male predominance, aberrant social interaction, and low functioning frontal cortex may be novel targets for autism prevention and treatment strategies.

1. Introduction

Autism spectrum disorders (ASDs) are a range of neurodevelopmental disorders typically characterized by repetitive and stereotyped behavior, limited social development, and impaired language skills. Autistic disorder, Asperger syndrome, and pervasive development disorder not otherwise specified (PDD-NOS) are the most commonly diagnosed ASDs and there are also a large number of cases that are considered idiopathic because the etiology is unclear [1]. Notably, the incidence of ASD diagnoses has increased substantially in the past twenty years, growing by as much as 5- or 10-fold, although, the approximate 4 : 1 ratio of affected males to female has been maintained [2]. Some of this increase has been driven by shifting diagnostic criteria, heightened awareness, and improved diagnostic techniques [3]. However, some of this increase could be attributable to an authentic increase in the frequency of ASDs. The identity of the factors fueling this increase remains somewhat elusive and the precise causes of ASD diagnoses remain unknown [4]. Although its basis is thought to be multifactorial, autism is known to be a highly heritable disorder [5]. To a certain extent, the observed inheritance patterns can be explained by typical genetic processes but, especially in light of studies noting discordance among monozygotic twins, this is unlikely to be the whole story [6]. Recently, the idea that epigenetic influences may be partly responsible for the development of ASDs in many patients has gained popularity.

Epigenetics refers to processes, notably the methylation of genes and modification of histones, that affect gene expression without altering the genetic code; a related term, epigenomics, concerns the study of the epigenome, which is a catalog of the heritable chemical changes made to DNA and histones. The effects of environment on phenotype are generally mediated through epigenetic processes [7]. Typical epigenetic mechanisms include the formation of 5-methylcytosine and acetylation of histones, thereby modifying the chromatin [8]. These epigenetic mechanisms can result in the silencing of particular genes and will ultimately impact the expressed phenotype [9]. Each individual's unique epigenome—the genome plus any epigenetic modifications—develops as a consequence of a variety of factors. The first, and probably most important, is the various effects exerted by the environment on the epigenome [10]. Second, the epigenome is itself heritable; a mother, for instance, can pass a methylated gene to her offspring [11]. Third, the epigenome—much like the genome—is subject to replication errors; however, whereas the typical error rate for gene replication is 1 : 1,000,000, the usual error rate for replicating epigenetic elements is closer to 1 : 1,000 [12]. Fourth, spontaneous changes to the epigenome, apart from changes driven by environmental causes, are thought to occur, known as epigenetic drift [13]. The latter two elements account for the stochastic nature of the epigenome that is the tendency of epigenomes to diverge despite having identical starting conditions.

This review examines the current state of knowledge concerning the impact of epigenetic mechanisms of the development of ASD and is organized in the following sections.

2. Epigenetic Protein-DNA Interactions: Proteins Mediating Epigenetic Signaling

2.1. MeCP2. Methyl CpG binding protein 2 (MeCP2) is active in CNS regulation and development of synaptic contacts [14]. MeCP2 is known to be involved in gene silencing and as a consequence in its role epigenetic regulation has been the focus of a significant amount of investigation [15]. The MeCP2 gene is located on the q arm of the X chromosome. Since the MeCP2 gene is located on the X chromosome, it is X-linked and subject to X inactivation. Until recently, it was widely thought that MeCP2 was only responsible for the silencing of genes [16]. However, gene silencing is inconsistent with the mode of action of the MeCP2 protein product. Like other members of the methyl-CpG binding domain (MBD) family, MeCP2 binds to methylated DNA [17] and, after binding, MeCP2 forms a complex with the enzyme histone deacetylase 1 (HDAC1) that removes acetyl groups from histones, thereby causing the chromatin structure to condense. The condensation of the chromatin is critical to gene inactivation. However, recent investigations suggest that MeCP2 may also be capable of acting as an activator of a variety of genes [18]. Although the mechanism of this activating action is not totally clear, the dual functionality of MeCP2 is amply demonstrated by studies showing that 63% of MeCP2-bound promoters are actively expressed [17]. It is not clear whether the role of MeCP2 in the epigenetic regulation of autism is related to its role as a gene silencer or promoter. Nevertheless, a correlation between reduced expression of MeCP2 and ASD is noted.

Using immunofluorescence, Nagarajan et al. quantified MeCP2 in the frontal cortex (Brodmann area 9) and fusiform gyrus (Brodmann area 37) [19]. The frontal cortex had previously been linked to autism and associated with high levels of MeCP2 expression, whereas the fusiform gyrus is associated with face processing [20, 21]. MeCP2 expression at these brain sites was measured for 14 autistic brains, each of which was compared to three age-matched controls. In 11 of the 14 cases, the autism brain samples showed significantly decreased MeCP2 expression compared to age-matched controls; in some cases the reduction was as much as twofold. Similarly, the proportion of cells that expressed high levels of MeCP2 was reduced in 11 out of the 14 autistic samples. Of the six fusiform gyrus samples examined by Nagarajan et al., five showed decreased expression of MeCP2 in the fusiform cortex and each of those five were among the samples that exhibited decreased MeCP2 expression in the frontal cortex. This concordance suggests that whatever is responsible for decreased MeCP2 expression in the brains of ASD subjects is likely exerting a generalized, nonlocalized effect. The autism patients whose brains were examined by Nagarajan et al. were classified as idiopathic, indicating that there was no known genetic cause for their ASD or for the decreased MeCP2 expression that appears to be linked to the ASD. Epigenetic regulation might help explain these findings. In order to test for methylation of the promoter region associated with the MeCP2 gene, Nagarajan et al. conducted bisulfite sequencing. The MeCP2 is on the X chromosome, and all the study subjects were males and, thus, actively expressing the X chromosome. Methylation of the 5′ portion of the MeCP2 regulatory region was observed for most autism samples and the autism group showed a statistically significant increase in methylation when compared to similarly aged control group samples. As expected, an inverse correlation was found between promoter region methylation and MeCP2 expression. These findings suggest that aberrant methylation may have resulted in decreased expression of MeCP2, which was associated with autism. It is also worth noting that there is a well-established relationship between MeCP2 defects and Rett syndrome (Rett is definitively diagnosed by evidence of such a defect) since, from a clinical standpoint, Rett is classified as an ASD.

3. Epigenetic DNA-Protein Interactions

3.1. Protein Kinase C Beta. Recent evidence suggests that a correlation exists between downregulation of the protein kinase C beta gene (PRKCB1) in the temporal lobe and ASDs [22]. In particular, this association appears to be linked to the alternative splicing of PRKCB1 isozymes fsI and betaII. In addition, PRKCB1 haplotypes are (statistically) significantly associated with autism. Moreover, whole genome expression analysis showed less coordinated expression of PKCB1-driven genes [22]. Phosphorylation of histone H3 at threonine 6 (H3T6) by protein kinase c beta-1 protein appears to prevent lysine-specific demethylase 1 (LSD1) from demethylating H3K4 during androgen receptor-dependent gene activation [23]. This finding may partly explain the male predominance of ASDs and might support the hypothesis that the higher fetal androgen levels in males than females produce greater arousal inputs to the amygdala which might sensitize boys to environmental stressors. Girls lack such androgen-facilitated arousal inputs to the amygdala and are protected from such high arousal inputs by estrogens, oxytocin, and the oxytocin receptor [24]. A role for an oxytocin receptor polymorphism in

ASDs is also reported in Chinese and Japanese cohorts [25, 26] and dysregulation of DNA methylation in the promoter region of the oxytocin receptor gene has been observed after acute psychosocial stress in an elderly German cohort [27].

3.2. Oxytocin Receptor. Epigenetic regulation of the oxytocin receptor gene (OXTR) has been implicated in the etiology of ASDs [28]. Oxytocin, along with vasopressin, has also been determined to have a prosocial function [29]. Insel was the first to suggest a link between oxytocin and ASDs [30]. Some evidence for this link comes from animal studies. *OXTR* and oxytocin-knockout mice have been shown to have limited social memory and a diminished ability to recognize other individuals, both of which are common ASD symptoms [31, 32]. Interestingly, the effect of OXTR-knockout on social functioning is thought to be sex-specific; both developmental compensation and the effects of vasopressin have been posited as possible explanations for the normal social development in female OXTR knockout mice [33]. These findings suggest that any defect of the oxytocin pathway, including a deficiency of oxytocin receptors, may in some cases contribute to the development of ASDs. A diminished number of oxytocin receptors can have a variety of causes, including both genomic and epigenetic. A study by Gregory et al. looked at a family in which the mother had a hemizygous deletion of the OXTR gene, which she passed down to one of her sons, but not the other; however, both sons were diagnosed with autism [34]. Kimura et al. hypothesized that the promoter region of the OXTR gene of the affected sibling without the deletion was hypermethylated. Prior studies had identified two CpG island regions of the OXTR gene that, as a consequence of variable methylation, are reported to be associated with differential OXTR expression in liver and myometrium [35]. The first CpG island overlaps with exons 1, 2, and 3 of OXTR gene and the second CpG island was localized to the third intron. The second CpG island, within intron 3, was found to be heavily methylated in all three family members studied, the mother and her two affected sons. On the other hand, the other CpG island—overlapping exons 1, 2, and 3—was methylated differently in each of the family members; specifically, the affected sibling without the deletion showed significantly more methylation than his brother or mother at three sites within the intron. This hypermethylation occurred at locations that have previously been shown to impact OXTR expression. Since both siblings were autistic, even though one had a genomic deletion and the other displayed hypermethylated promoter regions, the Gregory et al. study stands as an elegant demonstration of the idea that epigenetic and genetic mechanisms can have equivalent effects on phenotype. The Gregory et al. study went one step further in an attempt to demonstrate that OXTR gene silencing is not unique to the highlighted case and is, in fact, a common contributor to autism. Five differentially methylated CpG islands were examined in a group of 20 autistic and 20 phenotypically normal individuals and, as expected, the autism group showed a statistically significantly higher level of methylation at several examined loci. These observations were made in samples of both blood and cerebral cortex. Additionally, low levels of OXTR expression were found to be associated with increased methylation at a statistically significant level. This finding strengthens the idea that promoter region methylation causes gene silencing. Moreover, when the data were stratified by sex, two of the loci showed significant differences in methylation for males only, thereby implying that the different frequencies of autism in males and females might be driven by epigenetic mechanisms.

3.3. Bcl-2. Bcl-2 (B-cell lymphoma 2) is a protein responsible for the regulation of apoptosis [36]. The *Bcl-2* gene has been implicated in the etiology of several cancers and the abnormal expression of the gene has also been linked to diseases with social impacts such as schizophrenia and autism [37]. The Bcl-2 protein is reported to be decreased in both the cerebellum and frontal cortex of autistic subjects compared to age and gender-matched controls [38, 39].

Evidence linking *Bcl-2* gene expression to the development of ASD is still being assembled and thus the extent to which a causative relationship exists remains largely a matter of speculation. That said, a study by Nguyen et al. [40] examining lymphoblastoid cell lines from sets of monozygotic twins that were discordant for autism, and also comparing the twins' cell lines to those of their nonautistic, nontwin siblings, provides a basis for preliminary discussion.

3.4. RORA. The proposition that epigenetic regulation of the retinoic acid-related orphan receptor alpha (RORA) might cause autism is relatively new. Although the functions of RORA are largely unknown, RORA regulation of circadian rhythm and neuroprotection against oxidative stress and inflammation is reported [41, 42]. A link between RORA and autism makes intuitive sense because autism is thought to be associated with increased levels of oxidative stress and inflammation [43, 44]. The Nguyen et al. study was the first to give scientific grounding to this intuition by noting that—as was the case with Bcl-2—there were statistically significant differences in both RORA gene promoter region methylation and protein product expression between autistic subjects and their (non-twin) unaffected siblings [40]. This was the case in both lympoblastoid cell line and postmortem brain tissue. Interestingly, when the population was stratified by the various ASD subtypes, it turned out that reduced RORA expression was only observed in ASD subjects with severe language impairment. As a consequence, reduced RORA expression was not observed in all ASD subjects. The notion that RORA methylation might be largely responsible for the language deficits sometimes associated with ASD is a useful finding that helps clarify the etiology of autism and an important first step in determining the particular mechanism responsible for these symphtoms. Moreover, the connection between promoter region methylation and RORA expression was confirmed by treatment with global inhibition of methylation using 5-Aza, which increased gene expression in autistic subjects, but not in unaffected subjects. However, as with Bcl-2, the effects of 5-Aza on undiagnosed cotwins and unaffected subjects were not found to be statistically significant. This finding must be interpreted cautiously because there could be a variety of possible explanations.

3.5. β-Catenin. The β-catenin gene has been the subject of much investigation related to its potential as an oncogene but it can also act as the fulcrum in at least two relevant epigenetic processes related to the development of ASD. One epigenetic process of β-catenin involves estrogens. Estrogens are critical players in the sexual differentiation of the brain and it is likely that brain estrogen levels are increased in autistic subjects [45]. Estrogens, being steroid hormones, and their receptors—including estrogen receptor alpha (ERα)—are located in the nucleus and in the cytosol of target cells. One of the targets of cytosolic ERα is GSK3B, which is known to form a complex with β-catenin for degradation of β-catenin. ERα activation by estradiol is reported to release β-catenin from this complex, thereby increasing β-catenin availability [46]. An increase in the cytosolic concentration of estrogens is thought to result in increases in cytosolic and nuclear β-catenin during critical periods of prenatal and/or neonatal development wherein β-catenin binding to the LEC/TCF promoter has positive effects on Wnt pathway gene transcription. Such increased transcription in the Wnt pathway is strongly associated with the development of ASDs. The effect of ERα in this process is to cause the dissociation of β-catenin from a complex whose integral members include the proteins GSK3β, axin, and adenomatous polyposis coli tumor suppressor (APC). GSK3β, axin, and APC are negative regulators of the Wnt signaling pathway and the complex requires all of these constituents to initiate the destruction of β-catenin. The absence or downregulation of any of these components may increase the availability of cytosolic β-catenin, as well as in the various knockin effects discussed previously—increased nuclear β-catenin with greater Wnt pathway transcription. Lithium, used mostly as a mood stabilizing drug, exerts an inhibitory effect on GSK3β both directly and indirectly, by interrupting the dephosphorylation of phospo-GSK3β [47]. In either case, the effect is the same, and also the same as that of increased estrogen levels; that is, the complex responsible for initiating the degradation of β-catenin is made nonfunctional, and the concentration of cytosolic β-catenin increases.

3.6. The Neurexin-Neuroligin Pathway. SHANK3 is a scaffolding protein in the neurexin-neuroligin pathway that interacts with synaptic proteins. Recent research suggests that copy number variations or mutations of either of these proteins may be associated with the development of ASDs [48]. It appears that epigenetic mechanisms are used to control the expression of this gene. For instance, Beri et al. identified five CpG islands in the SHANK3 gene, the posttranslational methylation of which determines gene expression [49]. One specific locus—CpG island 2—appeared to particularly impact tissue SHANK expression. Further more, taking advantage of the fact that the SHANK3 gene is well conserved between humans and rodents, Uchino and Waga demonstrated that the neonatal expression of certain SHANK3 transcripts in mice temporarily decreases as the methylation of CpG island 2 peaks two weeks after birth [50]. This suggests that the expression of SHANK3 (and thus its effect on the development of ASD) is regulated by epigenetic mechanisms, though this connection has yet to be directly established in humans. Additionally, two genes responsible for the production of cell adhesion molecules in this pathway, NLGN3 and NLGN4, have also been associated with the development of ASD [48]. However, to date, epigenetic regulation of this gene is still unproven [51].

4. Role of Maternal Hypomethylation in Autism

Thus far, discussion of the contribution made by epigenetic mechanisms to the development of ASDs has focused on the genes and proteins of autistic patients. There is good reason for this. ASDs are known to possess a variety of genetic determinants, so investigations into the effects of gene silencing or promotion naturally focus on the silencing or promotion of the genes of the patient. However, epigenetic mechanisms do not exert their influence only by mechanisms of gene manipulation. For example, epigenetic influences on the maternal genome could alter the intrauterine environment such that the probability of the offspring developing ASDs is increased or decreased. DNA hypomethylation linked to variants in the maternal folate pathway has been linked to aberrant fetal development [52, 53]. Also, and more importantly, folate is the primary one carbon donor critical for methylation reactions. Because epigenetic mechanisms typically exert their influences by methylation of DNA, investigation of the folate pathway should provide insight into the availability of methylation precursors and also the extent of genomic methylation in mothers of both their autistic and their unaffected children.

A study by James et al. was performed, in part, to bolster the findings that mothers of autistic children often presented with aberrant DNA methylation [54]. Mothers of autistic children exhibited significantly lower levels of methylfolate and methionine—essential precursors for DNA methylation—than their counterparts in the control group. In addition, levels of the methylation-inhibiting proteins S-adenosylmethionine, adenosine, and homocysteine were all elevated in autism mothers. S-adenosylmethionine (SAM) is the primary methyl donor for the DNA methyltransferase reaction, which produces S-adenosylhomocysteine (SAH) and methylated DNA. Because SAM and SAH are linked by the transferase reaction, the SAM/SAH ratio is generally considered to be a good indicator of DNA methylation potential. Mothers of autistic children displayed a lower SAM/SAH ratio than the control group, which is indicative of a diminished capacity for methylation. Going one step further, in addition to having a lower capacity for methylation, the DNA of autism mothers is in fact less methylated than that of mothers of unaffected children; the ratio of 5-methylcytosine to total cytosine—a measure of overall genomic methylation—was significantly lower in the mothers of autistic children. Taken together, this evidence strongly suggests that hypomethylation of maternal DNA may be linked to ASDs. The significance of these findings about the influences of epigenetics on the development of autism is not entirely clear. However, it is not even clear that what is being observed is the effect of epigenetics. For example, although the ratio of 5-methycytosine to total cytosine was statistically correlated to the SAM/SAH ratio, it was more closely linked to the presence of an uncommon recessive allele in the gene that codes for reduced folate carrier protein. It is generally assumed that genes subjected to an atypical level of methylation are manifesting the effects of epigenetic influences. However, for this particular case of the SAM/SAH ratio, this assumption should be questioned. If, as the correlation data suggest, the differential methylation exhibited by mothers of autistic children is largely a consequence of a genetic polymorphism, then it is not likely to be epigenetics at work. If intrauterine conditions are altered by maternal hypomethylation, such changed conditions must impact fetal development pathways by specific mechanisms that remain to be elucidated.

5. Epigenetics and Nutritional Factors in Autism

The period of development in which the nutritional imbalance occurs is very important in determining which disease-related genes will be affected. Different organs have critical developmental stages, and the time point at which they are compromised will predispose individuals to specific diseases. Epigenetic modifications that occur during development may not be expressed until later in life depending on the function of the gene. While the majority of studies implicate prenatal periods as critical time windows, some research has shown that nutritional intake during adulthood can also affect the epigenome.

Genetic polymorphisms of cytochrome P450 enzymes have been linked to ASD, specifically the cytochrome P450 family 27 subfamily B gene (CYP27B1) that is essential for proper vitamin D metabolism. Epigenetic regulation of cytochrome P450 genes for hydroxylation and activation of vitamin D in has been shown in prostate cancer cells [55]. Vitamin D is important for neuronal growth and neurodevelopment, and defects in metabolism or deficiency have also been implicated in ASDs [56]. Mutations of MeCP2 associated with impaired methylation are known to be associated with ASDs and the related neurological disorder, Rett syndrome. One component of Rett syndrome is abnormal bone formation wherein abnormal vitamin D metabolism is associated with epigenetic dysregulation of cytochrome P450 genes [57] which could be a conceptual model for epigenetic interactions between MeCP2, vitamin D, and cytochrome P450 genes [56]. Abnormal folic acid metabolism may also play a role in the decreased capacity for methylation and DNA hypomethylation associated with significantly greater than normal levels of plasma homocysteine, adenosine, and SAH in mothers of subjects diagnosed with ASDs [58]. Changes in autism-related behaviors are reported to be strongly associated with vitamin-supplementation associated changes in plasma levels of biotin and vitamin K [59] and although biotin is a known cofactor in bioavailability of methyl groups for DNA methylation, a vitamin-K-related epigenetic mechanism has not been described.

6. Epigenetics and Toxic Factors in Autism

6.1. Valproic Acid. Valproic acid (VPA) is a therapeutic anticonvulsant and mood stabilizing drug that gained attention in the 1980s as a potential teratogen. VPA exposure is highly correlated with autism; as many as 60% of infants who exhibit the suite of symptoms associated with VPA teratogenicity also display two or more autistic characteristics [60]. Autism has also been shown to occur in 9% of cases of prenatal exposure to VPA [61]. The mechanisms underlying the pharmacological actions of VPA are also suggestive of a correlation between VPA and autism [62]. VPA is responsible for inhibiting two enzymes: myo-inositol-1-phosphate (MIP) synthase and the class 1 and 2 histone deacetylase (HDAC). HDAC1 is an important inhibitor of DNA transcription that works by associating with the LEC/TCF transcription factor. When HDAC1 is removed from the LEC/TCF complex, it leaves behind a primed (but inactive) promoter of gene transcription. The primed promoter then forms a complex with β-catenin, thus activating the promoter and increasing transcriptions rates of a variety of genes in the Wnt signaling pathway including cyclin D1, required for the transition from the G1 to S phases of mitosis, and MYC, a transcription enhancer for many genes throughout the genome [63]. Accordingly, the consequence of VPA-mediated inhibition of HDAC1 is to upregulate the transcription of Wnt pathway genes. In addition, VPA increases cellular levels of β-catenin, presumably in response to the increased availability of primed LEC/TCF promoters [64]. The effect of VPA on Wnt gene transcription is well understood but fails to explain the connection between VPA and autism. In order to complete this link, an increase in the number of neocortical minicolumns is highly correlated with autism [65]. This observation is supported by fMRI studies that report differences in how autism brains coordinate the processing of information [66]. It is reasonable to assume that processes which upregulate genes of the Wnt signaling pathway—such as prenatal exposure to VPA—may result in poorly regulated mitosis and cellular proliferation, one manifestation of which could be an increase in the number of neocortical minicolumns and macrocephaly. This mechanism has been observed at work in a slightly different context. Recall that MeCP2 inactivates genes by forming complexes with a variety of different molecules. One of these molecules is HDAC1 [67] and in the absence of HDAC1, or even if HDAC1 has merely been downregulated, the gene inactivating properties of MeCP2 is expected to have a diminished effect. One of the promoters on which MeCP2 typically exerts its regulatory effect is the LEC/TCF promoter, which, as mentioned previously, ultimately regulates the transcription rates of the Wnt signaling pathway. Although MeCP2 has effects on gene methylation, the function of HDAC1 concerns acetylation of histones. However, to transcriptionally deactivate genes, they must often be both

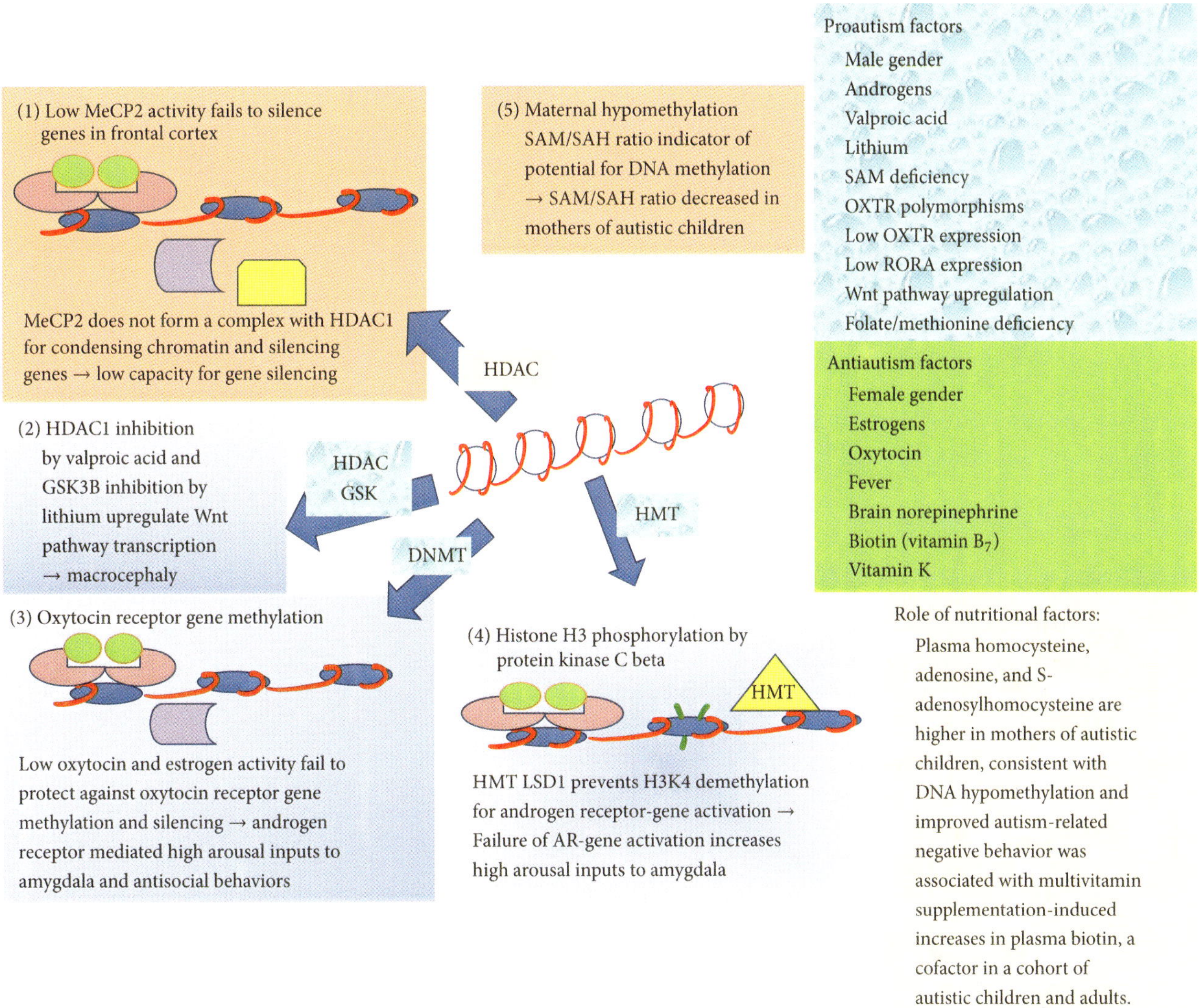

FIGURE 1: Main mechanisms of epigenetic alterations in autism. Each alteration involves many enzymes but the main players to cause methylation or acetylation are shown by arrows. These are not separate mechanisms and the enzymes do not act alone. Several enzymes act at a promoter simultaneously. (1) Low methyl CpG binding protein-2 (MeCP2) at CpG islands of frontal cortex reduces capacity for complexing with histone deacetylase 1 (HDAC1) for gene silencing. (2) HDAC1 inhibition by valproic acid exposure and glycogen synthetase kinase-3B (GSK3B) inhibition by lithium upregulate Wnt signaling pathway and activate transcription, associated with macrocephaly with increased number of cerebral cortical column. (3) DNA methyltransferase (DNMT) methylates oxytocin receptor gene produces low oxytocin and estrogen activity necessary for androgen receptor mediated high-arousal inputs to amygdala. (4) Histone H3 phosphorylation by protein kinase C beta activates the histone methyltransferase (HMT) lysine demethylase 1 (LSD1) which prevents demethylation of lysine-4 site of histone-3 (H3K4) that is also necessary for androgen receptor (AR) mediation of high arousal inputs to amygdala. (5) Maternal hypomethylation by dietary folic acid deficiency decreases availability of S-adenosyl methionine (SAM), associated with abnormal intrauterine growth.

methylated and deacetylated. Thus, VPA-induced inhibition of HDAC1 interferes with the functionality of MeCP2 which appears to increase the risk of developing ASDs.

7. Epigenetics and Other Illnesses Associated with Autism

Epigenetic effects may also manifest through aberrant methylation patterns of imprinted genes. The expression of imprinted genes, which are mostly found in clusters on chromosomes 6, 7, 11, 14, and 15, is controlled by a series of epigenetic marks (DNA methylation and histone modification). Imprinting defects may be primary or secondary. Primary imprinting defects cause changes in methylation patterns but leave the DNA sequences unaltered and thus may be classified as an epigenetic mechanism [68]. Angelman syndrome, which is caused by an absence of active maternal genes in the 15q11-1q13 region, may result from a primary imprinting defect (though the syndrome is more commonly caused by a deletion on the maternal chromosome or a paternal uniparental disomy). There is some basis to suspect a link between Angelman syndrome and ASDs. For instance, a study by Steffenburg et al. sought to ascertain the frequency of ASDs among children diagnosed with Angelman syndrome [69]. The study screened a series of mentally retarded children for Angelman syndrome and subsequently evaluated the children with Angelman syndrome for evidence of autism. Four out of the approximately 49,000 screened children were diagnosed with Angelman syndrome, and each of those four were found to demonstrate autistic behaviors. However, other studies place the rate of cooccurrence of ASDs and Angelman syndrome at a rate of as low as 2%. Taken together, it seems reasonable to assert that, to the extent that Angelman syndrome and ASDs are linked, the condition of some percentage of these patients will be related to an epigenetic primary imprinting defect. That said, the available evidence does not establish whether the epigenetic defect causing Angelman syndrome leads directly to autistic symptoms or if instead the relationship between Angelman syndrome and ASDs is merely correlative, and not causative.

On the other hand, secondary imprinting defects occur when a gene mutation results in improper epigenetic regulation. Such a defect may occur in Prader-Willi syndrome, which is characterized by the lack of a paternal contribution at the 15q11-q13 locus. The specific mutation most commonly responsible for secondary imprinting Prader-Willi syndrome is a cis-acting defect of the imprinting regulatory center of the Prader-Willi gene [70]. Prader-Willi patients present with autistic behavior more frequently than Angelman syndrome patients; studies suggest that the frequency of ASDs co-occurrence with Prader-Willi syndrome is between 18% and 38% [71], though the causative nature of this relationship has not been established.

Fragile X syndrome is the leading single-gene cause of autism accounting for as many at 5% of all cases [72]. As with Prader-Willi and Angelman syndromes, epigenetic mechanism can contribute to the development of the fragile X, which is characterized by the presence of 200 or more CGG repeats in the 5′ untranslated region of the FMR1 gene [73]. The resulting increased concentration of cytosine and guanine nucleotides causes the global methylation of not only the CGG-repeat region but also adjacent regions, which happen to include FMR1 promoter elements.

8. Conclusions

Figure 1 summarizes the main epigenetic mechanisms that may play roles in ASD. Low activity of methyl CpG binding protein 2 (MeCP2) at CpG islands in genes of frontal cortex is shown to reduce the capacity for inhibiting HDAC1 and chromatin condensation for gene silencing. HDAC1 inhibition by valproic acid and GSK3β inhibition by lithium are shown to upregulate the Wnt signaling pathway which causes accumulation of β-catenin in the cytoplasm and its translocation to the nucleus, acting as an activator of transcription and resulting in macrocephaly with increased numbers of cerebral cortical columns. DNMT is shown to methylate the oxytocin receptor gene and silence it, resulting in the low oxytocin and estrogen activity necessary for androgen receptor mediation of high arousal inputs to the amygdala, associated with antisocial behaviors after exposure to environmental stressors. Histone H3 phosphorylation by protein kinase C beta is shown to activate the LSD1, an HMT that prevents demethylation of H3K4, that is also necessary for androgen receptor mediation of high arousal inputs to the amygdala. Hypomethylation by decreased availability of S-adenosyl methionine (SAM) is shown to occur in mothers of autistic children. Environmental and nutritional conditions acting as pro- or antiautism factors by epigenetic mechanisms suggest strategies for decreasing the prevalence of ASD. This knowledge of putative epigenetic targets should motivate clinical practitioners and educators to develop novel treatment strategies based on the environment-gene interactions which could contribute to the core symptoms of ASD.

References

[1] R. F. Gillis and G. A. Rouleau, "The ongoing dissection of the genetic architecture of autistic spectrum disorder," *Molecular Autism*, vol. 2, no. 1, article 12, 2011.

[2] B. Kadesjö, C. Gillberg, and B. Hagberg, "Brief report: autism and asperger syndrome in seven-year-old children: a total population study," *Journal of Autism and Developmental Disorders*, vol. 29, no. 4, pp. 327–331, 1999.

[3] S. E. Levy, D. S. Mandell, and R. T. Schultz, "Autism," *The Lancet*, vol. 374, no. 9701, pp. 1627–1638, 2009.

[4] C. Stoltenberg, S. Schjølberg, M. Bresnahan et al., "The autism birth cohort: a paradigm for gene-environment-timing research," *Molecular Psychiatry*, vol. 15, no. 7, pp. 676–680, 2010.

[5] V. W. Hu, B. C. Frank, S. Heine, N. H. Lee, and J. Quackenbush, "Gene expression profiling of lymphoblastoid cell lines from monozygotic twins discordant in severity of autism reveals differential regulation of neurologically relevant genes," *BMC Genomics*, vol. 7, article 118, 2006.

[6] C. Ptak and A. Petronis, "Epigenetic approaches to psychiatric disorders," *Dialogues in clinical neuroscience*, vol. 12, no. 1, pp. 25–35, 2010.

[7] J. T. Bell and T. D. Spector, "A twin approach to unraveling epigenetics," *Trends in Genetics*, vol. 27, no. 3, pp. 116–125, 2011.

[8] B. F. Vanyushin, "Enzymatic DNA methylation is an epigenetic control for genetic functions of the cell," *Biochemistry*, vol. 70, no. 5, pp. 488–499, 2005.

[9] A. P. Feinberg, "Epigenomics reveals a functional genome anatomy and a new approach to common disease," *Nature Biotechnology*, vol. 28, no. 10, pp. 1049–1052, 2010.

[10] R. Jaenisch and A. Bird, "Epigenetic regulation of gene expression: how the genome integrates intrinsic and environmental signals," *Nature Genetics*, vol. 33, pp. 245–254, 2003.

[11] L. M. Hjelmeland, "Dark matters in AMD genetics: epigenetics and stochasticity," *Investigative Ophthalmology and Visual Science*, vol. 52, no. 3, pp. 1622–1631, 2011.

[12] A. D. Riggs, Z. Xiong, L. Wang, and J. M. LeBon, "Methylation dynamics, epigenetic fidelity and X chromosome structure," *Novartis Foundation Symposium*, vol. 214, pp. 214–232, 1998.

[13] A. Petronis, I. I. Gottesman, P. Kan et al., "Monozygotic twins exhibit numerous epigenetic differences: clues to twin discordance?" *Schizophrenia Bulletin*, vol. 29, no. 1, pp. 169–178, 2003.

[14] S. Luikenhuis, E. Giacometti, C. F. Beard, and R. Jaenisch, "Expression of MeCP2 in postmitotic neurons rescues Rett syndrome in mice," *Proceedings of the National Academy of Sciences of the United States of America*, vol. 101, no. 16, pp. 6033–6038, 2004.

[15] M. Chahrour, Y. J. Sung, C. Shaw et al., "MeCP2, a key contributor to neurological disease, activates and represses transcription," *Science*, vol. 320, no. 5880, pp. 1224–1229, 2008.

[16] S. Cohen, Z. Zhou, and M. E. Greenberg, "Activating a repressor," *Science*, vol. 320, no. 5880, pp. 1172–1173, 2008.

[17] D. H. Yasui, S. Peddada, M. C. Bieda et al., "Integrated epigenomic analyses of neuronal MeCP2 reveal a role for long-range interaction with active genes," *Proceedings of the National Academy of Sciences of the United States of America*, vol. 104, no. 49, pp. 19416–19421, 2007.

[18] M. F. Mehler, "Epigenetic principles and mechanisms underlying nervous system functions in health and disease," *Progress in Neurobiology*, vol. 86, no. 4, pp. 305–341, 2008.

[19] R. P. Nagarajan, A. R. Hogart, Y. Gwye, M. R. Martin, and J. M. LaSalle, "Reduced MeCP2 expression is frequent in autism frontal cortex and correlates with aberrant MECP2 promoter methylation," *Epigenetics*, vol. 1, no. 4, pp. e1–e11, 2006.

[20] J. M. LaSalle, J. Goldstine, D. Balmer, and C. M. Greco, "Quantitative localization of heterogeneous methyl-CpG-binding protein 2 (MeCP2) expression phenotypes in normal and Rett syndrome brain by laser scanning cytometry," *Human Molecular Genetics*, vol. 10, no. 17, pp. 1729–1740, 2001.

[21] K. Pelphrey, R. Adolphs, and J. P. Morris, "Neuroanatomical substrates of social cognition dysfunction in autism," *Mental Retardation and Developmental Disabilities Research Reviews*, vol. 10, no. 4, pp. 259–271, 2004.

[22] C. Lintas, R. Sacco, K. Garbett et al., "Involvement of the PRKCB1 gene in autistic disorder: significant genetic association and reduced neocortical gene expression," *Molecular Psychiatry*, vol. 14, no. 7, pp. 705–718, 2009.

[23] E. Metzger, A. Imhof, D. Patel et al., "Phosphorylation of histone H3T6 by PKCbeta(I) controls demethylation at histone H3K4," *Nature*, vol. 464, no. 7289, pp. 792–796, 2010.

[24] D. W. Pfaff, I. Rapin, and S. Goldman, "Male predominance in autism: neuroendocrine influences on arousal and social anxiety," *Autism Research*, vol. 4, no. 3, pp. 163–176, 2011.

[25] S. Wu, M. Jia, Y. Ruan et al., "Positive association of the oxytocin receptor gene (OXTR) with autism in the Chinese Han population," *Biological Psychiatry*, vol. 58, no. 1, pp. 74–77, 2005.

[26] X. Liu, Y. Kawamura, T. Shimada et al., "Association of the oxytocin receptor (OXTR) gene polymorphisms with autism spectrum disorder (ASD) in the Japanese population," *Journal of Human Genetics*, vol. 55, no. 3, pp. 137–141, 2010.

[27] E. Unternaehrer, P. Luers, J. Mill et al., "Dynamic changes in DNA methylation of stress-associated genes (OXTR, BDNF) after acute psychosocial stress," *Translational Psychiatry*, vol. 2, article e150, 2012.

[28] S. Jacob, C. W. Brune, C. S. Carter, B. L. Leventhal, C. Lord, and E. H. Cook Jr., "Association of the oxytocin receptor gene (OXTR) in Caucasian children and adolescents with autism," *Neuroscience Letters*, vol. 417, no. 1, pp. 6–9, 2007.

[29] J.-P. Gouin, C. S. Carter, H. Pournajafi-Nazarloo et al., "Marital behavior, oxytocin, vasopressin, and wound healing," *Psychoneuroendocrinology*, vol. 35, no. 7, pp. 1082–1090, 2010.

[30] T. R. Insel, "Oxytocin—a neuropeptide for affiliation: evidence from behavioral, receptor autoradiographic, and comparative studies," *Psychoneuroendocrinology*, vol. 17, no. 1, pp. 3–35, 1992.

[31] J. N. Ferguson, L. J. Young, E. F. Hearn, M. M. Matzuk, T. R. Insel, and J. T. Winslow, "Social amnesia in mice lacking the oxytocin gene," *Nature Genetics*, vol. 25, no. 3, pp. 284–288, 2000.

[32] Y. Takayanagi, M. Yoshida, I. F. Bielsky et al., "Pervasive social deficits, but normal parturition, in oxytocin receptor-deficient mice," *Proceedings of the National Academy of Sciences of the United States of America*, vol. 102, no. 44, pp. 16096–16101, 2005.

[33] L. Sun, L. Huang, P. Nguyen et al., "DNA methyltransferase 1 and 3B activate BAG-1 expression via recruitment of CTCFL/BORIS and modulation of promoter histone methylation," *Cancer Research*, vol. 68, no. 8, pp. 2726–2735, 2008.

[34] S. G. Gregory, J. J. Connelly, A. J. Towers et al., "Genomic and epigenetic evidence for oxytocin receptor deficiency in autism," *BMC Medicine*, vol. 7, article 62, 2009.

[35] T. Kimura, F. Saji, K. Nishimori et al., "Molecular regulation of the oxytocin receptor in peripheral organs," *Journal of Molecular Endocrinology*, vol. 30, no. 2, pp. 109–115, 2003.

[36] Y. Tsujimoto, L. R. Finger, and J. Yunis, "Cloning of the chromosome breakpoint of neoplastic B cells with the t(14;18) chromosome translocation," *Science*, vol. 226, no. 4678, pp. 1097–1099, 1984.

[37] L. A. Glantz, J. H. Gilmore, J. A. Lieberman, and L. F. Jarskog, "Apoptotic mechanisms and the synaptic pathology of schizophrenia," *Schizophrenia Research*, vol. 81, no. 1, pp. 47–63, 2006.

[38] S. H. Fatemi, J. M. Stary, A. R. Halt, and G. R. Realmuto, "Dysregulation of reelin and Bcl-2 proteins in autistic cerebellum," *Journal of Autism and Developmental Disorders*, vol. 31, no. 6, pp. 529–535, 2001.

[39] S. Hossein Fatemi and A. R. Halt, "Altered levels of Bcl2 and p53 proteins in parietal cortex reflect deranged apoptotic regulation in autism," *Synapse*, vol. 42, no. 4, pp. 281–284, 2001.

[40] A. Nguyen, T. A. Rauch, G. P. Pfeifer, and V. W. Hu, "Global methylation profiling of lymphoblastoid cell lines reveals epigenetic contributions to autism spectrum disorders and a novel autism candidate gene, RORA, whose protein product is reduced in autistic brain," *FASEB Journal*, vol. 24, no. 8, pp. 3036–3051, 2010.

[41] M. Akashi and T. Takumi, "The orphan nuclear receptor RORα regulates circadian transcription of the mammalian core-clock Bmal1," *Nature Structural & Molecular Biology*, vol. 12, no. 5, pp. 441–448, 2005.

[42] F. Boukhtouche, G. Vodjdani, C. I. Jarvis et al., "Human retinoic acid receptor-related orphan receptor α1 overexpression protects neurones against oxidative stress-induced apoptosis," *Journal of Neurochemistry*, vol. 96, no. 6, pp. 1778–1789, 2006.

[43] C. A. Pardo, D. L. Vargas, and A. W. Zimmerman, "Immunity, neuroglia and neuroinflammation in autism," *International Review of Psychiatry*, vol. 17, no. 6, pp. 485–495, 2005.

[44] A. Chauhan and V. Chauhan, "Oxidative stress in autism," *Pathophysiology*, vol. 13, no. 3, pp. 171–181, 2006.

[45] N. J. MacLusky, A. S. Clark, F. Naftolin, and P. S. Goldman-Rakic, "Estrogen formation in the mammalian brain: possible role of aromatase in sexual differentiation of the hippocampus and neocortex," *Steroids*, vol. 50, no. 4-6, pp. 459–474, 1987.

[46] P. Cardona-Gomez, M. Perez, J. Avila, L. M. Garcia-Segura, and F. Wandosell, "Estradiol inhibits GSK3 and regulates interaction of estrogen receptors, GSK3, and beta-catenin in the hippocampus," *Molecular and Cellular Neuroscience*, vol. 25, no. 3, pp. 363–373, 2004.

[47] R. S. Jope, "Lithium and GSK-3: one inhibitor, two inhibitory actions, multiple outcomes," *Trends in Pharmacological Sciences*, vol. 24, no. 9, pp. 441–443, 2003.

[48] Y. Liu, Y. Du, W. Liu et al., "Lack of association between NLGN3, NLGN4, SHANK2 and SHANK3 gene variants and autism spectrum disorder in a Chinese population," *PLoS ONE*, vol. 8, Article ID e56639.

[49] S. Beri, N. Tonna, G. Menozzi, M. C. Bonaglia, C. Sala, and R. Giorda, "DNA methylation regulates tissue-speci.c expression of Shank3," *Journal of Neurochemistry*, vol. 101, no. 5, pp. 1380–1391, 2007.

[50] S. Uchino and C. Waga, "SHANK3 as an autism spectrum disorder-associated gene," *Brain Development*, vol. 35, pp. 106–110, 2013.

[51] Y. Yasuda, R. Hashimoto, H. Yamamori et al., "Gene expression analysis in lymphoblasts derived from patients with autism spectrum disorder," *Molecular Autism*, vol. 2, no. 1, article 9, 2011.

[52] A. E. Beaudin, C. A. Perry, S. P. Stabler, R. H. Allen, and P. J. Stover, "Maternal Mthfd1 disruption impairs fetal growth but does not cause neural tube defects in mice," *American Journal of Clinical Nutrition*, vol. 95, no. 4, pp. 882–891, 2012.

[53] T. O. Scholl and W. G. Johnson, "Folic acid: influence on the outcome of pregnancy," *American Journal of Clinical Nutrition*, vol. 71, no. 5, pp. 1295S–1303S, 2000.

[54] S. Jill James, S. Melnyk, S. Jernigan, A. Hubanks, S. Rose, and D. W. Gaylor, "Abnormal transmethylation/transsulfuration metabolism and DNA hypomethylation among parents of children with autism," *Journal of Autism and Developmental Disorders*, vol. 38, no. 10, pp. 1966–1975, 2008.

[55] W. Luo, A. R. Karpf, K. K. Deeb et al., "Epigenetic regulation of vitamin D 24-hydroxylase/CYP24A1 in human prostate cancer," *Cancer Research*, vol. 70, no. 14, pp. 5953–5962, 2010.

[56] S. A. Currenti, "Understanding and determining the etiology of autism," *Cellular and Molecular Neurobiology*, vol. 30, no. 2, pp. 161–171, 2010.

[57] R. D. O'Connor, M. Zayzafoon, M. C. Farach-Carson, and N. C. Schanen, "Mecp2 deficiency decreases bone formation and reduces bone volume in a rodent model of Rett syndrome," *Bone*, vol. 45, no. 2, pp. 346–356, 2009.

[58] S. J. James, S. Melnyk, S. Jernigan et al., "A functional polymorphism in the reducedfolate carrier gene and DNA hypomethylation in mothers of children with autism," *American Journal of Medical Genetics, Part B*, vol. 153, no. 6, pp. 1209–1220, 2010.

[59] J. B. Adams, T. Audhya, S. McDonough-Means et al., "Effect of a vitamin/mineral supplement on children and adults with autism," *BMC Pediatrics*, vol. 11, article 111, 2011.

[60] S. J. Moore, P. Turnpenny, A. Quinn et al., "A clinical study of 57 children with fetal anticonvulsant syndromes," *Journal of Medical Genetics*, vol. 37, no. 7, pp. 489–497, 2000.

[61] A. D. Rasalam, H. Hailey, J. H. G. Williams et al., "Characteristics of fetal anticonvulsant syndrome associated autistic disorder," *Developmental Medicine and Child Neurology*, vol. 47, no. 8, pp. 551–555, 2005.

[62] J. A. Shimshoni, E. C. Dalton, A. Jenkins et al., "The effects of central nervous system-active valproic acid constitutional isomers, cyclopropyl analogs, and amide derivatives on neuronal growth cone behavior," *Molecular Pharmacology*, vol. 71, no. 3, pp. 884–892, 2007.

[63] A. N. Billin, H. Thirlwell, and D. E. Ayer, "β-Catenin-histone deacetylase interactions regulate the transition of LEF1 from a transcriptional repressor to an activator," *Molecular and Cellular Biology*, vol. 20, no. 18, pp. 6882–6890, 2000.

[64] Z. Wang, L. Xu, X. Zhu et al., "Demethylation of specific Wnt/β-catenin pathway genes and its upregulation in rat brain induced by prenatal valproate exposure," *Anatomical Record*, vol. 293, no. 11, pp. 1947–1953, 2010.

[65] E. L. Williams and M. F. Casanova, "Autism or autisms? Finding the lowest common denominator," *Boletín de la Asociación Médica de Puerto Rico*, vol. 102, no. 4, pp. 17–24, 2010.

[66] N. J. Minshew and D. L. Williams, "The new neurobiology of autism: cortex, connectivity, and neuronal organization," *Archives of Neurology*, vol. 64, no. 7, pp. 945–950, 2007.

[67] X. Nan, H.-H. Ng, C. A. Johnson et al., "Transcriptional repression by the methyl-CpG-binding protein MeCP2 involves a histone deacetylase complex," *Nature*, vol. 393, no. 6683, pp. 386–389, 1998.

[68] M. Gos, "Epigenetic mechanisms of gene expression regulation in neurological diseases," *Acta Neurobiologica Experimentalis*, vol. 73, pp. 19–37, 2013.

[69] S. Steffenburg, C. L. Gillberg, U. Steffenburg, and M. Kyllerman, "Autism in Angelman syndrome: a population-based study," *Pediatric Neurology*, vol. 14, no. 2, pp. 131–136, 1996.

[70] E. Dykens and B. Shah, "Psychiatric disorders in Prader-Willi syndrome: epidemiology and management," *CNS Drugs*, vol. 17, no. 3, pp. 167–178, 2003.

[71] M. W. M. Veltman, R. J. Thompson, S. E. Roberts, N. S. Thomas, J. Whittington, and P. F. Bolton, "Prader-Willi syndrome: a study comparing deletion and uniparental disomy cases with reference to autism spectrum disorders," *European Child and Adolescent Psychiatry*, vol. 13, no. 1, pp. 42–50, 2004.

[72] Y. McLennan, J. Polussa, F. Tassone, and R. Hagerman, "Fragile X syndrome," *Current Genomics*, vol. 12, no. 3, pp. 216–224, 2011.

[73] R. Willemsen, J. Levenga, and B. Oostra, "CGG repeat in the FMR1 gene: size matters," *Clinical Genetics*, vol. 80, no. 3, pp. 214–225, 2011.

11

Back to Basic: Do Children with Autism Spontaneously Look at Screen Displaying a Face or an Object?

Marie Guimard-Brunault,[1,2,3,4] Nadia Hernandez,[3] Laetitia Roché,[3] Sylvie Roux,[3] Catherine Barthélémy,[1,2,3] Joëlle Martineau,[2,3] and Frédérique Bonnet-Brilhault[1,2,3]

[1] *CHRU de Tours, Centre Universitaire de Pédopsychiatrie, 2 Boulevard Tonnellé, 37044 Tours Cedex 9, France*
[2] *Université François Rabelais de Tours, 60 rue du Plat D'Etain, 37020 Tours Cedex 1, France*
[3] *UMR Inserm U 930, Équipe 1: Imagerie et Cerveau, Université François Rabelais de Tours, Tours, France*
[4] *UMR Inserm U 930, Équipe 1: Imagerie et Cerveau, CHRU de Tours-Hôpital Bretonneau, 2 boulevard Tonnellé, Bât B1A, 1er Etage, 37044 Tours Cedex 9, France*

Correspondence should be addressed to Marie Guimard-Brunault; marie.guimard-brunault@univ-tours.fr

Academic Editor: Elizabeth Aylward

Eye-tracking studies on exploration of faces and objects in autism provided important knowledge but only in a constraint condition (chin rest, total time looking at screen not reported), without studying potential differences between subjects with autism spectrum disorder (ASD) and controls in spontaneous visual attention toward a screen presenting these stimuli. This study used eye tracking to compare spontaneous visual attention to a screen displaying a face or an object between children with autism and controls in a nonconstraint condition and to investigate the relationship with clinical characteristics in autism group. Time exploring screen was measured during passive viewing of static images of faces or objects. Autistic behaviors were assessed by the CARS and the BSE-R in autism group. In autism group, time exploring face screen and time exploring object screen were lower than in controls and were not correlated with degree of distractibility. There was no interaction between group and type of image on time spent exploring screen. Only time exploring face screen was correlated with autism severity and gaze impairment. Results highlight particularities of spontaneous visual attention toward a screen displaying faces or objects in autism, which should be taken into account in future eye-tracking studies on face exploration.

1. Introduction

Autism spectrum disorder (ASD) represents a significant public health concern and their prevalence is 60–70 per 10000 [1]. ASD is a developmental disorder characterized by impairments in communication and social interaction and by repetitive and stereotyped behavior and restricted interests [2].

Some authors suggest that social interaction impairment is linked to face processing impairment [3–5]. Face processing is one of the most studied areas of visual processing in ASD [6], and eye-tracking studies have made a large contribution to research in this field. Many eye-tracking studies focused on exploration strategies of faces in ASD. A consistent finding in eye-tracking studies is less visual exploration of the eyes by individuals with ASD compared to typically developing individuals [7–12], associated in some cases to greater exploration of the mouth [9–11].

Some other eye-tracking studies investigated both visual attention to faces and objects in ASD and control groups [13–15]. While the two first authors found no group differences in visual attention to faces versus objects [13, 14], Rice et al. reported a significantly reduced fixation on faces in ASD compared to controls [15].

Another major contribution of eye-tracking studies is that they allow studying associations between visual attention to both face and objects and the clinical characteristics of ASD [10, 14–16]. Klin et al. indeed found a significant correlation between fixation on mouths and objects and social functioning: increased focus on mouths predicted better social adjustment and less autistic social impairment, whereas more time on objects predicted the opposite [10]. In addition, Rice et al. found an association between higher fixation on the inanimate environment and greater social disability [15]. A recent study found that face processing skills were significantly correlated with measures of attention to faces [14]. In another clinical domain, Sasson et al. found that, within their autism group, overall severity of repetitive behavior symptoms correlated positively with exploration of object pictures and negatively with perseveration on social pictures [16].

Although these eye-tracking studies provide important knowledge about visual attention to faces and objects in autism, these results are subject to a potential bias that might limit the generalization of these findings and explain mixed results. These studies only assessed visual attention to stimuli in a constraint condition. Indeed, they either used a chin rest to ensure that children necessarily look at screen and/or only calculated time exploring stimuli by dividing the time spent looking at stimuli by the total amount of time looking at screen without reporting this latter measure. By focusing on exploration of faces and objects stimuli when subjects looked at screen, they do not take into account the potential difference between children with ASD and control subjects in terms of spontaneously visual attention toward a screen presenting faces or objects stimuli. In a nonconstraint condition, Martineau et al. have already highlighted a difference between ASD and controls in terms of pupil responses during visual scanning of face and object stimuli [17]. What about spontaneous visual attention to a screen displaying a face or an object in autism?

This study aimed to compare spontaneous visual attention to a screen displaying a face or an object between children with ASD and controls using an eye-tracking approach in a nonconstraint condition. We also aimed to study in autism group the link between spontaneous visual attention to a screen displaying a face or an object and clinical characteristics. We hypothesized that children with ASD would spend less time exploring screen than controls for both stimuli (face and object). We further hypothesized that there would be no interaction between group and type of image—face versus object—on time spent exploring the screen. Finally, we hypothesized that spontaneous visual attention to a screen displaying a face or an object would be inversely correlated to autism severity but not linked to age or distractibility.

2. Method

2.1. Participants. Seventy-two subjects—24 with autism and 48 controls—aged 3 to 16 years old participated in this study.

Children with ASD were recruited from the Department of Child Psychiatry, University Hospital Center of Tours, France. The diagnosis of autism was based on the clinical judgment of an expert based on the criteria of the Diagnostic and Statistical Manual of Mental Disorders, Fourth Edition (DSM-IV-TR) [2]. This assessment was conducted in a tertiary medical center expert in autism which uses the Autism Diagnostic Interview-Revised (ADI-R) [18] and/or the Autism Diagnostic Observation Schedule (ADOS) [19]. All children with ASD met criteria for autistic disorder.

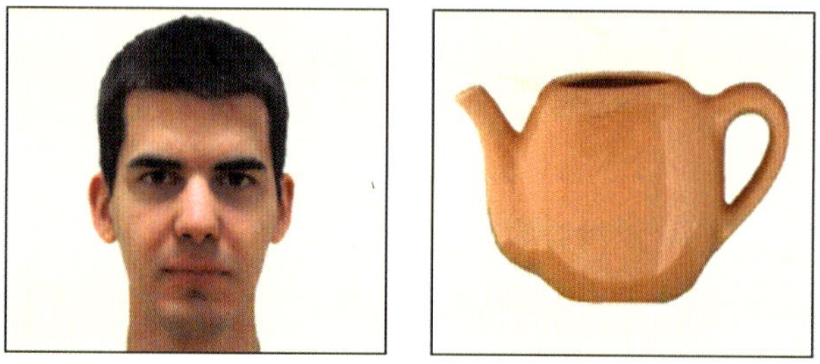

Figure 1: The two types of visual stimuli: neutral faces and objects.

Typical subjects were recruited from the local community. The exclusion criteria were a history of developmental disabilities, psychiatric, or neurological disorders. They all had a normal history of cognitive development and were progressing in age-appropriate education programs. Typical and autism groups did not differ in age (M age autism group = 9.53, SD = 3.71; M age typical group = 9.22, SD = 3.37; $F_{1,70} = 0.12$; $P = .73$).

For all participants, inclusion criteria consisted of normal or corrected vision ≥10/10 and no history of any eye disorder. None of the participants were taking any prescribed or over-the-counter medication. Written informed consent was obtained from all participants' parents. This study conformed to the Declaration of Helsinki.

2.2. Materials

2.2.1. Stimuli. Visual stimuli included 10 neutral faces—photographs of humans aged 18–35 years on a beige background—and 10 objects from daily life on a beige background (Figure 1). These stimuli have been previously used and validated elsewhere [8]. They were presented in color and matched on image size and luminosity.

2.2.2. Eye-Tracking System. We recorded gaze direction with an eye-tracking system described in detail elsewhere [8] including a computer equipped with two cameras which film the eyes of a subject looking at pictures presented on the computer screen. The software supporting the camera system captured cornean-illumination through infrared diodes, thus eliminating constraints on the subject, who remained free to move. The FaceLAB monitoring system determined eye direction, and Gaze Tracker software provided measurement and real-time analysis of the duration of exploration of the entire screen. The eye-tracking system recorded the eye position every 0.017 s. The size of the stimuli was 37.7 cm × 30 cm with a resolution of 1024 × 768 px (visual angle = 27°). We studied total time tracked defined as time spent on the screen during the stimulus projection.

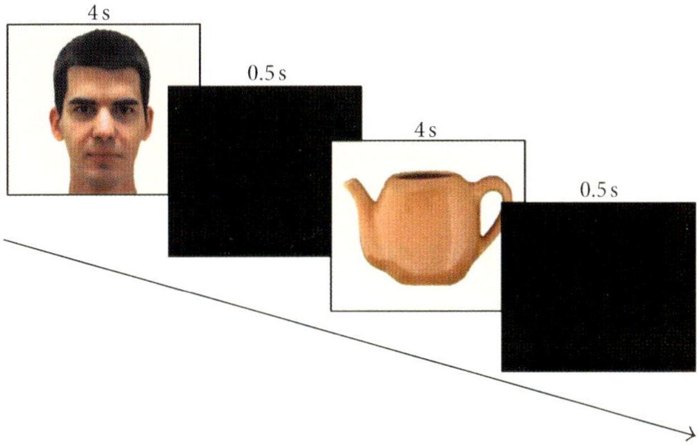

FIGURE 2: Procedure.

2.3. Procedure. Each of the 20 visual stimuli was successively projected on a 21 in. computer screen for 4 s with an inter-stimulus interval of 0.5 s consisting of a blank black slide (Figure 2). Gaze was spontaneously centered in the middle of the screen between each stimulus with this blank black slide. Central position of gaze was systematically checked by the experimenter for each patient and for each blank black slide during the experiment using the control screen of the gaze tracker system. The order of presentation of the stimuli was randomized between subjects. We wanted to study spontaneous visual attention towards stimuli, so there was no instruction before or during the experiment. Participants sat in a comfortable armchair, 90 cm from the computer screen, with no chin rest and in the darkness. After a brief calibration, gaze direction was recorded by the eye-tracking system during the entire session of visual stimuli projection.

2.4. Measures

2.4.1. Eye-Tracking Measures. For both groups (autism and control), the eye-tracking system measured the time spent exploring the entire screen in both "face screen" and "object screen" conditions. In both groups, the average time exploring the entire screen did not differ between the 10 stimuli in the same condition. There was no effect of the order of the stimuli. To achieve our statistical analyses, we therefore averaged the results of the 10 stimuli of each condition for each subject. We thus used two measures called "time exploring face screen" and "time exploring object screen." These two measures were the mean duration per each 4 s exposure time for each condition. We did not exclude any participant for these two measures.

2.4.2. Clinical Measures. Several clinical measures for the autism group were obtained during multidisciplinary assessment. All clinical measures were based on clinical observations conducted by clinicians expert in autism. Full-scale intelligence quotient (IQ) was estimated using reliable and appropriate scales. For each child, we chose the intelligence measure appropriate to mental age: the Brunet Lézine-R, a psychomotor developmental test for infants 1–30 months of age (Brunet and Lézine 1976, the French version of the Gesell scale, revised form 2001) [20], the EDEI-R (Echelles différentielles d'efficiences intellectuelles, Perron-Borelli 1978, revised form 1996), a cognitive test for children 30 months–9 years of age [21], and the Wechsler Intelligence Scale for Children, Third Edition (WISC-III), a cognitive test for children between the ages of 6 and 16 inclusive [22].

Children with ASD were also assessed with the Childhood Autism Rating Scale (CARS) [23] designed to assess the severity of autistic syndrome and with the Behavior Summarized Evaluation-Revised (BSE-R) [24] developed for the quantitative assessment of autistic behavior (Table 1). In particular, we studied Factor 1 of BSE-R "Interaction disorder" (13 items: aloneness, ignores people, poor social interaction, abnormal eye contact, does not make an effort to communicate using voice and words, lack of appropriate facial expression and gestures, lack of initiative, poor activity, inappropriate relating to inanimate objects or to dolls, stereotyped sensorimotor activity, unstable attention, easily distracted, bizarre responses to auditory stimuli, does not imitate the gestures or voices of others, and does not share emotion) reflecting relational defect and quantifying the severity of autistic behavior and BSE-R item scores reflecting functions associated with visual attention (item 4: abnormal eye contact, item 23: unstable attention, easily distracted). Previous studies already pulled items of BSE-R out of the scale to study correlations between neurophysiological variables and target autistic behaviors [25, 26].

2.5. Data Analysis. We used Statistica 6.1 software (StatSoft, Inc., Tulsa, OK). We used repeated measures ANOVA to study the effects of group and type of image on eye tracking measures. Before these tests, we checked for the homogeneity of variances with a Levene test. In autism group, Spearman correlations were used to assess the relationship between visual patterns and clinical variables. P value $\leq .05$ was considered significant for all statistical analyses. All analyses were two tailed.

3. Results

3.1. Clinical Assessments. Results for the autism group with the various scales assessed during multidisciplinary assessment are reported in Table 2.

3.2. Time Exploring Screen

3.2.1. Descriptive Statistics. The mean time exploring face screen was 1.28 s (SD = .91) for children with ASD and 3.04 s (SD = .77) for controls. The mean time exploring object screen was 1.13 s (SD = .67) for children with ASD and 2.85 s (SD = .91) for controls.

3.2.2. Autism Group versus Controls. The ANOVA showed a significant group effect on time exploring the screen ($F_{1,70}$ = 81.66; P < .0001) and a significant effect of the type of image ($F_{1,70}$ = 5.00; P = .03); their interaction was not significant ($F_{1,70}$ = 0.06; n.s.). Children with ASD spent

Table 1: Items of BSE-R scale.

Items of BSE-R scale
(1) Aloneness
(2) Ignores people
(3) Poor social interaction
(4) Abnormal eye contact
(5) Does not make an effort to communicate using voice and words
(6) Lack of appropriate facial expression and gestures
(7) Stereotyped vocal and verbal utterances, echolalia
(8) Lack of initiative, poor activity
(9) Inappropriate relating to inanimate objects or to doll
(10) Irresistible and/or ritual use of objects
(11) Intolerance of change and to frustration
(12) Stereotyped sensorimotor activity
(13) Agitation, restlessness
(14) Bizarre posture and gait
(15) Autoaggressiveness
(16) Heteroaggressiveness
(17) Mild anxiety signs
(18) Mood difficulties
(19) Disturbance of feeding behavior
(20) Does not try to be clean (stools or urine), plays with stools
(21) Individual bodily activities
(22) Sleep problems
(23) Unstable attention, easily distracted
(24) Bizarre responses to auditory stimuli
(25) Variability
(26) Does not imitate the gestures or voices of others
(27) Child too floppy, lifeless
(28) Does not share emotion
(29) Paradoxical sensitivity to touching and contact

Table 2: Clinical assessments in autism group.

	N	Mean ± SD	Range
Full IQ scale[1]	24	63.3 ± 20.1	19–99
CARS score[2]	16	30.0 ± 4.7	21.5–37.5
Factor 1 of BSE-R[3]	18	29.7 ± 10.7	16–46
Item 4 of BSE-R[3]	18	2.3 ± 1.2	1–5
Item 23 of BSE-R[3]	18	3.1 ± 1.1	1–5

[1]IQ: intelligence quotient.
[2]CARS: Childhood Autism Rating Scale.
[3]BSE-R: Behavior Summarized Evaluation-Revised.

less time than controls exploring screen whatever the type of image. All participants spent more time exploring face screen than object screen (Figure 3).

3.2.3. Clinical Correlates in Autism Group. Correlation tests between clinical variables and time exploring face or object screen are described in Table 3.

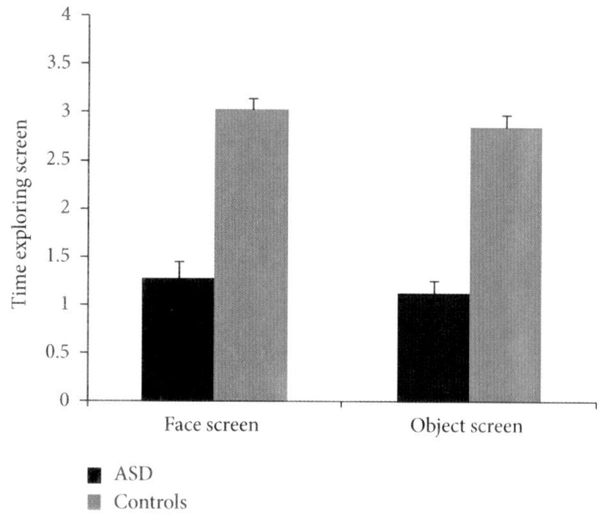

Figure 3: Time exploring face screen and time exploring object screen in children with ASD and controls.

Table 3: Clinical correlates in autism group.

	Time exploring face screen			Time exploring object screen		
	n	r	P	n	r	P
Chronological age	24	0.15	n.s.	24	0.06	n.s.
Full IQ[1] scale	24	0.19	n.s.	24	0.20	n.s.
CARS score[2]	16	−0.54	0.03	16	−0.31	n.s.
CARS score*	16	−0.54	0.03	16		
Factor 1 of BSE-R[3]	18	−0.32	n.s.	18	−0.13	n.s.
Item 4 of BSE-R[3]	18	−0.47	0.047	18	−0.16	n.s.
Item 23 of BSE-R[3]	18	−0.28	n.s.	18	0.03	n.s.

[1]IQ: intelligence quotient.
[2]CARS: Childhood Autism Rating Scale.
[3]BSE-R: Behavior Summarized Evaluation-Revised.
*Partial correlation adjusted for full IQ scale.
n.s.: nonsignificant.

In the autism group, there was no significant correlation between the time exploring face screen and chronological age, full-scale IQ, item 23 of BSE-R (distractibility), or factor 1 score of BSE-R. There was a significant negative correlation between the time exploring face screen and CARS score: the higher the score CARS was, the less time was spent exploring face screen (Figure 4). This correlation remained significant after adjustment with full-scale IQ (Figure 4). We also found a significant negative correlation between the time exploring face screen and score for item 4 of BSE-R (abnormal eye contact): the more impaired the gaze, the less time was spent exploring face screen. There was no significant correlation between the time exploring object screen and any of the clinical variables (chronological age, full-scale IQ, score CARS, item 23 of BSE-R (distractibility), factor 1 score of BSE-R, or item 4 of BSE-R (abnormal eye contact).

3.2.4. Maturation Effect on Time Exploring Screen. In controls, there was a correlation between chronological age and

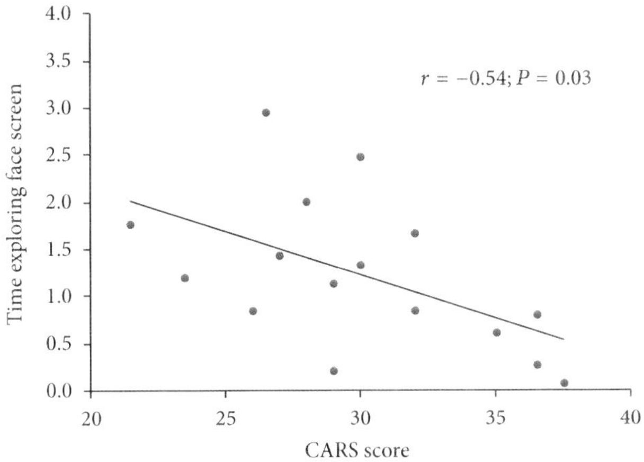

[1]CARS: childhood autism rating scale

FIGURE 4: Correlation between time exploring face screen and CARS score[1] in autism group.

the time exploring face screen ($n = 48$; $r = .32$; $P = .02$): as age increased, the time exploring face screen increased. There was no correlation between chronological age and time exploring object screen ($n = 48$; $r = .25$; n.s.). In the autism group, there was no correlation between chronological age and the time exploring face screen ($n = 24$; $r = .15$; n.s.) nor between chronological age and the time exploring object screen ($n = 24$; $r = .06$; n.s.).

4. Discussion

In this study, we report that children with ASD spent significantly less time than controls exploring a screen presenting a face or an object. In addition, we found no interaction between group and type of image—face versus object—on the time spent exploring screen. The low screen exploration by the autism group was not associated with the degree of distractibility. Finally, the time exploring face screen was specifically associated with autism severity and gaze impairment; this was not the case for the time exploring object screen.

First, supporting our original hypothesis, children with ASD spent significantly less time than controls spontaneously exploring the screen, regardless of whether the screen showed a face or an object. Two main hypotheses can be drawn to explain this low spontaneous visual attention in autism: deficits in visual attention and enhanced perception processing strategies [27–38]. Deficits in visual attention have been reported in autism, including "subselecting" important stimuli and/or hyperselecting irrelevant stimuli [27–29], a low attention engagement [30, 31], a disengagement and visual attention shift disorder [32–34], and abnormal visual orientation skills [32, 34, 35]. The use of more specific attention tests would help explore the various components of visual attention potentially involved in this low spontaneous visual attention in autism. The hypothesis of enhanced perceptual function in autism [36–38] could also explain why children with ASD spent less time exploring the screen displaying stimuli: they might capture the information provided by the stimuli more quickly.

Consistent with our prediction, there was no interaction between group and type of image—face versus object—on time spent exploring the screen. This finding is in line with previous studies [13, 14] which were conducted using a constraint condition. This may reflect a global alteration of spontaneous visual attention in autism [39–41], which would not be specific to visual attention toward faces stimuli.

Our final hypothesis was that spontaneous visual attention to a screen displaying a face or an object would be inversely correlated to autism severity but not linked to age or distractibility. We partly confirmed this final hypothesis. First, we confirmed that the time exploring a screen (projecting a face or an object) was not related to the degree of distractibility, as assessed by item 23 of BSE-R. Second, we found no association between time exploring screen for both stimuli and the severity of developmental delay. However, this result should be tempered by the lack of IQ assessment in controls needed to further explore this hypothesis. The low screen exploration in ASD compared to controls could be explained by a difference in cognitive abilities. Third, we found no association between age and time exploring screen for both stimuli in autism group. We found developmental maturation of the time exploring face screen in controls, consistent with previous descriptions of the development of expertise in face processing during typical development [42]. There was no evidence of such developmental maturation of the time exploring face screen in the autism group. Indeed, we did not find any correlation between chronological age and time exploring face screen in the autism group. Neither the autism group nor controls showed developmental maturation for the time exploring object screen. These results are in line with particularities of visual attention to faces, differing between children with ASD and controls, not present for visual attention to objects. Finally, in the autism group, the time exploring face screen was inversely correlated with the CARS score and was therefore related to the severity of autistic behaviors. This study is the first demonstration, as far as we are aware, of a significant association between time spent exploring screen toward faces and autism severity in a nonconstraint condition. However, the time exploring face screen was not correlated with the Factor 1 score of the BSE-R. The differences between these two scales may explain this result. Careful analysis of the details of the various scale items indicates that the CARS is more focused than the BSE-R on eyes, attention to others, and visual perception. Moreover, item 4 of BSE-R score, specifically related to abnormal eye contact, was inversely correlated with time exploring face screen: the more impaired the gaze of children with ASD, the shorter time spent exploring the screen with a face. To refine the results and the specificity of these behavioral patterns, we studied the time exploring object screen. In contrast to our predictions, for such images of objects, we did not find the same clinical correlations. Time exploring object screen was not correlated with any of the clinical variables that were tested or with the severity of autistic behaviors. This result highlights specific peculiarities in spontaneous visual attention toward a screen displaying a face compared to spontaneous visual attention toward a screen displaying an object in autism.

This study has some limitations. A larger sample would have allowed more detailed study of each age and an improvement in statistical power, especially for correlations. It would also have been interesting to assess the subjects using attention tests to better investigate the involvement of visual attention abnormalities in the atypical processing of faces in autism. As another limitation of our study, the screen contained only 1 image surrounded by a beige background. This approach could be considered as a potential constraint, and it would be interesting to propose simultaneously several images on the screen with the same methodology. Such study could assess ocular preference between several images by determining first whether subjects do or do not spontaneously look at the screen. Our results should also be tempered by the lack of IQ assessment in controls, which could be a potential confounding factor that might explain low exploration in ASD, since most of them had low IQ. Finally, we used photographs of faces, such that they were not animated, and they were not in any sort of natural environment; this may have influenced our findings [43].

In conclusion, this eye-tracking study demonstrates a lower spontaneous visual attention towards both a screen displaying an object and a screen displaying a face in autism. In autism group, spontaneous visual attention for both stimuli was not associated with age and degree of distractibility. Only spontaneous visual attention to face screen was associated with autism severity. The mechanisms underlying this specificity need to be investigated.

Our study has research and practical implications. As for research implication, we confirmed our hypothesis of a difference between children with ASD and control subjects in terms of spontaneously visual attention towards a screen presenting faces or objects stimuli. As far as we are aware, this study is the first to demonstrate this difference. Previous eye-tracking studies on face and object exploration did not take into account this difference since they either used a chin rest to ensure that children necessarily look at screen, and/or only calculated time exploring stimuli by dividing the time spent looking at stimuli by the total amount of time looking at screen without reporting this latter measure. Our study highlights the need to take into account this difference in the interpretation of eye-tracking studies in face and object exploration in autism, by stating whether the investigators used a constraint or a nonconstraint condition and by reporting the total amount of time spontaneously looking at screen in addition to previously used measures. Another implication of this work is a clinical one. Indeed, it would be interesting to apply this nonconstraint protocol during treatment. Treatment followup with the BSE-R may help to characterize the development of social and nonsocial behavior, including spontaneous visual attention to faces and objects, and this could be used to adjust the treatment plan and thereby improves the social prognosis of children with ASD.

Acknowledgments

The authors thank the Fondation Pour la Recherche Médicale and the Fondation Planiol for their financial support and greatly appreciate the support of Inserm Unit 930, the University Hospital of Tours and François Rabelais University of Tours. They thank all the participants for their cooperation.

References

[1] E. Fombonne, "Epidemiology of pervasive developmental disorders," *Pediatric Research*, vol. 65, no. 6, pp. 591–598, 2009.

[2] American Psychiatric Association, *Diagnostic and Statistical Manual of Mental Disorders: DSM-IV-TR*, American Psychiatric Association, Washington, DC, USA, 4th edition, 2000.

[3] G. Dawson, S. J. Webb, and J. McPartland, "Understanding the nature of face processing impairment in autism: insights from behavioral and electrophysiological studies," *Developmental Neuropsychology*, vol. 27, no. 3, pp. 403–424, 2005.

[4] R. T. Schultz, D. J. Grelotti, A. Klin et al., "The role of the fusiform face area in social cognition: implications for the pathobiology of autism," *Philosophical Transactions of the Royal Society B*, vol. 358, no. 1430, pp. 415–427, 2003.

[5] R. T. Schultz, "Developmental deficits in social perception in autism: the role of the amygdala and fusiform face area," *International Journal of Developmental Neuroscience*, vol. 23, no. 2-3, pp. 125–141, 2005.

[6] D. R. Simmons, A. E. Robertson, L. S. McKay, E. Toal, P. McAleer, and F. E. Pollick, "Vision in autism spectrum disorders," *Vision Research*, vol. 49, no. 22, pp. 2705–2739, 2009.

[7] K. M. Dalton, B. M. Nacewicz, T. Johnstone et al., "Gaze fixation and the neural circuitry of face processing in autism," *Nature Neuroscience*, vol. 8, no. 4, pp. 519–526, 2005.

[8] N. Hernandez, A. Metzger, R. Magné et al., "Exploration of core features of a human face by healthy and autistic adults analyzed by visual scanning," *Neuropsychologia*, vol. 47, no. 4, pp. 1004–1012, 2009.

[9] W. Jones and A. Klin, "Altered salience in autism: developmental insights, consequences and questions," in *Autism: An Integrated View From Neurocognitive, Clinical and Intervention Research*, E. McGregor, M. Núñez, K. Cebula, and J. C. Gómez, Eds., pp. 62–82, Blackwell, Oxford, UK, 2008.

[10] A. Klin, W. Jones, R. Schultz, F. Volkmar, and D. Cohen, "Visual fixation patterns during viewing of naturalistic social situations as predictors of social competence in individuals with autism," *Archives of General Psychiatry*, vol. 59, no. 9, pp. 809–816, 2002.

[11] A. Klin and W. Jones, "Altered face scanning and impaired recognition of biological motion in a 15-month-old infant with autism," *Developmental Science*, vol. 11, no. 1, pp. 40–46, 2008.

[12] K. A. Pelphrey, N. J. Sasson, J. S. Reznick, G. Paul, B. D. Goldman, and J. Piven, "Visual scanning of faces in autism," *Journal of Autism and Developmental Disorders*, vol. 32, no. 4, pp. 249–261, 2002.

[13] J. C. McPartland, S. J. Webb, B. Keehn, and G. Dawson, "Patterns of visual attention to faces and objects in autism spectrum disorder," *Journal of Autism and Developmental Disorders*, vol. 41, no. 2, pp. 148–157, 2011.

[14] J. Parish-Morris, C. Chevallier, N. Tonge, J. Letzen, J. Pandey, and R. T. Schultz, "Visual attention to dynamic faces and objects is linked to face processing skills: a combined study of children with autism and controls," *Frontiers in Psychology*, vol. 4, article 185, 2013.

[15] K. Rice, J. M. Moriuchi, W. Jones, and A. Klin, "Parsing heterogeneity in autism spectrum disorders: visual scanning of dynamic social scenes in school-aged children," *Journal of the American Academy of Child and Adolescent Psychiatry*, vol. 51, no. 3, pp. 238–248, 2012.

[16] N. J. Sasson, L. M. Turner-Brown, T. N. Holtzclaw, K. S. L. Lam, and J. W. Bodfish, "Children with autism demonstrate circumscribed attention during passive viewing of complex social and nonsocial picture arrays," *Autism Research*, vol. 1, no. 1, pp. 31–42, 2008.

[17] J. Martineau, N. Hernandez, L. Hiebel, L. Roché, A. Metzger, and F. Bonnet-Brilhault, "Can pupil size and pupil responses during visual scanning contribute to the diagnosis of autism spectrum disorder in children?" *Journal of Psychiatric Research*, vol. 45, no. 8, pp. 1077–1082, 2011.

[18] C. Lord, M. Rutter, and A. L. Couteur, "Autism diagnostic interview-revised: a revised version of a diagnostic interview for caregivers of individuals with possible pervasive developmental disorders," *Journal of Autism and Developmental Disorders*, vol. 24, no. 5, pp. 659–685, 1994.

[19] C. Lord, S. Risi, L. Lambrecht et al., "The Autism Diagnostic Observation Schedule-Generic: a standard measure of social and communication deficits associated with the spectrum of autism," *Journal of Autism and Developmental Disorders*, vol. 30, no. 3, pp. 205–223, 2000.

[20] O. Brunet and L. Lézine, *Brunet-Lézine Psychomotor Development Test*, ECPA, Paris, France, 2001.

[21] M. Perron-Borelli, *Échelles différentielles d'efficiences intellectuelles, forme révisée*, EAP, Issy-les-Moulineaux, France, 1996.

[22] D. Wechsler, *Échelle d'intelligence de Wechsler pour enfants (WISC-III)*, ECPA, Paris, France, 3rd edition, 1996.

[23] E. Schopler, R. J. Reichler, R. F. DeVellis, and K. Daly, "Toward objective classification of childhood autism: childhood autism rating scale (CARS)," *Journal of Autism and Developmental Disorders*, vol. 10, no. 1, pp. 91–103, 1980.

[24] C. Barthélémy, S. Roux, J. L. Adrien et al., "Validation of the revised behavior summarized evaluation scale," *Journal of Autism and Developmental Disorders*, vol. 27, no. 2, pp. 139–153, 1997.

[25] N. Bruneau, F. Bonnet-Brilhault, M. Gomot, J.-L. Adrien, and C. Barthélémy, "Cortical auditory processing and communication in children with autism: electrophysiological/behavioral relations," *International Journal of Psychophysiology*, vol. 51, no. 1, pp. 17–25, 2003.

[26] M. Gomot, R. Blanc, H. Clery, S. Roux, C. Barthelemy, and N. Bruneau, "Candidate electrophysiological endophenotypes of hyper-reactivity to change in autism," *Journal of Autism and Developmental Disorders*, vol. 41, no. 6, pp. 705–714, 2011.

[27] S. E. Bryson, J. A. Wainwright-Sharp, and I. M. Smith, "Autism: a developmental spatial neglect syndrome?" in *The Development of Attention: Research and Theory*, J. Enns, Ed., pp. 405–427, Elsevier, Amsterdam, The Netherlands, 1990.

[28] J. A. Burack, "Selective attention deficits in persons with autism: preliminary evidence of an inefficient attentional lens," *Journal of Abnormal Psychology*, vol. 103, no. 3, pp. 535–543, 1994.

[29] K. Pierce, K. S. Glad, and L. Schreibman, "Social perception in children with autism: an attentional deficit?" *Journal of Autism and Developmental Disorders*, vol. 27, no. 3, pp. 265–282, 1997.

[30] J. N. van der Geest, C. Kemner, G. Camfferman, M. N. Verbaten, and H. van Engeland, "Eye movements, visual attention, and autism: a saccadic reaction time study using the gap and overlap paradigm," *Biological Psychiatry*, vol. 50, no. 8, pp. 614–619, 2001.

[31] Y. Kawakubo, H. Maekawa, K. Itoh, O. Hashimoto, and A. Iwanami, "Spatial attention in individuals with pervasive developmental disorders using the gap overlap task," *Psychiatry Research*, vol. 125, no. 3, pp. 269–275, 2004.

[32] B. J. Casey, C. T. Gordon, G. B. Mannheim, and J. M. Rumsey, "Dysfunctional attention in autistic savants," *Journal of Clinical and Experimental Neuropsychology*, vol. 15, no. 6, pp. 933–946, 1993.

[33] J. Townsend and E. Courchesne, "Parietal damage and narrow "spotlight" spatial attention," *Journal of Cognitive Neuroscience*, vol. 6, no. 3, pp. 220–232, 1994.

[34] J. Wainwright-Sharp and S. E. Bryson, "Visual orienting deficits in high-functioning people with autism," *Journal of Autism and Developmental Disorders*, vol. 23, no. 1, pp. 1–13, 1993.

[35] P. Renner, L. G. Klinger, and M. R. Klinger, "Exogenous and endogenous attention orienting in autism spectrum disorders," *Child Neuropsychology*, vol. 12, no. 4-5, pp. 361–382, 2006.

[36] L. Mottron and J. A. Burack, "Enhanced perceptual functioning in the development of autism," in *The Development of Autism: Perspectives From Theory and Research*, J. A. Burack, T. Charman, N. Yirmiya, and P. R. Zelazo, Eds., pp. 131–148, Lawrence Erlbaum Associates, Mahwah, NJ, USA, 2001.

[37] L. Mottron, M. Dawson, I. Soulières, B. Hubert, and J. Burack, "Enhanced perceptual functioning in autism: an update, and eight principles of autistic perception," *Journal of Autism and Developmental Disorders*, vol. 36, no. 1, pp. 27–43, 2006.

[38] K. Plaisted, "Reduced generalization in autism: an alternative to weak central coherence," in *The Development of Autism: Perspectives From Theory and Research*, J. A. Burack, T. Charman, N. Yirmiya, and P. R. Zelazo, Eds., pp. 149–169, Lawrence Erlbaum Associates, Mahwah, NJ, USA, 2001.

[39] M. Behrmann, G. Avidan, G. L. Leonard et al., "Configural processing in autism and its relationship to face processing," *Neuropsychologia*, vol. 44, no. 1, pp. 110–129, 2006.

[40] I. Comte-Gervais, "Recherches actuelles sur l'intelligence sociale et les troubles envahissants du développement," *Annales Médico-Psychologiques*, vol. 167, no. 7, pp. 550–562, 2009.

[41] S. Davies, D. Bishop, A. S. R. Manstead, and D. Tantam, "Face perception in children with autism and Asperger's syndrome," *Journal of Child Psychology and Psychiatry and Allied Disciplines*, vol. 35, no. 6, pp. 1033–1057, 1994.

[42] S. Carey, R. Diamond, and B. Woods, "Development of face recognition: a maturational component?" *Developmental Psychology*, vol. 16, no. 4, pp. 257–269, 1980.

[43] L. Speer, A. Cook, W. McMahon, and E. Clark, "Face processing in children with autism: effects of stimulus contents and type," *Autism*, vol. 11, no. 3, pp. 265–277, 2007.

12

Parent Training Interventions for Toddlers with Autism Spectrum Disorder

Audrée Jeanne Beaudoin, Guillaume Sébire, and Mélanie Couture

Université de Sherbrooke, Sherbrooke, QC, Canada J1H 5N4

Correspondence should be addressed to Mélanie Couture; melanie.m.couture@usherbrooke.ca

Academic Editor: Manuel F. Casanova

Background. Now that early identification of toddlers with autism spectrum disorder (ASD) is possible, efforts are being made to develop interventions for children under three years of age. Most studies on early intervention have focused on intensive and individual interventions. However, parent training interventions that help parents interact and communicate with their toddlers with ASD might be a good alternative to promote the development of their child's sociocommunicative skills. *Objective.* This review aims to systematically examine (1) the use of parent training interventions for children with ASD under three years of age and (2) their effects on children's development, parents' well-being and parent-child interactions. *Methods.* Systematic searches were conducted to retrieve studies in which at least one parent was trained to implement ASD-specific techniques with their toddlers (0–36 months old) with a diagnosis of or suspected ASD. *Results.* Fifteen studies, involving 484 children (mean age: 23.26 months), were included in this review. Only two of them met criteria for conclusive evidence. Results show that parents were able to implement newly learned strategies and were generally very satisfied with parent training programs. However, findings pertaining to the children's communication and socioemotional skills, parent-child interactions, and parental well-being were inconclusive.

1. Introduction

Autism spectrum disorder (ASD) is characterized by difficulties in social interaction and communication and by repetitive and stereotyped behaviors. With an estimated prevalence of up to 1/88 children in the US [1], ASD is amongst the most frequent and severe developmental disorders. In the United States, ASD is associated with an estimated annual cost between 35 and 90 billion dollars [2, 3].

In response to parents' concerns about their child's development that are present as early as 12 months of age [4], knowledge about and strategies to identify young toddlers with ASD are emerging [5]. It is now possible to identify a child with ASD in the first two years of life based on sociocommunicative behaviors [6].

Now that early identification of toddlers with ASD is possible, efforts must be made to develop interventions for these young children. In 1987 and 1993, Lovaas and colleagues first described the potential efficacy of early intervention for children with ASD by reporting less restrictive school placement and higher IQ in the group of children who received an intensive behavioral intervention compared to children in the control group [7, 8]. More recently, early interventions have been associated with greater developmental gains and more reduction in autistic symptoms than interventions provided later on [9, 10]. Reilly and colleagues [11] reported that typically developing children between 12 and 24 months of age go through an important period of development that results in more advanced social communication abilities. Interventions in this time frame are crucial to prevent an increase in the gap between children with ASD and their typically developing peers [12]. Also, the significant neuroplasticity in young children emphasizes the importance of very early intervention [13]. In fact, many clinical studies [14–20] have described the interaction between infants' brains and their social environment and its impact on the development of infants' social and language brain circuitry [12]. Knowing that each experience influences the brain structure and function of young children, interventions with toddlers with ASD have the potential to influence their developmental trajectories towards a more typical and behavioral development [12, 13, 21].

Most research on early intervention focused on early intensive and individual interventions (20 to 40 hours per week). Despite their demonstrated efficacy for preschoolers with ASD [8, 22], intensive individual interventions are expensive and time-consuming and were originally developed for children between three and five years of age who have different learning needs than younger children. Infants from 12 to 36 months of age have specific developmental abilities and learning capacities, which require interventions that are tailored to them. Parent training interventions may be an effective alternative to support the learning capacities of toddlers with ASD [23]. Moreover, parent training interventions are based on language development in very young children, which has been demonstrated to be dependent on the language used by their parents [24]. Thus, teaching parents how to interact and communicate with their toddlers with ASD through parent training interventions might promote the development of their child's sociocommunicative skills.

Few researchers have reviewed the effect of parent training interventions specifically for young children with ASD. At this time, most of the literature on early parent training interventions for children with ASD focuses on children under seven [25–27] or nine years of age [28]. No review focusing on parent training interventions for toddlers under 3 years of age has been published to date. Given the previously described potential benefits of very early parent-mediated interventions, there is a need to understand if this type of intervention is effective specifically for those young children. This review aimed to systematically examine the use of parent training interventions for children from 0 to 36 months of age at risk of or with a diagnosis of ASD and their effects on children and parents. In particular, the following questions were addressed.

(1) What are the parent training programs used for children from 0 to 36 months of age with a diagnosis of or suspected ASD?

(2) What are the effects of parent training programs on (a) child development, (b) parental well-being, and (c) parent-child interactions?

2. Method

2.1. Search Procedures. Systematic searches were conducted in May and June 2013 in four electronic databases: CINAHL, ERIC, PubMed/Medline, and PsycINFO. The search was limited to articles published in English or French in peer-reviewed journals. Searches were conducted using combinations of the three keywords (and synonyms): "autism spectrum disorder" (e.g., autism, pervasive developmental disorder), "toddlers" (e.g., infants, preschoolers, and early intervention), and "parent training" (e.g., parent coaching, parent-mediated intervention, and caregiver-mediated intervention). We also searched in the Cochrane Database of Systematic Reviews, looked in Google Scholar, and examined bibliographies of systematic and nonsystematic reviews found in any of the six databases. Reference lists of articles that met inclusion criteria were also examined to identify articles that had not been found through electronic searches. We found eleven additional studies using these alternative procedures.

2.2. Inclusion and Exclusion Criteria. To be included in the review, studies had to meet four inclusion criteria as follows:

(1) all children had to be at risk of or have had a diagnosis of ASD (including pervasive developmental disorder, autistic disorder, Asperger syndrome, and pervasive developmental disorder not otherwise specified);

(2) more than 50% of the children had to be 36 months of age or less at the time of recruitment (if this information was not available, the mean age of participants at recruitment had to be under 36 months) and all children in the study had to be 5 years old or less;

(3) at least one parent (referring to fathers, mothers, foster parents, grandparents, or other relatives) had to be trained by an education or health professional to use ASD-specific techniques to promote the child's development. Parents must have received ongoing supervision and support from the professional. The training could involve individual and/or group coaching at home and/or in a clinic environment. Studies that assessed different types of interventions (e.g., individual intensive interventions) were excluded from the review if they did not report effects of parent training interventions separately from other types of interventions;

(4) effects of the intervention had to be reported by quantitative data. Quantitative data from mixed methods studies could be included if they reported intervention effects.

2.3. Data Extraction and Coding. Studies included in this review were summarized in terms of (a) participant characteristics, (b) dependent variables and measurement tools, (c) intervention characteristics (including program type, strategies, setting, frequency, duration, and goals), (d) intervention outcomes (directly after intervention and at followup, when appropriate) on children, parents, and parent-child interactions, and (e) certainty of the evidence.

Parent training outcomes (effects on children, parents, and parent-child interactions) were summarized as reported in the original paper (i.e., pre-post change, statistical significance, or effect size). Considering that a systematic review is a scientific tool that can be used by healthcare providers, consumers, researchers, and policy makers [29] to "evaluate existing or new technologies and practices efficiently and consider the total available data" [30], outcomes in each article were then classified into four categories (positive, mixed, no, and negative effects) according to the magnitude of changes due to parent training interventions. Previous systematic reviews used the three first categories [31–33]. Results were classified as "positive" if visual analysis of the results of single case studies showed an increase in abilities for all participants between baseline and intervention or if there was a statistically significant between-group difference in experimental designs. "Mixed" results were defined as improvement in some but not all participants in single-case designs or a trend short of statistical significance in between-group designs. If no participants in single-case studies benefited from the intervention or if there was no statistically significant improvement in between-group designs, results were classified as "no effects." Finally, the research team added a fourth category to the original 3-level classification, namely, "negative" effects. Results were classified as "negative" if visual analysis of the results of single-case studies demonstrated deterioration in abilities in most participants between baseline and intervention or if there was a statistically significant between-group difference in favor of the control group in experimental designs. However, none of the studies reviewed reported negative effects of the intervention.

The studies' methodological rigor could be assessed based on several classification systems. The research team used a 3-level classification system (suggestive, preponderant, and conclusive evidence) used in previous reviews [31, 32] to summarize the level of evidence for each study reviewed. "Suggestive" evidence was the lowest level of evidence. Studies classified at this level did not use a true experimental design. They might have used pre- or quasi-experimental designs including an AB-design or pre-post intervention design without a control group. The next level of certainty was "preponderant" evidence, which means that there was a strong, but not irrefutable, conclusion. Studies included in this second level of certainty needed to (a) use a true experimental design, (b) have adequate interobserver agreement (i.e., at least 80% fidelity) for at least 20% of evaluation sessions, (c) have an operationally defined dependent variable, and (d) provide sufficient details about the intervention for replication of procedures. The strongest form of evidence was "conclusive." To provide conclusive evidence, studies had to comply with all the attributes of the preponderant level plus contain (a) design features that provided at least some control for alternative explanations for intervention outcomes and (b) a measure of treatment fidelity to assess the degree of implementation of treatment-specific strategies by parents and/or therapists throughout the program.

3. Results

3.1. Description of Studies. Six hundred sixty-nine (669) articles were retrieved from the electronic searches. After removing duplicates and elimination based on the title, 174 abstracts remained. Based on these 174 abstracts, we eliminated 86 articles. The remaining 91 full-text articles were further assessed for eligibility. At this point, 75 articles were excluded because they described intervention models rather than assessing their effects ($n = 7$), children had developmental disabilities other than ASD ($n = 4$), children were older than 36 months ($n = 60$), studies reported exclusively qualitative data ($n = 1$), studies did not report results specifically for the parent training intervention ($n = 1$), or studies focused exclusively on a specific component of parent training rather than the whole intervention ($n = 2$). Of the remaining 16 articles, Vismara et al.'s paper [34] concerned the single participant included in a previous case study [35]. Therefore, we excluded the single case study [35] to avoid redundancy. The research team also contacted Gerald Mahoney, who ascertained that most children in Mahoney and Perales' studies [36, 37] were different. Despite a little overlap, these two studies were included in the review. A total of 15 studies were analyzed for this review. Table 1 describes the main features of each of these 15 articles.

3.1.1. Participants. A total of 484 children with a mean age of 23.26 months were included in this review. Those children were diagnosed with ASD ($n = 248$; [34, 36–40, 42–45]) or identified as being at risk of ASD based on either the presence of early markers ($n = 156$; [10, 41, 46]) or because they were infant siblings of probands with ASD ($n = 80$; [47, 48]).

Two hundred seventy-seven (57%) parent-child dyads received a parent training intervention, whereas the remaining 207 children were controls. Gender was reported for 253 of the 277 toddlers involved [10, 36, 37, 39–45, 47]; 192 children were male (76%) and 61 were female (24%).

Primary caregiver gender was detailed in seven of the 15 studies reviewed [36, 37, 40–42, 45, 47]. Most primary caregivers who participated in parent training programs in these studies were female ($n = 95$; 99%), compared to only one male primary caregiver (1%). Two papers reported training of relatives other than mothers or fathers. Kasari and colleagues [43] included a grandparent as the primary caregiver for two children. Also, Vismara et al. [34] included a grandmother as an observer during parent training sessions rather than as an active participant, who was the child's mother in this case. The mean age of parents (or other caregivers) receiving training ranged from 27.3 [41] to 36 years [40].

3.1.2. Intervention Types. Parent training interventions for children with a diagnosis of or suspected ASD may be classified based on their theoretical paradigms or their targeted goals.

Based on their theoretical paradigms, interventions may be positioned on a continuum from pure behavioral interventions to sociopragmatic interventions [49]. Interventions based on a behavioral paradigm stem from Lovaas [7] and colleagues' work and are characterized by a high level of structure in which a therapist prompts the child's behavior. When the child responds correctly, the therapist reinforces the behavior. At the other end of the continuum, sociopragmatic interventions are represented by the DIR Floortime model [50]. Sociopragmatic interventions are characterized by following the child's lead through spontaneous play activities and using those activities to enhance the child's learning. Eight of the 15 articles reviewed used interventions mainly based on the sociopragmatic paradigm [36–39, 41, 44, 45, 47] and two articles reported more behaviorally based interventions [40, 48]. The remaining five articles incorporated strategies from both paradigms [10, 34, 42, 43, 46]. For example, the Early Start Denver Model parent training program used by Vismara and colleagues [34] and Rogers and colleagues [10] integrates behavioral techniques,

Table 1: Description of studies.

(a)

Studies	Participant characteristics: n total (intervention group)	Age (months) mean (min–max)	Diagnosis	Methods	Control condition (if applicable)
Drew et al., 2002 [38]	24 (intervention = 12)	22.5	Childhood autism (ICD-10)	Randomized controlled trial	Local services: mixture of services
Mahoney and Perales, 2003 [36]	20	32.1	Autistic disorder or PDD	Preexperimental design: pre/postintervention	n/a
Mahoney and Perales, 2005 [37]	20	32.6	ASD	Preexperimental design: pre/postintervention	n/a
Wetherby and Woods, 2006 [39]	17	18.2 (12–24)	Provisional clinical diagnosis of ASD	Quasi-experimental design: pre/postintervention	Contrast group: no treatment
Rocha et al., 2007 [40]	3	31.7 (26–42)	Autistic disorder	Single subject multiple baseline across pairs of participants	n/a
Schertz and Odom, 2007 [41]	3	26.3 (22–33)	Strong early markers of ASD	Mixed methods: multiple-baseline design	n/a
Vismara et al., 2009 [34]	8	27.5 (10–36)	Autistic disorder (DSM-IV)	Case study: nonconcurrent multiple-baseline design	n/a
Gulsrud et al., 2010 [42]	34	30.6 (21–36)	ASD	Quasi-experimental design	n/a
Kasari et al., 2010 [43]	38 (intervention = 19)	30.8 (21–36)	Autistic disorder (DSM-IV)	Randomized waitlist control design	Waitlist: mixture of services
Oosterling et al., 2010 [44]	67 (intervention = 36)	32.9	Autistic disorder or PDD	Randomized controlled trial	Care-as-usual: daycare with speech and language therapy, motor therapy, music therapy, play therapy, and support for parents
Wong and Kwan, 2010 [45]	17 (intervention = 9)	26.5 (17–30)	ASD (DMS-IV)	Randomized waitlist control design	Waitlist: no intervention
Carter et al., 2011 [46]	55 (intervention = 29)	20.3 (15–25)	At risk of ASD	Randomized controlled trial	Control group: business as usual
Rogers et al., 2012 [10]	98 (intervention = 49)	21.0 (14–24)	At risk of ASD	Randomized controlled trial	Community group; mixture of services
Green et al., 2013 [47]	77 (intervention = 7)	8.4 (8–10)	Infant siblings of autistic probands	Case series with comparison groups; high risk (n = 37) and low risk (n = 33)	Comparison groups: no intervention
Steiner et al., 2013 [48]	3	12	Infant siblings of probands with ASD	Case series	n/a

(b)

Studies	Type	Setting	Intervention characteristics Recommended frequency and duration	Hours of intervention	Children's targeted behaviors/abilities
Drew et al., 2002 [38]	Social-pragmatic joint attention-focused parent training	Home	3 h/6 weeks over 1 year	27 hours	Declarative acts combined with eye contact, nonverbal requests, object-function play, imitation of actions, and turn-taking.
Mahoney and Perales, 2003 [36]	Relationship-focused parent training	Clinic or home	1 h/week over 1 year	31 hours	Cognition, communication, socioemotional functioning, and motivation
Mahoney and Perales, 2005 [37]	Relationship-focused parent training (responsive teaching)	Clinic or home	1 h/week over 1 year	32.6 hours	Cognition, communication, socioemotional functioning, and motivation
Wetherby and Woods, 2006 [39]	Parent-child playgroup Naturalistic comprehensive parent training	Clinic Home	2x/week for 12 months 1x/week over 9 weeks	Not specified Not specified	Individualized social communication goals
Rocha et al., 2007 [40]	Joint attention-focused parent-implemented intervention using natural behavior analytic strategies	Clinic	3x/week for 75 minutes over 6 weeks	At least 17 hours	Response of joint attention
Schertz and Odom, 2007 [41]	Joint attention-focused parent training	Home	1x/week for 9 to 26 weeks	Mean = 14 hours	Focus on faces, turn-taking, responding to joint attention, and initiating joint attention
Vismara et al., 2009 [34]	Comprehensive parent training incorporating behavioral and developmental strategies	Clinic	1 h/week over 12 weeks	12 hours	Attention and motivation, sensory social routines, dyadic engagement, nonverbal communication, imitation, joint attention, speech, and behavior
Gulsrud et al., 2010 [42]	Joint attention-focused caregiver training incorporating behavioral and developmental strategies	Clinic	3x/week for 30 minutes over 8 weeks	12 hours	Initiation and response of joint attention
Kasari et al., 2010 [43]	Joint attention-focused caregiver training incorporating behavioral and developmental strategies	Clinic	3x/week for 30 minutes over 8 weeks	12 hours	Initiation and response of joint attention
Oosterling et al., 2010 [44]	Social-pragmatic joint attention-focused parent training	Clinic Home	2 plenary sessions 2 h/week over 4 weeks + 3 h/6 weeks over 11 months	Not specified 32 hours	Declarative acts combined with eye contact, nonverbal requests, object-function play, imitation of actions, and turn-taking
Wong and Kwan, 2010 [45]	Communication-focused intervention with the child Communication-focused parent training	Clinic	5x/week for 30 minutes for 2 weeks (10 sessions)	5 hours	Eye contact, gesture, and vocalization/words

(b) Continued.

Studies	Type	Setting	Intervention characteristics Recommended frequency and duration	Hours of intervention	Children's targeted behaviors/abilities
Carter et al., 2011 [46]	Communication-focused parent group training	Clinic	1x/week over 8 weeks	Not specified	Two-way interaction, mature and conventional ways of communication
	Communication-focused parent training	Home	3x	Not specified	Communication for social purposes, understanding of language
Rogers et al., 2012 [10]	Comprehensive parent training incorporating behavioral and developmental strategies	Clinic	1x/week for 1 hour over 12 weeks	12 hours	Attention and motivation, sensory social routines, dyadic engagement, nonverbal communication, imitation, joint attention, speech, and behavior
Green et al., 2013 [47]	Developmental video-aided autism-specific parent training	Home	12 sessions of 1.5 hours over 5 months	18 hours	Social engagement and reciprocity
Steiner et al., 2013 [48]	Behavioral parent training	Clinic	8 sessions of 1 hour over 3 months	8 hours	Communication
		Home	2 sessions of 1 hour over 3 months	2 hours	

such as repetition and the ABC structure of activities with sociopragmatic strategies, including intervention through activities chosen by the child in natural settings [51].

Interventions can also be classified as either ability-focused or comprehensive. Focused interventions are individual instructional strategies used to develop specific abilities in children with ASD [52]. Ten papers used focused interventions [38, 40–48]. Abilities targeted in these interventions included communication [45, 46, 48], joint attention [38, 40–44], and parent-child relationship [47]. On the other hand, comprehensive treatment models were studied in five articles [10, 34, 36, 37, 39]. These interventions use sets of practices with multiple components for a broader developmental impact on core deficits in ASD [53]. They may include development of communication, social interaction, cognition, play, and autonomy. Notwithstanding the type of intervention, development of communication was a main goal of all 15 papers. In fact, difficulties with communication are a core deficit in ASD and frequently the main concern of parents.

Eight of the 15 articles used a comparison group, which allows for a better estimate of the effect of the intervention on children and parent outcomes. Interventions received by the 233 participants in comparison groups varied widely. Ninety-six of these participants (41%) from three studies [39, 45, 47] did not receive any treatment while, in the other five studies, 137 participants (59%) received treatment "as usual" [44, 46] or a mixture of interventions [10, 38, 43].

3.1.3. Setting. All 15 articles reported individual parent sessions, six of which took place in the family home [38, 39, 41, 44, 46, 47], at a clinic in six studies [10, 34, 40, 42, 43, 45], and either at home or in a clinic in three studies [36, 37, 48]. Mahoney and Perales [36, 37] gave families the choice of setting (clinic- or home-based) for the parent training program. Steiner and colleagues [48] varied the setting of the parent training: 8 sessions took place in a clinic and 3 at home. In this paper, clinic-based sessions were focused on teaching new strategies while home-based sessions focused on generalization of the newly acquired techniques at home. Also, two studies used some parent group classes that took place in a clinical setting [39, 46].

3.1.4. Intensity. Total time of interventions received varied between five and 32 hours (mean = 18 hours). Most studies involved parent training sessions for a total time between 10 and 20 hours [10, 34, 40–43, 47, 48] over a period of two to six months [10, 34, 39, 41–43, 46–48]. Intervention programs that offered more than 20 hours of intervention lasted at least 12 months [36–38, 44]. Only one paper assessed the effects of a shorter, but intensive, parent training program. Wong and Kwan [45] studied an intensive 2-week parent training intervention during which parents attended ten 30-minute sessions.

3.1.5. Teaching Strategies. Studies incorporated a range of strategies to teach parents new skills. Some articles reported the use of only one [42, 43, 47] or two [46] teaching strategies. However, most studies used many different teaching strategies to enhance parents' learning; the mean number of strategies described in the articles reviewed was 4.4 (from 1 to 9). Wetherby and Woods' [39] article reported the most varied use of teaching strategies. Unlike every other study, therapists in this study did not use all of the teaching strategies in the intervention program. They rather personalized the teaching strategies used based on therapists' and parents' preferred teaching and learning styles, respectively.

The most commonly used teaching strategy was didactic teaching by the therapist. Only two studies [39, 47] did not report therapists verbally explaining new techniques to caregivers. Rather than using traditional lectures by the trainer, Wetherby and Woods [39] used video clips to introduce new skills to parents. Other popular teaching strategies included demonstration or modeling of intervention techniques by the trainer [10, 34, 38–40, 44, 48], guided practices of new skills by parents with support and/or feedback from the therapist [10, 34, 38–40, 44, 48], written materials given to parents [10, 34, 39–41, 44], discussion between the trainer and parents on activities to develop targeted child skills [36–39, 41, 44], review of previous techniques [10, 34, 36, 37, 41], and parents having to implement new skills in daily living routines [38, 40, 41, 44, 45].

Other teaching strategies used in some studies included discussions about short-term objectives [38, 39, 44], about generalization of newly acquired skills in family daily routines [10, 34, 39, 44] and about family concerns that were not included in the parent training program [39, 41]. To ensure good comprehension by parents, they were encouraged to ask questions [39, 40], to provide good and poor examples of implementing a strategy [40], and to demonstrate their use of the strategy [45] Also, video feedback [46, 47] and fading of prompts [40] were used in recent studies to help parent implement strategies with their children.

3.2. Effects of Interventions. Only four of the 15 studies included a follow-up assessment in their study design [34, 40, 41, 46]. Timing of follow-up assessments varied from one [34] to four months [46] after the end of the intervention. Table 2 summarizes the effects of interventions for both postintervention and follow-up assessments.

3.2.1. Child Outcomes. Thirteen of the 15 articles reported the effects of a parent training program on children's abilities directly at the end of the intervention (postintervention), and three of these 13 papers reported effects on children's development at followup. However, the results of the 13 studies diverged, partly because of the heterogeneity of the intervention programs proposed and the diverse research methodology used.

As reported in Table 2, some gains in general communication outcomes were reported by Wong and Kwan [45]. More precisely, studies reported a significant increase in the number of words understood [39] and expressed [34], frequency of communication [48], imitative behaviors [34], joint attention [39], and eye contact [39, 41] after a parent training intervention.

However, these gains were not consistently reported across the studies reviewed. In fact, five of the six randomized controlled trials reported few [38, 43] or no [10, 44, 46] gains in sociocommunicative outcomes for children with ASD after a parent training intervention. Although Wong and Kwan [45] reported similar mixed results concerning expressive and receptive communication skills, their study was the only randomized controlled trial that reported positive effects on children's social communication. In fact, parents reported statistically better social relationships with people ($P = 0.007$) for their child after the Wong and Kwan's 2-week parent training program that targeted eye contact, gestures, and vocalizations. Also, both studies that met methodological criteria for conclusive evidence reported divergent results. On the one hand, Carter and colleagues [46] reported no main effect of the intervention on changes in child communication outcomes after the intervention (ES < 0.001). On the other hand, Kasari and colleagues [43] reported significant improvements in engagement states (object engagement ES: 1.09; joint engagement ES: 0.87), frequency of joint attention responses (ES: 0.74), and quality of functional play (ES: 0.88), whereas they did not observe significant improvements in frequency of attention initiations and quality of symbolic play following the 8-week parent training intervention.

Effects of interventions at follow-up assessments were similar to postintervention results. Among the three studies that examined children's communication trajectories after the end of the intervention program, one reported no intervention effects [46], one reported mixed results [40], and one reported positive results [34]. Again, if we examine the results of these studies in light of their certainty of evidence, the only randomized controlled trial available [46] did not report any significant effect of the intervention on children's communication four months after the end of the Hanen *More Than Words* parent education program (ES: [−0.19; 0.16]), as opposed to both case studies [34, 41] that reported more positive long-term outcomes.

No major difference was found between parent-reported results and direct observation measures. In fact, proportions of categorical outcomes (no, mixed, and positive effects) are similar between results from caregiver-reported assessments (no effect: 27%; mixed effects: 36%, positive effect: 36%) and direct observation measures (no effect: 27%; mixed effects: 20%; positive effect: 53%). Furthermore, two studies used both types of measures to assess intervention effects on the same variable and they both reported similar results from parent-reported and professional observation data. More precisely, Oosterling and colleagues [44] did not report any significant improvement in expressive communication after their 1-year parent training program or in the parent-reported MacArthur Communication Developmental Inventory [54] nor in the direct observation rating on item A1 (level of nonechoed language) of the Autism Diagnosis Observation Schedule (ADOS; [55]). Also, Wong and Kwan [45] reported significant gains after their 2-week intensive parent training intervention in parent ratings of their child's communication ($P = 0.010$) on the Language subscale of the Ritvo-Freeman Real Life Rating Scale [56] and in blind assessors' ratings on the Communication and Language subscale of the ADOS ($P = 0.007$).

3.2.2. Parent Outcomes. Considering that parents are the main actors in parent-mediated interventions, it is very important to evaluate the effects of parent training interventions on both parent and child behavior [57, 58]. However, in the articles reviewed, parent outcomes received much less attention than their child's sociocommunicative development (see Table 2).

In general, parents of toddlers at risk of ASD who participated in a parent training program reported a high level of satisfaction with the intervention [41, 46, 48]. These parents also tended to have a high level of fidelity of strategy implementation [10, 34, 40, 43, 48] that was maintained four weeks after the end of the intervention [34]. However, Rocha and collaborators [40] reported higher fidelity of strategy implementation when interventions took place in clinics (mean = 92.7%), compared to the family home, which represented a generalization context (86.8%).

The scientific literature strongly supports the notion that parents of children with ASD often experience higher stress than parents with typically developing children or children with other disabilities [59–63]. Therefore, parent training may be an important strategy for reducing parental stress [64]. However, few ($n = 2$) studies examined the effect of parent training on this very important parental variable. In addition, the results available differ from one study to the next. Wong and Kwan [45] reported a significant decrease in parental stress as measured by the total score on the Parental Stress Index- (PSI-) Short Form ($P = 0.004$) after a 2-week intervention comprising a child-therapist therapy targeting eye contact, gestures, and vocalizations and a program teaching parents how to use corresponding techniques at home. Interestingly, no significant decrease was observed in this study when analyzing parental stress separately for the three subscales of the PSI-Short Form (P's from 0.025 to 0.069). In the other study, the social-pragmatic joint attention-focused parent training program evaluated by Drew and colleagues [38], which lasted longer but was less intensive (i.e., once every six weeks) than Wong and Kwan's program, did not significantly decrease parental stress in comparison to the local services control group ($P > 0.05$).

The effects of parent training programs on other parental variables have received very little attention. Based on data available at this time, parent training interventions seem to be well accepted by parents [47] and may facilitate the establishment of a good therapeutic relationship [10]. Parental variables such as parental competence, self-efficacy, and empowerment were not explored in the studies included in this review.

3.2.3. Parent-Child Interactions Outcomes. As reported in Table 2, 10 of the 15 studies reviewed assessed effects of interventions on parent-child interactions. However, no study reported parent-child interactions with a global measure for the parent-child dyad. Instead, analyses of parent-child interactions were based on the engagement of each partner

Table 2: Effects of interventions.

(a)

Studies	Time of followup after intervention assessment	Certainty of evidence	Child outcomes: Communication: Expressive	Child outcomes: Communication: Receptive	Child outcomes: Socioemotional functioning	Child outcomes: Other
Drew et al., 2002 [38]	n/a	Preponderant	Mixed	Mixed	—	*Symptom severity*: none *Nonverbal IQ*: none
Mahoney and Perales, 2003 [36]	n/a	Suggestive	—	—	Mixed	—
Mahoney and Perales, 2005 [37]	n/a	Suggestive	—	—	Mixed	*Global development*: **positive**
Wetherby and Woods, 2006 [39]	n/a	Suggestive	Mixed	**Positive**	—	—
Rocha et al., 2007 [40]	3 months	Preponderant	—	PI: **positive** FU: mixed	—	—
Schertz and Odom, 2007 [41]	5 weeks	Suggestive	—	—	—	—
Vismara et al., 2009 [34]	Weekly over 4 weeks	Suggestive	PI: **positive** FU: **positive**	—	—	—
Gulsrud et al., 2010 [42]	n/a	Suggestive	—	—	Mixed	—
Kasari et al., 2010 [43]	n/a	Conclusive	—	—	—	*Play*: mixed
Oosterling et al., 2010 [44]	n/a	Preponderant	None	None	—	—
Wong and Kwan, 2010 [45]	n/a	Preponderant	Mixed		**Positive**	*Play*: mixed
Carter et al., 2011 [46]	4 months	Conclusive	PI: none FU: none	—	—	—
Rogers et al., 2012 [10]	n/a	Preponderant	None	None	—	*Adaptive behaviors*: none *Global development*: none *Symptom severity*: none
Green et al., 2013 [47]	n/a	Suggestive	Mixed	None	—	*Symptom severity*: none *Global development*: mixed *Visual attention*: mixed
Steiner et al., 2013 [48]	n/a	Suggestive	**Positive**	—	—	—

(b)

Studies	Fidelity of implementation	Parent outcomes: Stress	Parent outcomes: Satisfaction	Other	Parent-child interactions: Parent's engagement with child	Parent-child interactions: Child's engagement with parent
Drew et al., 2002 [38]	—	None	—	—	—	—
Mahoney and Perales, 2003 [36]	—	—	—	—	Mixed	**Positive**
Mahoney and Perales, 2005 [37]	—	—	—	—	Mixed	**Positive**
Wetherby and Woods, 2006 [39]	—	—	—	—	—	—
Rocha et al., 2007 [40]	Clinic PI: **positive** Home PI: mixed	—	**Positive**	—	PI: **positive** FU: none	PI: mixed FU: mixed
Schertz and Odom, 2007 [41]	—	—	**Positive**	—	—	PI: mixed FU: mixed
Vismara et al., 2009 [34]	PI: **positive** FU: **positive**	—	—	—	—	PI: mixed FU: mixed
Gulsrud et al., 2010 [42]	—	—	—	—	**Positive**	—
Kasari et al., 2010 [43]	**Positive**	—	—	—	—	Mixed
Oosterling et al., 2010 [44]	—	—	—	—	None	None
Wong and Kwan, 2010 [45]	—	Mixed	—	—	—	—
Carter et al., 2011 [46]	—	—	**Positive**	—	PI: mixed FU: none	PI: none FU: none
Rogers et al., 2012 [10]	Mixed	—	—	*Therapeutic relationship*: **positive**	—	—
Green et al., 2013 [47]	—	—	—	*Social validity*: **positive**	Mixed	—
Steiner et al., 2013 [48]	**Positive**	—	**Positive**	—	—	—

PI:postintervention.
FU: followup.

in the interaction separately. Thus, authors of the ten articles assessing parent-child interactions used either one [34, 41–43, 47] or both [36, 37, 40, 44, 46] of the following outcomes: parent's engagement with the child and child's engagement with the parent.

Seven studies assessed the parent's engagement in interactions with their child using different scales that were all based on observing an interaction period lasting a few minutes during which the parent and child played together. Four of these studies reported mixed results of intervention programs on parental engagement. More precisely, the studies reported a moderate increase in the parent's responsivity [36, 37, 46, 47] and positive effect [36, 37] after the intervention. However, no significant change was reported in directiveness [36, 37, 47] and achievement orientation, which refers to the parent's encouragement of the child's achievement and the quality of praise provided to the child [36, 37] after intervention. Both studies that assessed parent engagement with their child at followup reported that gains observed in the intervention period were not maintained [40, 46].

Eight studies analyzed the child's engagement with the parent during play. Mahoney and Perales [36, 37] reported significant improvement in children's social interactive behavior generally with their parents. However, most studies targeted specific components of children's engagement and reported mixed results. For example, children's responsivity to parents' joint attention bids [40, 43] and children initiating joint attention bids in parent-child interactions [34, 36, 37, 40] increased moderately in most studies. However, Kasari and colleagues [43] did not report greater initiations of joint attention in children who received the parent training intervention compared to a waitlist control group. Kasari and colleagues [43] also assessed the effects of interventions on the types of engagement and found that children increased their joint engagement with their parents and reduced their engagement in object-focused play. An increase in attention toward parents was also reported in three other studies [34, 36, 37]. Interestingly, changes in children's engagement were less significant in generalization contexts such as with the therapist instead of the parent [34] or at home instead of at the clinic where intervention sessions were conducted [40].

Finally, only two studies assessed maintenance of children's improved engagement with their parent and they both reported mixed results. More precisely, the increase in children's engagement with their parents was maintained for most, but not all, children [34, 40].

4. Discussion

To sum up, 15 studies on parent training interventions for toddlers with ASD were included in this systematic review. There was substantial heterogeneity between these 15 studies, particularly with respect to the intervention programs and assessment measures used. Consequently, the results could not be compiled in a quantitative analysis such as a meta-analysis. Nevertheless, the research team used two classification systems that described the magnitude of change (positive, mixed, no, or negative effects) and the certainty of evidence (suggestive, preponderant, or conclusive evidence) to summarize the meaningfulness of the differences found in each study. However, most studies on parent training interventions included in the review had low levels of certainty of evidence (as a result of methodological limitations) and the magnitudes of changes were hard to judge (few effect size data available). Thus, despite the use of two classification systems, the results must be interpreted with caution because of the substantial variability and methodological limitations that make comparison between studies difficult.

Despite these limitations, most studies in the present review demonstrated that positive changes can be obtained in young children with ASD following a parent training intervention. In fact, the 15 studies reviewed reported substantial but inconsistent gains in this group of children in communication, socioemotional functioning, symptom severity, and play. These results are consistent with the work of McConachie and Diggle [27], who concluded that there is a good reason to think that the training of specific skills for parents may produce positive changes in children under seven years of age diagnosed with ASD. However, the current lack of experimental studies with large sample sizes that take place in the clinical real world (rather than a university-based clinic) makes it impossible to reach firm conclusions regarding the effectiveness of parent training interventions in supporting the development of toddlers with ASD.

Furthermore, parents' attitudes and skills showed great improvement following parental training interventions. In fact, parents who participated in these interventions for toddlers with ASD consistently reported a high degree of satisfaction. Similarly, a qualitative study exploring the experience of parents of children with ASD from 28 to 37 months of age who participated in the *More Than Words* (MTW) parent education program reported that parents viewed the MTW program as a good starting point for learning how to help their child with ASD [65].

In general, parents also showed high rates of fidelity of strategy implementation after the training period. The ability of parents to learn how to implement strategies adapted to their child and their satisfaction with the parent training show the feasibility of using parent-mediated interventions with parents of toddlers at risk of or diagnosed with ASD. These results are consistent with previous reviews of parent-mediated interventions for older children with ASD [66–68]. For instance, a systematic review of parent training interventions that targeted the communication skills of children 10 years of age and younger with ASD [67] reported similar results. Parents included in that review reported high levels of satisfaction and acceptability with the intervention programs. In addition, they were able to implement communication interventions more accurately following training [67]. Finally, Lang and colleagues' review [67] also reported that parents were still able to implement interventions correctly in six of the seven studies that looked at maintenance data [67]. This was also reported in the only study in our review that included follow-up data on implementation [34].

Also, that review reported mixed effects of parent training interventions on parental stress, which is consistent with the inconclusive results reported by Oono and colleagues [25].

However, this contradicts the hypothesis that parental stress decreases in low-intensity treatments while it increases in high-intensity interventions [69, 70]. Thus, parent training interventions may reduce the number of hours of intervention with a therapist. However, parents in the parent training group rated their workload as higher than those assigned to the intensive early intervention implemented by a therapist [71]. Considering that the workload perceived by parents may be an important factor related to stress levels, future parent training programs should take into account the reality of parents of children with ASD, who are significantly more stressed than parents of children with typical development or with other neurodevelopmental disabilities [72, 73]. Effective parent training programs for toddlers with ASD should therefore limit parents' workload. The high level of stress in families of children with ASD may also explain why, even though parent training is associated with a decrease in stress and an increase in the sense of competence of parents of preschoolers with attention deficit hyperactivity disorder [74], the effects of such interventions are different for parents of children with ASD. Future studies should include an assessment of the effects of parent training interventions on parental stress and other well-being outcomes such as self-competence and empowerment.

Overall, the results of this review are consistent with those of a meta-analytic review of parent training programs for toddlers with behavior problems but without developmental disabilities [26]. The meta-analysis found greater effect sizes for parental outcomes than for children's outcomes. In fact, considering that parent-mediated interventions are by definition multilevel and involve the transfer of an intervention from the trainer to the parent and then from the parent to the child [58], parents have a role as change agents for their child's development. The assumption that parental outcomes are more direct than child outcomes explains the greater and more consistent effects on parental outcomes in Kaminski and colleagues' meta-analysis. Similarly, parent training interventions are likely to have greater effects on proximal parental outcomes such as knowledge about ASD, use of specific strategies, and attitudes than on more distal parental outcomes such as stress levels. Also, it is important to consider that parents need to first learn the different strategies; then it may take some time before they begin to implement the strategies in their everyday activities and in different settings [75], and still more time is needed before the effects on the children's behavior or skills are observable [76]. Consequently, effects of parent-mediated interventions may only become apparent weeks after the end of the intervention, giving time for changes to happen at the child level. To capture possible improvements after interventions, followup seems to be an important aspect of parent training study design that has been poorly assessed.

Finally, few studies looked specifically at parent-child interactions outcomes and most of them reported mixed results. The lack of scientific evidence prevents us from drawing definitive conclusions about the effects of parent training interventions on parent-child interactions. However, a review of parent-mediated interventions for children with ASD under 7 years of age reported strong and statistically significant positive changes in patterns of parent-child interactions [25]. Knowing that parent-mediated interventions are based on the assumption that the effects of the intervention depend on parents implementing the strategies in their interaction with their child and consequently on parents' responsiveness to their child [36], parent-child interactions are a very important outcome to assess. Future studies should include an assessment of parent training effects on parent-child interactions as a potential mediator of the effectiveness of parent-mediated interventions for toddlers with ASD.

5. Conclusion

This review shows that parent training interventions are a promising way to foster children's development by enhancing parent-child interactions. In fact, parents who received parent training interventions for their young child with ASD were able to learn and implement strategies to foster their child's development and were very satisfied with the program. However, poor evidence concerning children's skills, parents' well-being, and parent-child interactions outcomes prevents us reaching definitive conclusions regarding the effects of parent training interventions.

References

[1] J. Baio, "Prevalence of Autism spectrum disorders: autism and developmental disabilities monitoring network, 14 sites, United States, 2008," *Morbidity and Mortality Weekly Report*, vol. 61, no. 3, pp. 1–19, 2012.

[2] M. L. Ganz, "The lifetime distribution of the incremental societal costs of autism," *Archives of Pediatrics & Adolescent Medicine*, vol. 161, no. 4, pp. 343–349, 2007.

[3] M. Knapp, R. Romeo, and J. Beecham, "Economic cost of autism in the UK," *Autism*, vol. 13, no. 3, pp. 317–336, 2009.

[4] L. Zwaigenbaum, S. Bryson, C. Lord et al., "Clinical assessment and management of toddlers with suspected autism spectrum disorder: insights from studies of high-risk infants," *Pediatrics*, vol. 123, no. 5, pp. 1383–1391, 2009.

[5] L. Zwaigenbaum, "Advances in the early detection of autism," *Current Opinion in Neurology*, vol. 23, no. 2, pp. 97–102, 2010.

[6] L. Zwaigenbaum, S. Bryson, T. Rogers, W. Roberts, J. Brian, and P. Szatmari, "Behavioral manifestations of autism in the first year of life," *International Journal of Developmental Neuroscience*, vol. 23, no. 2-3, pp. 143–152, 2005.

[7] O. I. Lovaas, "Behavioral treatment and normal educational and intellectual functioning in young autistic children," *Journal of Consulting and Clinical Psychology*, vol. 55, no. 1, pp. 3–9, 1987.

[8] J. J. McEachin, T. Smith, and O. I. Lovaas, "Long-term outcome for children with autism who received early intensive behavioral treatment," *American Journal on Mental Retardation*, vol. 97, no. 4, pp. 359–372, 1993.

[9] R. L. Koegel, Y. Bruinsma, and L. K. Koegel, "Developmental trajectories in early intervention," in *Pivotal Response Treatmentsfor Autism*, R. L. Koegel and L. K. Koegel, Eds., pp. 131–140, Brookes, Baltimore, Md, USA, 2006.

[10] S. J. Rogers, A. Estes, C. Lord et al., "Effects of a brief Early Start Denver Model (ESDM)-based parent intervention on toddlers at risk for autism spectrum disorders: a randomized controlled trial," *Journal of the American Academy of Child & Adolescent Psychiatry*, vol. 51, no. 10, pp. 1052–1065, 2012.

[11] S. Reilly, E. L. Bavin, L. Bretherton et al., "The early language in Victoria study (ELVS): a prospective, longitudinal study of communication skills and expressive vocabulary development at 8, 12 and 24 months," *International Journal of Speech-Language Pathology*, vol. 11, no. 5, pp. 344–357, 2009.

[12] G. Dawson, "Early behavioral intervention, brain plasticity, and the prevention of autism spectrum disorder," *Development and Psychopathology*, vol. 20, no. 3, pp. 775–803, 2008.

[13] G. Dawson, E. J. Jones, K. Merkle et al., "Early behavioral intervention is associated with normalized brain activity in young children with autism," *Journal of the American Academy of Child & Adolescent Psychiatry*, vol. 51, no. 11, pp. 1150–1159, 2012.

[14] G. Dawson, L. Carver, A. N. Meltzoff, H. Panagiotides, J. McPartland, and S. J. Webb, "Neural correlates of face and object recognition in young children with autism spectrum disorder, developmental delay, and typical development," *Child Development*, vol. 73, no. 3, pp. 700–717, 2002.

[15] G. Dawson, S. J. Webb, E. Wijsman et al., "Neurocognitive and electrophysiological evidence of altered face processing in parents of children with autism: implications for a model of abnormal development of social brain circuitry in autism," *Development and Psychopathology*, vol. 17, no. 3, pp. 679–697, 2005.

[16] M. Elsabbagh and M. H. Johnson, "Getting answers from babies about autism," *Trends in Cognitive Sciences*, vol. 14, no. 2, pp. 81–87, 2010.

[17] D. J. Grelotti, I. Gauthier, and R. T. Schultz, "Social interest and the development of cortical face specialization: what autism teaches us about face processing," *Developmental Psychobiology*, vol. 40, no. 3, pp. 213–225, 2002.

[18] M. H. Johnson, R. Griffin, G. Csibra et al., "The emergence of the social brain network: evidence from typical and atypical development," *Development and Psychopathology*, vol. 17, no. 3, pp. 599–619, 2005.

[19] P. K. Kuhl, "Is speech learning "gated" by the social brain?" *Developmental Science*, vol. 10, no. 1, pp. 110–120, 2007.

[20] P. K. Kuhl, S. Coffey-Corina, D. Padden, and G. Dawson, "Links between social and linguistic processing of speech in preschool children with autism: behavioral and electrophysiological measures," *Developmental Science*, vol. 8, no. 1, pp. F1–F12, 2005.

[21] M. H. Johnson, "Functional brain development in infants: elements of an interactive specialization framework," *Child Development*, vol. 71, no. 1, pp. 75–81, 2000.

[22] S. J. Rogers and L. A. Vismara, "Evidence-based comprehensive treatments for early autism," *Journal of Clinical Child and Adolescent Psychology*, vol. 37, no. 1, pp. 8–38, 2008.

[23] S. Rogers and K. Wallace, "Intervention for infants and toddlers with autism spectrum disorders," in *Autism Spectrum Disorders*, D. Amaral, G. Dawson, and D. Geshwind, Eds., pp. 1182–1195, Oxford University Press, 2011.

[24] M. Carpenter, K. Nagell, and M. Tomasello, "Social cognition, joint attention, and communicative competence from 9 to 15 months of age," *Monographs of the Society for Research in Child Development*, vol. 63, no. 4, pp. 1–143, 1998.

[25] I. P. Oono, E. J. Honey, and H. McConachie, "Parent-mediated early intervention for young children with autism spectrum disorders (ASD)," *The Cochrane Database of Systematic Reviews*, no. 4, Article ID CD009774, 2013.

[26] J. W. Kaminski, L. A. Valle, J. H. Filene, and C. L. Boyle, "A meta-analytic review of components associated with parent training program effectiveness," *Journal of Abnormal Child Psychology*, vol. 36, no. 4, pp. 567–589, 2008.

[27] H. McConachie and T. Diggle, "Parent implemented early intervention for young children with autism spectrum disorder: a systematic review," *Journal of Evaluation in Clinical Practice*, vol. 13, no. 1, pp. 120–129, 2007.

[28] H. Meadan, M. M. Ostrosky, H. Y. Zaghlawan, and S. Yu, "Promoting the social and communicative behavior of young children with autism spectrum disorders: a review of parent-implemented intervention studies," *Topics in Early Childhood Special Education*, vol. 29, no. 2, pp. 90–104, 2009.

[29] J. P. T. Higgins and S. Green, *Cochrane Handbook for Systematic Reviews of Interventions 4.2.6*, John Wiley & Sons, Chichester, UK, 2006.

[30] S. Green, "Systematic reviews and meta-analysis," *Singapore Medical Journal*, vol. 46, no. 6, pp. 270–274, 2005.

[31] A. Palmen, R. Didden, and R. Lang, "A systematic review of behavioral intervention research on adaptive skill building in high-functioning young adults with autism spectrum disorder," *Research in Autism Spectrum Disorders*, vol. 6, no. 2, pp. 602–617, 2012.

[32] R. Lang, M. O'Reilly, O. Healy et al., "Sensory integration therapy for autism spectrum disorders: a systematic review," *Research in Autism Spectrum Disorders*, vol. 6, no. 3, pp. 1004–1018, 2012.

[33] W. Machalicek, M. F. O'Reilly, N. Beretvas et al., "A review of school-based instructional interventions for students with autism spectrum disorders," *Research in Autism Spectrum Disorders*, vol. 2, no. 3, pp. 395–416, 2008.

[34] L. A. Vismara, C. Colombi, and S. J. Rogers, "Can one hour per week of therapy lead to lasting changes in young children with autism?" *Autism*, vol. 13, no. 1, pp. 93–115, 2009.

[35] L. A. Vismara and S. J. Rogers, "The early start denver model: a case study of an innovative practice," *Journal of Early Intervention*, vol. 31, no. 1, pp. 91–108, 2008.

[36] G. Mahoney and F. Perales, "Using relationship-focused intervention to enhance the social-emotional functioning of young children with autism spectrum disorders," *Topics in Early Childhood Special Education*, vol. 23, no. 2, pp. 74–86, 2003.

[37] G. Mahoney and F. Perales, "Relationship-focused early intervention with children with pervasive developmental disorders and other disabilities: a comparative study," *Journal of Developmental and Behavioral Pediatrics*, vol. 26, no. 2, pp. 77–85, 2005.

[38] A. Drew, G. Baird, S. Baron-Cohen et al., "A pilot randomised control trial of a parent training intervention for pre-school children with autism: preliminary findings and methodological challenges," *European Child & Adolescent Psychiatry*, vol. 11, no. 6, pp. 266–272, 2002.

[39] A. M. Wetherby and J. J. Woods, "Early social interaction project for children with autism spectrum disorders beginning in the second year of life: a preliminary study," *Topics in Early Childhood Special Education*, vol. 26, no. 2, pp. 67–82, 2006.

[40] M. L. Rocha, L. Schreibman, and A. C. Stahmer, "Effectiveness of training parents to teach joint attention in children with autism," *Journal of Early Intervention*, vol. 29, no. 2, pp. 154–172, 2007.

[41] H. H. Schertz and S. L. Odom, "Promoting joint attention in toddlers with autism: a parent-mediated developmental model," *Journal of Autism and Developmental Disorders*, vol. 37, no. 8, pp. 1562–1575, 2007.

[42] A. C. Gulsrud, L. B. Jahromi, and C. Kasari, "The co-regulation of emotions between mothers and their children with autism," *Journal of Autism and Developmental Disorders*, vol. 40, no. 2, pp. 227–237, 2010.

[43] C. Kasari, A. C. Gulsrud, C. Wong, S. Kwon, and J. Locke, "Randomized controlled caregiver mediated joint engagement intervention for toddlers with autism," *Journal of Autism and Developmental Disorders*, vol. 40, no. 9, pp. 1045–1056, 2010.

[44] I. Oosterling, J. Visser, S. Swinkels et al., "Randomized controlled trial of the focus parent training for toddlers with autism: 1-year outcome," *Journal of Autism and Developmental Disorders*, vol. 40, no. 12, pp. 1447–1458, 2010.

[45] V. C. N. Wong and Q. K. Kwan, "Randomized controlled trial for early intervention for autism: a pilot study of the Autism 1-2-3 project," *Journal of Autism and Developmental Disorders*, vol. 40, no. 6, pp. 677–688, 2010.

[46] A. S. Carter, D. S. Messinger, W. L. Stone, S. Celimli, A. S. Nahmias, and P. Yoder, "A randomized controlled trial of Hanen's "more than words" in toddlers with early autism symptoms," *Journal of Child Psychology and Psychiatry and Allied Disciplines*, vol. 52, no. 7, pp. 741–752, 2011.

[47] J. Green, M. W. Wan, J. Guiraud et al., "Intervention for infants at risk of developing autism: a case series," *Journal of Autism and Developmental Disorders*, vol. 43, no. 11, pp. 2502–2514, 2013.

[48] A. M. Steiner, G. W. Gengoux, A. Klin, and K. Chawarska, "Pivotal response treatment for infants at-risk for autism spectrum disorders: a pilot study," *Journal of Autism and Developmental Disorders*, vol. 43, no. 1, pp. 91–102, 2013.

[49] B. M. Prizant and A. M. Wetherby, "Understanding the continuum of discrete-trial traditional behavioral to social-pragmatic developmental approaches in communication enhancement for young children with autism/PDD," *Seminars in Speech and Language*, vol. 19, no. 4, pp. 329–424, 1998.

[50] S. I. Greenspan and S. Wieder, *Engaging Autism: Using the Floortime Approach to Help Children Relate, Communicate, and Think*, Da Capo Press, 2006.

[51] S. J. Rogers and G. Dawson, *Early Start Denver Model for Young Children with Autism: Promoting Language, Learning, and Engagement*, Guilford Press, 2010.

[52] S. L. Odom, L. Collet-Klingenberg, S. J. Rogers, and D. D. Hatton, "Evidence-based practices in interventions for children and youth with autism spectrum disorders," *Preventing School Failure*, vol. 54, no. 4, pp. 275–282, 2010.

[53] S. L. Odom, B. A. Boyd, L. J. Hall, and K. Hume, "Evaluation of comprehensive treatment models for individuals with autism spectrum disorders," *Journal of Autism and Developmental Disorders*, vol. 40, no. 4, pp. 425–436, 2010.

[54] L. Fenson, P. S. Dale, J. S. Reznick et al., *The MacArthur Communicative Development Inventories: User's Guide and Technical Manual*, Paul H. Brookes, Baltimore, Md, USA, 1993.

[55] C. Lord, M. Rutter, P. DiLavore, and S. Risi, *Autism Diagnostic Observation Schedule (ADOS) Manual*, Western Psychological Services, Los Angeles, Calif, USA , 2001.

[56] B. J. Freeman, E. R. Ritvo, A. Yokota, and A. Ritvo, "A scale for rating symptoms of patients with the syndrome of autism in real life settings," *Journal of the American Academy of Child Psychiatry*, vol. 25, no. 1, pp. 130–136, 1986.

[57] R. L. Koegel, A. Bimbela, and L. Schreibman, "Collateral effects of parent training on family interactions," *Journal of Autism and Developmental Disorders*, vol. 26, no. 3, pp. 347–359, 1996.

[58] B. Ingersoll and A. Wainer, "Initial efficacy of projet ImPACT: a parent-mediated social communication intervention for young children with ASD," *Journal of Autism and Developmental Disorders*, vol. 43, no. 12, pp. 2943–2952, 2013.

[59] A. Dabrowska and E. Pisula, "Parenting stress and coping styles in mothers and fathers of pre-school children with autism and Down syndrome," *Journal of Intellectual Disability Research*, vol. 54, no. 3, pp. 266–280, 2010.

[60] N. O. Davis and A. S. Carter, "Parenting stress in mothers and fathers of toddlers with autism spectrum disorders: associations with child characteristics," *Journal of Autism and Developmental Disorders*, vol. 38, no. 7, pp. 1278–1291, 2008.

[61] J. E. Dumas, L. C. Wolf, S. N. Fisman, and A. Culligan, "Parenting stress, child behavior problems, and dysphoria in parents of children with autism, Down syndrome, behavior disorders, and normal development," *Exceptionality*, vol. 2, no. 2, pp. 97–110, 1991.

[62] K. Mori, T. Ujiie, A. Smith, and P. Howlin, "Parental stress associated with caring for children with Asperger's syndrome or autism," *Pediatrics International*, vol. 51, no. 3, pp. 364–370, 2009.

[63] A. Estes, J. Munson, G. Dawson, E. Koehler, X.-H. Zhou, and R. Abbott, "Parenting stress and psychological functioning among mothers of preschool children with autism and developmental delay," *Autism*, vol. 13, no. 4, pp. 375–387, 2009.

[64] A. Estes, V. Hus, and L. Elder, "Family adaptive functioning in autism," in *Autism Spectrum Disorders*, D. Amaral, G. Dawson, and D. Geshwind, Eds., pp. 1182–1195, Oxford University Press, 2011.

[65] S. Y. Patterson and V. Smith, "The experience of parents of toddlers diagnosed with autism spectrum disorder in the more than words parent education program," *Infants & Young Children*, vol. 24, no. 4, pp. 329–343, 2011.

[66] M. L. Matson, S. Mahan, and J. L. Matson, "Parent training: a review of methods for children with autism spectrum disorders," *Research in Autism Spectrum Disorders*, vol. 3, no. 4, pp. 868–875, 2009.

[67] R. Lang, W. Machalicek, M. Rispoli, and A. Regester, "Training parents to implement communication interventions for children with autism spectrum disorders (ASD): a systematic review," *Evidence-Based Communication Assessment and Intervention*, vol. 3, no. 3, pp. 174–190, 2009.

[68] S. Y. Patterson, V. Smith, and P. Mirenda, "A systematic review of training programs for parents of children with spectrum disorders: single subject contributions," *Autism*, vol. 16, no. 5, pp. 498–522, 2012.

[69] L. Brookman-Frazee, "Using parent/clinician partnerships in parent education programs for children with autism," *Journal of Positive Behavior Interventions*, vol. 6, no. 4, pp. 195–213, 2004.

[70] D. V. Keen, F. D. Reid, and D. Arnone, "Autism, ethnicity and maternal immigration," *The British Journal of Psychiatry*, vol. 196, no. 4, pp. 274–281, 2010.

[71] T. Smith, A. D. Groen, and J. W. Wynn, "Randomized trial of intensive early intervention for children with pervasive developmental disorder," *American Journal on Mental Retardation*, vol. 105, no. 4, pp. 269–285, 2000.

[72] L. Abbeduto, M. M. Seltzer, P. Shattuck, M. W. Krauss, G. Orsmond, and M. M. Murphy, "Psychological well-being and coping in mothers of youths with autism, Down syndrome, or fragile X syndrome," *American Journal of Mental Retardation*, vol. 109, no. 3, pp. 237–254, 2004.

[73] M. J. Baker-Ericzén, L. Brookman-Frazee, and A. Stahmer, "Stress levels and adaptability in parents of toddlers with and without autism spectrum disorders," *Research and Practice for Persons with Severe Disabilities*, vol. 30, no. 4, pp. 194–204, 2005.

[74] S. Pisterman, P. Firestone, P. McGrath et al., "The role of parent training in treatment of preschoolers with ADDH," *American Journal of Orthopsychiatry*, vol. 62, no. 3, pp. 397–408, 1992.

[75] L. K. Cordisco, P. S. Strain, and N. Depew, "Assessment for generalization of parenting skills in home settings," *Journal of the Association for Persons With Severe Handicaps*, vol. 13, no. 3, pp. 202–210, 1988.

[76] T. Diggle, H. R. McConachie, and V. R. Randle, "Parent-mediated early intervention for young children with autism spectrum disorder," *The Cochrane Database of Systematic Reviews*, no. 1, Article ID CD003496, 2003.

13

Early Intervention with a Parent-Delivered Massage Protocol Directed at Tactile Abnormalities Decreases Severity of Autism and Improves Child-to-Parent Interactions

Louisa M. T. Silva,[1] Mark Schalock,[1] Kristen R. Gabrielsen,[1] Sarojini S. Budden,[2] Martha Buenrostro,[1] and Gretchen Horton[3]

[1] *Teaching Research Institute, Western Oregon University, 345 N. Monmouth Avenue, Monmouth, OR 97361, USA*
[2] *Providence Neurodevelopmental Center for Children, St. Vincent's Hospital, Portland, OR, USA*
[3] *Sikhara Group, 3434 NW Savier Street, Portland, OR 97210, USA*

Correspondence should be addressed to Louisa M. T. Silva; lmtsilva@qsti.org

Academic Editor: Herbert Roeyers

Tactile abnormalities are severe and universal in preschool children with autism. They respond well to treatment with a daily massage protocol directed at tactile abnormalities (QST massage for autism). Treatment is based on a model for autism proposing that tactile impairment poses a barrier to development. Two previous randomized controlled trials evaluating five months of massage treatment reported improvement of behavior, social/communication skills, and tactile and other sensory symptoms. This is the first report from a two-year replication study evaluating the protocol in 103 preschool children with autism. Parents gave daily treatment; trained staff gave weekly treatment and parent support. Five-month outcomes replicated earlier studies and showed normalization of receptive language (18%, $P = .03$), autistic behavior (32%, $P = .006$), total sensory abnormalities (38%, $P = .0000005$), tactile abnormalities (49%, $P = .0002$), and decreased autism severity (medium to large effect size, $P = .008$). In addition, parents reported improved child-to-parent interactions, bonding, and decreased parenting stress (44%, $P = .00008$). Early childhood special education programs are tasked with addressing sensory abnormalities and engaging parents in effective home programs. Until now, they have lacked research-based methods to do so. This program fulfills the need. It is recommended to parents and ECSE programs (ages 3–5) at autism diagnosis.

1. Introduction

Autism spectrum disorder (ASD) is the most rapidly growing childhood developmental disability in the United States [1]. Currently, it is estimated to affect one in 68 children [2]. To date, there is no known cause, no known cure, and no known explanation for why symptoms emerge prior to the age of two. In 2013, the diagnostic criteria for ASD were updated and abnormal sensory responses were included [3]. Today, ASD is diagnosed by a dyad of persistent symptoms that arise before the age of two: deficits of social interaction and restricted, repetitive behaviors, including sensory abnormalities. Symptoms occur on a spectrum of severity that is characterized on the basis of communication deficits and inflexibility of behavior.

Abnormal sensory responses were included in the diagnostic criteria for autism in 2013 because there was mounting evidence that they are directly related to severity of autism [4]. They occur early in life, encompass a range of hypo- and hyperreactivity, and are highly prevalent in children with autism [5]. Since early in the research literature, abnormal sensory responses have been widely thought to be due to disordered processing of sensory information [6–10]. Of all the sensory abnormalities, abnormal tactile responses are the most prevalent, with reported rates over 95% by parent report and direct observation [11, 12]. They are described in terms that are remarkably severe and unusual [13] but have never been subjected to full neurological evaluation.

The neurological evaluation of tactile symptoms proceeds by evaluating sensory nerve function relative to touch, pain, temperature, vibration, and position in symptomatic areas and then ruling out central pathology [14]. Ruling out peripheral sensory impairment is done first because sensory loss early in development results in both disordered sensory processing and changes in brain structure [15, 16]. Surprisingly enough, this evaluative sequence has not been followed in autism, and to date only three small studies evaluating partial aspects of touch have been published [17–19]. As such, a primary impairment of touch has not been ruled out, and a full neurological evaluation of the sense of touch has been urgently called for [20]. The missing information is extraordinarily germane because touch is the primary sense informing the bonding and preverbal communication that is required for social and language development [21, 22], and impairment of the sense of touch early in development can readily account for the social/language delay and disordered sensory processing that has been so well documented in autism.

Over the course of 14 years and 10 peer-reviewed research studies, our research group has investigated a model and treatment for autism proposing that autism symptoms are due in some part to tactile impairment [12, 23–27] and are treatable with a massage protocol based on Chinese medicine. Loss/damage to the sense of touch is proposed to block the child's perception of soothing and affectionate parent touch and interfere with social/language and self-regulatory development. This can first be observed when soothing touch fails to soothe the child, and affectionate touch fails to stimulate the social response, simultaneous orienting, eye contact, and listening [28]. The tactile barrier to soothing is proposed to result in prolonged episodes of elevated sympathetic tone [29, 30] and account for the remaining sensory abnormalities on the basis of poorly regulated sympathetic tone disorganizing sensory thresholds [31, 32].

For the purposes of our research we developed a checklist of common sensory symptoms in children with autism that could be used to identify skin areas in need of massage treatment and to measure tactile and other sensory outcomes [33]. The checklist also identifies delays of early touch-stimulated self-regulation milestones, including self-soothing, attention, sleep, digestion, and behavioral self-regulation [34]. The validation study distinguished children with autism from typical and otherwise developmentally delayed groups by a multifocal tactile abnormality characterized by signs of painful withdrawal from noninjurious touch (allodynia/pain) and lack of response to injury (hypoesthesia/numbness) [33]. Ninety-three percent of the ASD group had signs of pain with touch on the face and in the mouth, 93% on the scalp, and 88% on the fingers and toes. Sixty-five percent had signs of numbness in response to injury. In addition, there was global delay of first-year self-regulation milestones. Pain and numbness are typical of the clinical presentation of small fiber neuropathy, a common disorder of small sensory fibers in the skin [35].

Experimental data from two randomized controlled trials (RCT) evaluating five months of daily massage treatment support our model for autism [24, 25]. The protocol is called Qigong Sensory Treatment (QST) massage for autism. The protocol is designed to increase circulation to the skin, normalize the child's perception of touch, and allow touch-stimulated social and self-regulatory development to unfold naturally in the context of the care and feeding of the child. The outcomes of the two studies, one evaluating a program of five months of dual parent- and therapist-delivered treatment (n = 46, QST Dual program) and the other evaluating the parent component (n = 47, QST Home program), showed increased social and self-regulatory abilities, reduced autistic behavior, and reduced tactile and other sensory symptoms. The intervention was effective in both high- and low-functioning children and ten-month follow-up indicated that continued treatment resulted in continued improvement [25]. Longer-term studies to determine the endpoint of treatment have not yet been conducted.

From the start of the research, it was evident that treatment outcomes were highly dependent on parent fidelity with daily treatment. However, children's initial resistance to touch, the range of tactile responses seen, the complexity of adjusting treatment to changing responses, and the need for long-term daily treatment called for a manual with flexible procedures and a program of ongoing parent training and support. Thus a five-month parent training program was developed, comprised of a parent handbook [36] and an initial 3-hour training, followed by 20 one-on-one support visits with a trained professional. This proved to be adequate to ensure fidelity with the intervention in the first five months of treatment.

The present study is part of a three-year, multisite RCT replicating and extending previous studies and evaluating the efficacy of the QST Dual massage intervention on tactile abnormalities and severity of autism in a larger group. In the first two years, treatment outcomes for 103 children under the age of six will be evaluated. In year three, treatment outcomes for 35 children between the ages of 6–11 will be evaluated. We will also seek further evaluation of tactile abnormalities with skin biopsy.

The three-year study will test two hypotheses.

(1) Treatment of 103 preschool children with autism with the QST Dual massage intervention will result in decreased severity of autism across language, behavioral, and other sensory aspects of autism compared to the control condition. Treatment will be effective in both lower- and higher-functioning children. In addition, treatment will improve tactile and other sensory abnormalities and early self-regulation milestones and reduce parenting stress.

(2) Treatment outcomes will be independent of severity of autism.

The objectives of this portion of the study are to evaluate initial 5-month treatment outcomes on severity of autism and on parent-child interaction and bonding. As compared to previous studies, this study will add new measures evaluating the overall severity of autism and receptive/expressive language level, as well as qualitative analysis of parent comments on parent-child bonding and interactions. The main outcomes are on measures of severity of autism, autistic

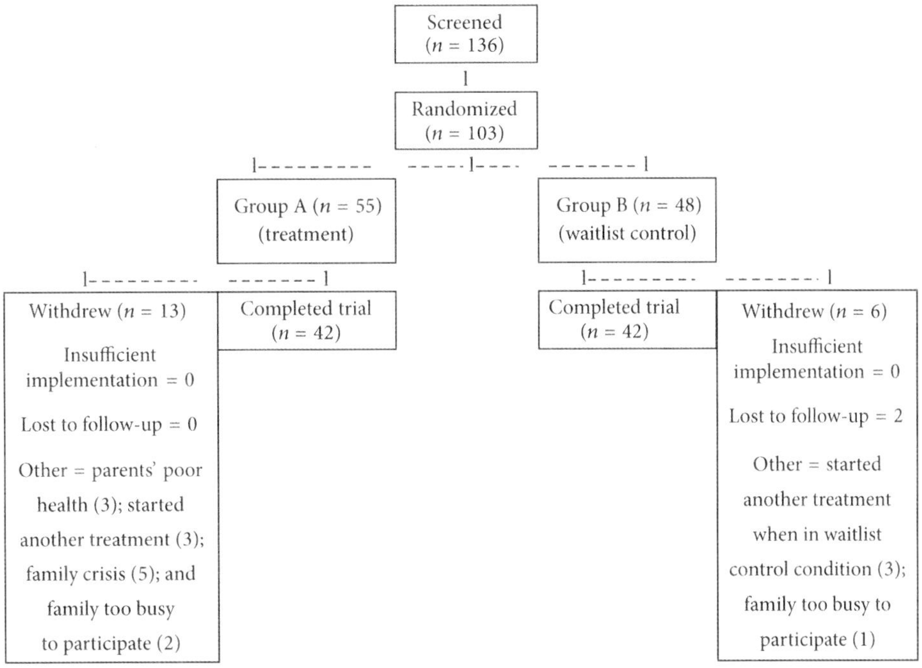

Figure 1: Participant flow diagram.

behavior, and language development. The secondary outcomes are tactile and other sensory abnormalities, self-regulatory delay, parenting stress, and general development. In addition, qualitative data on parent comments will be presented and analyzed.

2. Materials and Methods

2.1. Study Design. This study was a multisite, randomized, single-blind, controlled trial of the QST Dual massage intervention in 103 preschool children with autism. Blinded professional examiners evaluated baseline and interval measurements. Baseline and interval reports were collected from parents. This is a replication and extension study of previously published studies; therefore, it was not possible for parents to remain blind to group. However, parents are known to be accurate reporters of current, observable child behavior [37] and parent information was treated as reliable and accurate. Children were randomized to treatment and control groups using a random number generator. Both groups were enrolled in early intervention programs. The treatment group received five months of daily parent-delivered massage and 20 sessions of therapist-delivered massage. Fidelity was assured with a formalized training program and ongoing support. The control group was in the waitlist condition and received treatment after five months. Treatment was directed towards normalizing responses to touch. Pre- and posttesting were done by the same professional examiners who were blind to group. Additional data was collected from parents. The study was conducted with Institutional Review Board approval and registered with the U.S. National Institutes of Health clinical trials registry (# NCT01801696).

2.2. Participants and Recruitment. Recruitment was accomplished via distribution of brochures, emails, listserv messages, website postings, presentations, social media, TV, radio, and word of mouth. In addition, invitation letters were sent to parents of children aged 2 to 5 receiving autism services from state-funded, early childhood special education and early intervention programs in eight counties in Oregon. Criteria for entry into the study included age of 2 to 5 years; diagnosis of autism; no additional chronic disability; no psychoactive medication or pharmaceutical chelation therapy; and not receiving more than fifteen hours per week of intensive behavioral treatment for autism. This criterion was chosen because there is no research evidence that low-intensity ABA treatment produces therapeutic outcomes [38, 39]. Only two study participants were identified as receiving ABA treatment; they were receiving 8 and 10 hours/week, respectively. Parents agreed to give their children the daily massage treatment for the duration of the study; to follow through with all training and support visits; and not to begin additional interventions for autism during the study. Parents provided records documenting their child's autism diagnosis. The majority of diagnoses had been previously made at autism evaluation centers using instruments such as the ADI and/or the ADOS. Children subsequently underwent a second diagnosis with such instruments prior to acceptance into early intervention autism programs. Prior to acceptance into the study, records were reviewed and the previous diagnosis of autism was confirmed. In addition, a developmental pediatrician reviewed the pretreatment testing and reconfirmed the autism diagnosis using DSM-IV criteria.

2.3. Study Completion. Figure 1 provides an overview of participant flow. One hundred thirty-six children were screened for the study during the period of September 2012 through April 2014 by the principal investigator and the project director. An additional 39 parents indicated interest in enrolling their children but did not submit enrollment documents. One hundred three children from 10 different counties in Oregon were determined to be eligible for the study, of which 55 were randomized to the treatment group and 48 to the waitlist control group. During the study period, 19 participants withdrew from the study for a total participant completion rate of 82% and a final $n = 42$ for both study and control groups.

2.4. Randomization Procedures. Children and their families from each geographical area who met study criteria were randomly assigned into either the treatment or control group condition based on age in months to reduce bias on developmental measures. A random number generator was used. One pair of siblings was assigned into the same group by necessity. Odd numbers of participants in each site resulted in uneven initial group sizes when randomized.

2.5. The Massage Protocol. The QST massage protocol is a whole-body massage that takes about 15 minutes to give and is usually done at bedtime. It is formalized in a parent training handbook with flexible constraints [36]. The parent does not avoid areas that are uncomfortable but instead works with them by attuning the massage techniques to the child's responses, within the comfort zone of the child. Over the course of treatment, tactile responses undergo predictable changes from hyposensitive to hypersensitive to normosensitive [36]. The protocol requires adjustment of the manual technique with each transition. The protocol also aims to sequentially stimulate social and self-regulatory activity, first by stimulating awareness and receptivity to massage, then by stimulating eye contact and smile, and finally by stimulating deep relaxation with touch.

The protocol has 12 parts that follow the acupuncture channels down the front and back of the body. Massage is carried out in a downward direction towards the hands and feet in the direction of capillary blood flow. Both patting and pressure are used according to the child's response. Generally, a quicker, lighter, patting technique is used to begin with, but in areas where the child withdraws from touch or is ticklish, slower pressing techniques are used. Additional options are available when neither patting nor pressure resolves the difficulty. For a summary of the massage movements, go to http://qsti.org/wp-content/uploads/2014/06/12Movements-Autism.pdf.

Therapists providing the parent training and support program benefitted from a 60-hour training. A total of 19 therapists participated in the study. Parent training unfolded with a group training followed by weekly one-on-one support. At each visit, therapists inquired about fidelity with daily massage, provided ongoing support and training, and gave children a massage treatment.

There are four time periods when parents are at risk for discontinuing the program. These are (1) upon initiating the program and not knowing how to deal with the child's resistance to massage; (2) during the transition period when the sensory system switches from hyposensitive to hypersensitive and massage techniques must be modified; (3) the transition period when the child moves into the autonomy phase of development and parenting techniques must be modified; and (4) the period after which the child has come to relax and enjoy the massage, progress is no longer dramatic, and daily massage can fall off the priority list. Therapists were instructed to watch for these at-risk periods and provide the necessary support.

2.6. Measures. Demographic information was obtained from participants and is shown in Table 1. Treatment and control groups were comparable. Overall, the percentage of boys (89%) was higher than the national average. Lower income families were identified as being at or below 100% and 150% of federal poverty guidelines for 2014 [40]. Representation of lower income families (53%) and culturally diverse families (44%) was higher than state demographics (Hispanic 34%, American Indian/Alaska Native 7%, and Native Hawaiian/Pacific Islander 3%). Eighty percent of parents involved had no previous experience with massage or Chinese medicine. Families who withdrew from the study did not have different demographics.

The following measures were used to evaluate five-month treatment outcomes.

(1) Childhood Autism Rating Scale, 2nd Edition, Standard Version (CARS2-ST) [41]. The CARS2 standard version is validated for children younger than 6. It has been found to be stable in the face of change over 12 months and not generally used as an outcomes measure. Total CARS scores range from 15 to 60. A score of 30 serves as the cutoff for a diagnosis of autism on the mild end of the autism spectrum; 30 to 36 is scored as mild to moderate; 36 and higher is scored as severe. The pretreatment median score of 39 was used as the criteria in the analyses to determine effects on language development by level of severity. Internal consistency is reported at .93, interrater correlation at .95, and test-retest stability at .88. The CARS2-ST was administered by professionals who were blind to group.

(2) Preschool Language Scale, 5th Edition (PLS-5) [42]. The PLS-5 has standardized subscales which evaluate relative ability in receptive and expressive language in children under 7. The test-retest stability coefficients ranged between .97 and .98 for the subscale scores and .97 to .98 for the total score. Internal consistency (split-half reliability) ranges from .91 to .93 for the subscale scores and .95 for the total score. The PLS-5 was administered by blinded professionals.

(3) Vineland Adaptive Behavior Scales, 2nd Edition (Vineland-II) [43]. The Vineland-II is a validated parent interview that assesses socialization, communication, motor skills, and daily living skills. Internal consistency split-half reliability coefficients were .97 for the composite scale and ranged from .83 to .95 for the domains. Test-retest coefficients were .94 for the composite scale and ranged from .88 to .92 for the domains.

TABLE 1: Participant demographics.

	Tx active	Tx dropped	Tx total	Control active	Control dropped	Control total	Total active	Total dropped
Total number	42	13	55	42	6	48	103	19
Gender								
Male	36	12	48	39	5	44	92	17
Female	6	1	7	3	1	4	11	2
Race*								
AI/AN	4	1	5	1	1	2	7	2
Asian	4	0	4	5	0	5	9	0
NH/PI	0	1	1	2	0	2	3	1
Black	1	2	3	3	1	4	6	3
White	40	10	50	39	6	45	95	16
Other	4	2	6	1	0	1	7	2
Ethnicity								
Hispanic/Latino	11	4	15	7	2	9	24	6
Not Hisp./Lat.	31	9	40	35	4	39	79	13
Poverty level								
100%	9	1	10	9	1	10	20	2
150%	16	3	19	16	1	17	36	4
Did not share income level	4	3	7	6	0	6	13	3

Tx = treatment.
Tx drop = those participants who were in the treatment group condition that dropped out.
Control drop = those participants who were in the waitlist control group condition that dropped out.
AI/AN = American Indian/Alaska native.
NH/PI = native Hawaiian/Pacific Islander.
*Note: parents could select more than one ethnicity/race. So the numbers add up to more than the number of subjects.

Raw scores were used in the statistical analysis while age equivalent scores are used to illustrate the magnitude of the changes in development over the treatment period. The social and daily living subscales were administered by blinded professionals.

(4) Autism Behavior Checklist (ABC) [44]. The ABC is a validated measure of autism and a component of the Autism Screening Instrument for Educational Planning. The ABC is used as a measure of change in response to the classroom program and as an outcomes measure in research. It measures behaviors typical of autism in five domains: sensory, relating, body and object use, language, and social and self-help. Adequate reliability and an alpha coefficient of .89 are established. Parents completed the ABC to report outcomes in the home setting at baseline and 5 months. The mean value for typically developing children is reported at 17.81 [45].

(Note: we were particularly interested to see whether we could replicate previous results in individuals with low functioning autism as there is little available evidence-based treatment for that group. Thus, we used two outcomes measures of autism severity: the CARS, a highly stable measure that is stable over a 12-month interval, and the ABC, a more sensitive questionnaire that is currently used in conjunction with a direct observation measure for evaluating educational outcomes [44]. Both the CARS and the ABC measure current functioning relative to similar aspects of autism but differ as to the length of time over which the measurement is taken. One is a direct-observer measure taken at a single point in time; the second is a questionnaire that solicits information describing the child at the present time. Thus, because child behavior can differ from day to day, measures were analyzed together in order to get a more balanced view of present functioning.)

(5) Sense and Self-Regulation Checklist (SSC) [33]. The SSC is a validated parent/caregiver measure of sensory difficulties and self-regulatory delays in children with autism under the age of 6. It is used as an outcomes measure in clinical practice and research. Scores can be generated for sensory and self-regulation domains. An overall internal consistency alpha of .87 has been demonstrated. Sensory items have an internal consistency alpha of .83; self-regulation items have an internal consistency alpha of .78. The SSC significantly differentiates children with autism from otherwise developmentally delayed (other DD) and typically developing (typical) children. The means and standard deviations for abnormal sensory response for ASD, other DD, and typically developing children are 39.6 (SD 10.6), 30.6 (SD 7.9), and 18.4 (SD 9.5), respectively. The mean oral/tactile scores for ASD, other DD, and typical children are 29.2 (SD 7.9), 22.8 (SD 6.7), and 13.5 (SD 7.2), respectively. The mean self-regulatory difficulty scores for ASD, other DD, and typical children are 56.8 (SD 14.1), 44.0 (SD 13.4), and 25.8 (SD 11.3), respectively. The SSC

was completed by parents and used in data exploration of intervening variables affecting treatment outcomes.

(6) Autism Parenting Stress Index (APSI) [46]. The APSI is a validated parent/caregiver measure of parenting stress relative to autism symptoms. It is intended to measure the level of difficulty experienced by parents in successfully parenting the various physical and behavioral manifestations of autism, as well as factors impacting parenting stress such as lack of feeling close to the child, and concerns about the future of the child. It is used as an outcomes measure in clinical practice and research. Current data indicate adequate internal consistency (.83) and test-retest stability (.89). A validation study comparing scores from children with ASD with normally developing and otherwise developmentally delayed peers showed that the scales differentiate significantly between groups, with mean scores for ASD, other DD, and typical children of 23 (SD 10.4), 11.74 (SD 6.7), and 5.4 (SD 5.1), respectively. The APSI was completed by parents and used to measure changes in parenting stress relative to autism symptoms.

(7) Beach Center Family-Professional Partnership Scale [47]. The partnership scale is a validated tool that assesses satisfaction with services received. It contains two subscales: child-focused relationships and family-focused relationships. This 27-item scale is designed to be used as a research tool. Cronbach's alpha is 0.93. Parents completed the partnership scale at posttesting.

(8) Fidelity and Social Validation Testing. Therapists monitored parent fidelity with massage procedures by testing parents at weeks one and two with a checklist. The principal investigator monitored therapist fidelity with the parent training and support program. Parents completed a daily log recording fidelity with daily massage, reasons for missing the massage, and problems or concerns. In addition, parents completed a posttreatment survey consisting of a series of open-ended questions exploring their reactions to treatment and outcomes. See Table 2 for posttreatment survey questions.

Table 2: Parent posttreatment questions.

Question
(1) What has the massage done for you and your child?
(2) Compared to before starting this program, do you use touch more, less, or the same when your child is having behavior problems?
(3) What changes have you seen in your child since beginning the massage?
(4) When you compare the massage to other treatments, how does it differ?
(5) If you could sum up your experience in a way that would be helpful for another parent considering this treatment, what would it be?

2.7. Data Collection. Pre- and postintervention data collection was conducted within a one-month window both prior to beginning of treatment and after the 20-week intervention for children in both the treatment and control conditions. Parents completed an online set of surveys and background questionnaires that included the Autism Parenting Stress Index, the Sense and Self-Regulation Checklist, and the Autism Behavior Checklist. The Vineland-II, CARS2-ST, and PLS-5 were administered in the home by trained, blind-to-condition professionals. Treatment fidelity was monitored throughout the 20-week intervention by assigned therapists.

2.8. Data Analysis. Initial analyses were conducted to detect any potential attrition bias using 2-way ANOVA and MANOVA on preassessment outcome measures. This was followed with analyses to confirm equivalence of treatment and control groups on preassessment outcome measures using 2-way ANOVA and MANOVA. Descriptive and paired t-tests on outcome measures were conducted for both treatment and control groups. Main treatment effects were tested using 2-way repeated measure ANOVAs and MANOVAs. Testing whether treatment outcomes were independent of language ability and severity of autism was also conducted using 2-way repeated measure ANOVAs and MANOVAs.

3. Results

3.1. Sample Size Justification and Power Analysis. A power analysis to determine sample size for this study was conducted using pooled data from all children under the age of six who had participated in our previous studies and received the QST intervention. The primary outcome used was the composite score from the Pervasive Developmental Disorders Behavior Inventory [48]. An n of 45 for both the treatment and control group, with 12% attrition, yielded a final n of 40 for each group. Allowing for attrition, a final n of 40 in each group, and a $P < .05$, a power analysis yielded a power of .99 on parent measures.

3.2. Potential Attrition Bias. Participants in the control and treatment condition withdrew at a proportional rate X^2 $(1, N = 100) = .841$, $P = .359$. Two-way ANOVA and MANOVA indicate no differences between completers and noncompleters on outcome measures. F values range from .018 to 3.57 with associated P values ranging from .894 to .062. There was a difference in age between completers and noncompleters, with noncompleters being on average six months younger than completers $F(1, 98) = 4.58$, $P = .035$.

3.3. Equivalence of Treatment and Control Groups. Participants in the treatment and control conditions did not differ on outcome measures or age. Two-way ANOVA and MANOVA indicate no differences between groups on outcome measures and age. F values ranged from .619 to 1.56 with associated P values ranging from .528 to .216.

3.4. Preassessment to Postassessment Changes. Table 3 displays descriptive pre- and postoutcomes for both treatment

TABLE 3: Preassessment to postassessment results for the QST massage.

	Treatment group (n = 42)						Control group (n = 42)					
	Preassessment mean (SD)	Postassessment mean (SD)	Diff.	% norm	t	P	Preassessment mean (SD)	Postassessment mean (SD)	Diff.	% norm	t	P
Parent measures												
Parenting stress	24.3 (9.51)	15.8 (8.9)	−8.5	44%	−6.49	.0000001	22.5 (9.33)	21.0 (9.6)	−1.5	9%	−1.39	.171
ABC	82.4 (25.9)	61.5 (26.6)	−20.9	32%	−5.64	.000001	83.1 (25.9)	75.7 (28.6)	−7.4	—	−2.48	.018
Abnormal sensory response	39.7 (9.1)	30.4 (9.8)	−9.3	38%	−6.68	.00000005	41.3 (10.3)	38.6 (11.6)	−2.7	11%	−3.00	.005
Tactile/oral abnormalities	29.6 (6.8)	22.4 (8.0)	−7.2	49%	−6.14	.0000003	29.6 (7.7)	27.7 (8.6)	−1.9	11%	−2.59	.013
Self-regulatory difficulties	57.6 (11.2)	45.1 (11.5)	−12.5	34%	−7.64	.000000001	57.4 (13.4)	54.0 (14.5)	−3.4	9%	−2.35	.024
Blinded assessor measures												
Vineland daily living skills	34.3 (17.7)	42.7 (19.1)	8.4		5.21	.00001	37.5 (20.0)	45.9 (22.7)	8.4		5.50	.000002
Vineland socialization	36.0 (14.4)	45.7 (16.3)	9.7		5.54	.000003	40.7 (17.4)	48.6 (21.0)	7.9		5.82	.000002
CARS	39.7 (6.6)	38.2 (6.6)	−1.5		−2.61	.013	38.0 (7.8)	37.7 (7.8)	−0.3		−1.13	.266
PLS-5 auditory communication	25.9 (12.1)	30.6 (12.1)	4.7		6.07	.0000004	29.2 (13.5)	31.8 (14.3)	2.6		5.16	.00001
PLS-5 expressive communication	26.5 (11.1)	30.0 (11.1)	3.5		6.22	.0000002	28.2 (11.6)	31.3 (13.1)	3.1		5.54	.000002

Note: SD = standard deviation; Diff. = the change from pre- to postscore; % norm = the percentage reduction in parenting stress, autistic behavior, abnormal sensory responses, and self-regulatory difficulties toward typically developing children.

TABLE 4: Treatment effects for QST massage (repeated measures Anova/Manova).

Variable	Group main intervention effect				
	F	(Degrees of freedom)	P	η_P^2	
Univariate analysis					
Stress	17.2	(1,82)	.00008	.173	Large
Receptive language (PLS-5 auditory)	4.81	(1,82)	.031	.055	Medium
Expressive language (PLS-5 expressive)	0.18	(1,82)	.667	.002	Small
Multivariate analyses					
Severity	5.17	(2,81)	.008	.113	Medium-large
Post-hoc					
ABC	8.11	(1,82)	.006	.090	
CARS	3.34	(1,82)	.071	.039	
Sensory and self-regulation	7.40	(3,80)	.00002	.217	Large
Post-hoc					
Sensory	15.16	(1,82)	.00002	.156	
Tactile/oral	14.92	(1,82)	.00002	.154	
Self-regulation	17.92	(1,82)	.00006	.179	
General development	0.42	(2,81)	.656	.010	Small
Post-hoc					
Vineland daily living skills		No post-hoc analyses			
Vineland socialization					

and control groups. Paired t-test results are also shown. Treatment group participants experienced significant improvement on all measures. Control group participants also experienced significant improvements on a number of measures, although typically these changes were not as large as for the treatment group. Because mean scores for text typically developing children are well above zero, an additional column calculating percent (%) change toward typical norm has been added to Table 3 to show the percent (%) normalization of the reported change. Children in the treatment group experienced a 38% decrease in abnormal sensory response toward normalization. These children experienced a 49% decrease in abnormal oral/tactile response toward normalization. The decrease in self-regulatory difficulties represented 34% improvement toward normalization. Autistic behavior decreased 32% towards normalization. Parents of these children experienced a 44% decrease in stress toward normalization.

3.5. Intervention Effects on Main and Secondary Outcomes. Main outcomes include severity of autism, language, and general development. Secondary outcomes include sensory, self-regulation, and parenting stress. Table 4 presents results from the 2-way repeated measures ANOVA and MANOVA analyses. Equality of error variances were confirmed for all analyses. There was an overall treatment effect in reducing the overall severity of autism in the treatment group as measured by the CARS and ABC. Effect size was in the medium to large range. Post-hoc univariate analyses found a significant effect on the ABC but not the CARS. The correlation between the ABC and CARS was low (.273), indicating that they measure different things.

Separate 2-way repeated measure ANOVAs were conducted on receptive and expressive language. A significant treatment effect was found on receptive language with an effect size in the medium range. No treatment effect was found on expressive language.

A 2-way repeated measures MANOVA was conducted on general development of social and living skills. No treatment effect was found on general development. Both groups experienced increases in raw scores equivalent to 4–8-month increases in mental age on living skills and 4–6 months on socialization.

A 2-way repeated measures MANOVA was conducted on sensory and self-regulation. An overall significant treatment effect was found with a large effect size. Post-hoc univariate analyses found a significant effect on the sensory abnormalities, tactile/oral abnormalities, and the self-regulatory difficulties.

Finally, a 2-way repeated measure ANOVA was conducted on parenting stress. A significant treatment effect was found with a large effect size.

3.6. Effectiveness of Treatment by Severity of Autism. To further test whether the effectiveness of the treatment was independent of severity of autism, the treatment group was split into mild/moderate (a score of less than 39 on the CARS) and severe (a score of 39 and higher on the CARS) autism subgroups. Paired t-tests were performed on the outcome measures for the subgroups.

As can be seen in Table 4, there was an overall significant treatment effect on receptive language. Further, children with both mild/moderate and severe autism experienced significant improvements in receptive language as measured by the PLS-5 Auditory Language (t values are −4.26 and −4.29, respectively, with associated P values of .0001 and .0003).

The results in Table 4 show overall significant multivariate and post-hoc univariate treatment effects on abnormal sensory response and self-regulation. Again, children with mild/moderate and severe autism both experienced significant reductions in abnormal sensory response and self-regulatory difficulties as well as tactile/oral abnormalities (t values ranged from −4.24 to −5.88, with respective P values ranging from .0004 to .00001).

The overall significant treatment effect on reducing parenting stress is shown in Table 4. Parents of children with mild/moderate and severe autism experienced significant reductions in stress (t values were −5.135 and −4.448, with associated P values of .0001 and .0002).

3.7. Parent Satisfaction and Reactions to the Treatment and Outcomes. The Beach Center Family-Partnership Scale survey showed that 95% of the treatment group parents were very satisfied with their experience with the intervention, and 5% were somewhat satisfied.

Table 5 lists examples of parent responses to posttreatment survey questions about the parent experience of changes in their child. The table has additional columns reporting the survey question referenced (see Table 2). The table illustrates the normalization of touch and relationship that all parents experienced in one way or another with their child and gives examples of the accompanying sensory and behavioral changes that they observed.

Table 6 lists the types of responses parents had to posttreatment questions 4 and 5: "When you compare the massage to other treatments, how does it differ?" and "If you could sum up your experience in a way that would be helpful for another parent considering this treatment, what would it be?" Themes that emerged were improved bonding (18), parent empowerment to actively help their child (12), treatment supporting overall development (5), and ability to easily give the treatment at home (3).

3.8. Fidelity. Therapists tested parents on the 12 massage movements after the first and second week of treatment using a checklist. At the end of the second week, 75% of parents demonstrated complete fidelity with massage procedures. The other 25% needed correction on one or two of the 12 parts of the massage. For those that did not complete all 12 movements correctly, therapists checked on fidelity each of the following weeks until all 12 movements were correct. Twenty-nine of the 42 sets of parents provided the treatment daily throughout the 5-month treatment period. The balance, 13, provided the treatment less than daily during some periods, usually due to sickness of the child or the parent. All therapists provided 20 training and support visits.

3.9. Adverse Effects. There were no adverse effects reported in children. One parent with severe wartime PTSD found that he was unable to give the massage due to excessive anxiety triggered by his child's resistance to touch. Once he stopped giving the massage, he experienced no further anxiety relative to the massage.

4. Discussion

This is the first evidence-based intervention for tactile abnormalities in children with autism that effectively treats them with a massage protocol rather than making environmental accommodations to them. Before treatment, the mean tactile abnormality score for the treatment group was more than twice that of the typically developing group. After treatment, scores normalized by 49%. Parents reported that the massage helped to build a stronger bond and improved the experience of touch and relationship. Children sought out touch and affection from their parents, and parents felt closer and more connected. Child-to-parent attachment difficulties are described in the autism literature [49], and the profound degree to which they impact the parenting experience is illustrated in the parent comments, the very large decrease (44%) in parenting stress, and the very high parent satisfaction rate (95%) when they improve. Attachment theory has had difficulty in accounting for attachment difficulties in autism because they exist despite evidence of normal parent-to-child bond and sensitivity [50]. We suggest that normal attachment requires child sensitivity as well and that tactile abnormalities interfere with child-to-parent bonding. The very good news is that tactile abnormalities are reversible with treatment.

We were particularly interested in the 5-month treatment outcomes on receptive language. Concordant with increased diagnosis of high functioning autism (HFA) [51], this study had a higher proportion of children with HFA than previous studies. In children with low functioning autism (LFA), receptive language delay stands in the way of the development of speech; in children with HFA, receptive language delay manifests as echolalia or as monologues on topics of interest, for example, dinosaurs or robots. As it turned out, receptive language improved in both groups by a mean value of 18%. We ascribe the improvement to the effect of normalization of touch on foundational social and nonverbal communication abilities: the ability to be receptive to another person, make eye contact, give face-to-face attention, and listen. All of these are normally stimulated by touch in the first year of life in typically developing children but tend to be absent in young children with autism.

This was a replication and extension study, a necessary step before an intervention can be more widely recommended. Results replicated earlier studies with regard to overall decrease in severity of autism, improvements in autistic behavior, communication, sensory symptoms, and parenting stress. As shown previously, treatment was effective in both low- and high-functioning children. We were particularly interested to see whether we could replicate previous results in individuals with LFA, as there is little available evidence-based treatment for that group. We used two outcomes measures of autism severity: a highly stable measure that is stable

Table 5: Parent comments on changes in the child and changes in relationship.

ID #	Changes in the child	Q	Changes in relationship	Q
1	She is a lot more cuddly. Her sensory issues have improved a little	1	This has brought us closer together. She is more friendly with family members.	4
2	Increased calm, less tantrums, increased communication/speech. He is now potty trained!!!!	1		2
3	He doesn't have the long tantrums he used to have.	3	We've become closer and he's developed a stronger bond with both his parents. His speech development has made dramatic progress. He's using full sentences now, often to our amazement and gratitude.	1
4	He tolerates touching and the massage a great deal more. He now cries when he's hurt. He makes eye contact more often, and displays spontaneous affection way more than he used to!	3	We have developed a closer relationship, his development accelerated, and he is much more social than he was.	1
5	Meltdowns are fewer and less severe when they do occur, and he is using his words much more frequently.	3	He has become more interactive in class, even interacting with a few other students. He has taken the initiative to ask other kids to play with him at our local park.	3
6	We are able to cut his finger and toe nails with very little fuss! We've also seen some progress in potty training.	1, 3		
7	He wants us to touch him more. He's more talkative, learning to use the toilet more, gained a bunch of new skills.	3	He loves his massage. It calms him down, he likes spending the time with me. It makes him nice and sleepy before bed.	1
8	Touch seems comforting to my child after starting the program. Easy transition, less tantrum.	3	The most obvious one is the child get a lot closer to family members.	1
9	Some of his sensory issues are starting to shift for the better. More eye contact. He's more aware of what is going on around him. More tantrums from being more aware.	1	He is more cuddly and affectionate than before. Now he hugs and kisses his stuffed animals, as well as gives his dad and I more hugs and kisses.	3
10	He has started to self soothe. He tries new thing and is interested in more things than just matchbox cars. He has grown up so much. It is amazing to see the transformation. It's like the frustrated little boy who couldn't get his point across has finally come out and has so much to say and do.	1	I feel like it bonds the parent to the child. I think it opens the child up and they understand they are safe.	3
11	He makes better eye contact and will make eye contact when asked. He has developed some self-soothing techniques and has improved in his toileting.	3	He is socializing more with other children and will ask his sister to play. He uses his words to communicate a lot better than he had before the massage. He has better patience and self-control.	
12	She made a lot of eye contact, improving every week. Likes hugs and massages, calms her down.	1	Connection between father and daughter at night time.	1
13	Better interactions. Better for her as far as being comfortable being touched. Sleep has improved.	1	Better interactions. Massage builds a better bond.	4
14	I gave my child a haircut without a single scream. This is a huge change. He now will sit in a chair at home, wear a cape, verbally say "you cut my hair mommy" and then sit and hold still and giggle when the clippers tickle his neck.	3	He has made huge leaps and bounds in his social interaction with the world since starting the massage, He is beginning to notice other people and appropriately interact with them and reciprocate language. His ability to communicate his own needs has also increased an amazing amount. He is now requesting for items in full sentences the majority of the time as opposed to one or two word requests 60% of the time. I loved that the massage focused on him being comfortable in his own body.	1
15	Well right after we started we had an extremely difficult time for about 4 weeks with our son. My husband stuck with doing his massage and it seems to have paid off. Brenner asks for it! He also does the "massage" to us. That is huge in itself. Overall there is consistent improvement.	1	He likes massage with me (mom), super silly for dad. He communicates better. He does not react towards people as bad as he did before.	3

Table 5: Continued.

ID #	Changes in the Child	Q	Changes in Relationship	Q
16			More joyful content pride self esteem.	3
17	He can feel pain now! It amazes me to see him cry for even the tiniest scratch or bump. He also has stopped biting me. He looks forward to the massage.	3	He actively hugs me if he thinks that I am sad.	3
18	He's more present. Massage helps me calm him.	3	Massage strengthens our connection.	1
19	He's more aware of his body, more eye contact. Massage gives tools to help calm him. We can use the massage to get him to sleep if we need to. Potty training progress.	3	Social games, increase in spontaneous language and longer sentences. Massage makes an emotional and spiritual connection between us.	3, 4
20	He is able to sleep during the night. . .his language has catapulted and he is less aggressive!	3	Massage is calming and brings you closer to your child.	4
21	He does more eye contact. He gets more concentred [sic]. He slept through all the night.	3	Massage get [sic] you and your kid closer. It's like time to relax and show love with each other.	4
22	I has [sic] been able to calm him down a little bit.	1	Had some great momma and son time.	1
23	It's probably improved his eye contact somewhat. He eats better and is not as sensitive to touching sticky things as he used to be. He is able to calm himself down much easier. He rarely has major tantrums. If he starts one, it's usually over within a couple of seconds. He also seems to be sleeping better and it's easier for me to clip his finger and toe nails than it used to be.	3	It's been a good time of connection. About half the time, the massage seems to help calm him down before bed.	1
24	It helped him transition before during and after the move.	1	It helped him get a bit more calmed after massage and he wanted to cuddle right after.	1
25	I can cut her nails while she's awake, She has tried some new foods that she used to eat when she was younger, her bowel movements are not as hard - there's practically no pushing on her end. She uses pronouns properly now, she uses a ton more words.	3	It's done by me and my husband, no outsider can do it better than we can. Every other improvement seems to be because of some professional, this is because of our touch.	4
26	His ability to calm himself or request aid in calming himself is unmatched, started taking an interest in potty training. Improved verbal and communication skills.	3	Brought us closer. We both really enjoy the time we spend doing the massage together. It's been a great bonding experience for us. It also is a good time for both of us to de-stress and calm down together.	4
27	Well I could not pinpoint one in particular.	3	Got me more in tune with my son's body language.	1
28	He moves his fingers and toes, explores them, and is responsive and ok with the feeling or sensations in them. He is toe walking less. He reacts to pain when he gets hurt. He sleeps most nights now. It used to be a couple hours. He is noticing when he is wet or poopy and will come to us to change him. He has more self awareness and self confidence. He is more engaged and will look at us more. Sometimes he will respond to his name being called. Often he will initiate a game with eye contact. He gets frustrated less often because he is able to physically do more things successfully. Seems to be interested in more foods.	3	Overall, he is so much happier, calmer, and life is so much more enjoyable and livable. He talks more, babbles all the time, and we can understand some words, once in a while will use one with purpose or meaning.	3
29	He is much calmer and affectionate. Overall he seems happier and is communicating much better. He is 100% potty trained and is much more social with children he sees frequently.	3	He has always cuddled with his dad, but has been very selective cuddling with me. Now he approaches me, wants me, asks for me, and it feels like he loves me whereas before it did not.	1, 2
30	Lots of big hugs, back patting, and hand holding - it helps with attention.	2	I feel like he has become more oppositional, but I think it's more that we're getting to know his limits and body language. At the same time, he's more cuddly than ever and wants to be held and hugged when he has an owie. At times he wants us to pat him to get the "jellybeans" out.	3

Table 5: Continued.

ID #	Changes in the Child	Q	Changes in Relationship	Q
31	He is more present daily and seems to be opening up. He is sleeping much better. He is less over stimulated, he can handle going into crowed places and does not run away.	1	He is more receptive. We have bonded more. He will now spontaneously give us hugs and show affection. His speech is coming along.	3
32	Most changed would be he understands more.	3	With the massage he is more manageable daily to live with.	1
33	It has built more trust when it comes to touch.	3	She seems to be trying to talk more - making more verbal noises. Interested in what we are doing, trying to involve herself.	3
34	Happier and less fighting with other children. Has lowered violence at school.	1	Seems friendlier and more willing to interact.	1
35	We saw change right away upon beginning the massage. His language increased as well as his awareness of what was happening in his environment. He began to understand much more of what we were communicating to him & also began communicating more effectively with us as his language skills & comprehension grew stronger. His frustrations & tantrums decreased due to this improved communication & understanding. He has more eye contact & is much more responsive to questions and/or instructions. He seems to be more motivated to work harder at communicating with us & others. His focus has improved greatly.	3	He has developed a relationship with his sister. He has become very empathetic towards others. He is extremely protective of his sister, making sure she isn't too far behind and has even become very worried when she has a dirty diaper in public. The relationship he has with his older brother has gotten stronger. He addresses people that he knows well by name. He does "hi" and "bye" greetings often now.	3
36	He is becoming more comfortable with physical affection and comfort. All around vast improvements in every area that I can think of. Improvements in eating, sleeping, interactions with everyone around him, understanding and expression, toileting, concentration, appropriate play.	3	I feel it has brought us closer together both physically and emotionally. Before doing the massage therapy his dad and I made a point of being affectionate with him. We hugged him, kissed him, snuggled him as much as we could. He generally responded by "allowing" us to "assault" him. . .or at least that's how it felt. He would generally stare off away from us and he rarely responded in kind. After several months of massage he is reciprocating and will even seek hugs and comfort. I feel that is the most significant change, for us, since starting massage therapy.	1
37	I truly feel it has helped him be more "present" and aware of his surroundings. His speech has come incredibly far and potty training is starting to take off right now.	3	It has given us a way to encourage different kinds of touch. Added in a positive way to our bed-time routine.	
38	More eye contact and more verbal (more spontaneous communication but not a lot). Follows directions better and seems to pay attention and listen longer when I'm talking.	3	It's a practical way to engage and help your child.	3
39	She's able to self feed and won't spit out new foods.	3	Bonding	5
40	He is happier.	3	Massage will help parents and kids somehow get closer together.	3
41	In the beginning he made huge gains in speech especially (he never before seemed to be present at speech therapy or seem like he understood what was going on) and also things like being touched. I often reach for his head and his chest now to calm him. I often will just hold him when he's acting out.	3	That it helps the parents to actually bond with our kids and to pay close attention to small gains.	4
42	He is beginning to gained the ability to tolerate touch.	3	Got us closer, and I was able to understand him more.	1

Table 6: Parent comments on the intervention.

ID #	Parent comment on the intervention
1	This has brought us closer together.
2	More "active" form of therapy. Continue to stick with the massage and you will see improvements in your child.
3	I feel that it's accelerated his progress more than anything else.
4	This is something I can do at home at any time, and it's easy to do. It's also tailor-able to his individual issues. It really does make a difference, and it's so worth the time you put into it!
5	So far Qigong is the only treatment he's had that showed a significant difference in behavior.
6	Relaxing
7	Less invasive, less medical, more natural feeling
8	I would strongly encourage other parents to try it.
9	This is the only treatment he's received to date.
10	I feel like it bonds the parent to the child. I think it's opens them up and they understand they are safe.
11	He has had outpatient speech and occupational therapy as a toddler as well as services while in school. I think the massage has complimented these services.
12	Relaxes her to the point it is easy transition for bedtime.
13	Hands on builds stronger bond
14	I loved that the massage focused on strengthening his skills and working on him being comfortable in his own body.
15	That it is about touch and energy and doing something for him, not asking him to "do" something for us, that is, speech therapy.
16	More fun
17	He is non-verbal so the massage does not help with specific speech sounds. He pats his legs to show me he is ready for massage at bedtime. Qigong works!
18	I feel more empowered
19	Emotional and spiritual sort of connection. parent driven and consistent (daily). Awareness to body.
20	The massage is parent delivered. . .all the other methods for his autism are done by others. . .it is intimate and therefore I feel like I am taking an active part!
21	Massage gets you and your kid closer. It's like time to relax and show love with each other.
22	I can almost do his massage anywhere. We love our massage time.
23	We haven't really tried other treatments but what I like about the massage is that there is really no way to harm him by giving it to him. It's gentle, safe and fosters our relationships with him.
24	Well it was great that someone knowledgeable was performing it. My son beneficiated more from that than other massages where someone just tells you what to do but no one oversees your implementation.
25	It's done by me and my husband, no outsider can do it better than we can. Every other improvement seems to be because of some professional, this is because of our touch.
26	This is the first actual hands on treatment we have been offered. It's not more vitamins or shots, it's something he is involved in and really enjoys. It's not a "job" like ABA or the stuff he does at school, it's far less like traditional treatment.
27	Personal help. It's been eye opening
28	It is easy and something that I can do at home. It has been what makes all the other therapies work. It has done more for him than Speech and OT. It was like they didn't work until we started the massage.
29	It is easier, more calm and more bonding since you are touching your child the whole time. It is also more consistent.
30	Qigong massage gets you and your child in touch with their body and their needs. It gives you a way to communicate with your child about their needs.
31	It is something I can do for him and see the changes daily
32	We like it because we don't use pills. At first it is hard to do because it is something new. Stick with it because all you see is results.
33	This is really the only other treatment we have tried.
34	Lets you connect to your child and open up their senses and awareness.
35	This treatment gives our child a chance to relax & spend one-on-one time with us comfortably at home, as opposed to spending time with a therapist in a different setting.

Table 6: Continued.

ID #	Parent comment on the intervention
36	It helped us break down the barrier between us and him. There was always this disconnect and none of the therapies we tried got us closer to him. Now he seeks us out for comfort and just to be close. If we sleep in on a weekend he'll come in and lay with us in bed rather than playing in his room alone. He comes pattering into our room and climbs into bed with us and will lay there until we get up or, if he decides it's been long enough, he'll start slapping our cheeks and saying, "Mama wake up, daddy wake up." It's the most irritating thing in the world and we love it.
37	I like that the massage is every day like a medicine and it's easy to put into a routine. It has been a positive experience from start to finish and has given us nothing but rewards.
38	It's relaxing and It's a practical way to engage and help your child.
39	It's not pricey
40	Much less intrusive, more physical.
41	It's family oriented, it's long term, it's inexpensive, it has no risks. It makes you feel like you have some control in an uncontrollable situation.
42	That it helps the parents to actually bond with our kids and to pay close attention to small gains

over a 12-month interval (the CARS) and a more sensitive questionnaire currently used in conjunction with a direct observation measure for evaluating educational outcomes (the ABC). Thus it was quite remarkable that the CARS confirmed the findings of the ABC in showing significant decrease in severity of autism in the LFA group over the relatively short treatment period of five months. The CARS did not reflect the improvement seen on the ABC in the HFA group. We think this is most likely because the CARS was not standardized on individuals with HFA, has a compressed range of scores for HFA, and is less sensitive in that group [52]. We await the one- and two-year results to see whether the CARS will confirm the ABC results in the HFA group after a longer intervention period.

Taken altogether, these results represent a breakthrough in autism treatment. It is the first research-based intervention to be effective for the individual sensory, behavioral, and language components of autism as well as severity overall; it is the first intervention to be effective in both lower- and higher-functioning children. And it is the first time a model for autism revolving around tactile abnormalities is presented and supported with experimental data. The intervention was powerfully effective with children, because parent touch is critical to early social and self-regulatory development and because the intervention normalized children's sense of touch. As a result, behavior improved, social and self-regulatory gaps in the developmental foundation are filled in, and development was better supported.

Early intervention policy is to involve parents of children with autism in the direct care of their child's disability and offer them training and support in research-based home interventions. Parents desperately need effective tools to help their children. Two parent-delivered interventions are commonly recommended to parents of newly diagnosed children with autism by occupational therapists: the Wilbarger brushing protocol and joint compression [53, 54]. There is little research demonstrating efficacy on autism symptoms for either method. Since there is now replicated research to show efficacy for QST massage for autism, we recommend that parents be offered training and support in QST massage at the time of their children's autism diagnosis.

Over the past 14 years, our research has been conducted in collaboration with state-sponsored, early intervention programs for autism. School administrators are well aware of the importance of early identification and treatment of hearing and vision impairment to educational outcomes for children. A randomized controlled trial conducted in children with autism in early intervention classrooms has already shown that classroom behavior and social communication skills improved in the classroom with QST massage [25]. As the tactile abnormality in autism comes to be better understood and QST massage comes to be better known, we anticipate that tactile abnormalities will also be recognized as important to educational outcomes and that QST massage will be recommended. In our view, all children with autism should be evaluated for the need for hearing aids, glasses, and QST massage at the time of diagnosis. The results presented here support earlier recommendations to implement the QST program at the time of autism diagnosis concurrent with the early intervention program in order to prepare the child for school. If tactile and other sensory symptoms can be remediated prior to entering school, educational outcomes can only be enhanced.

5. Conclusions

The QST Dual program for autism directed at tactile abnormalities was effective in decreasing severity of individual sensory, behavioral, and language components of autism as well as severity of autism overall. The intervention works by decreasing tactile and other sensory abnormalities and removing the sensory barriers to learning social/language skills and regulating behavior. Child-to-parent bonding improved, and the experience of touch and relationship normalized for parent and child. Children were better able to make eye contact, focus, and listen, and parenting stress decreased. This program can be recommended to parents and early intervention programs at the time of autism diagnosis. It can be expected to improve educational outcomes for children and reduce stress in the preschool classroom environment.

Acknowledgments

This study was supported by Grant R40 MC 24945 from the Maternal and Child Health Research Program, Maternal and Child Health Bureau, Health Resources and Services Administration, and Department of Health and Human Services. The authors wish to thank the project's QST therapists and blind-to-group assessors for all of the time and effort they put into the project.

References

[1] C. A. Boyle, S. Boulet, L. A. Schieve et al., "Trends in the prevalence of developmental disabilities in US children, 1997–2008," *Pediatrics*, vol. 127, no. 6, pp. 1034–1042, 2011.

[2] Centers for Disease Control and Prevention, "Prevalence of autism spectrum disorder among children aged 8 years—autism and developmental disabilities monitoring network, 11 sites, United States, 2010," *Morbidity and Mortality Weekly Report*, vol. 63, no. SS02, pp. 1–21, 2014.

[3] American Psychiatric Association, *Diagnostic and Statistical Manual of Mental Disorders*, American Psychiatric Association, Washington, DC, USA, 5th edition, 2013.

[4] A. Ben-Sasson, L. Hen, R. Fluss, S. A. Cermak, B. Engel-Yeger, and E. Gal, "A meta-analysis of sensory modulation symptoms in individuals with autism spectrum disorders," *Journal of Autism and Developmental Disorders*, vol. 39, no. 1, pp. 1–11, 2009.

[5] E. P. Hazen, J. L. Stornelli, J. A. O'Rourke, K. Koesterer, and C. J. McDougle, "Sensory symptoms in autism spectrum disorders," *Harvard Review of Psychiatry*, vol. 22, no. 2, pp. 112–124, 2014.

[6] O. I. Lovaas, L. Schreibman, R. Koegel, and R. Rehm, "Selective responding by autistic children to multiple sensory input," *Journal of Abnormal Psychology*, vol. 77, no. 3, pp. 211–222, 1971.

[7] M. A. Kientz and W. Dunn, "A comparison of the performance of children with and without autism on the sensory profile," *The American Journal of Occupational Therapy*, vol. 51, no. 7, pp. 530–537, 1997.

[8] G. Dawson and R. Watling, "Interventions to facilitate auditory, visual, and motor integration in autism: a review of the evidence," *Journal of Autism and Developmental Disorders*, vol. 30, no. 5, pp. 415–421, 2000.

[9] G. Iarocci and J. McDonald, "Sensory integration and the perceptual experience of persons with autism," *Journal of Autism and Developmental Disorders*, vol. 36, no. 1, pp. 77–90, 2006.

[10] E. J. Marco, L. B. N. Hinkley, S. S. Hill, and S. S. Nagarajan, "Sensory processing in autism: a review of neurophysiologic findings," *Pediatric Research*, vol. 69, no. 5, part 2, pp. 48R–54R, 2011.

[11] S. D. Tomchek and W. Dunn, "Sensory processing in children with and without autism: a comparative study using the short sensory profile," *The American Journal of Occupational Therapy*, vol. 61, no. 2, pp. 190–200, 2007.

[12] L. Silva and M. Schalock, "Prevalence and significance of abnormal tactile responses in young children with autism," *North American Journal of Medicine and Science*, vol. 6, no. 3, pp. 121–127, 2013.

[13] A. Ben-Sasson, S. A. Cermak, G. I. Orsmond et al., "Extreme sensory modulation behaviors in toddlers with autism spectrum disorders," *The American Journal of Occupational Therapy*, vol. 61, no. 5, pp. 584–592, 2007.

[14] R. Baron, "Neuropathic pain: a clinical perspective," in *Handbook of Experimental Pharmacology*, B. J. Canning, D. Spina, F. B. Hofmann et al., Eds., vol. 194 of *Sensory Nerves*, pp. 3–30, Springer, New York, NY, USA, 2009.

[15] D. K. Shibata, "Differences in brain structure in deaf persons on MR imaging studied with voxel-based morphometry," *The American Journal of Neuroradiology*, vol. 28, no. 2, pp. 243–249, 2007.

[16] O. Collignon, G. Dormal, G. Albouy et al., "Impact of blindness onset on the functional organization and the connectivity of the occipital cortex," *Brain*, vol. 136, no. 9, pp. 2769–2783, 2013.

[17] S.-J. Blakemore, T. Tavassoli, S. Calò et al., "Tactile sensitivity in Asperger syndrome," *Brain and Cognition*, vol. 61, no. 1, pp. 5–13, 2006.

[18] B. Güçlü, C. Tanidir, N. M. Mukaddes, and F. Ünal, "Tactile sensitivity of normal and autistic children," *Somatosensory and Motor Research*, vol. 24, no. 1-2, pp. 21–33, 2007.

[19] C. Cascio, F. McGlone, S. Folger et al., "Tactile perception in adults with autism: a multidimensional psychophysical study," *Journal of Autism and Developmental Disorders*, vol. 38, no. 1, pp. 127–137, 2008.

[20] J. H. Foss-Feig, J. L. Heacock, and C. J. Cascio, "Tactile responsiveness patterns and their association with core features in autism spectrum disorders," *Research in Autism Spectrum Disorders*, vol. 6, no. 1, pp. 337–344, 2012.

[21] A. Montagu, *Touching: The Human Significance of the Skin*, Harper, New York, NY, USA, 1986.

[22] T. Field, *Touch*, The MIT Press, Cambridge, Mass, USA, 2001.

[23] L. Silva and M. Schalock, "Treatment of tactile impairment in young children with autism: results with qigong massage," *International Journal of Therapeutic Massage & Bodywork*, vol. 6, no. 4, pp. 12–20, 2013.

[24] L. M. Silva, M. Schalock, and K. Gabrielsen, "Early intervention for autism with a parent-delivered qigong massage program: a randomized controlled trial," *The American Journal of Occupational Therapy*, vol. 65, no. 5, pp. 550–559, 2011.

[25] L. M. T. Silva, M. Schalock, R. Ayres, C. Bunse, and S. Budden, "Qigong massage treatment for sensory and self-regulation problems in young children with autism: a randomized controlled trial," *The American Journal of Occupational Therapy*, vol. 63, no. 4, pp. 423–432, 2009.

[26] L. M. T. Silva, R. Ayres, and M. Schalock, "A model and treatment for autism at the convergence of Chinese medicine and Western science: first 130 cases," *Chinese Journal of Integrative Medicine*, vol. 17, no. 6, pp. 421–429, 2011.

[27] L. M. T. Silva, R. Ayres, and M. Schalock, "Outcomes of a pilot training program in a Qigong massage intervention for young children with autism," *The American Journal of Occupational Therapy*, vol. 62, no. 5, pp. 538–546, 2008.

[28] S. W. Porges, *The Polyvagal Theory: Neurophysiological Foundations of Emotions, Attachment, Communication, and Self-Regulation*, WW Norton & Company, New York, NY, USA, 2011.

[29] X. Ming, P. Julu, M. Brimacombe, S. Connor, and M. Daniels, "Reduced cardiac parasympathetic activity in children with autism," *Brain and Development*, vol. 27, no. 7, pp. 509–516, 2005, Erratum in: *Brain and Development*, vol. 34, no. 8, p. 704, 2012.

[30] A. Kushki, J. Brian, A. Dupuis, and E. Anagnostou, "Functional autonomic nervous system profile in children with autism spectrum disorder," *Molecular Autism*, vol. 4, no. 5, article 39, 2014.

[31] H. G. Schaible, "Peripheral and central mechanisms of pain generation," in *Handbook of Experimental Pharmacology*, vol. 177, pp. 3–28, Springer, 2007.

[32] M. M. Loman and M. R. Gunnar, "Early experience and the development of stress reactivity and regulation in children," *Neuroscience & Biobehavioral Reviews*, vol. 34, no. 6, pp. 867–876, 2010.

[33] L. M. T. Silva and M. Schalock, "Sense and self-regulation checklist, a measure of comorbid autism symptoms: initial psychometric evidence," *The American Journal of Occupational Therapy*, vol. 66, no. 2, pp. 177–186, 2012.

[34] M. I. Posner and M. K. Rothbart, "Toward a physical basis of attention and self-regulation," *Physics of Life Reviews*, vol. 6, no. 2, pp. 103–120, 2009.

[35] G. Devigili, V. Tugnoli, P. Penza et al., "The diagnostic criteria for small fibre neuropathy: from symptoms to neuropathology," *Brain*, vol. 131, part 7, pp. 1912–1925, 2008.

[36] L. Silva, *Qigong Massage for Your Child with Autism: A Home Program from Chinese Medicine*, Singing Dragon, London, UK, 2011.

[37] J. K. Squires, L. Potter, D. D. Bricker, and S. Lamorey, "Parent-completed developmental questionnaires: effectiveness with low and middle income parents," *Early Childhood Research Quarterly*, vol. 13, no. 2, pp. 345–354, 1998.

[38] B. Reichow, "Overview of meta-analyses on early intensive behavioral intervention for young children with autism spectrum disorders," *Journal of Autism and Developmental Disorders*, vol. 42, no. 4, pp. 512–520, 2012.

[39] N. Peters-Scheffer, R. Didden, H. Korzilius, and P. Sturmey, "A meta-analytic study on the effectiveness of comprehensive ABA-based early intervention programs for children with Autism Spectrum Disorders," *Research in Autism Spectrum Disorders*, vol. 5, no. 1, pp. 60–69, 2011.

[40] Centers for Medicaid and CHIP Services and Children and Adults Health Program, *2014 Poverty Guidelines*, 2014, http://www.medicaid.gov/medicaid-chip-program-information/by-topics/eligibility/downloads/2014-federal-poverty-level-charts.pdf.

[41] E. Schopler, R. J. Reichler, and B. R. Renner, *Childhood Autism Rating Scale, Standard Version*, Western Psychological Services, Los Angeles, Calif, USA, 2nd edition, 2013.

[42] I. Zimmerman, V. Steiner, and R. Pond, *Preschool Language Scale*, Pearson Education, San Antonio, Tex, USA, 5th edition, 2011.

[43] S. Sparrow, D. Cicchetti, and D. Balla, *Vineland Adaptive Behavior Scales*, Pearson, San Antonio, Tex, USA, 2nd edition, 2005.

[44] D. Krug, J. Arick, and P. Almond, *Autism Screening Instrument for Educational Planning*, Pro-Ed, Austin, Tex, USA, 3rd edition, 2008.

[45] M. Marteleto and M. Pedromônico, "Validity of autism behavior checklist (ABC): preliminary study," *Revista Brasileira de Psiquiatria*, vol. 27, no. 4, pp. 295–301, 2005.

[46] L. M. T. Silva and M. Schalock, "Autism parenting stress index: initial psychometric evidence," *Journal of Autism and Developmental Disorders*, vol. 42, no. 4, pp. 566–574, 2012.

[47] J. A. Summers, J. G. Marquis, H. Mannan et al., *Relationship of Perceived Adequacy of Services, Family-Professional Partnerships, and Family Quality of Life in Early Childhood Service Programmes*, Taylor & Francis, Oxford, UK, 2007.

[48] I. L. Cohen and V. Sudhalter, *PDD Behavior Inventory*, Psychological Assessment Resources, Lutz, Fla, USA, 2005.

[49] A. H. Rutgers, M. J. Bakermans-Kranenburg, M. H. van Ijzendoorn, and I. A. van Berckelaer-Onnes, "Autism and attachment: a meta-analytic review," *Journal of Child Psychology and Psychiatry*, vol. 45, no. 6, pp. 1123–1134, 2004.

[50] M. H. van Ijzendoorn, A. H. Rutgers, M. J. Bakermans-Kranenburg et al., "Parental sensitivity and attachment in children with autism spectrum disorder: comparison with children with mental retardation, with language delays, and with typical development," *Child Development*, vol. 78, no. 2, pp. 597–608, 2007.

[51] J. Blumberg, M. Bramlett, M. Kogan, L. Schieve, J. Joes, and M. Lu, "Changes in prevalence of parent-reported autism spectrum disorder in school-aged U.S. children: 2007 to 2011-2012," National Health Statistics Reports, Centers for Disease Control and Prevention, Atlanta, Ga, USA, 2013.

[52] S. D. Mayes, S. L. Calhoun, M. J. Murray et al., "Comparison of scores on the Checklist for Autism Spectrum Disorder, Childhood Autism Rating Scale, and Gilliam Asperger's Disorder Scale for children with low functioning autism, high functioning autism, Asperger's disorder, ADHD, and typical development," *Journal of Autism and Developmental Disorders*, vol. 39, no. 12, pp. 1682–1693, 2009.

[53] National Autism Resources, *The Wilbarger Protocol: Helping People Sensitive to Touch*, 2014, http://www.nationalautismresources.com/wilbarger-protocol.html.

[54] M. Zimmer and L. Desch, "Sensory integration therapies for children with developmental and behavioral disorders," *Pediatrics*, vol. 129, no. 6, pp. 1186–1189, 2012.

14

Computer Vision Tools for Low-Cost and Noninvasive Measurement of Autism-Related Behaviors in Infants

Jordan Hashemi,[1] Mariano Tepper,[1] Thiago Vallin Spina,[2] Amy Esler,[3] Vassilios Morellas,[4] Nikolaos Papanikolopoulos,[4] Helen Egger,[5] Geraldine Dawson,[6] and Guillermo Sapiro[7]

[1] *Department of Electrical and Computer Engineering, Duke University, Durham, NC 27708, USA*
[2] *Institute of Computing, University of Campinas, 13083 Campinas, SP, Brazil*
[3] *Department of Pediatrics, University of Minnesota, Minneapolis, MN 55455, USA*
[4] *Department of Computer Science and Engineering, University of Minnesota, Minneapolis, MN 55455, USA*
[5] *Department of Psychiatry and Behavioral Sciences, Duke University, Durham, NC 22708, USA*
[6] *Department of Psychiatry and Behavioral Sciences and School of Medicine, Duke University, Durham, NC 27708, USA*
[7] *Department of Electrical and Computer Engineering, Department of Computer Science, and Department of Biomedical Engineering, Duke University, Durham, NC 27708, USA*

Correspondence should be addressed to Jordan Hashemi; jordan.hashemi33@gmail.com

Academic Editor: Herbert Roeyers

The early detection of developmental disorders is key to child outcome, allowing interventions to be initiated which promote development and improve prognosis. Research on autism spectrum disorder (ASD) suggests that behavioral signs can be observed late in the first year of life. Many of these studies involve extensive frame-by-frame video observation and analysis of a child's natural behavior. Although nonintrusive, these methods are extremely time-intensive and require a high level of observer training; thus, they are burdensome for clinical and large population research purposes. This work is a first milestone in a long-term project on non-invasive early observation of children in order to aid in risk detection and research of neurodevelopmental disorders. We focus on providing low-cost computer vision tools to measure and identify ASD behavioral signs based on components of the Autism Observation Scale for Infants (AOSI). In particular, we develop algorithms to measure responses to general ASD risk assessment tasks and activities outlined by the AOSI which assess visual attention by tracking facial features. We show results, including comparisons with expert and nonexpert clinicians, which demonstrate that the proposed computer vision tools can capture critical behavioral observations and potentially augment the clinician's behavioral observations obtained from real in-clinic assessments.

1. Introduction

The analysis of children's natural behavior is of key importance for the early detection of developmental disorders such as autism spectrum disorder (ASD). For example, several studies have revealed behaviors indicative of ASD in early home videos of children that were later diagnosed with ASD [1–5]. These studies involved video recording infant behavior and then coding and analyzing the data a posteriori, using frame-by-frame viewing by an observer who typically trains for several weeks to achieve interrater reliability. Hours of labor are required, thereby making such analyses burdensome for clinical settings as well as for big data studies aiming at the discovery or improvement of behavioral markers. While clinical tools for early screening of ASD are available, they require administration and interpretation by specialists. Many families in low resource communities lack easy access to specialists in ASD. This work examines the potential benefits that computer vision can provide for research in early detection of ASD risk behaviors. It is a first milestone in a long-term project aimed at developing low-cost, automatic, and quantitative analysis tools that can be used by general practitioners in child development and in general environments to identify children at risk for ASD and other developmental disorders.

Although much is unknown about the underlying causes of ASD, some neuropathological studies indicate that ASD may have its origins in abnormal brain development early in prenatal life [6]. Moreover, Zwaigenbaum et al. [7] argue that many children with ASD exhibit several specific behavioral markers as early as in the first year of life. In high-risk siblings of children who later developed ASD, some of these symptoms can be observed during activities involving visual attention and are often expressed as difficulties in disengagement and shifting of attention [8, 9]. In addition, high-risk infant siblings have been shown to demonstrate impaired visual attention development between the ages of 7 and 14 months [10]. With this said, there is still much research needed to be done in determining potential risk indices. For example, a study performed by Nadig et al. [11] found that there is no significant difference in response-to-name disengagement between at-risk and low-risk infants.

Despite the fact that autism symptoms often emerge early and the syndrome can be diagnosed in toddlers, the average age of ASD diagnosis in the USA is close to 5 years [12]. Recently, research has demonstrated the benefit of early detection and diagnosis to allow for early intensive intervention. Early intervention, initiated in preschool and sustained for at least 2 years, can substantially improve child outcomes [13]. Detecting ASD risk and starting interventions before the full set of behavioral symptoms appears to may ultimately have an even greater impact, preventing difficult behaviors and delayed developmental trajectories from taking hold [14]. Although the diagnosis of ASD involves much more than the detection of symptoms, improving availability of cost-effective and accessible methods for identifying which children might be at risk and in need of further evaluation would potentially be of value. Towards this end, we have focused on developing semiautomatic computer vision video analysis techniques to aid in measuring ASD-related behaviors which can be used in early detection research.

More specifically, the main objectives in this paper are to use and validate computer vision tools to capture reliably two critical visual attention behaviors, Disengagement of Attention and Visual Tracking, belonging to the Autism Observation Scale for Infants (AOSI) [15], a behavioral observation tool for gathering information on early ASD risk signs [16]. (In this paper we refer to the AOSI and the scoring based on the DSM-IV. Research is needed to assess how measures of early signs of autism derived from automated video coding, such as those from the AOSI, relate to later diagnosis of ASD based on the newly established DSM-5 criteria. This is the subject of on-going efforts in our team.) Thus, the aim of the study is to examine the correspondence between the measures derived from the computer vision tools and the clinical assessment given by one trained expert. To demonstrate the validity of our tools, we compare our computer vision methods' results to those of the AOSI trained expert who performed the assessments and three nonexperts. Towards this end, other objectives of our work are to demonstrate the accurate and objective measurements provided by our low-cost methods and their potential to be used in the research of ASD risk marker identification. The work with such a specific population of infants and toddlers is unique in the computer vision community, making this a novel application for the psychology community. While the data is obtained from actual clinical assessments, the tasks pulled from the assessment are easy to administer and/or involve recordings of the child's natural behavior, thereby opening the door to broad behavioral studies, considering that the actual analysis is automatically done as introduced here.

These tools could potentially aid the practitioner and researcher in the risk marker identification task by providing accurate and objective measurements. These measurements can further provide means for improving the shareability of clinical records without compromising anonymity. In addition and particularly for research, automatic analysis will permit researchers to analyze vast amounts of naturally recorded videos, opening the door for data mining towards the improvement of current assessment protocols and the discovery of new behavioral features. This project is being developed by a multidisciplinary group bringing together professionals from psychology, computer vision, and machine learning. As an alternative to other research strategies [17–19], which require laboratory assessments, one of our main goals is to provide nonintrusive capturing systems that do not necessarily induce behavioral modification in the children. In other words, hardware must not constrain the testing environment; for example, the children are not asked to wear any type of sensors [20, 21].

2. Methods

2.1. Procedures for AOSI Tasks. The AOSI consists of a set of tabulated tasks that are designed for assessing specific behaviors, where each task consists of a certain number of presses and the child's responses receive scores. According to the AOSI, Disengagement of Attention is characterized as the "ability to disengage and move eyes/attention from one of two competing visual stimuli" [15, 22], while Visual Tracking is characterized as the "ability to visually follow a moving object laterally across the midline" [15, 22]. During the AOSI assessment, the clinician performs three trials for the Disengagement of Attention task and two trials for the Visual Tracking task, per participant. Every trial receives an AOSI-tabulated score, according to the following guidelines.

Disengagement of Attention. This activity consists of (1) shaking a noisy toy to one side of the infant until his/her attention is engaged and then (2) shaking a second noisy toy on the opposite side, while continuing to shake the first object. A delayed response in high-risk infants has been shown to be associated with a later ASD diagnosis [7, 15]. A trial is considered "passed" if the child looks to the second object in less than 1s, considered "delayed" if the child looks after a 1-2 s delay, and considered "stuck" if the child looks after more than 2 s.

Visual Tracking. To evaluate this activity, the following is performed: (1) a rattle or other noisy toy is used to engage the infant's attention, (2) the rattle is positioned to one side of the infant, and (3) the rattle is then moved silently at eye level across the midline to the other side. In high-risk infants, an interrupted, delayed, or partial gaze tracking has been shown to be associated with a later ASD diagnosis [15]. Depending on how continuously and smoothly the participant is able to track the object, the trial is considered "passed," "delayed or interrupted," or "partial or no tracking."

The clinician makes a "live" judgment about these time frames or may look at videos of this task if available. Finally, an overall score for each task is computed by merging the individual trials. We followed the protocol of comparing the assessments done by (1) an expert psychologist examiner who has been trained in the AOSI as well as ASD diagnosis in children, (2) a child/adolescent's psychiatrist, (3) two psychology students with no particular autism training, and (4) the results of our new computational tools. The child/adolescent's psychiatrist and two psychology students assigned their scores by following the AOSI guidelines, without prior training, while watching the same videos used by the automatic method. This setup allows us to contrast the automatic method's findings with human assessments across the full range of expertise.

2.2. Computer Vision Algorithms for Assessing Visual Attention. To analyze the child's reactions in the Visual Attention activities, we automatically estimate the changes of two head pose motions: yaw (left and right motion) and pitch (up and down motion). For the Visual Tracking and Disengagement of Attention tasks, which involve lateral motions, we focus on the yaw motion. We develop computer vision algorithms for estimating these head motions from low-cost cameras. The algorithms track specific facial features: the left ear, left eye, and nose (see right image of Figure 1). From their positions we estimate the participant's yaw and pitch motions. The only user input in our algorithm is during initialization. On the first frame, the user places a bounding box around the left ear, left eye, and nose (Figure 7). This could potentially be avoided by standard feature detection techniques. We marked the play objects by hand, although this also can be done automatically from prior knowledge of their visual and sound features (e.g., color or squeaking noise). Additional technical details are available in Appendices A and B (Figure 6 presents the data flow of our visual attention analysis system). We should note that we exploit and extend computer vision techniques that form the basis of virtual all automatic face analysis systems, and therefore have been extensively validated in the literature.

Scoring for our automatic method is based on automatic visual inspection of the estimated head motion measurements. After marking when the second object is presented in the Disengagement of Attention task, our method is able to automatically determine when the participants start and complete disengagement from the first object to the second. We assign the disengagement delay based on how many frames/seconds it takes the participant's head motion to completely transition to the second object (note that we are recording the video at 30 frames per second). We incorporate $a + (1/3)$ of a second margin for each delay to accommodate human error of making a live judgment. The scoring for the Visual Tracking task is determined by visual inspection of the head motion measurements as the object is moving laterally in front of the participants. More specifically, the scores are assigned based on whether or not the measurements exhibit full lateral head motion and also depend on the rate of change of the measurements. A "pass" is assigned if the head motion measurements exhibit full lateral head motion and a smooth rate of change. If there is an instance where the measurements exhibit a plateau or the rate of change changes direction for a short period of time but the measurements still display full lateral head motion, an "interrupted" score is assigned. For trials where the measurements do not exhibit full lateral head motion, a "partial" or "no tracking" score is assigned. Examples of our method's measurements for a "pass," "interrupted," and "partial" or "no tracking" tracking scores are shown in Figure 3. The developed automatic technique operates at a much higher resolution and accuracy than the standard 1-second intervals used by the expert clinician during live testing.

2.3. Participants. The purpose of the study was not to examine the correspondence between early assessments and outcome but rather the ability of our tools to accurately capture individual differences in behavior. We sought to include a sample in which a diversity of responses to the AOSI would be expected; thus the sampled population of this study involves 12 at-risk participants being examined in a clinic, including both males and females ranging in age from 5 to 18 months. Approval for this study was obtained from the Institutional Review Board at the University of Minnesota, and we have gathered our data from a series of ASD evaluation sessions of an ongoing concurrent study performed on a group of at-risk infants, at the Department of Pediatrics of the University of Minnesota.

All at-risk participants were infant siblings of a child diagnosed with ASD, a premature infant, or as a participant showing developmental delays. Table 1 presents a summary of this information. Note that, the participants are not clinically diagnosed until they are 36 months of age and only participant number 3 has presented conclusive signs of ASD.

2.4. Hardware. In our clinical setup, we use a low-cost GoPro Hero HD color camera (with a resolution of 1080 p at 30 fps), placed freely by the clinician in the center of the table between 2 and 4 feet away from the participant to ensure that it remains still throughout each trial and captures both the clinician and the participant (e.g., left image of Figure 1). The displayed images here are downsampled, blurred, and/or partially blocked to preserve anonymity (processing was done on the original videos).

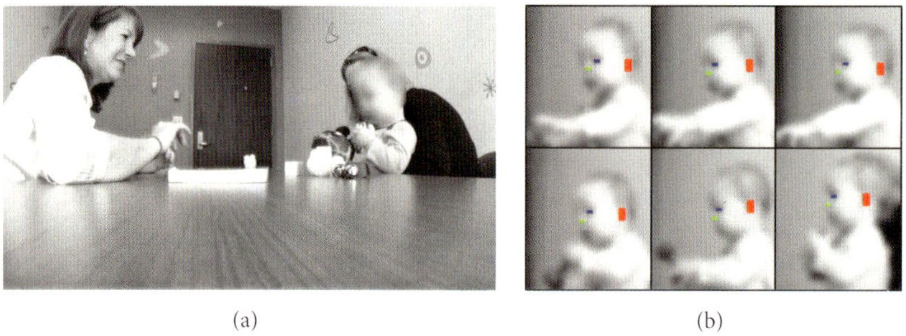

FIGURE 1: (a) General scene capturing the AOSI evaluation session. (b) Example of our algorithm automatically tracking three facial features: the left eye, left ear, and nose. In this paper, all figures have been blurred to protect the participants' privacy.

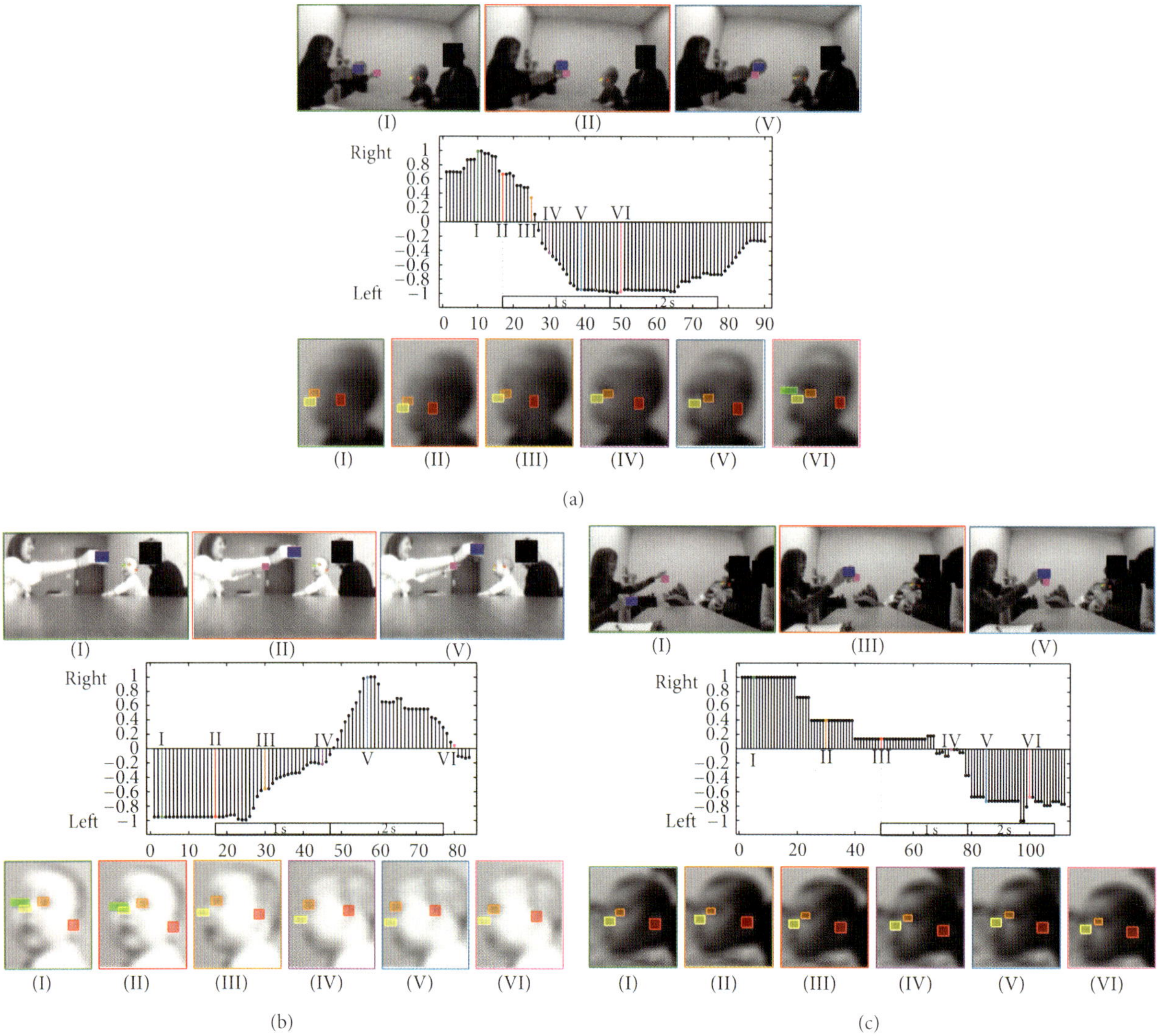

FIGURE 2: (a) First example of the Disengagement of Attention task. Top: when the clinician is holding one object, when the second object appears, and when the child recognizes the second object. Middle: changes in the yaw motion ($\widehat{yaw}$ values in the y-axis; see Appendices A and B) for every frame (x-axis). The dotted line represents when the second object is presented, followed by boxes representing 1 and 2 seconds after the object is presented. Bottom: 6 examples of the infant's face during the task. All facial features are automatically detected and tracked (as indicated by the colored boxes around the nose, eyes, and ear). Colors and roman numerals identify corresponding images and spikes in the graph. (b, c) Two examples of the Disengagement of Attention task.

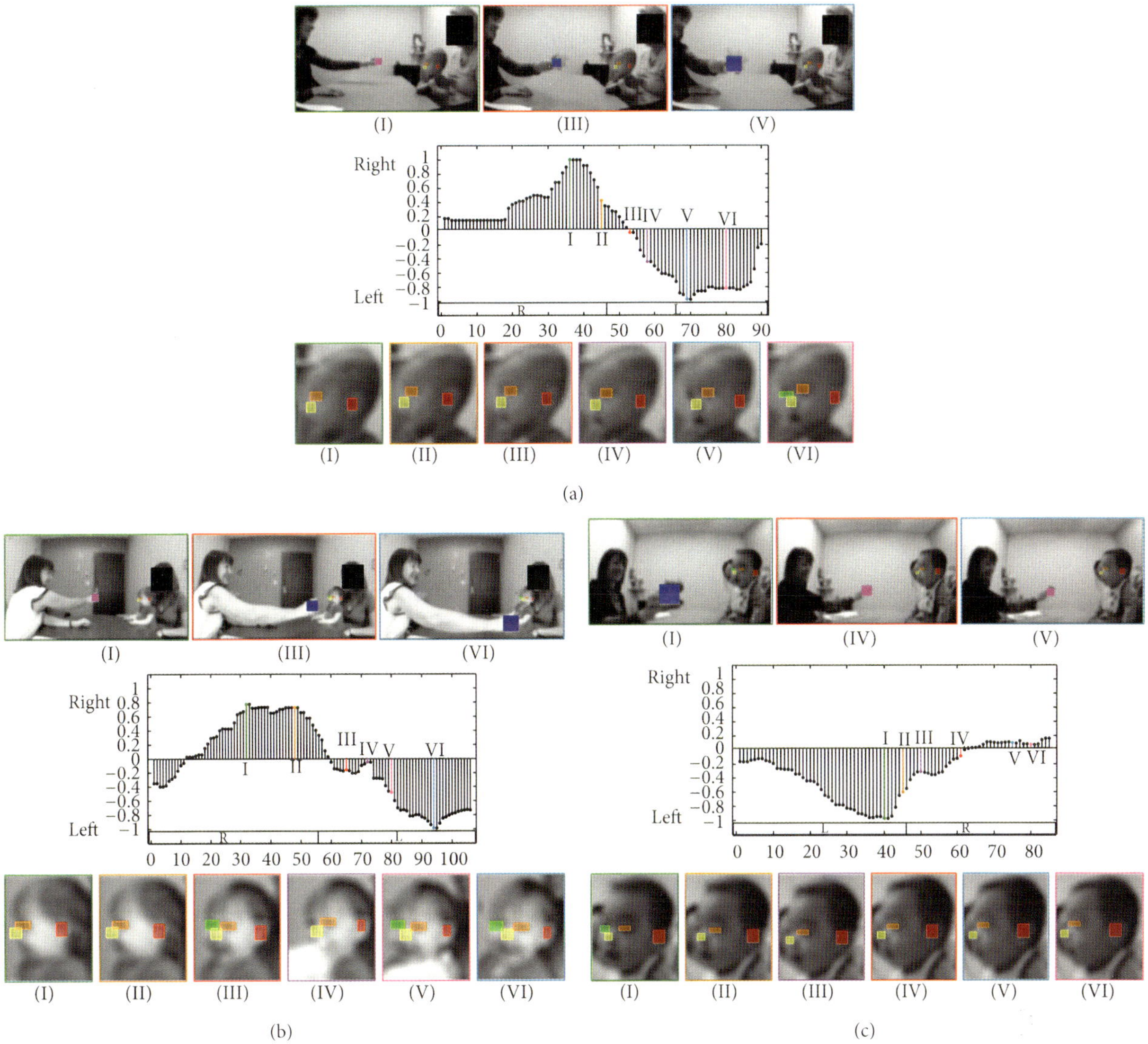

FIGURE 3: (a) First example of the Visual Tracking task. Top: when the clinician is holding the object, when the object is at one extreme side (right or left), and when the object is at the other extreme side. Middle: changes in the yaw motion ($\widehat{yaw}$ values in the y-axis; see Appendices A and B) for every frame (x-axis). The boxes labeled "R" and "L" represent when the object is to the right and left of the participant, respectively. The gray shaded areas represent when the object is not moving and at an extreme side (either right or left). Bottom: 6 examples of the infant's face during the task. Colors and roman numerals identify corresponding images and spikes in the graph. (b, c) Two examples of the Visual Tracking task.

3. Results

3.1. Disengagement of Attention. Table 2 summarizes the results of our method, the clinical assessments, and the ratings by a child/adolescent's psychiatrist and two psychology students for the Disengagement of Attention task. (See all video results in supplementary video files available online at http://dx.doi.org/10.1155/2014/935686.) Since the current set up for the visual attention tasks only involves a single camera placed nonintrusively, there are trials that our current method cannot handle (this could be easily solved in the future with a second low-cost camera). These trials include instances when the participant left the camera's field of view or when a toy or object obstructed it. (Standard face detection algorithms, such as the ones used in digital cameras, can be used to automatically alert the clinician of such cases for repositioning of the camera if needed.) For Table 2, the trials with blank spaces and a horizontal line correspond to such cases. Out of the 24 trials that the clinician assigned a "pass" score, our method agreed on 23 of them and scored a "delayed" for the other trial. And out of the 3 trials the clinician scored "delayed" our method agreed on 2 trials, scoring one as a "pass." The clinician did not assign a score for number 2, stating that it was a "spoiled" trial due to the

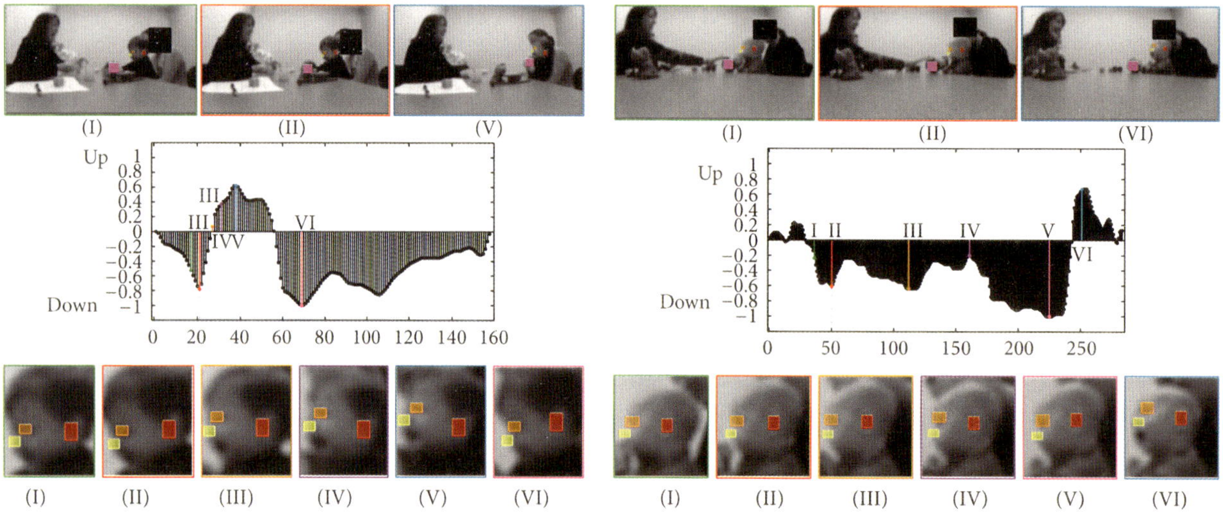

FIGURE 4: Two examples of the ball playing activity. Top: when the ball contacts the child, when the child looks down at the ball, and when the child looks up at the clinician. Middle: changes in the pitch motion (y-axis) for each frame (x-axis). The dotted line represents when the ball contacts the participant. Bottom: 6 examples of the infant's face during the administration. All facial features are automatically detected and tracked. Colors and roman numerals identify corresponding images and spikes in the graph.

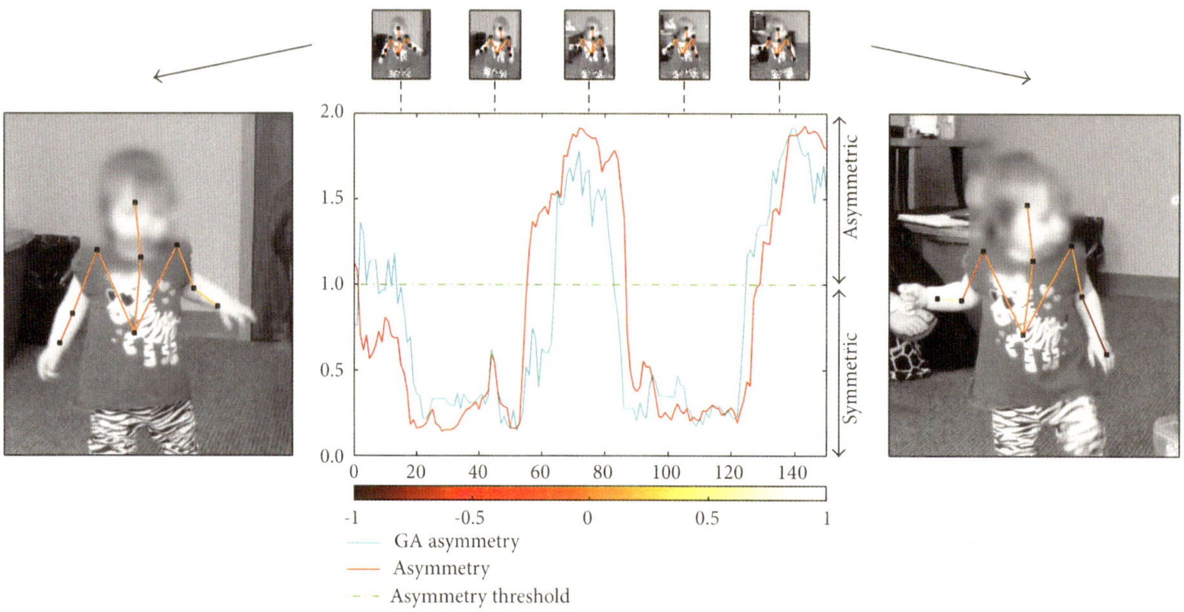

FIGURE 5: Comparison of arm-asymmetry scores between automatic method and ground truth in a video segment containing participant number 1. The cyan line represents normalized results from our method, while the red line represents the ground truth (GT) of the normalized arm differences. See [28] for more information on arm-asymmetry calculations and analysis. The normalized color scale visually displays the angle difference between the right and left forearms, where symmetric arm positions have similar overlaying colors.

participant being afraid of the toys. However, we show our method's results to exemplify a possible Disengagement of Attention score.

To further clarify our results, Figure 2 displays examples of our method's results and important cases for the Disengagement of Attention task. In Figure 2(a), the participant is able to disengage from the first object and look at the second within 0.7 s (21 frames) of the second object being presented. This would be scored as "passed" on the AOSI test. The participant in Figure 2(b) disengages to the second object within 1.3 s (40 frames), which would be scored as "delayed" on the AOSI test.

3.2. Visual Tracking. Table 3 summarizes the results of our method, the clinical assessments, and the ratings by a child/adolescent's psychiatrist and two psychology students for the Visual Tracking task. As in Table 2, the trials with

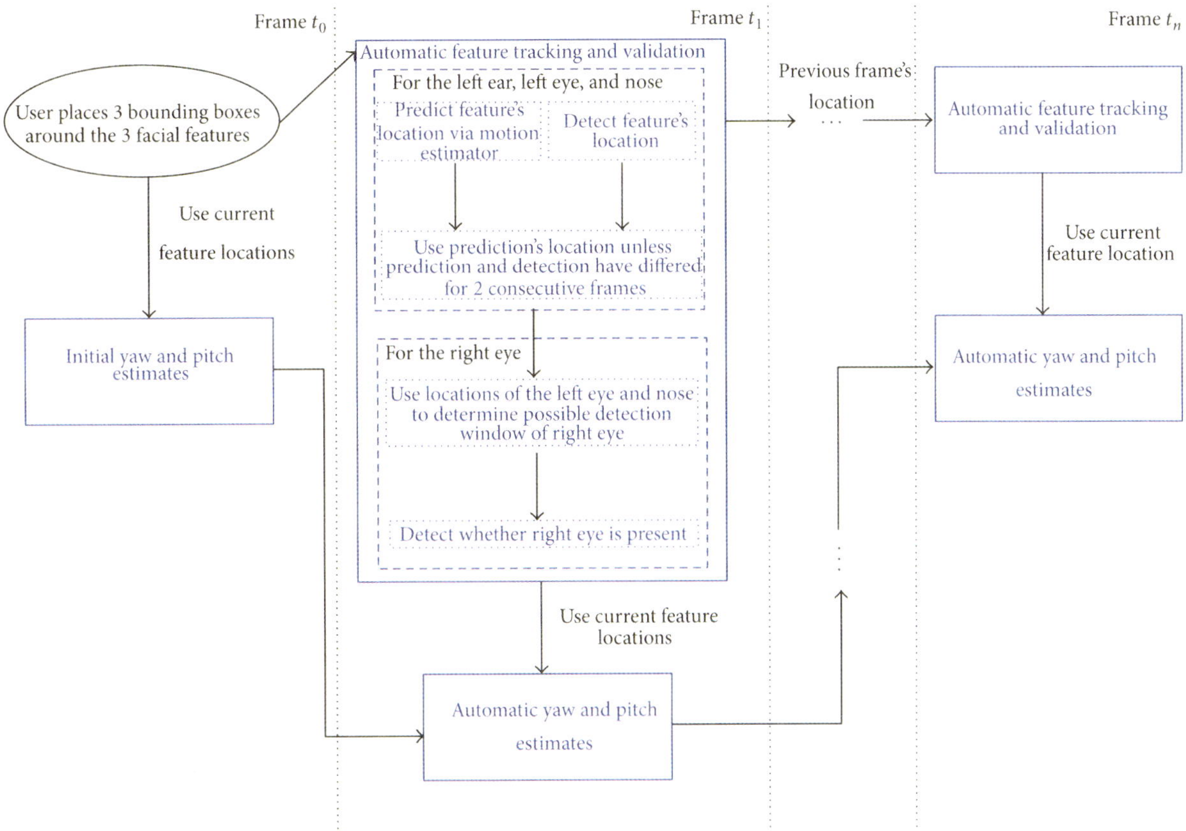

FIGURE 6: Data flow of the system for estimating yaw and pitch motions. We only require the user to place a bounding box around the left ear, left eye, and nose in the first frame of the video segment (black ellipse at time t_0). All the subsequent steps occur in a fully automatic fashion (blue blocks).

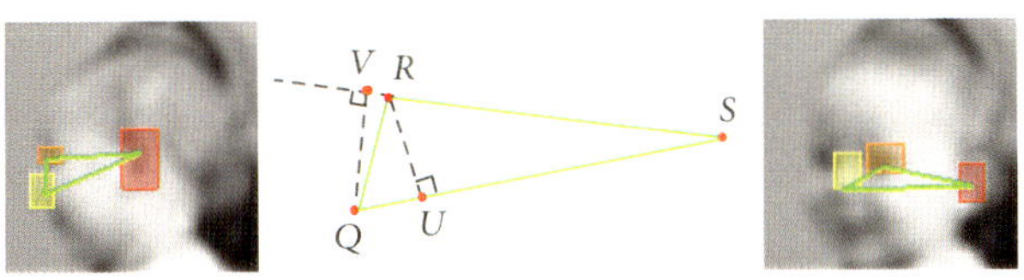

FIGURE 7: The triangle created by the left ear, left eye, and nose. The leftmost and rightmost images depict the triangle when the infant is looking right and more towards the camera, respectively. The middle image shows the points used for calculating $\widehat{yaw}$.

blank spaces and a horizontal line could not be used by our automatic method. Out of the 14 trials that the clinician assessed as "pass", our method agreed with 13 of them and scored an "interrupted" for 1 of the trials. For all the 4 trials the clinician assessed as "interrupted," our automatic method was in agreement. The clinician scored two trials as "partial," our method scored one of them as "partial" and the other as "interrupted."

Figure 3 shows important examples of our results for the Visual Tracking task. Figure 3(a) demonstrates a participant that received a "passed" on the AOSI's Visual Tracking task, since the participant was able to smoothly track the object with minimal delay as the object approached the participant's right. In Figure 3(b), the participant exhibited "interrupted" tracking motion. The participant's tracking of the object was interrupted as the object moved across the clinician's face.

TABLE 1: Information on participants involved in this study. Each participant was chosen for a different reason: being a baby sibling of someone with ASD, a premature infant, or showing developmental delays.

Part number	Age (months)	Gender	Risk degree
Number 1	14	F	Showing delays
Number 2	5	F	Baby sibling
Number 3	16	M	Showing delays
Number 4	15	M	Showing delays
Number 5	8	M	Premature infant
Number 6	9	F	Premature infant
Number 7	10	F	Premature infant
Number 8	9	M	Premature infant
Number 9	7	M	Premature infant
Number 10	6	M	Baby sibling
Number 11	9	M	Premature infant
Number 12	18	M	Showing delays

Table 2: Results of Disengagement of Attention task. Scores from the clinician (Clin.), automatic method (Automatic), a psychiatrist (Psy.), and two students (St. 1 and St. 2) for each trial. A trial is considered either as "passed" (Pass), "delayed" (Del), or "stuck" (Stck) depending on whether the child disengages from the first object in less than 1 s, between 1 and 2 s, or more than 2 s, respectively. We also present the automatically computed delay that the child takes to disengage. Note that we consider $a + (1/3)$ of a second margin for each delay to accommodate human error of making a live judgment.

Part number	Clin.	Automatic Score	Automatic Delay (s)	Psy.	St. 1	St. 2
			First trial score			
Number 1	Pass	Pass	0.9	Pass	Del	Del
Number 2	N/A	Del	1.87	N/A	N/A	N/A
Number 3	Pass	Pass	0.5	Pass	Del	Del
Number 4	Pass	Pass	0.23	Pass	Pass	Pass
Number 5	Del	Pass	1.07	Del	Del	Del
Number 6	Pass	Pass	1.03	Pass	Del	Pass
Number 7	Pass	Pass	0.83	Pass	Del	Del
Number 8	—	—	—	—	—	—
Number 9	—	—	—	—	—	—
Number 10	Pass	Pass	0.87	Del	Del	Del
Number 11	Pass	Pass	0.83	Pass	Del	Pass
Number 12	Pass	Pass	0.93	Pass	Pass	Pass
			Second trial score			
Number 1	Pass	Pass	0.7	Pass	Pass	Pass
Number 2	—	—	—	—	—	—
Number 3	—	—	—	—	—	—
Number 4	Pass	Pass	1.1	Pass	Pass	Pass
Number 5	Del	Del	1.77	Del	Stck	Del
Number 6	Pass	Del	1.43	Pass	Pass	Pass
Number 7	Pass	Pass	0.97	Del	Del	Del
Number 8	Pass	Pass	1.33	Pass	Del	Del
Number 9	—	—	—	—	—	—
Number 10	Pass	Pass	1.3	Pass	Pass	Pass
Number 11	Pass	Pass	0.63	Pass	Pass	Pass
Number 12	Pass	Pass	0.9	Pass	Del	Del
			Third trial score			
Number 1	Pass	Pass	0.37	Pass	Pass	Pass
Number 2	—	—	—	—	—	—
Number 3	—	—	—	—	—	—
Number 4	Pass	Pass	0.3	Pass	Pass	Pass
Number 5	Pass	Pass	0.5	Pass	Del	Pass
Number 6	Pass	Pass	0.7	Del	Del	Del
Number 7	Pass	Pass	1.13	Pass	Del	Del
Number 8	—	—	—	—	—	—
Number 9	Del	Del	1.37	Pass	Del	Stck
Number 10	Pass	Pass	1.33	Del	Del	Del
Number 11	Pass	Pass	0.87	Pass	Pass	Pass
Number 12	Pass	Pass	0.87	Pass	Pass	Pass

Instead of tracking the object as it moved across the clinician's face, the participant stopped tracking the object and looked at the clinician for 0.46 s (14 frames) before continuing to track the object as it moved to the participant's left. Such short behaviors can be detected by an automatic system. In Figure 3(c), the participant displays a "partial" tracking score on the AOSI. As the object crosses the clinician's face, the participant completely stops tracking the object and instead looks straight at the clinician.

3.3. Comparisons between Ratings by Automatic Computer Vision Method, Nonexpert Clinical Raters, and Expert Clinician. We next compared ratings made by nonexpert clinical raters (child/adolescent's psychiatrist and two psychology students) and by the computer vision methods with ratings made by an expert clinician. The results obtained by the child/adolescent's psychiatrist and two psychology students are presented in Tables 2 and 3. Out of the 27 Visual Disengagement trials (Table 2), the two psychology students agreed with the clinician on 13 and 16 of the trials, respectively, while the child/adolescent's psychiatrist agreed on 22 trials. The computer vision system agreed with the expert clinician in 25 out of the 27 cases. Similarly for the 22 Visual Tracking trials (Table 3), the two psychology students agreed with the expert clinician on 13 and 14 of the trials, respectively, while the child/adolescent's psychiatrist agreed on 16 trials. The computer vision system agreed on 19 of the 22 cases. Table 4 shows the interrater reliability value for each individual compared with the expert clinician, based on weighted Cohen's kappa with a range of 0-1, where 1 means complete agreement.

4. Discussion

In addition to providing a broadly deployable low-cost tool for ASD risk assessment, if validated in future research, the potential benefits of an automated method for head motion estimation are threefold. First, it would provide accurate quantitative measurements for tasks assessing infant visual attention, such as the AOSI tasks, improving the shareability of clinical records while not compromising anonymity. Second, it could also prove beneficial in the discovery of new behavioral patterns by easily collecting large amounts of data and mining it. Third, it could increase the granularity of the analysis by providing data at a finer scale. As the results demonstrate, the computer vision method performed very well when compared to the expert clinician and outperformed the three other nonexperts. Using unweighted kappa, Bryson et al. [15] reported a combined average interrater reliability score of 0.80 for both the Disengagement of Attention and Visual Tracking. Although our combined average weighted score of 0.75 is not as high as reported by the original authors, it is still considered excellent (greater than 0.65) according to them.

4.1. Disengagement of Attention. Compared to the expert clinician's results, the computer vision method achieved high accuracy. In Table 2, the method obtained one false positive by scoring one trial "delayed" that the clinician scored as "pass" (participant number 6) and missed one "delayed" trial

TABLE 3: Results of Visual Tracking task. Scores from the clinician (Clin.), automatic method (Automatic), a psychiatrist (Psy.), and two students (St. 1 and St. 2) for each trial. A trial is considered "passed" (Pass), "delayed" (Del), "interrupted" (Int), "partial" (Prt), or "no tracking" depending on how smoothly the child visually tracks the object.

Part number	First trial score					Second trial score				
	Clin.	Automatic	Psy.	St. 1	St. 2	Clin.	Automatic	Psy.	St. 1	St. 2
Number 1	Pass	Pass	Pass	Pass	Pass	Pass	Int	Int	Int	Int
Number 2	Int	Int	Pass	Int	Pass	Int	Int	Pass	Pass	Pass
Number 3	Del	Pass	Pass	Pass	Pass	Pass	Pass	Pass	Pass	Pass
Number 4	Pass	Pass	Pass	Pass	Pass	Pass	Pass	Pass	Pass	Pass
Number 5	Prt	Int	Pass	Int	Pass	Prt	Prt	Del	Prt	Prt
Number 6	Pass	Pass	Pass	Pass	Pass	—	—	—	—	—
Number 7	—	—	—	—	—	Int	Int	Int	Prt	Prt
Number 8	Pass	Pass	Pass	Del	Pass	Pass	Pass	Pass	Pass	Pass
Number 9	Pass	Pass	Pass	Del	Pass	Pass	Pass	Pass	Pass	Pass
Number 10	Pass	Pass	Pass	Pass	Pass	Int	Int	Int	Prt	Prt
Number 11	Pass	Pass	Pass	Pass	Pass	Int	Int	Int	Prt	Prt
Number 12	Pass	Pass	Pass	Pass	Pass	Pass	Pass	Pass	Pass	Pass

TABLE 4: Number of agreements with the autism expert for each participant in the two visual attention tasks and overall interrater reliability using weighted Cohen's kappa. See Tables 2 and 3.

Task	Trials	Automatic	Psychiatrist	Student 1	Student 2
Disengagement	27	**25**	22	13	16
tracking	22	**19**	16	13	14
Total	49	**44**	38	26	30
Interrater score	—	**0.75**	0.37	0.27	0.27

(participant number 11). In the current project, the temporal resolution is 30 frames per second, allowing for discovery of possible latent head motion patterns. Figure 2(c) provides an interesting pattern in the participant's head movement. Not only does it take the third participant over 1 s to look at the second object (which is "delayed" on the AOSI), but the participant displays piece-wise constant lateral head movements compared to the other two examples (which presented a much smoother motion), a pattern virtually impossible to detect with the naked eye. Again, such automatic and quantitative measurements could potentially add critical information that could aid in risk detection, such as new ways of scoring the AOSI. With a study on a larger population, new time intervals (and their variability) for scoring may be discovered, and these false positives could be analyzed not as a strict "pass" or "delayed" but as something in between.

4.2. Visual Tracking. Again, compared to the expert clinician's results, the automated method achieved high accuracy. As shown in Table 3, the clinician scored one trial belonging to the only participant that has been positively diagnosed as "delayed"; however, based on our nonintrusive camera placement (as selected by the practitioner), it was not possible to continuously extract the object's location accurately enough to assign "delayed" scores. In future studies, it would be possible to extend the setup to include an overhead camera to accurately record the playing objects' positions. Another aspect of the method is that it provides accurate and quantitative measurements of the participant's head motions; thus, one is able to automatically determine the delays between when the participant looks at the object or how long the participant stops his/her tracking.

5. Concluding Remarks

This work is the first milestone in a long-term project focused on the development of noninvasive early observation of children in order to aid in risk detection and research of neurodevelopmental disorders. With the goal of aiding and augmenting the visual analysis capabilities in evaluation and developmental monitoring of ASD, we proposed (semi-) automatic computer vision tools to observe specific important behaviors related to ASD elicited during AOSI, providing both new challenges and opportunities in video analysis. The proposed tools, if validated in future research, could significantly reduce the effort by only requiring interactive initialization in a single frame. The eventual goal is to minimize the need for extensive training and add both accuracy of quantitative measurements and objectivity. We focused on two visual attention activities performed during the AOSI. We developed specific computer vision algorithms for these activities, obtaining encouraging results that correlated with an expert's judgment. The automated method proved to be more consistent with the expert clinician's rating that those produced by less expert human observers; it should be noted that these human observers still have higher levels of expertise than normally available in most school settings.

The improvement and extension of the proposed methods is an ongoing work and we plan to provide code for the method. Current limitations of our methods include requiring the participant's face to be present throughout the video, estimating the yaw and pitch motions independently of one another, and we have only tested on relatively high-definition video sequences (from low-cost GoPro Hero cameras). Although the present study included 12 at-risk infants and toddlers, some limitations of our study include the use of only a single expert examiner as well as the small and relatively unimpaired sample size (although as mentioned before, the exploited tools have been extensively validated in the literature). For the visual attention tasks, we plan to complement the estimation of the child's motions with estimating the red examiner's behaviors. The work presented demonstrates the validity of the tools with a specific examiner's assessments. To expand these tools to broader clinical and naturalistic settings that involve different examiners and examiners with different levels of training, the quality of interaction, engagement, and variability between the examiners must also be considered. These examiner-related behaviors include how far away from the participant the examiner positions the toy(s), the displacement velocity of the toy(s) throughout the assessment, audio cues from the examiner, and head position of the examiner in the sense of whether he/she is looking at the participant or away. A study on the variability of examiner's performance in both clinical and naturalistic settings, such as at the participant's home, is an important topic for future research and should be considered before any data mining analyses are carried out. A method that examines the examiner's behaviors would also allow the examiner to receive immediate feedback on whether a trial or press needs to be redone. Notice that this could also lead to an automatic method for training examiners. Based on the set-up of the AOSI tasks discussed in this work, we assume that the participant's head motion is directly correlated to his/her gaze direction. This assumption is known as "center bias" and has been well established in gaze estimation and saliency detection literature [23, 24]. To further research and broaden the scope of this method, we plan to validate the assumption of the direct relationship between the head motion and eye movements in a specific population of infants and children at risk for ASD or with ASD; see also [25] for some early results in this direction.

5.1. Extensions of Computer Vision Tools for ASD Behavioral Observations. There are additional potential behavioral risk indices for ASD, both included in and beyond the scope of AOSI, such as facial expression in first birthday home videos [26] and mounting a camera near the examiner's face to estimate the participant's gaze [27], which are not addressed by the current method but we aim to address in the future, both in terms of the technical methods and the assessment of their validity and reliability. Computer vision tools hold promise as a novel and cost-efficient method for capturing behavior that could be used in both the clinical and research settings. Using the methods in this work, we also provide initial data suggesting that these methods might be useful in less structured situations, such as tracking a participant's head motion during a ball playing activity (Figure 4), providing information regarding the participant's interaction with the examiner such as the time it takes for a participant to look up after receiving a ball.

In addition, computer vision tools are not restricted to only aiding visual attention related markers. Our group has also been developing nonintrusive tools for aiding the assessment of motor patterns [28]. Through a meticulous process of hand fitting stickman to the participants in every frame, Esposito et al. [29] have found that toddlers with ASD often presented asymmetric arm positions in early life. Using computer vision, we were able to automatically estimate the 2D body pose of the toddlers in the video segments (Figure 5) as well as estimate arm angles relative to the ground with little user intervention (see mentioned reference for technical details and evaluations). The only required user intervention consisted of interactively creating a segmentation mask in the initial frame of the video segment. By creating nonintrusive and semiautomatic computer vision tools, such as these, large datasets can be analyzed, potentially leading to the discovery of new and/or improved behavioral markers.

Appendices

A. Tracking and Validating Facial Features

This section provides technical details about the algorithm for tracking facial features and computing head motions from them. The large variability of the data and the lack of control about the camera positioning call for using very simple and robust features and algorithms.

We assume that, in the first frame, we have bounding boxes of three facial features: the left ear, left eye, and nose (see, e.g., Figure 2). These bounding boxes are in practice selected by hand on the first frame. It is possible to achieve a fully automatic initialization, but this was not the objective of the present work. The user intervention is nonetheless minimal.

We aim at tracking these three facial features. Following a scheme loosely based on the TLD tracker [30], we use dense motion estimation coupled with a validation step that employs an offline-trained facial feature detector. The dense motion estimator [31] tracks the features with high accuracy in most cases, but when the child's head moves quickly, illumination changes can sometimes cause the tracker to lag behind the features. Thus, we validate the output of the tracker using facial feature detectors in every frame (Figure 6).

To validate the features we train left eye, right eye, left ear, and nose detectors. For this, we adapt the widely used method by Dalal and Triggs [32], proposed for pedestrian detection, to our particular setting (see also [33, 34]). Our method employs the popular multiscale Histograms of Orientated Gradients (HOG) using 8 × 8 pixel blocks and 9 orientation bins as descriptors to represent each facial feature and then classifies these descriptors using a support vector machine (http://www.csie.ntu.edu.tw/~cjlin/libsvm/) with a radial basis function kernel (see [32] for further technical details). As positive training samples, we use hand labeled facial patches from children in our experimental environment. As negative training samples, we extract random patches from around multiple children's faces. Our classifier was trained a single time before any experiment was carried out. Then, we used it for all experiments with no need for retraining or parameter setting.

For each frame, search areas for the facial feature detectors are defined around the bounding boxes given by the tracker. The left eye, left ear, and nose are present in every frame for the given camera position and their final detected positions are determined by the locations that exhibit a maximal response from the classifier (i.e., extrema of each feature's classifier output). The tracker's bounding boxes are validated if their centers are within the bounding boxes returned by the detectors; however, if the tracker's centers are outside of the detector's bounding boxes for two consecutive frames, then the corresponding bounding box for the tracker is reset to a new location within the detector's bounding box. Determining the presence of the right eye aids in the estimation of the yaw motion. The rectangular search area for the right eye, which is not tracked since it appears and disappears constantly due to the camera position, is based on the location of the detected nose and the horizontal and vertical distances between the detected left eye and nose. More specifically, the search area is between the detected nose's location plus/minus the horizontal and vertical distances between the detected left eye and nose. Also employed as a right eye search area restriction is that the nose must be between the left and right eyes.

Thus, using our method, we are able to track the facial features via a dense motion estimator, and validate their positions via the facial feature detectors. To estimate head motion, see the following, we use the facial feature locations given by the dense motion estimators. The dense motion estimator provides smoother and more precise locations than the detector.

B. Yaw and Pitch Motion Estimation from Facial Features

As a way to provide an accurate motion estimation of the pitch angle, we cumulatively sum the vertical coordinate changes of the left eye and nose with respect to the left ear every frame. We expect a positive sum when the child is looking up and a negative sum when the child is looking down, with the magnitude representing how much the child is looking up or down.

For estimating the yaw motion, we calculate two ratios based on the triangle created by the left ear, left eye, and nose (Figure 7); we also use information about the presence of the right eye. Let Q, R, and S denote the locations of the nose, left eye, and left ear, respectively. For the first ratio $r_{\mathrm{NoseToEye}}$, we project R into the line defined by QS, thus defining the point U; we then define $r_{\mathrm{NoseToEye}} = |US|/|QS|$, where $|\cdot|$ is the Euclidian distance. For the second ratio, we project Q into the line defined by RS, defining $r_{\mathrm{EyeToEar}} = |VR|/|RS|$.

The two ratios r_{EyeToEar} and $r_{\mathrm{NoseToEye}}$ are inversely proportional. Looking at Figure 7, we can observe that when the face is looking in profile view, r_{EyeToEar} will be large and $r_{\mathrm{NoseToEye}}$ will be small, conversely when the face is in frontal view (looking more towards the camera). To combine these two ratios into one value, we calculate the normalized difference between them, $\widehat{\mathrm{yaw}} = (r_{\mathrm{EyeToEar}} - r_{\mathrm{NoseToEye}})/(r_{\mathrm{EyeToEar}} + r_{\mathrm{NoseToEye}})$. Thus, as the child is looking to his/her left, $\widehat{\mathrm{yaw}}$ goes to -1; and, as the child is looking to his/her right, $\widehat{\mathrm{yaw}}$ goes to 1. The presence of the right eye further verifies that the infant is looking left.

We incorporate whether the right eye is present or not to verify that the infant is looking left or right at the maximum and minimum $\widehat{\mathrm{yaw}}$ values.

Authors' Contribution

J. Hashemi, M. Tepper, and T. V. Spina equally contributed to this work.

Acknowledgments

The authors would like to thank the participants and their families for their participation. This work was partially supported by NSF Grants 1039741 and 1028076, CAPES (BEX 1018/11-6) and FAPESP (2011/01434-9) Ph.D scholarships from Brazil, ONR, NGA, ARO, and AFOSR.

References

[1] J. L. Adrien, M. Faure, A. Perrot et al., "Autism and family home movies: preliminary findings," *Journal of Autism and Developmental Disorders*, vol. 21, no. 1, pp. 43–49, 1991.

[2] J. L. Adrien, A. Perrot, D. Sauvage et al., "Early symptoms in autism from family home movies. Evaluation and comparison between 1st and 2nd year of life using I.B.S.E. scale," *Acta Paedopsychiatrica*, vol. 55, no. 2, pp. 71–75, 1992.

[3] G. Losche, "Sensorimotor and action development in autistic children from infancy to early childhood," *Journal of Child Psychology and Psychiatry and Allied Disciplines*, vol. 31, no. 5, pp. 749–761, 1990.

[4] G. T. Baranek, "Autism during infancy: a retrospective video analysis of sensory-motor and social behaviors at 9-12 months of age," *Journal of Autism and Developmental Disorders*, vol. 29, no. 3, pp. 213–224, 1999.

[5] F. Muratori and S. Maestro, "Early signs of autism in the first year of life," in *Signs of Autism in Infants: Recognition and Treatment*, pp. 46–62, Karnac, London, UK, 2007.

[6] P. M. Rodier, "Converging evidence for brain stem injury in autism," *Development and Psychopathology*, vol. 14, no. 3, pp. 537–557, 2002.

[7] L. Zwaigenbaum, S. Bryson, T. Rogers, W. Roberts, J. Brian, and P. Szatmari, "Behavioral manifestations of autism in the first year of life," *International Journal of Developmental Neuroscience*, vol. 23, no. 2-3, pp. 143–152, 2005.

[8] R. Landry and S. E. Bryson, "Impaired disengagement of attention in young children with austism," *Journal of Child Psychology and Psychiatry and Allied Disciplines*, vol. 45, no. 6, pp. 1115–1122, 2004.

[9] M. Elsabbagh, A. Volein, K. Holmboe et al., "Visual orienting in the early broader autism phenotype: disengagement and facilitation," *Journal of Child Psychology and Psychiatry and Allied Disciplines*, vol. 50, no. 5, pp. 637–642, 2009.

[10] M. Elsabbagh, J. Fernandes, S. Jane Webb, G. Dawson, T. Charman, and M. H. Johnson, "Disengagement of visual attention in infancy is associated with emerging autism in toddlerhood," *Biological Psychiatry*, vol. 74, no. 3, pp. 189–194, 2013.

[11] A. S. Nadig, S. Ozonoff, G. S. Young, A. Rozga, M. Sigman, and S. J. Rogers, "A prospective study of response to name in infants at risk for autism," *Archives of Pediatrics and Adolescent Medicine*, vol. 161, no. 4, pp. 378–383, 2007.

[12] P. T. Shattuck, M. Durkin, M. Maenner et al., "Timing of identification among children with an autism spectrum disorder: findings from a population-based surveillance study," *Journal of the American Academy of Child and Adolescent Psychiatry*, vol. 48, no. 5, pp. 474–483, 2009.

[13] J. S. Howard, C. R. Sparkman, H. G. Cohen, G. Green, and H. Stanislaw, "A comparison of intensive behavior analytic and eclectic treatments for young children with autism," *Research in Developmental Disabilities*, vol. 26, no. 4, pp. 359–383, 2005.

[14] G. Dawson, "Early behavioral intervention, brain plasticity, and the prevention of autism spectrum disorder," *Development and Psychopathology*, vol. 20, no. 3, pp. 775–803, 2008.

[15] S. E. Bryson, L. Zwaigenbaum, C. McDermott, V. Rombough, and J. Brian, "The autism observation scale for infants: scale development and reliability data," *Journal of Autism and Developmental Disorders*, vol. 38, no. 4, pp. 731–738, 2008.

[16] K. Downing, K. Concannon, V. Vogel-Farley, C. A. Nelson, and H. Tager-Flusberg, "Can the AOSI at nine months discriminate between infants at high or low risk for ASD?" in *International Meeting for Autism Research (IMFAR '11)*, San Diego, Calif, USA, 2011.

[17] W. Jones, K. Carr, and A. Klin, "Absence of preferential looking to the eyes of approaching adults predicts level of social disability in 2-year-old toddlers with autism spectrum disorder," *Archives of General Psychiatry*, vol. 65, no. 8, pp. 946–954, 2008.

[18] M. Freeth, T. Foulsham, and P. Chapman, "The influence of visual saliency on fixation patterns in individuals with autism spectrum disorders," *Neuropsychologia*, vol. 49, no. 1, pp. 156–160, 2011.

[19] A. Klin, W. Jones, R. Schultz, F. Volkmar, and D. Cohen, "Visual fixation patterns during viewing of naturalistic social situations as predictors of social competence in individuals with autism," *Archives of General Psychiatry*, vol. 59, no. 9, pp. 809–816, 2002.

[20] M. S. Goodwin, S. S. Intille, F. Albinali, and W. F. Velicer, "Automated detection of stereotypical motor movements," *Journal of Autism and Developmental Disorders*, vol. 41, no. 6, pp. 770–782, 2011.

[21] F. A. Boujarwah, S. Sadler, A. Mogus, G. D. Abowd, and R. I. Arriaga, "Understanding the challenges and opportunities for richer descriptions of stereotypical behaviors of children with ASD: a concept exploration and validation," in *Proceedings of the 12th International ACM SIGACCESS Conference on Computers and Accessibility (ASSETS '10)*, pp. 67–74, Orlando, Fla, USA, October 2010.

[22] S. E. Bryson, L. Zwaigenbaum, J. Brian et al., "A prospective case series of high-risk infants who developed autism," *Journal of Autism and Developmental Disorders*, vol. 37, no. 1, pp. 12–24, 2007.

[23] S. Mannan, K. H. Ruddock, and D. S. Wooding, "Automatic control of saccadic eye movements made in visual inspection of briefly presented 2-D images," *Spatial vision*, vol. 9, no. 3, pp. 363–386, 1995.

[24] Y. Li, A. Fathi, and J. Rehg, "Learning to predict gaze in egocentric video," in *Proceedings of the International Conference on Computer Vision (ICCV '13)*, Sydney, Australia, 2013.

[25] H. Bloch and I. Carchon, "On the onset of eye-head coordination in infants," *Behavioural Brain Research*, vol. 49, no. 1, pp. 85–90, 1992.

[26] J. Osterling and G. Dawson, "Early recognition of children with autism: a study of first birthday home videotapes," *Journal of Autism and Developmental Disorders*, vol. 24, no. 3, pp. 247–257, 1994.

[27] Z. Ye, Y. Li, A. Fathi et al., "Detecting eye contact using wearable eye-tracking glasses," in *Proceedings of the 14th International Conference on Ubiquitous Computing (UbiComp '12)*, pp. 699–704, Pittsburgh, Pa, USA, September 2012.

[28] T. V. Spina, J. Hashemi, M. Tepper et al., "Automatically aiding the assessment of atypical motor patterns for autism spectrum disorder diagnosis," in *Proceedings of the 59th AACAP Meeting*, San Fransisco, Calif, USA, 2012.

[29] G. Esposito, P. Venuti, F. Apicella, and F. Muratori, "Analysis of unsupported gait in toddlers with autism," *Brain and Development*, vol. 33, no. 5, pp. 367–373, 2011.

[30] Z. Kalal, K. Mikolajczyk, and J. Matas, "Face-TLD: tracking-learning-detection applied to faces," in *Proceedings of the 17th IEEE International Conference on Image Processing (ICIP '10)*, pp. 3789–3792, Hong Kong, September 2010.

[31] M. Tepper and G. Sapiro, "Decoupled coarse-to-fine matching and nonlinear regularization for efficient motion estimation," in *Proceedings of the 19th IEEE International Conference on Image Processing (ICIP '12)*, pp. 1517–1520, Orlando, Fla, USA, October 2012.

[32] N. Dalal and B. Triggs, "Histograms of oriented gradients for human detection," in *Proceedings of the IEEE Computer Society Conference on Computer Vision and Pattern Recognition (CVPR '05)*, pp. 886–893, San Diego, USA, June 2005.

[33] M. Everingham, J. Sivic, and A. Zisserman, ""Hello! My name is... Buffy"—automatic naming of characters in TV video," in *Proceedings of the British Machine Vision Conference (BMVC '06)*, Edinburgh, UK, 2006.

[34] T. Vatahska, M. Bennewitz, and S. Behnke, "Feature-based head pose estimation from images," in *Proceedings of the 7th IEEE-RAS International Conference on Humanoid Robots (HUMANOIDS '07)*, pp. 330–335, Pittsburgh, Pa, USA, December 2007.

15

Mild Dermatoglyphic Deviations in Adolescents with Autism Spectrum Disorders and Average Intellectual Abilities as Compared to Typically Developing Boys

Esther I. de Bruin,[1,2] John H. Graham,[3] Anneke Louwerse,[4] and Anja C. Huizink[5]

[1] *Research Institute of Child Development and Education (RICDE), University of Amsterdam, 1018 WS Amsterdam, The Netherlands*
[2] *Research Priority Area Yield, University of Amsterdam, 1018 WS Amsterdam, The Netherlands*
[3] *Department of Biology, Berry College, Mount Berry, GA 30149, USA*
[4] *Department of Child and Adolescent Psychiatry/Psychology, Erasmus MC-Sophia, 3015 CN Rotterdam, The Netherlands*
[5] *Department of Developmental Psychology, Faculty of Psychology & Education, VU University Amsterdam, 1081 BT Amsterdam, The Netherlands*

Correspondence should be addressed to Esther I. de Bruin; e.i.debruin@uva.nl

Academic Editor: Robert F. Berman

Dermatoglyphics, ridge constellations on the hands and feet, are permanently formed by the second trimester of pregnancy. Consequently, they are considered "fossilized" evidence of a specific prenatal period. A high frequency of dermatoglyphic anomalies, or a high rate of dermatoglyphic asymmetry (discordance), is an indication of developmental instability (prenatal disturbances) prior to 24-week gestation. Most dermatoglyphic studies in psychiatry focus on adult schizophrenia. Studies on dermatoglyphic deviances and autism are sparse, include severely disturbed and intellectually retarded patients with autism, and are carried out mainly in non-Western European populations. In this study, finger print patterns, atd-angles, and palmar flexion crease patterns (PFCs) are compared between Western European adolescent teenage males, of average intellect, with Autism Spectrum Disorders (ASD; $n = 46$) and typically developing adolescent teenage males (TD; $n = 49$). Boys with ASD had a higher rate of discordance in their finger print patterns than TD boys. Thus, the hypothesized prenatal disturbances that play a role in the etiology of schizophrenia and severe autism might not be specific to these severe psychiatric disorders but might also be involved in the etiology of varying degrees of ASD.

1. Introduction

Dermatoglyphics are the ridge constellations found on the hand palms and foot soles. They have been studied for nearly 120 years [1]. Dermatoglyphics are formed from the 10th week of pregnancy [2] and from the 24th week they remain unchanged and therefore can be considered as fossils of a specific period of prenatal development [3, 4]. The most commonly studied dermatoglyphic indices include finger and palmar ridge counts, palmar atd-angle, ridge patterns on the fingertips, and palmar flexion crease patterns (PFCs). Unusual and atypical dermatoglyphic ridge patterns are often associated with mental disorders such as schizophrenia [5]. This is unsurprising, given the involvement of the nervous system in the timing and development of dermal ridge patterns [6]. Other disorders of neural development, such as autism, which is marked by defective synaptic function and aberrant neural connectivity [7, 8], might also display unusual dermatoglyphic ridge patterns. This study will focus on the association between autism and dermatoglyphic indices.

Dermatoglyphic patterns are highly variable. This phenotypic variation can be subdivided into factorial and stochastic components [9, 10]. The factorial component is the variation among individuals, which can be further subdivided into genetic, macro- and microenvironmental, and ontogenetic components. Dermatoglyphic variation has a strong genetic component (e.g., $h^2 = 0.70$ for fingerprint ridge counts, [11]), but it can also be affected by environmental stressors such as infections, pollution, parasites, or the abuse of alcohol or drugs by the mother [12]. The stochastic component is the variation within individuals and it represents developmental instability or developmental noise.

Developmental instability reflects an individual's inability to either correct developmental fluctuations (stability) or to buffer perturbations (resilience). If perturbations are small and constant, one can estimate the stability and resilience of a developmental system by examining its fluctuations [9]. This is usually accomplished by measuring deviations from perfect symmetry of bilateral traits, such as dermatoglyphic traits on left and right sides of the body or brain. There are three types of asymmetry: fluctuating asymmetry, directional asymmetry, and antisymmetry [13, 14]. Of the three, fluctuating asymmetry is regarded as the most relevant when studying associations with mental health outcomes [15]. Fluctuating asymmetry represents random deviations from perfect symmetry between the left and right sides of a bilateral trait [16–20]. These deviations are symmetrically distributed around a mean of zero [9]. Fluctuating asymmetry generally increases as a result of environmental and genetic stress, though the patterns are often inconsistent. In general, it provides an indication of a population's overall state of adaptation and coadaptation [9, 21].

For dermatoglyphic traits, high fluctuating asymmetry can be used to infer prenatal stress and instability, which can have an impact on postnatal development and behavior. Individuals with schizophrenia, for example, have higher dermatoglyphic fluctuating asymmetry [22, 23]. In addition, higher dermatoglyphic asymmetry has been reported for developmentally delayed individuals [24].

In addition to fluctuating asymmetry, dermatoglyphic anomalies have also been used as a marker of developmental instability in psychiatric disorders, mainly adult schizophrenia. In particular, a lowered a-b palmar ridge count has been shown in patients with schizophrenia [4, 25], although this has not been replicated in all studies (e.g., [3, 26]). A meta-analysis showed an overall effect-size (Cohen's d) of 0.39 for the reductions of palmar a-b ridge count in schizophrenic patients as compared to unaffected individuals [27]. With respect to finger print patterns, a higher percentage of discordance, as a measure of fluctuating asymmetry, was shown in schizophrenic patients as compared to controls (e.g., [25, 28]). Some other studies, however, failed to find significant differences [3]. With respect to abnormal PFCs, such as the Simian and the Sydney creases, an association with schizophrenia has been shown in different studies (e.g., [26]). Furthermore, deviant PFC patterns, particularly the Simian crease, have been strongly linked with chromosomal anomalies and genetic disorders, such as Down syndrome; the Sydney crease, although rarer, is associated with conditions such as fetal alcohol syndrome and craniofacial syndrome (e.g., [29]).

Mainly older dermatoglyphic studies are available for people with Autism Spectrum Disorders (ASD), disorders of neural development that have a complex genetic basis [30, 31]. ASD in this paper is used as an umbrella term and refers to autistic disorder, Asperger syndrome, and Pervasive Developmental Disorder Not Otherwise Specified (PDD-NOS). Children with ASD were found to have more arches and fewer whorls than typically developing (TD) children [32]. A study of children with intellectual disability (ID) also found more arches, the simplest fingerprint pattern, and more abnormal PFC patterns [33]. Palmar atd-angles are smaller in patients with ASD compared to TD children (e.g., [32]). Not all studies, however, agree on this finding [34]. Arrieta and colleagues [35] found larger atd-angles in girls with ASD than in boys. A few descriptions of dermatoglyphic variables in people with ASD in Eastern European countries (Croatia, Romania, and Serbia) have recently become available. Miličić and colleagues [36] found a smaller atd-angle in patients with ASD as compared to nonaffected TD individuals. Another study showed that boys with ASD had more arches on their fingertips as compared to TD children, as well as a lower total and a-b ridge count and a wider atd-angle [37]. It must be noted, however, that participants in all of these studies were extremely low functioning children with autistic disorder. Although autistic disorder was the primary classification, approximately one-third of the patients in the Eastern European study suffered from profound ID (IQ < 35), whereas more than 50% were diagnosed with mild ID (IQ 35–50). It is therefore unknown whether these dermatoglyphic deviances, as a proxy marker of deviations in early prenatal development, would also show up in children with milder forms of ASD, such as PDD-NOS.

In the current study, we compared (discordance of) fingerprint patterns, atd-angles, and PFC patterns of northern European boys of average intellect and ASD (mainly PDD-NOS), with TD boys. If boys with ASD show, for instance, a higher rate of discordance, this could indicate that disturbances in prenatal development may play a role in the later development of high-functioning ASD.

2. Methods

2.1. Participants. The 46 male patients (mean age = 16.16, SD = 1.67) were recruited at the Child and Adolescent Psychiatry outpatient department of the Erasmus MC-Sophia, the Netherlands. All patients were diagnosed with a subtype of ASD according to DSM-IV-TR-criteria [38]; more specifically, $n = 1$ Asperger syndrome, $n = 8$ autistic disorder, and $n = 37$ PDD-NOS. Classifications were made by highly ASD-experienced child psychiatrists and validated by administering the Autism Diagnostic Observation Schedule-Generic (ADOS-G; [39]) and the Autism Diagnostic Interview-Revised (ADI-R; [40]). The Diagnostic Interview Schedule for Children (DISC-parent informant; [41]) was used to assess comorbid psychiatric disorders. Of the adolescents diagnosed with ASD, 41% fulfilled diagnostic criteria for an internalizing disorder (i.e., anxiety disorder or depression) and 50% fulfilled criteria for an externalizing disorder (24% met diagnostic criteria for Attention Deficit Hyperactivity Disorder [ADHD], 13% for Oppositional Defiant Disorder [ODD], and 13% fulfilled diagnostic criteria for ADHD and ODD). IQ scores for the total sample (assessed with the

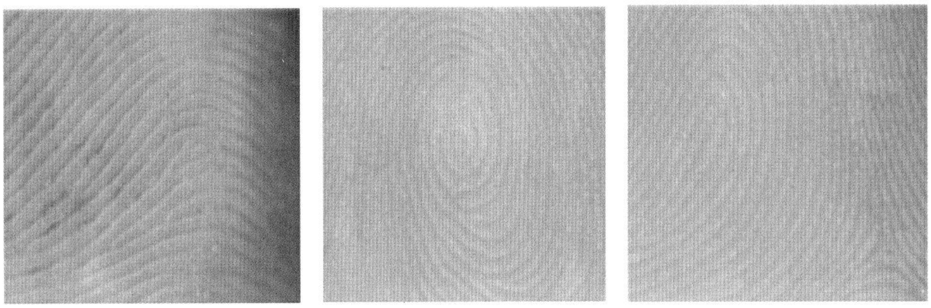

FIGURE 1: Examples of finger ridge patterns: 1 = arch; 2 = whorl; 3 = loop.

Wechsler Abbreviated Scale of Intelligence [42]) were Total Intelligence Quotient (TIQ), M = 103.04 (SD = 14.12), Verbal Intelligence Quotient (VIQ), M = 100.87 (SD = 15.07), and Performance Intelligence Quotient (PIQ), M = 104.57 (SD = 13.45). More specific ASD subtype IQ scores were the following: autistic disorder (n = 8), TIQ = 111.50 (SD = 13.07), VIQ = 107.63 (SD = 15.99), and PIQ = 113.50 (SD = 9.21); Asperger syndrome (n = 1), TIQ = 108, VIQ = 98, and PIQ = 118; PDD-NOS (n = 37), TIQ = 106.63 (SD = 14.83), VIQ = 105.70 (SD = 14.40), and PIQ = 106.23 (SD = 15.70). IQ scores did not differ significantly between groups.

The 49 TD adolescent males (mean age = 15.98, SD = 2.26) were recruited from two different high schools in the Netherlands. Although no IQ tests were administered to the control boys, the level of high school (higher general secondary education and preuniversity secondary education) indicates that IQ scores were most likely above average. To ensure no boys with psychiatric disorders were included in the TD group, the Youth Self Report (YSR) [43] was administered and adolescents who scored above the clinical cutoff point were excluded. The patients and TD adolescent males did not differ in mean age, $t = 0.47$, $df = 93$, $P = 0.64$.

2.2. Procedure. Digital hand scans were made at 1800 dpi with a Hewlett-Packard Scanjet 4600 scanner. Fingerprint patterns were classified according to the three-pattern system (loops, arches, and whorls) [44]. Fingerprint patterns have cores and triradii and the classification is based on the number of triradii present; see also Figure 1. Atd-angles were measured with the Image J software program [45]. PFC patterns were rated as normal or abnormal (Simian or Sydney creases). An interrater reliability (IRR) study was carried out for a subsample of the total sample of $n = 95$. Two independent raters rated a random set of $n = 28$ pairs of hands. Cohen's kappa (κ) was 1 for all finger print patterns in all fingers, apart from the little finger of the left hand (for which $\kappa = 0.87$) and the middle finger of the right hand (for which $\kappa = 0.91$). Kappa theoretically ranges from 0 to 1 and the values in this study fall within the highest range of agreement according to kappa interpretation guidelines [46]. Further, Spearman's correlations were calculated for the agreement on the continuous variable atd-angle. Correlations were nearly perfect, $r = 0.96$ for the left hand and $r = 0.98$ for the right hand, and thus agreement between raters was extremely high. Moreover, dermatoglyphic analyses were conducted by research assistants who were blind to group membership. Informed consent was obtained prior to participation from parents, caretakers, and adolescents. The Medical Ethics Committee of the Erasmus MC approved the study.

Fingerprint discordance was evaluated finger-by-finger. For example, if an individual's right and left index fingers have different patterns (say loop and arch), they are classified as discordant. If both index fingers have the same pattern, they are classified as concordant. Consequently, fingerprint discordance ranges from 0 (all fingers concordant) to 4 (all fingers discordant, thumb was not included).

2.3. Statistical Analyses. Analysis of variance (ANOVA) was used to compare fingerprint patterns, fingerprint discordance, mean atd-angle, and atd-angle asymmetry of boys with ASD and TD boys. Because fingerprint patterns on right and left hands have a Poisson distribution (counts of randomly occurring objects), we used the Anscombe transformation, $2\sqrt{(x + 3/8)}$, to stabilize their variances. Moreover, we only examined whorls and arches because a third variable (loops) is redundant; knowing the numbers of whorls and arches completely determines the number of loops. Previous studies [33, 47] have used contingency tables of fingerprint patterns, but this approach violates the independence assumption of chi-square. The ten fingers of a single individual are not independent observations. The unit of observation is the individual person, not each finger, and this cannot be accommodated in a contingency table analysis. The mean atd-angles $(R + L)/2$ were log transformed to stabilize their variances. Unsigned asymmetry of atd-angles was $|\log_{10} \text{LH} - \log_{10} \text{RH}|$. Cohen's d was estimated as a measure of effect size. Chi-square tests were used to assess the association between group (ASD, TD) and PFC pattern (normal, abnormal).

3. Results

As can be seen in Table 1, boys with ASD did not differ from TD boys in the number of arches, $F_{1,91} = 1.44$, $P = 0.23$, or whorls, $F_{1,91} = 0.11$, $P = 0.75$. Nevertheless, boys with ASD showed more discordant finger pairs than TD boys, $F_{1,91} = 6.86$, $P = 0.01$. Average atd-angle ($\log_{10}$) did not differ between boys with ASD and TD boys, $F_{1,45} = 1.62$, $P = 0.21$. In addition, there was no difference in unsigned asymmetry of atd-angle between the two groups, $F_{1,45} = 0.99$, $P = 0.33$. And no associations were found between group

TABLE 1: Fingerprint pattern counts, number of discordant finger pairs, atd-angles, and fluctuating asymmetry of atd-angles for boys with ASD and typically developing boys.

Trait	Character	ASD boys M (SD)	Control boys M (SD)	*P* value	ES (Cohen's *d*)
Fingerprint patterns (Anscombe transformation of counts)	Number of whorls (LH + RH)	2.52 (1.43)	2.42 (1.42)	0.75	0.07
	Number of arches (LH + RH)	1.53 (0.56)	1.74 (1.04)	0.23	−0.25
	Number of discordant finger pairs	2.24 (0.88)	1.80 (0.72)	0.01	0.55
Atd-angles ($\log_{10}$ degrees)	$(\log_{10} LH + \log_{10} RH)/2$	1.61° (0.033°)	1.62° (0.048°)	0.21	−0.38
	$\lvert\log_{10} LH - \log_{10} RH\rvert$	0.03° (0.05°)	0.02° (0.02°)	0.33	0.30

ASD = Autism Spectrum Disorders; ES = effect size; LH = left hand; M = mean (SD = standard deviation); RH = right hand.

TABLE 2: Palmar flexion creases (PFCs) as a percentage of all palms for boys with ASD and typically developing boys.

Hand	Pattern	ASD boys	Control boys	χ^2	*P* value
Left	Normal	100% (46)	97.9% (47)	0.97	0.33
	Simian	0% (0)	2.1% (1)		
	Sydney	0% (0)	0% (0)		
Right	Normal	97.8% (45)	93.8% (45)	1.96	0.38
	Simian	0% (0)	4.2% (2)		
	Sydney	2.2% (1)	2.1% (1)		
Discordance between LH and RH		2.2% (1)	4% (2)	0.30	0.58

ASD = Autism Spectrum Disorders; LH = left hand; RH = right hand.
Exact counts of palms are in parentheses. Chi-square tests the hypothesis that there is no association between PFC patterns and group membership.

and abnormal PFCs for the left hand, $\chi^2 = 0.97$, $df = 1$, $P = 0.33$, or the right hand, $\chi^2 = 1.96$, $df = 2$, $P = 0.38$. In addition, there was no association between PFC discordance and group, $\chi^2 = 0.30$, $df = 1$, $P = 0.58$. Both TD and boys with ASD showed very low basal rates of abnormal patterns (Simian or Sydney) in their palmar creases. See Table 2 for all PFC information.

4. Discussion

This study showed that Western European boys with ASD and average intellect had a significantly higher rate of discordance in their fingerprint pairs than TD boys. They did not differ, however, in the numbers of whorls, the numbers of arches, mean atd-angle, or atd-angle asymmetry. A higher rate of discordance, reflecting greater fluctuating asymmetry, is considered a proxy marker of developmental instability during the second trimester, when the finger ridges form. Thus, the hypothesized altered neurodevelopment that plays a role in schizophrenia and severe autistic disorder might not be specific to these severe psychiatric disorders but might also be involved in the etiology of more broadly defined autism, that is, ASD.

A higher number of arches, as was found in other studies of patients with autism [32, 36, 37], was not found in the boys with ASD in our sample. Arches are the simplest form of fingerprint pattern and seem to be associated with lower intellectual functioning (i.e., [24]). Perhaps this partly explains the (non-)finding in this study. Although the boys in this study were diagnosed with ASD (of which around 80% with PDD-NOS), they were patients with average intellectual abilities (IQ around 100). Patients with ASD in previous studies were profoundly retarded (IQ < 35) and this often coincided with other (i.e., usually chromosomal) disorders. For instance Walker [32] described his patients as suffering from "a profound inability to relate to people, or establish any positive human contact," which obviously refers to severely disturbed patients, very different from the current study sample.

With respect to the PFCs, no association with ASD was found. This might be related to the extremely low basal rate of the abnormal Simian and Sydney patterns in our sample (i.e., only one Sydney pattern in the right hand was found in the boys with ASD). We know from the literature that these deviant patterns are strongly associated with chromosomal anomalies and genetic disorders, such as Down syndrome [29]. Our sample did not include such patients, which might explain the low basal rate. Further, Sharma and Sharma [48] showed an overview of prevalence of the Simian crease across different populations in the world, and the prevalence in the Netherlands was very low (1.5%) compared to other populations (for instance 14.4% in India).

In summary, a higher rate of discordance, which is an indicator of developmental instability, was found in high-functioning adolescent males with ASD. They showed no other dermatoglyphic deviances. Dermatoglyphic deviances do not seem specific for severely impaired patients with ASD or those with schizophrenia or genetic anomalies (i.e., aneuploidy, deletion, and duplication), but also in the milder forms of ASD (i.e., PDD-NOS), prenatal disturbances might have occurred, which could be reflected in these deviances in the fingerprints. An important note is that to diagnose ASD based on fingerprint asymmetry is not the conclusion that should be drawn from these findings. However, inspection of dermatoglyphics in clinical psychiatric practice could possibly function as an additional observation.

Acknowledgment

Part of this study was supported financially by a grant from the Netherlands Organization for Scientific Research (NWO/ZonMw/Implementation Impuls 100002106).

References

[1] F. Galton, *Finger Prints*, Macmillan and Company, London, UK, 1892.

[2] M. Okajima, "Development of dermal ridges in the fetus," *Journal of Medical Genetics*, vol. 12, no. 3, pp. 243–250, 1975.

[3] M. Fatjó-Vilas, D. Gourion, S. Campanera et al., "New evidences of gene and environment interactions affecting prenatal neurodevelopment in schizophrenia-spectrum disorders: a family dermatoglyphic study," *Schizophrenia Research*, vol. 103, no. 1–3, pp. 209–217, 2008.

[4] P. Fearon, A. Lane, M. Airie et al., "Is reduced dermatoglyphic a-b ridge count a reliable marker of developmental impairment in schizophrenia?" *Schizophrenia Research*, vol. 50, no. 3, pp. 151–157, 2001.

[5] F. M. Ahmed-Popova, M. J. Mantarkov, S. T. Sivkov, and V. H. Akabaliev, "Dermatoglyphics—a possible biomarker in the neurodevelopmental model for the origin of mental disorders," *Folia Medica*, vol. 56, no. 1, pp. 5–10, 2014.

[6] M. Kücken, "Models for fingerprint pattern formation," *Forensic Science International*, vol. 171, no. 2-3, pp. 85–96, 2007.

[7] N. Krumm, B. J. O'Roak, J. Shendure, and E. E. Eichler, "A *de novo* convergence of autism genetics and molecular neuroscience," *Trends in Neurosciences*, vol. 37, no. 2, pp. 95–105, 2014.

[8] J. O. Maximo, E. J. Cadena, and R. K. Kana, "The implications of brain connectivity in the neuropsychology of autism," *Neuropsychology Review*, vol. 24, no. 1, pp. 16–31, 2014.

[9] J. H. Graham, S. Raz, H. Hel-Or, and E. Nevo, "Fluctuating asymmetry: methods, theory, and applications," *Symmetry*, vol. 2, no. 2, pp. 466–540, 2010.

[10] D. L. Lajus, J. H. Graham, and A. V. Kozhara, "Developmental instability and the stochastic component of total phenotypic variance," in *Developmental Instability: Causes and Consequences*, pp. 343–363, Oxford University Press, Oxford, UK, 2003.

[11] D. Loesch, "Genetics of dermatoglyphic patterns on palms," *Annals of Human Genetics*, vol. 34, no. 3, pp. 277–290, 1971.

[12] N. M. Durham and C. C. Plato, *Trends in Dermatoglyphic Research*, Kluwer Academic Publishers, Dordrecht, The Netherlands, 1990.

[13] A. R. Palmer and C. Strobeck, "Fluctuating asymmetry: measurement, analysis, patterns," *Annual Review of Ecology and Systematics*, vol. 17, pp. 391–421, 1986.

[14] L. Van Valen, "A study of fluctuating asymmetry," *Evolution*, vol. 16, pp. 125–142, 1962.

[15] R. Thornhill and A. P. Møller, "Developmental stability, disease and medicine," *Biological Reviews*, vol. 72, no. 4, pp. 497–548, 1997.

[16] K. Mather, "Genetical control of stability in development," *Heredity*, vol. 7, no. 3, pp. 297–336, 1953.

[17] T. A. Markow, *Developmental Instability: Its Origins and Evolutionary Implications: Proceedings of the International Conference, Tempe, Arizona, USA, 14-15 June 1993*, Kluwer Academic, Dordrecht, The Netherlands, 1994.

[18] A. P. Møller and J. P. Swaddle, *Asymmetry, Developmental Stability and Evolution*, Oxford University Press, New York, NY, USA, 1997.

[19] M. Polak, *Developmental Instability: Causes and Consequences*, Oxford University Press, New York, NY, USA, 2003.

[20] V. M. Zakharov and J. H. Graham, *Developmental Stability in Natural Populations*, Finnish Zoological Publishing Board, Helsinki, Finland, 1992.

[21] J. S. Jones, "An asymmetrical view of fitness," *Nature*, vol. 325, no. 6102, pp. 298–299, 1987.

[22] T. A. Markow and I. I. Gottesman, "Fluctuating dermatoglyphic asymmetry in psychotic twins," *Psychiatry Research*, vol. 29, no. 1, pp. 37–43, 1989.

[23] T. A. Markow and K. Wandler, "Fluctuating dermatoglyphic asymmetry and the genetics of liability to schizophrenia," *Psychiatry Research*, vol. 19, no. 4, pp. 323–328, 1986.

[24] C. T. Naugler and M. D. Ludman, "A case-control study of fluctuating dermatoglyphic asymmetry as a risk marker for developmental delay," *American Journal of Medical Genetics*, vol. 66, no. 1, pp. 11–14, 1996.

[25] L. Fananas, J. van Os, C. Hoyos, J. McGrath, C. S. Mellor, and R. Murray, "Dermatoglyphic a-b ridge count as a possible marker for developmental disturbance in schizophrenia: replication in two samples," *Schizophrenia Research*, vol. 20, no. 3, pp. 307–314, 1996.

[26] J. L. Reilly, P. T. Murphy, M. Byrne et al., "Dermatoglyphic fluctuating asymmetry and atypical handedness in schizophrenia," *Schizophrenia Research*, vol. 50, no. 3, pp. 159–168, 2001.

[27] E. Bramon, M. Walshe, C. McDonald et al., "Dermatoglyphics and schizophrenia: a meta-analysis and investigation of the impact of obstetric complications upon a-b ridge count," *Schizophrenia Research*, vol. 75, no. 2-3, pp. 399–404, 2005.

[28] F. Shakibaei, G. A. Asadollahi, and A. Tabibi, "Dermatoglyphics in patients with schizophrenia," *Journal of Research in Medical Sciences*, vol. 16, no. 8, pp. 1055–1061, 2011.

[29] B. A. Schaumann and J. M. Opitz, "Clinical aspects of dermatoglyphics," *Birth Defects: Original Article Series*, vol. 27, no. 2, pp. 193–228, 1991.

[30] B. S. Abrahams and D. H. Geschwind, "Connecting genes to brain in the autism spectrum disorders," *Archives of Neurology*, vol. 67, no. 4, pp. 395–399, 2010.

[31] D. H. Geschwind, "Genetics of autism spectrum disorders," *Trends in Cognitive Sciences*, vol. 15, no. 9, pp. 409–416, 2011.

[32] H. A. Walker, "A dermatoglyphic study of autistic patients," *Journal of Autism and Childhood Schizophrenia*, vol. 7, no. 1, pp. 11–21, 1977.

[33] A. Rosa, B. Gutiérrez, A. Guerra, B. Arias, and L. Fañanás, "Dermatoglyphics and abnormal palmar flexion creases as markers of early prenatal stress in children with idiopathic intellectual disability," *Journal of Intellectual Disability Research*, vol. 45, no. 5, pp. 416–423, 2001.

[34] S. R. Wolman, M. Campbell, M. L. Marchi, S. I. Deutsch, and T. D. Gershon, "Dermatoglyphic study in autistic children and controls," *Journal of the American Academy of Child and Adolescent Psychiatry*, vol. 29, no. 6, pp. 878–884, 1990.

[35] M. I. Arrieta, B. Martinez, B. Criado, A. Simon, L. Salazar, and C. M. Lostao, "Dermatoglyphic analysis of autistic Basque children," *American Journal of Medical Genetics*, vol. 35, no. 1, pp. 1–9, 1990.

[36] J. Miličić, Z. B. Petković, and J. Božikov, "Dermatoglyphs of digito-palmar complex in autistic disorder: family analysis," *Croatian Medical Journal*, vol. 44, no. 4, pp. 469–476, 2003.

[37] M. Stošljevic and M. Adamovic, "Dermatoglyphic characteristics of digito-palmar complex in autistic boys in Serbia," *Vojnosanitetski Pregled*, vol. 70, no. 4, pp. 386–390, 2013.

[38] APA, *Diagnostic and Statistical Manual of Mental Disorders: DSM-IV-TR*, American Psychiatric Association, Washington, DC, USA, 2000.

[39] C. Lord, S. Risi, L. Lambrecht et al., "The Autism Diagnostic Observation Schedule-Generic: a standard measure of social and communication deficits associated with the spectrum of autism," *Journal of Autism and Developmental Disorders*, vol. 30, no. 3, pp. 205–223, 2000.

[40] A. Le Couteur, C. Lord, and M. Rutter, *The Autism Diagnostic Interview—Revised (ADI-R)*, Western Psychological Services, Los Angeles, Calif, USA, 2003.

[41] D. Shaffer, P. Fisher, and C. Lucas, *NIMH DISC-IV. Diagnostic Interview Schedule for Children*, Columbia University Press, New York, NY, USA, 1998.

[42] D. Wechsler, *Wechsler Abbreviated Scale of Intelligence*, Psychological Corporation, San Antonio, Tex, USA, 1999.

[43] T. M. Achenbach, *Manual for the Youth Self-Report and 1991 Profile*, Department of Psychiatry, University of Vermont, Burlington, Vt, USA, 1991.

[44] T. Reed and R. Meier, *Taking Dermatoglyphic Prints: A Self-Instruction Manual*, American Dermatoglyphic Association, Bloomington, Ind, USA, 1990.

[45] C. A. Schneider, W. S. Rasband, and K. W. Eliceiri, "NIH Image to ImageJ: 25 years of image analysis," *Nature Methods*, vol. 9, no. 7, pp. 671–675, 2012.

[46] D. G. Altman, "Mathematics for Kappa," in *Practical Statistics for Medical Research*, D. Altman, Ed., pp. 406–407, Chapman & Hall, London, UK, 1st edition, 1991.

[47] N. M. Scott, S. M. Weinberg, K. Neiswanger et al., "Dermatoglyphic fingerprint heterogeneity among individuals with nonsyndromic cleft lip with or without cleft palate and their unaffected relatives in China and the Philippines," *Human Biology*, vol. 77, no. 2, pp. 257–266, 2005.

[48] D. K. Sharma and V. Sharma, "Prevalences of Simian, Sydney and Suwon creases and their association with each other, body sides, handedness, sex and anomalies/diseases/syndromes in a population of Central india," *International Journal of Morphology*, vol. 29, no. 3, pp. 1069–1075, 2011.

16

Longitudinal Study of Sensory Features in Children with Autism Spectrum Disorder

Lucia Perez Repetto,[1,2] Emmanuelle Jasmin,[1,2,3] Eric Fombonne,[4] Erika Gisel,[5,6] and Mélanie Couture[1,2,3]

[1] *École de Réadaptation, Faculté de Médecine et des Sciences de la Santé, Université de Sherbrooke, Sherbrooke, QC, Canada J1H 5N4*
[2] *Axe Mère-Enfant, Centre de Recherche du Centre Hospitalier Universitaire de Sherbrooke (CRCHUS), Sherbrooke, QC, Canada J1H 5N4*
[3] *Axe le Développement de l'Enfant dans sa Famille et sa Communauté, Institut de Première Ligne en Santé et Services Sociaux, CIUSSS de l'Estrie-CHUS, Sherbrooke, QC, Canada J1H 4C4*
[4] *Department of Psychiatry and Institute for Development and Disability, Oregon Health & Science University, Portland, OR 97239, USA*
[5] *Center for Interdisciplinary Research in Rehabilitation, Montreal, QC, Canada H2H 2N8*
[6] *School of Physical & Occupational Therapy, Faculty of Medicine, McGill University, Montreal, QC, Canada H3G 1Y5*

Correspondence should be addressed to Mélanie Couture; melanie.m.couture@usherbrooke.ca

Academic Editor: Valsamma Eapen

Background. Between 45 and 95% of children with Autism Spectrum Disorder (ASD) present sensory features that affect their daily functioning. However, the data in the scientific literature are not conclusive regarding the evolution of sensory features in children with ASD. The main objective of this study was to analyze the sensory features of children within the age of 3-4 (T1) when they received their ASD diagnosis and two years later (T2) when they started school. *Methods.* We conducted a prospective cohort study to assess sensory features in 34 children with ASD over time. The data were collected using a standardized assessment tool, the Sensory Profile. *Results.* Our analyses show that sensory features in children with ASD are stable from the age of three to six years. The stability of sensory scores is independent of correction by covariates, such as cognitive level and autism severity scores. *Conclusions.* Children with ASD have sensory features that persist from the time of diagnosis at the age of 3 to 4 years to school age. This persistence of sensory features from an early age underscores the need to support these children and their parents. Sensory features should be detected early and managed to improve functional and psychosocial outcomes.

1. Introduction

Autism Spectrum Disorder (ASD) affects more than 1% of children [1]. Common characteristics associated with ASD are difficulties in communication and social interaction, as well as rigidity or repetitiveness in interests and behaviors [2]. Some restricted or repetitive interests and behaviors of people with ASD may be related to sensory features [3], such as difficulties in sensory processing and sensory integration [4–6].

Sensory processing is the process by which peripheral and central nervous systems receive, interpret, and respond to sensory information [7, 8]. The nature of the sensory input can vary (smell, touch, proprioception, etc.) and the organization of this information contributes to the development of muscle tone, motor skills, self-awareness, interactions with others, and everyday functioning [9–11]. According to Dunn's model of sensory processing [12], four sensory processing patterns characterize the perceptual process. These patterns are thought to arise from individual differences in neurological thresholds for stimulation (high-low) and self-regulation strategies (active-passive). Crossing these dimensions gives four sensory processing styles: sensory sensitivity, sensory avoiding, low registration, and sensory seeking [12, 13].

With advances in research, difficulties in sensory processing in children with ASD are becoming increasingly evident. Between 45 and 95% of children with ASD have sensory features that affect their functioning in everyday life [14, 15]. However, the data available in the scientific literature shed little light on the evolution of sensory features in children with ASD, making it impossible to provide appropriate services adapted to their specific needs. In addition, few longitudinal studies have been conducted on the sensory development of children with ASD [16, 17] and none studied ASD children prospectively for more than one year under stable conditions, that is, with every child in the study having the same age at the beginning of the study, as well as using the same assessment instruments.

To illustrate the aforementioned lack of conclusive evidence, we briefly reviewed the studies that documented the evolution of overall sensory features (including all senses) of children with ASD. First, a recent prospective study by McCormick et al. (2016) [17] found that 29 children aged 2 to 8 with ASD showed no significant change in sensory processing over time. The main limitations of this study are as follows: (1) only the Short Sensory Profile (SSP) [18] was used, limiting the interpretation of the subcategories (sections and quadrants) and not allowing interpretation according to the quadrants in Dunn's model of sensory processing [12]; and (2) the time between the two evaluations varied, which added a maturation bias.

A second longitudinal study by Ausderau et al. (2014) [16] analyzed the sensory features of 884 children with ASD aged 2 to 12 over one year. This study found no statistically significant differences in the sensory features of these children over time. However, no subdivisions in the wide age range (10 years) of the study participants were analyzed, which limits the interpretation of the results.

A third longitudinal study by Green et al. (2012) [19] included 149 participants with ASD from 18 to 30 months old at the beginning of the study and reevaluated them one year later. The evaluation tool used for this study, the Infant Toddler Social Emotional Assessment (ITSEA) [20], has a sensory component but was not specifically designed to assess sensory features. The ITSEA mainly examines emotional responses, sensory overresponsiveness, and anxiety. Sensory overresponsiveness in the study sample was found to be stable over time.

The findings of these three papers are in contradiction with those of the meta-analysis by Ben-Sasson et al. [21], which analyzed 14 cross-sectional studies involving children with ASD at different ages. This review revealed an increase in the frequency of overall sensory features up to 6–9 years of age (and a decrease thereafter) in children with ASD.

The weaknesses of this meta-analysis are as follows: (1) the inclusion of studies with heterogeneous groups of participants with age ranging from 7 months to 56 years; (2) use of a variety of evaluation tools; (3) diagnoses not all made alike as only 4 of the 14 studies reviewed used gold standard diagnostic tools for ASD; and (4) few studies reviewed including covariates in the analyses.

Other longitudinal studies exist. However, some focused on a single sensory system (e.g., vision) [22] while others targeted populations with a variety of developmental disorders who exhibited syndromic elements of ASD, such as fragile X syndrome [23] or Angelman syndrome [24], without studying children with ASD in particular.

This literature review reveals gaps in the current evidence on sensory processing in children with ASD over time and underlines the need for further research on the subject. The main objective of this study was to analyze the evolution of sensory features in children with ASD between the age of 3-4 years (T1) and two years later (T2) when they started school (5-6 years). Our general hypothesis was that overall sensory features of children with ASD would remain stable with age. Our second hypothesis was that the classification of children among the different subcategories of the Sensory Profile would not change between T1 and T2.

2. Methods

Three interrelated studies formed the basis of this study. First, between 2007 and 2008, parents of children at the Autism Clinic of the Montreal Children's Hospital were invited to participate in a major pan-Canadian longitudinal study, "Pathways for Better Outcomes" (also known as the Canadian Institutes of Health Research "CIHR-" funded TRAJ project). If they agreed, an ancillary study was conducted only in Montreal to document sensory-motor difficulties and their impact on daily functioning [25]. Additional funding from the FRQSC *(Fonds de Recherche du Québec-Société et Culture)* was obtained for a 2-year follow-up of participants in the sensory-motor study (2010). In the present study, we undertook a secondary analysis of data from both sensory-motor prospective studies (2008–2010). This study was approved by the ethics committee of the *CIUSSS de l'Estrie-CHUS* of the *Université de Sherbrooke* in October 2016.

2.1. Participants. Sixty-eight children aged 3 to 4 years diagnosed with ASD who were patients at the Autism Clinic of the Montreal Children's Hospital participated in the sensory-motor study at T1 (2008). Of the original 68, 39 participated in the follow-up two years later (T2). Complete data for the two-time points were available for 34 participants.

The diagnosis was based on the DSM-IV-TR [26] diagnostic criteria, expert clinical judgement, and scores from gold standard diagnostic tools: the Autism Diagnostic Interview, Revised (ADI-R) [27] and the Autism Diagnostic Observation Schedule-Generic (ADOS-G) [28].

2.2. Measures. The families' sociodemographic characteristics (child's gender and age, family income, mother's education, marital status, and ethnicity) were collected using a sociodemographic questionnaire designed for this purpose. To characterize the children's cognitive level and language skills and to measure sensory processing over time, the following standardized assessment tools were used:

(1) The Merrill-Palmer-Revised Scales of Development (M-P-R) [29] can be used to assess children's development in five domains: cognitive, language, motor, self-reliance, and socioemotional. In this paper, only

the standardized score for the cognitive component was used to evaluate cognitive level at T1 (controlled variable). The M-P-R has very good psychometric properties, including internal consistency ($\alpha = 0.90$) and test-retest reliability (intraclass correlation coefficient: ICC = 0.87–0.90) [29].

(2) The Preschool Language Scale, Fourth Edition (PLS-4) [30] is an interactive assessment of developmental language skills, including auditory comprehension and expressive communication for children aged 0–7 years [30]. In our study, standard scores were considered for the statistical analyses. Psychometric properties of the test include high interrater reliability (ICC = 0.99) [31].

(3) Autism severity scores [32] were calculated using the ADOS severity scores [33]. These calibrated scores range from 1 to 10 and are useful in comparing assessments across modules and over time [33].

(4) The Sensory Profile (SP) [34], children's version 3–10 years, is a questionnaire measuring children's response to sensory events that influence their functioning in everyday life. It is completed by parents and includes 125 items. The parent scores the items on a Likert scale (from 1 to 5) depending on the observed frequency of behavior. The questionnaire is divided into subcategories involving sections and quadrants. Sections reflect the different sensory systems (auditory processing, visual processing, etc.) and quadrants refer mainly to the different types of sensory processing (seeking, avoidance, sensitivity, and low registration), which correspond to Dunn's model of sensory processing [12], thus identifying the sensory system(s) that affect daily functioning [35].

More specifically, for each subcategory (sections and quadrants), the SP makes it possible to compare children's results with standardized values in order to classify their performance in three categories: typical performance, probable difference (one standard deviation below the mean), and definite difference (two standard deviations below the mean) [34]. However, the SP does not yield a total score. Finally, the SP has robust psychometric properties for both internal consistency (α = 0.89–0.95) [36] and test-retest reliability (ICC = 0.80–0.90) [36].

The Short Sensory Profile (SSP) [18] is a screening tool derived from the SP that has a similar structure to its longer counterpart. Its 38 items are related to the construct of sensory processing and were extracted from the SP. Interestingly, further validation analyses have been done with the SSP, allowing a validated total score to be calculated, which is an asset for quantitative statistical analyses. The SSP allows the calculation of a total score and has acceptable construct validity and its internal consistency is excellent, with α = 0.70–0.90 [18].

2.3. Procedure. At T1, a lengthy evaluation took place at the Montreal Children's Hospital within the framework of the TRAJ project. An experienced child psychiatrist confirmed the ASD diagnosis, and assessments of cognitive level and language skills were conducted by certified therapists trained in the administration of these tests.

Sensory features were assessed using the caregiver questionnaires. The SP was completed by either parent at the hospital, with the help of two certified occupational therapists, who had more than five years of clinical experience and were also in charge of obtaining signed informed consent from the parents and answering any questions they had.

A nonrandomized convenience sample was used for the families who agreed to participate in the follow-up at T2. After the evaluation was completed at T1, the parents received a report and were invited to participate in a second evaluation of their child's sensory features using the SP two years later (T2). The mean interval between T1 and T2 was 27.7 months (SD = 6.0). In our study, the SSP itself was not administered; instead its 38 items were extracted directly from the responses to the SP. A score was calculated for each subcategory of the SP and a total score was determined for the SSP at both T1 and T2.

2.4. Analyses. We analyzed data over time using SPSS 24© software to generate descriptive and inferential statistical analyses. Descriptive analyses for the continuous variables (means and standard deviations) and ordinal variables (frequencies and percentages) were performed on the sociodemographic variables and some of the sensory measurement categories. We verified the normality of the data using the Shapiro-Wilk test and the equality of the variances with Mauchly's sphericity test.

For the inferential analyses, we employed three tests: (1) a repeated measures ANOVA (T1 versus T2) for a single group, with matched measurements, to evaluate the effect of time on the SSP total score and the scores for different SP categories; (2) a repeated measures ANCOVA with the same purpose as the ANOVA, but adding two covariates: cognitive level and autism severity scores (from ADOS-2) [37]; (3) McNemar's tests which were applied to analyze matched categorical data for both time points, as performances on the SSP total score and SP subcategory scores were categorized as either typical for those within the "normal performance" range or atypical for those within the "probable differences" or "definite differences" range. The significance threshold for all tests was set at 0.05.

3. Results

Study population characteristics are presented in Table 1. The sample had a mean age of 45 months at T1 and 72 months at T2; most of the children were boys (82%) with English as their mother language (68%). Most mothers were Caucasian (68%) and had attended university (71%). A large percentage of the mothers (85%) lived with a partner (married, common-law, etc.), and in 77% of the cases, family income was above 40,000 CAD per year (30,000 USD).

Most children had cognitive and language delays as well as a moderately severe level of autism. Seventy-one percent (71%, n = 24) presented a significant cognitive delay

Table 1: General characteristics of participants.

	n	%	Mean (SD)
Gender			
Boys	28	82.4	
Girls	6	17.6	
Chronological age			
T1 (months)	34		44.7 (4.9)
T2 (months)	34		72.4 (5.4)
ADOS comparison score (CSS[a])	34		7.4 (2.1)
Cognitive functioning			
M-P-R SS[b]	32		60.1 (25.8)
Significant cognitive delay	24	70.6	
Language skills			
PLS-4 auditory SS	33		63.4 (21.9)
Significant auditory delay	20	58.8	
PLS-4 expressive SS	33		70.6 (19.9)
Significant expressive delay	24	70.6	
Mother's education			
University	24	70.6	
No university	10	29.4	
Mother's ethnicity			
Caucasian	23	67.6	
Non-Caucasian	11	32.4	
Mother's marital status			
Single	5	14.7	
Married/common-law	29	85.3	
Family income			
>40,000 CAD	26	76.5	
<40,000 CAD	8	23.5	
Mother tongue			
English	23	67.6	
French	4	11.8	
Other	7	20.6	

ASD rated from 1 to 10, with 10 being the most severe; [a]CSS is calibrated severity scores; [b]SS is standard score; M-P-R: Merrill-Palmer-Revised Scales of Development; PLS-4: Preschool Language Scale, Fourth Edition.

(standard score < 70), 59% ($n = 20$) had an expressive language delay (standard score < 70), and 71% ($n = 24$) had a receptive language delay. The mean ADOS severity score of the sample was 7.4 (SD = 2.1), which is between a moderately severe and severe level of autism.

Table 2 presents the mean raw scores and results of the repeated measures ANOVAs for the SSP and various SP subcategories at T1 and T2. The effect of time on the SSP total score was not significant ($F(1, 33) = 0.970$; $p = 0.330$). The same was true for all SP quadrants and sections. Quadrant 4 (sensory avoiding) ($F(1, 29) = 1.717$; $p = 0.199$) was the only mean score to fall within a "typical" range at T2.

In the repeated measures ANCOVAs, there was a nonsignificant effect of time on the SSP score after controlling for the ADOS severity score ($F(1, 28) = 0.087$; $p = 0.771$) as well as when controlling for cognitive level ($F(1, 28) = 0.530$; $p = 0.473$). The effect of time on the SP subcategories was also not significant (results available upon request).

Our study included 34 pairs of measurements. Our data indicate that the difference in response of matched pairs has a standard deviation of $\sigma = 15.34$. We detected a true difference in the mean response of matched pairs of −7.596 or 7.596 with a probability of 0.8 ($\alpha = 0.05$). Therefore, the observed stability of scores or absence of a difference between T1 and T2 could be attributed to a lack of power due to the small sample size. However, the magnitude of the difference is so small that it can reasonably be judged to be clinically nonsignificant (smaller than 1/4 SD). However, a larger sample would have allowed for the detection of smaller size effects that could not be detected in our study. Had our study had a larger sample (e.g., $n = 300$), we would have found the clinically nonsignificant differences between T1 and T2 to be statistically significant.

Table 3 presents the findings of the exact McNemar's tests on the classification into two categories of typical-atypical scores for the SSP total score and SP subcategory scores at T1 and T2. Thirty children ($n = 30$, 89%) at T1 and 28 children (82%) at T2 had sensory features (namely, at least one atypical score on the SP or SSP). The exact McNemar's tests determined that there was no statistically significant difference in the proportion of children with at least one atypical score from T1 to T2 ($p = 0.688$). Twenty-two children ($n = 22$; 65%) at T1 and 20 children (59%) at T2 had at least one score in the definite difference category ($p = 0.754$). The percentage of children classified in the atypical category according to the SSP total score increased from 50% (T1) to 56% (T2) but this difference was not statistically significant ($p = 0.754$). The same was true for the SP quadrants and sections. For example, 15 of the 34 participants (44%) had atypical responses for Quadrant 4 (sensory avoiding) at T1 and 13 (38%) at T2 ($p = 0.774$).

We found no statistically significant differences in the SP subcategories (atypical versus typical) when comparing T1 and T2. However, we saw a nonsignificant trend toward improvement over time in 7 (78%) of the 9 SP subcategories while 2 (22%) subcategories deteriorated between T1 and T2.

4. Discussion

As discussed in the Introduction, we had hypothesized that overall sensory features of children with ASD would remain stable with age. According to our results, the scores (SP and SSP) remained stable over time. The SSP mean score was in the atypical range at T1 and T2, indicating general sensory features in our study population at both time points. Our results are comparable to other studies which yielded prospective results [16, 17, 19]. Our findings are also in agreement with those in the longitudinal studies by McCormick et al. [17], Ausderau et al. [16], and Green et al. [19], who found that sensory features in children with ASD were stable, and in disagreement with the findings of Ben-Sasson's meta-analysis [21]. Furthermore, since children with typical development (TD) improve their sensory skills with age due to maturation [17, 38], the lack of improvement

TABLE 2: Repeated measures ANOVA results comparing T1 and T2.

	Mean raw score T1 (SD)	Mean raw score T2 (SD)	F^a	p value[b]
SSP total score	**153.9 (12.6)**	**151.4 (16.6)**	0.970	0.330
SP quadrants				
(Q1) Low registration	**63.3 (6.5)**	**63.9 (7.8)**	0.180	0.674
(Q2) Sensory seeking	**98.2 (13.7)**	**99.2 (19.3)**	0.180	0.674
(Q3) Sensory sensitivity	**78.6 (9.1)**	**78.8 (10.8)**	0.006	0.940
(Q4) Sensory avoiding	**112.0 (14.9)**	115.6 (11.9)	1.717	0.199
SP sections				
(A) Auditory processing	**28.5 (6.2)**	**29.8 (5.1)**	2.463	0.126
(B) Visual processing	37.2 (5.4)	38.4 (5.1)	2.023	0.164
(C) Vestibular processing	**47.1 (3.7)**	**47.5 (5.9)**	0.188	0.667
(D) Touch processing	73.1 (9.1)	74.3 (10.6)	0.681	0.415
(E) Oral sensory processing	46.9 (8.7)	**44.9 (10.6)**	1.510	0.228

[a]Repeated measures ANOVAs (tests of within-subjects effects); [b]$p < 0.05$. *Note.* Means in the atypical range are shown in bold.

TABLE 3: McNemar sensory results at T1 and T2.

Variable	ASD atypical responses T1		ASD atypical responses T2		χ^2 McNemar
	n	%	n	%	p value[a,b]
SSP total score	17	50.0	19	55.9	0.754
At least one "atypical category"	30	88.8	28	82.4	0.688
At least one "definite difference"	22	64.7	20	58.8	0.754
SP quadrants					
(Q1) Low registration	14	41.2	13	38.2	1.000
(Q2) Sensory seeking	20	58.8	18	52.9	0.727
(Q3) Sensory sensitivity	16	47.1	17	50.0	1.000
(Q4) Sensory avoiding	15	44.1	13	38.2	0.774
SP sections					
(A) Auditory processing	18	52.9	16	47.1	0.774
(B) Visual processing	4	11.8	3	8.8	1.000
(C) Vestibular processing	16	47.1	15	44.1	1.000
(D) Touch processing	14	41.2	13	38.2	1.000
(E) Oral sensory processing	12	35.3	16	47.1	0.344

[a]2-tailed binomial distribution used; [b]$p < 0.05$.

in sensory skills in children with ASD could mean a relative increase in sensory problems over time in these children.

Despite methodological differences between the longitudinal studies, the conclusion remains the same: sensory features in children with ASD are stable over time. The studies by McCormick et al. [17] and Ausderau et al. [16] also addressed general sensory features even if they used different measuring tools or had more variability in the initial ages than in our study. On the other hand, the study by Green et al. [19] did not measure sensory features in general but sensory overresponsiveness.

Lastly, among the conclusions in Ben-Sasson's study [21] regarding sensory features, they found an increase in the difference between children with ASD and typically developing children up to the age of 9 and a decrease thereafter. This could also be interpreted as an increase in the gap between ASD and TD children over time. Given that the sensory processing skills of typically developing children are expected to improve with age [17, 38], Ben-Sasson's results do not necessarily imply an increase in sensory features in children with ASD. Hence, it is not clear whether this increase was due to a deterioration in sensory features in children with ASD or to an improvement in typical developing children's sensory features. Consequently, our results are not necessarily in conflict with those of Ben-Sasson et al. but could be congruent: sensory features of children with ASD could have remained stable while the increase in the difference could be due to an improvement in sensory skills in children with TD.

We also hypothesized that the classification of children among the SP's different quadrants and sections would not change between T1 and T2. As verified by the ANOVA test, the means of each of the nine subcategories remained stable from T1 to T2, which is a novel finding. Secondly, McNemar tests were run on each SP subcategory, comparing the percentage of children classified as atypical for each subcategory at T1 and T2, further suggesting that the stability of the classification was reinforced.

Our study population was similar to comparable studies [16, 17]: most of the children were Caucasian English-speaking boys from families with a middle-class income and whose mothers had some university education on average. Most children in our study had significant sensory features at an early age, namely, the age of 3-4 years (88%), and these difficulties remained high and stable at least until the age of 6, which suggests that aging does not influence the presence of sensory features. Moreover, the few children with ASD but no sensory features at an early age (12%) did not seem to acquire them two years later, which had not been reported previously. In conclusion, the high frequency of sensory features highlights the need for early interventions addressing these features.

Additionally, the percentage of children classified as having "atypical" scores according to the SSP was stable between T1 (50%) and T2 (56%). Furthermore, if we take into consideration the children who had at least one atypical sensory score between T1 (88.2%) and T2 (82.4%), these percentages were also stable. This was also the case for the "definite difference" category (64.7% at T1 to 58.8% at T2).

Previous studies had pointed to the importance of follow-up periods longer than one year [16, 19]. Therefore, our time of 2 years between measures is an interesting contribution to the scientific literature evaluating the stability of general sensory features. An even longer follow-up period and a larger sample would probably be useful in assessing whether these results continue to be maintained over time. We deliberately designed the study to obtain a fairly high level of homogeneity in age at the beginning of the study and achieved a mean age of 44.7 months (SD = 4.9). Other studies had similar initial homogeneity in age, ranging from 26 to 41 months and from 18 to 33 months, respectively, for McCormick et al. (2016) [17] and Green et al. (2012) [19]. The study by Ausderau et al. (2014) [16] had a wider initial age range, namely, from the age of 2 to 12 years. Changes in the initial T1 age of the study may have important implications on the variation between the two measurements. Younger children aged 2-3 years may have more changes in their sensory information processing skills than older children, say, between 7 and 8 years of age.

We also tested the potential effect of two covariates on the measurement of sensory features over time: the ADOS severity scores and cognitive level (M-P-R). We considered other longitudinal studies [16, 17] that had controlled for different covariates: cognitive level, ASD severity, chronological age, gender, family income, mother's education, and so forth. Based on the literature, we included two previously tested covariates: cognitive level and ASD severity. Like previous studies, we found that the stability of the scores is independent of these two covariates.

Since the results of the present study show that children with ASD display early sensory features that persist, we believe that early detection, diagnosis, and management of ASD and its accompanying sensory features are important. Early treatment is advantageous given younger children's greater neuronal plasticity, which may contribute to improving outcomes [39–41]. Indeed, several studies have provided sufficient evidence in support of interventions targeting ASD [42], including behavioral interventions [43], the cognitive behavioral intervention package, language training, modeling, parent training [44], and the peer training package [42]. To date, there is no single guideline on how best to support children with sensory features. There is a growing amount of promising but still contradictory evidence regarding the efficacy of treatments to improve sensory features in children with ASD [6, 35, 45–48], and no specific strategy can be recommended as yet. However, parents often seek out OT services to better understand their child's sensory processing skills and to be able to modify tasks or structure the environment differently to facilitate the sensory processing of their child. Therefore, if children with ASD have true stable sensory processing difficulties despite the very marginal early interventions received and not specific to this area of their development, we believe it is still appropriate to recommend early intervention targeting specifically strategies to compensate by modifying the environment, tasks, or expectations (e.g., avoiding noisy places for a child with auditory hypersensitivity) to improve the quality of life of the child and the family.

5. Conclusions

Children with ASD have sensory features starting at an early age, namely, before 3-4 years, and continue to have these difficulties two years later when they start school (at the age of 5-6 years). We showed that the SP quadrants and sections were also remarkably stable over time, with no independent effect of time once we controlled for cognitive level and autism severity. Furthermore, the expected improvement in sensory skills in children with TD is not seen in children with ASD, which could mean an increase in their sensory features. Further research should seek to address our study's limitations by increasing follow-up time, adding a control group, controlling for the treatment received, and increasing the size of the sample to detect smaller effects size.

In conclusion, sensory features in children with ASD begin early in life and persist. Knowing that sensory features have a negative impact on daily life skills [25], anxiety [19], and social integration of children with ASD [46], we believe that efforts should be made to ensure early recognition and management of these sensory features to improve their functional and psychosocial outcomes.

Acknowledgments

The authors thank the families that participated in the study as well as the different funding organizations that made the study possible: Faculty of Medicine and Health

Sciences, *Université de Sherbrooke (bourse Maurice-Leclair)*, CNRIS *(Consortium National de Recherche sur l'Intégration Sociale)*, Mother-Child Axis, *Université de Sherbrooke*, and CRDITED *(Centre de Réadaptation en Déficience Intellectuelle et en Troubles Envahissants du Développement)*. Also, they appreciate the help they received from the statistics centre at the *Université de Sherbrooke*. Dr. Eric Fombonne was at McGill University when the research was conducted and he was supported by a CIHR-funded Canada Research Chair in Child Psychiatry and the Monique H. Bourgeois Chair on Pervasive Developmental Disorders.

References

[1] Centers for Disease Control and Prevention (CDC), "Prevalence of autism spectrum disorder among children aged 8 years-autism and developmental disabilities monitoring network, 11 sites, United States, 2010," *Morbidity and Mortality Weekly Report: Surveillance Summaries*, vol. 63, no. 2, p. 1, 2014.

[2] American Psychiatric Association, *Diagnostic and statistical manual of mental disorders (DSM-5)*, American Psychiatric Publishing, 2013.

[3] R. C. Schaaf and A. E. Lane, "Toward a Best-Practice Protocol for Assessment of Sensory Features in ASD," *Journal of Autism and Developmental Disorders*, vol. 45, no. 5, pp. 1380–1395, 2015.

[4] Y.-H. Chen, J. Rodgers, and H. McConachie, "Restricted and repetitive behaviours, sensory processing and cognitive style in children with autism spectrum disorders," *Journal of Autism and Developmental Disorders*, vol. 39, no. 4, pp. 635–642, 2009.

[5] E. P. Hazen, J. L. Stornelli, J. A. O'Rourke, K. Koesterer, and C. J. McDougle, "Sensory symptoms in autism spectrum disorders," *Harvard Review of Psychiatry*, vol. 22, no. 2, pp. 112–124, 2014.

[6] R. C. Schaaf and J. Case-Smith, "Sensory interventions for children with autism," *Journal of Comparative Effectiveness Research*, vol. 3, no. 3, pp. 225–227, 2014.

[7] A. C. Bundy, S. J. Lane, and E. A. Murray, *Sensory Integration: Theory and Practice*, FA Davis, 2002.

[8] L. J. Miller and S. Lane, "Toward a Concensus in Termonology in Sensory Integration Theory and Practice: Part 1: Taxonomy of Neurophysiological Processes History of Sensory Integration Terminology," *Sensory Integration Special Interest Section Quarterly*, vol. 23, no. 1, pp. 1–4, 2000.

[9] J. Ayres, *Sensory Integration and Praxis Tests (SIPT)*, Western Psychological Services, 1988.

[10] J. Ayres, *Sensory Integration and Learning Disorders*, Western Psychological Services, 1972.

[11] J. Ayres, *Southern California Postrotary Nystagmus Test Manual*, Western Psychological Services, 1979.

[12] W. Dunn, "The Impact of Sensory Processing Abilities on the Daily Lives of Young Children and Their Families: A Conceptual Model," *Infants & Young Children*, vol. 9, no. 4, pp. 23–35, 1997.

[13] W. Dunn, J. Saiter, and L. Rinner, "Asperger Syndrome and Sensory Processing: A Conceptual Model and Guidance for Intervention Planning," *Focus on Autism and Other Developmental Disabilities*, vol. 17, no. 3, pp. 172–185, 2002.

[14] L. M. Little, A. C. Freuler, M. B. Houser et al., "Psychometric validation of the sensory experiences questionnaire," *The American Journal of Occupational Therapy*, vol. 65, no. 2, pp. 207–210, 2011.

[15] S. D. Tomchek and W. Dunn, "Sensory processing in children with and without autism: a comparative study using the short sensory profile," *The American Journal of Occupational Therapy*, vol. 61, no. 2, pp. 190–200, 2007.

[16] K. K. Ausderau, M. Furlong, J. Sideris et al., "Sensory subtypes in children with autism spectrum disorder: Latent profile transition analysis using a national survey of sensory features," *Journal of Child Psychology and Psychiatry and Allied Disciplines*, vol. 55, no. 8, pp. 935–944, 2014.

[17] C. McCormick, S. Hepburn, G. S. Young, and S. J. Rogers, "Sensory symptoms in children with autism spectrum disorder, other developmental disorders and typical development: A longitudinal study," *Autism*, vol. 20, no. 5, pp. 572–579, 2016.

[18] D. McIntosh, L. Miller, V. Shyu, and W. Dunn, *Overview of the Short Sensory Profile (SSP) - The Sensory Profile: Examiner's Manual*, 1999.

[19] S. A. Green, A. Ben-Sasson, T. W. Soto, and A. S. Carter, "Anxiety and sensory over-responsivity in toddlers with autism spectrum disorders: Bidirectional effects across time," *Journal of Autism and Developmental Disorders*, vol. 42, no. 6, pp. 1112–1119, 2012.

[20] A. Carter, M. Briggs-Gowan, and S. Jones, "The infant–toddler social and emotional assessment (ITSEA): Factor structure, reliability, and validity," *Journal of Abnormal Child Psychology*, vol. 31, no. 5, pp. 495–514, 2003.

[21] A. Ben-Sasson, L. Hen, R. Fluss, S. A. Cermak, B. Engel-Yeger, and E. Gal, "A meta-analysis of sensory modulation symptoms in individuals with autism spectrum disorders," *Journal of Autism and Developmental Disorders*, vol. 39, no. 1, pp. 1–11, 2009.

[22] L.-A. R. Sacrey, S. E. Bryson, and L. Zwaigenbaum, "Prospective examination of visual attention during play in infants at high-risk for autism spectrum disorder: A longitudinal study from 6 to 36 months of age," *Behavioural Brain Research*, vol. 256, no. 2013, pp. 441–450, 2013.

[23] S. J. Rogers, E. A. Wehner, and R. Hagerman, "The behavioral phenotype in fragile X: Symptoms of autism in very young children with fragile X syndrome, idiopathic autism, and other developmental disorders," *Journal of Developmental and Behavioral Pediatrics*, vol. 22, no. 6, pp. 409–417, 2001.

[24] S. U. Peters, L. Horowitz, R. Barbieri-Welge, J. L. Taylor, and R. J. Hundley, "Longitudinal follow-up of autism spectrum features and sensory behaviors in Angelman syndrome by deletion class," *Journal of Child Psychology and Psychiatry and Allied Disciplines*, vol. 53, no. 2, pp. 152–159, 2012.

[25] E. Jasmin, M. Couture, P. McKinley, G. Reid, E. Fombonne, and E. Gisel, "Sensori-motor and daily living skills of preschool children with autism spectrum disorders," *Journal of Autism and Developmental Disorders*, vol. 39, no. 2, pp. 231–241, 2009.

[26] American Psychiatric Association, *Diagnostic and Statistical Manual of Mental Disorders*, vol. 1, American Psychiatric Association, Arlington, Va, USA, 4th edition, 2000.

[27] A. Le Couteur, C. Lord, and M. Rutter, *Autism Diagnostic Interview, Revised (ADI-R)*, Western Psychological Services, Los Angeles, Calif, USA, 2003.

[28] C. Lord, S. Risi, L. Lambrecht et al., "The Autism Diagnostic Schedule – Generic: A standard measures of social and communication deficits associated with the spectrum of autism," *Journal of Autism and Developmental Disorders*, vol. 30, no. 3, pp. 205–223, 2000.

[29] G. H. Roid and J. L. Sampers, *Merrill-Palmer-Revised Scales of Development*, Stoelting, 2004.

[30] I. L. Zimmerman, V. G. Steiner, and R. E. Pond, *Preschool Language Scale*, Pearson Education, Inc, 4th edition, 2002.

[31] I. L. Zimmerman and N. F. Castilleja, "The role of a language scale for infant and preschool assessment," *Mental Retardation and Developmental Disabilities Research Reviews*, vol. 11, no. 3, pp. 238–246, 2005.

[32] K. Gotham, A. Pickles, and C. Lord, "Standardizing ADOS scores for a measure of severity in autism spectrum disorders," *Journal of Autism and Developmental Disorders*, vol. 39, no. 5, pp. 693–705, 2009.

[33] A. De Bildt, I. J. Oosterling, N. D. J. Van Lang et al., "Standardized ADOS scores: Measuring severity of autism spectrum disorders in a Dutch sample," *Journal of Autism and Developmental Disorders*, vol. 41, no. 3, pp. 311–319, 2011.

[34] W. Dunn, *Sensory Profile: User's Manual*, Psychological Corporation, San Antonio, Tex, USA, 1999.

[35] R. C. Schaaf, T. Benevides, Z. Mailloux et al., "An intervention for sensory difficulties in children with autism: A randomized trial," *Journal of Autism and Developmental Disorders*, vol. 44, no. 7, pp. 1493–1506, 2014.

[36] A. Ohl, C. Butler, C. Carney et al., "Test-retest reliability of the sensory profile caregiver questionnaire," *American Journal of Occupational Therapy*, vol. 66, no. 4, pp. 483–487, 2012.

[37] C. Lord, M. Rutter, P. C. DiLavore, S. Risi, K. Gotham, and S. Bishop, *Autism Diagnostic Observation Schedule*, Western Psychological Services, Los Angeles, Calif, USA, 2nd edition, 2012.

[38] P. P. P. Cheung and A. M. H. Siu, "A comparison of patterns of sensory processing in children with and without developmental disabilities," *Research in Developmental Disabilities*, vol. 30, no. 6, pp. 1468–1480, 2009.

[39] L. Zwaigenbaum, S. Bryson, T. Rogers, W. Roberts, J. Brian, and P. Szatmari, "Behavioral manifestations of autism in the first year of life," *International Journal of Developmental Neuroscience*, vol. 23, no. 2-3, pp. 143–152, 2005.

[40] J. Mceachin, T. Smith, and O. I. Lovaas, "Long-Term Outcome for Children With Autism Who Received Early Intensive Behavioral Treatment," *American Journal of Mental Retardation*, vol. 97, no. 4, pp. 359–372, 1993.

[41] S. J. Rogers and L. A. Vismara, "Evidence-based comprehensive treatments for early autism," *Journal of Clinical Child and Adolescent Psychology*, vol. 37, no. 1, pp. 8–38, 2008.

[42] National Autism Center, *Findings and Conclusions: National Standards Project, Phase 2*, 2015.

[43] K. K. DeBoth and S. Reynolds, "A systematic review of sensory-based autism subtypes," *Research in Autism Spectrum Disorders*, vol. 36, pp. 44–56, 2017.

[44] A. J. Beaudoin, G. Sébire, and M. Couture, "Parent Training Interventions for Toddlers with Autism Spectrum Disorder," *Autism Research and Treatment*, vol. 2014, no. 839890, pp. 1–15, 2014.

[45] G. Baranek, "Efficacy of sensory and motor interventions for children with autism," *Journal of Autism and Developmental Disorders*, vol. 32, no. 5, pp. 397–422, 2002.

[46] R. Watling and S. Hauer, "Effectiveness of ayres sensory integration® and sensory-based interventions for people with autism spectrum disorder: A systematic review," *American Journal of Occupational Therapy*, vol. 69, no. 5, Article ID 2436568, pp. 1–12, 2015.

[47] T. A. May-Benson and J. A. Koomar, "Systematic review of the research evidence examining the effectiveness of interventions using a sensory integrative approach for children," *The American Journal of Occupational Therapy*, vol. 64, no. 3, pp. 403–414, 2010.

[48] B. A. Pfeiffer, K. Koenig, M. Kinnealey, M. Sheppard, and L. Henderson, "Effectiveness of sensory integration interventions in children with autism spectrum disorders: a pilot study," *American Journal of Occupational Therapy*, vol. 65, no. 1, pp. 76–85, 2011.

17

Autism Spectrum Disorder Screening Instruments for Very Young Children

Patricia O. Towle[1,2] and Patricia A. Patrick[1,2,3]

[1] *Westchester Institute for Human Development, Valhalla, NY, USA*
[2] *School of Health Sciences & Practice, New York Medical College, Valhalla, NY, USA*
[3] *Department of Pediatrics, New York Medical College, Valhalla, NY, USA*

Correspondence should be addressed to Patricia O. Towle; ptowle@wihd.org

Academic Editor: Bennett L. Leventhal

Research on ASD in infancy has provided a rationale for developing screening instruments for children from the first year of life to age of 18 months. A comprehensive literature search identified candidate screening tools. Using methodological probe questions adapted from the Quality Assessment of Diagnostic Accuracy Studies (QUADAS), two Level 1 and three Level 2 screening instruments were reviewed in detail. Research evidence conclusions were that instrument development was in beginning phases, is not yet strong, and requires further development. Clinical recommendations were to continue vigilant developmental and autism surveillance from the first year on but to use the screening instruments *per se* only for high-risk children rather than for population screening, with considerations regarding feasibility for individual settings, informing caregivers about strengths and weaknesses of the tool, and monitoring new research.

1. Introduction

Autism spectrum disorder (ASD), a neurodevelopmental condition that significantly affects social functioning, communication, and patterns of interests and behavior, is most often a life-long disorder that requires extensive educational, vocational, and community support [1, 2]. There is increasing evidence for the efficacy of early intervention [3–5], from which follows the assumption that the cost to society and to families can be mitigated to some degree by alleviating early symptoms and building early skills, leading to reduced symptom severity and greater independence later in life. Early detection based on this reasoning, as well as the high prevalence rates (1 in 68 children [6]), is currently being emphasized from clinical, advocacy, and public health sectors [7–10]. Early detection is increasingly accomplished through systematic developmental surveillance, which is a combined effort on several fronts by several systems and their components. Healthcare professionals are strongly encouraged to understand the importance of developmental screening, to know and inquire about developmental milestones, and to respond to caregiver concerns in specific and actionable ways (referring for more in-depth evaluations, as well as to early intervention systems, continuing to monitor the child) [11–13].

One important component of this general effort is the use of formal screening instruments that focus on specific questions and aid in decision-making about further steps for referral and evaluation. For example, the "Learn the Signs. Act Early." campaign of the Centers for Disease Control and Prevention's National Center on Birth Defects and Developmental Disabilities (NCBDDD) calls for, in addition to systematic developmental surveillance, autism-specific screening at 18 and 24 months [8]; a similar protocol is endorsed by the American Academy of Pediatrics [14].

Autism screening instruments have been available for this age range since the late 1990s [15]. Currently, there are a number of screeners that apply to children *starting* from age of 18–24 months and up to 30–36 months [11, 16]. The most well-used such instrument in the United States as well as in Europe [17] is the Modified Checklist for Autism in Toddlers (M-CHAT) [18], which has now been revised as the M-CHAT-R/F [19]. The M-CHAT-R/F is considered a Level 1 screener because it is intended to screen at a population level, that is, all children regardless of their risk level for developmental disabilities, including ASD.

There are Level 2 screening instruments for this age range as well. A second-level screener is to be applied to children at risk, such as those who have come to the attention of their parents or pediatrician in order to see if they are more likely to have ASD than another type of delay or disability and in this way route them more efficiently to relatively high-cost comprehensive evaluation procedures. An example of a Level 2 screening instrument with demonstrated predictive validity is the Screening Test for Autism in Two-Year-Olds (STAT) [20, 21], which is intended for children 24–36 months administered by a clinician who first goes through a training program to become a reliable administrator.

Over the last decade, however, several screening instruments have been developed to identify children with autism spectrum disorder *under* the age of 18 months, primarily during the 12–15-month period, sometimes extending down to 6–8 months and sometimes extending to 24 months. Several research, theoretical, and clinical trends have led to interest in developing such tools. In research, there are at least two different relevant areas of research—each demonstrating that symptoms of ASD can be seen quite early in life—that have led to these efforts. The first is the retrospective analysis of home movies of infants and toddlers later diagnosed with ASD, and the second is prospective studies of high-risk (for ASD) children from birth to three years of age. Both of these study methods have shown that a number of autism spectrum symptoms in the social, communication, behavioral, motor, and temperament realms can be seen as early as 12 months and sometimes younger.

Zwaigenbaum and colleagues [22], in a review that included home-movie research studies, concluded that behaviors that consistently differentiated children with ASD versus children who are typically developing (TD) at 12 months of age are the following: less or atypical orienting to people and their faces, reduced responding to name, reduced display of positive affect and social smiling, less eye contact, and less use of gestures used for communication, including pointing. Yet when focusing on studies that utilized a control group of infants with non-ASD developmental disabilities (DDs), a smaller list of behaviors emerged. Two studies found differences at 9–12 months between infants with ASD and DD for response to name and looking at faces (children with ASD showed these behaviors less than children with DDs), but not for frequency and type of gesture [23, 24]. Clearer differentiations between participants with ASD versus DDs have been found as the study age approaches 24 months [22]. In addition, there are also important distinctions between groups of infants that have differential timing patterns of symptom emergence. These retrospective home-movie analyses helped to confirm that some children with ASD have relatively typical first-year social/linguistic development and then change during their second year, while others show a prodromal phase of autistic symptomology during their first year, some by at least six months of age [25]. The early-home-movie method of inquiry has made it clear that an appreciable subset of children who will go on to be diagnosed with ASD will show social-communication and behavioral deficits and differences by the end of their first and beginning of their second year of life [22, 26].

The second influence was from the consortium of "infant sibling" studies, wherein newborn siblings of children diagnosed with ASD are enrolled for study prospectively. The rationale for this approach was that a genetics-based etiology would result in a higher incidence of ASD in these young children than in the population at large and thus would be an efficient means of studying the very early development of ASD. In fact, Ozonoff and colleagues [27] documented that the recurrence rate of ASD for these high-risk children was nearly 20%, with male gender and more than one older sibling diagnosed with ASD conferring additional risk.

Several study sites within the infant siblings consortium specifically track early social communication, social interaction, and other types of developmental behaviors so that possible patterns of very early emerging symptoms in these behavioral areas could be documented for those eventually confirmed as having ASD at age of 3 years [28]. These multisite studies began in the early 2000s and thus there are several reviews that document early social-communicative difference and presence of various repetitive behaviors [29–32]. The reviews report that very few behavioral differences could be seen at the 6-month mark, but it is from 6–9 months on to 24 months that the skill levels in key areas diverge for those infants later diagnosed with ASD versus those who were not [30–33]. The behaviors that distinguish these two groups from 12 months on were in fact very similar to those coded in the home-movie studies—reduced shared positive affect, social responsivity, communicative gesturing, and response to name [31, 33–35]. While significant group differences were found, that does not mean that every single infant who was later diagnosed with ASD had these early symptoms. Similar to the home-movie studies, there were subgroups based on timing of symptom emergence [31]. Landa and colleagues [36] demonstrated that some infants eventually diagnosed with ASD (at three years of age) maintained more typical social skills up until about age of 14 months (slightly over half, 16/30) and then began to lose them, compared to a group who was fairly symptomatic at 14 months (slightly less than half, 14/30).

The increased understanding about very early emergence of autism spectrum symptoms has led researchers to theorize about primary and secondary causes of delay and disorder in ASD, in order to concurrently elucidate etiology and suggest directions for intervention. A number of studies, both within the infant siblings general paradigm and apart from it, have focused on investigating the earliest postnatal neurologic and information-processing divergences from typical development such as in the areas of eye tracking, attention to faces, attentional regulation to objects versus social stimuli, visual and auditory processing, brain-based sensory integration systems, and interconnectivity within cerebral cortex [37]. Documenting very early brain organization and information-processing differences underpins frameworks for understanding such as the "developmental cascade," that is, earlier foundations that support continued development and, if disturbed, lead to failures of, or atypicality in, later developmental capabilities [38, 39]. For example, Chawarska et al. [40] demonstrated differences in attention to faces in 6-month-olds who would go on to receive an ASD diagnosis and hypothesized that "A limited attentional bias towards people early in development is likely to have a detrimental impact on the specialization of social brain networks and the emergence of social interaction patterns." In fact, a number of studies have demonstrated significant disturbances in fundamental social engagement precursors and processes during the first year of life, as studied through eye-tracking paradigms, fMRI, behavioral tasks, and EEG protocols [39].

Experts who advocate "the earlier, the better" point to these findings as well as three other tenets of early intervention, that is, the neuroplasticity of the developing brain and the associated notion of critical periods, that is, that there are functional and timing/phase-bound periods of rapid development when intervention is optimized [41, 42], and the interactive-specialization hypothesis—the widely held theory that children's brains and capabilities develop through the ongoing, iterative transaction of neuromaturation with environmental experiences [43, 44].

Therefore, the findings that observable *behavioral* ASD markers become more evident from about 12 months on (see above) can be viewed as both the result of earlier, derailed neurocognitive processes and also a disturbed foundation that may produce further ASD symptoms. For example, since children's early learning language and gesture learning is highly dependent upon frequent, ongoing communicative exchanges with an adult, then a child who is not interested in faces, does not easily become socially engaged, and is not responsive to language input is very vulnerable to delay in language acquisition as well as in development of social cognition and conventional play skills [45, 46]. In addition, the rapid emergence of language and social communication from 9–18 months constitutes its own critical period for these specific skills [47].

It is in this context that researchers have become very interested in a downward age extension in autism-specific screening tools that can be applied clinically. Earlier detection means earlier intervention and the possibility of preventing the secondary effects of atypical development, in other words, a more fully developed autism profile. There has been some success with screening instruments that target children from 18 to 24 months of age and older [22–25]. The goal of this paper is to review the extant screening instruments for children under 18 months of age.

To be included in the review, the screeners needed to have peer-reviewed published reports of sensitivity and specificity from prospective study designs. The instruments' development, method of administration, reliability and validity, receiver operator characteristics, and feasibility of use are described. The review also seeks to draw conclusions regarding methodological and substantive challenges highlighted by this close examination, recommended use of such screeners, and directions for future research.

2. Methods

2.1. Literature Review. This more focused review is part of a larger review conducted for the New York State Department of Health Clinical Practice Guidelines for Autism Spectrum Disorder for children ages birth to three years. For this larger, evidence-based review of autism screening instruments, a set of search terms were developed and refined and then applied to a broad set of databases such as PsycInfo and Medline. The resulting 2,188 abstracts returned were then sorted through for articles that met the inclusion criteria set for the review. The target was screening instruments in peer-reviewed journals, published in English, and that had reported receiver operator characteristics (ROC) or performance measures of sensitivity and specificity and/or positive predictive and negative predictive values.

Adequate ROC are considered a definitive test of predictive validity and utility for screeners because they inform about percentages of individuals that will be detected or missed by the screening procedures. Other ways of assessing the validity of tests use statistics applied to groups based on probability theory and can produce highly significant results but still have a relatively low effect size or account for a relatively small amount of variance. Therefore, significance can be high, but precision may still be low.

Once the screeners were identified, the authors did search for all the peer-reviewed articles that were relevant to the development, reliability, and validity of the instruments. This way each one could be critically evaluated in terms of its development, the constructs measured, psychometric properties, and performance. Examining these details yielded insights into methodological issues that will be important to consider as attempts to identify very young children with ASD continue.

2.2. Features of Studies Testing the Predictive Validity of an ASD Screening Instrument. Studies are conducted differently depending on whether the instrument is intended to be a Level 1 (population level) or Level 2 (for high-risk children) screener. How this affects the recruitment, inclusion criteria, and number of participants is covered in the sections below. Nonetheless, every study compares the screening results to a reference standard or "gold standard," which consensus dictates to be the true test of whether the child actually has the condition or not. For autism spectrum disorder, this invariably entails a "Best Estimate Diagnosis" by an experienced practitioner who is drawing from a variety of information gathered about the child (e.g., history, caregiver interview, standardized tests, and direct observation of the child).

When a child fails a screening test, he/she is shown to be at increased risk for the condition, and the result is called positive. When the child passes the screener, the result is called negative; the child is not considered at increased risk for the condition. The screener results, characterized as positive or negative, are then compared to the reference standard, which is also determined as positive or negative for each child. When a child is positive for the condition on the screener and is shown to have the condition on the reference standard, then it counts as a true positive. If the child did not turn out to have the condition, then it was a false positive. The negatives follow in the same fashion.

Sensitivity (Se) and specificity (Sp) are calculated with proportional formulae using true and false positives and negatives. In explanatory terms, Se represents the degree to which the screener accurately detects the condition. The measure runs from 0 to 1.0, with 1.0 being perfect detection. However, the predictive validity of the screener is only understood by considering both Se and Sp together. Sensitivity can be very high if the screener has included almost everyone, and in doing so, of course, it included children with ASD. Specificity represents the extent to which the screener distinguished the targeted condition from other or no disabilities. Therefore, Sp balances out the Se by showing that it did not include too many extra children who in fact had a different developmental disorder or had no developmental problems at all.

Acceptable levels of Se and Sp depend on the outcome or condition of interest. More specifically, for the detection of a preventable communicable disease, investigators may tolerate lower specificity (greater proportion of false positives) for higher sensitivity (greater proportion of true positives). Nevertheless, it is suggested that the threshold values for acceptable levels of sensitivity and specificity should be at least .80 or greater, although accuracy levels of .90 or above are considered optimal [48–50].

Positive predictive value (PPV) is a measure that reflects the percentage of children who screened positive and who did actually have the condition based on the gold standard testing. Negative predictive value (NPV) is the inverse—the percentage of children who screened negative and who did not have the condition. Positive and negative predictive values are directly related to the prevalence of the condition under study within the population; these measures are not intrinsic to the instrument. In other words, a screening instrument that has high sensitivity and specificity may have low PPV if the prevalence of the condition is low—a positive result is less likely to be accurate if a condition is rare.

The ideal procedure for examining the predictive validity of a screening instrument involves a direct route between screener administration and diagnostic outcomes, with the most knowledge available about scoring outcomes for every child who was given the screener. This can be challenged by attrition during the various phases of the study, and, as will be seen, many studies include additional steps and criteria for a child to advance from one phase of screening and testing to the next. After thorough review of the initial group of studies, several were excluded from in-depth reporting because of this feature; they were no longer considered a test of the targeted screener because other, sequential procedures obscured the findings.

2.3. Types of Screeners (Administration). ASD screening tools (or any type of behavioral screeners) generally take two forms: a caregiver-rated checklist or a clinician observation. A variant is to have the clinician administer the checklist to the parent.

2.4. Screening Instrument Reviews. For this review, each screening instrument was described and then critiqued in the following way. The extant literature on the instrument is summarized in the Background section. In the next sections, the instrument's development, how it is administered and scored, and the constructs it measures are described. The Research Summary section follows an adaptation of the Quality Assessment of Diagnostic Accuracy Studies (QUADAS-2) [51]. This research quality assessment method follows a typical evidence-based procedure whereby experts are gathered, probe questions from a pool are chosen for a given diagnostic or screening question/tool, the questions' utility is field tested, and reliability of ratings is established. The QUADAS and QUADAS-2 are very widely used for both diagnostic and screening tests in both the behavioral [52–54] and medical [55–57] fields. This rating system was not applied formally (i.e., assigning numerical ratings) but instead adapted in the following way: (1) the four domains of Participants, Index Test (the screening tool), the Reference Standard (the "gold standard"), and Timing and Flow were used as units of review with the additional domains of Evaluation and Performance; (2) probe questions were developed for each of the domains; and (3) the probe questions were applied to each study and conclusions were summarized.

Table 1 shows the probe questions developed for this review and their significance. For the Participants domain, different questions are needed for Level 1 versus Level 2 instruments. The differential parameters are discussed more in depth in the Results section. For the Screening Instrument domain, it is important to note if there is anything about how the instrument was administered in the study that would differ from how it would be used in the community. Examples are provided in the table and in the results.

For the Reference Standard domain, the extent to which the participants each had face-to-face evaluations using Best Estimate Diagnosis as well as how this was supported with standardized procedures and other disciplinary evaluations was noted. As part of the inclusion criteria, only studies that used Best Estimate Diagnosis based on DSM-IV or DSM-IV-TR [58] criteria were included. A second very important question was whether or not those who conducted the diagnostic evaluations were blind to the screener status of the children, that is, if they were screen negative or positive, since expectation bias could be introduced in this way. Finally, it was important to note what outcome categories the study considered, so that information about ASD severity level of children and differentiation from other types of disabilities could be known.

The Timing and Flow domain has a number of features. Two important questions—was the screener done prospectively and was the time interval between the screening and diagnosis adequate—were not included because conditions were met for all studies reviewed. The probe question used refers to conditions moving children from screening to diagnosis that could obscure interpretation directly from the screening tool being examined. It was this probe question that led to understanding that a number of the studies had multistep screening protocols without sufficient analysis of

Table 1: Review domains and related probe questions.

(a)

Domain	Level 1 screener probe questions	Level 2 screener probe questions
Sample/participants	*Was the sample appropriate in size and scope?* *How representative was the sample?* *Were there exclusion criteria based on other disabilities?*	*Was the sample appropriate in size and scope?* *Did investigators use a sample matched for developmental level?*

(b)

	Level 1 and 2 screener probe questions
Screening instrument	*Was there anything about how the screener was administered that would be different from its intended use in a nonresearch, community setting?* *Were there any issues regarding the way it is scored in the study?*
Reference standard	*Did all children receive a BED from in-person evaluations? How extensive was the information available to the clinician making the Best Estimate Diagnosis?* *Were the reference standard evaluators blind to the screener risk status of the children?* *What diagnostic outcome categories were used to test prediction from screener to reference standard?*
Timing and flow (including attrition)	*Was there excessive attrition through any phase of screening and evaluation?* *Were there conditions besides attrition that filtered the negative and positive screens from the original screening to the reference standard diagnostic testing phase?*
Evaluation	*How were performance/predictive values calculated?* *Was performance/prediction for younger versus older children explored?*
Performance	*What were the performance/predictive values?* *What was the developmental level of children detected?* *Of the false positives for ASD, what proportion had other developmental or learning disabilities?*

Se and Sp for each step, and therefore such studies were eliminated from more in-depth critique.

In addition, two other probe questions were used to evaluate the results *per se* of the instrument. The first was what developmental characteristics of the children identified as having ASD were presented. This will allow a comparison across screeners for which children were detected in terms of overall developmental level. The second referred to what extent the false positives detected other types of disabilities.

2.5. Methodological and Content Themes. As the screening studies were reviewed, themes were extracted related to methodology and content issues. Finally, conclusions were drawn as to recommendations for use, themes regarding this body of research as a whole, and recommendations for future research and development of these types of screeners.

3. Results

3.1. Level 1 Early Screening Instruments for Autism Spectrum Disorder

3.1.1. Features of Autism-Specific Level 1 Screening. Level 1, or first-level screening, is meant to be applied at a population level—for example, to all children coming through a pediatrician's or family physician's office. These are "low-risk" or "unselected" samples. In developmental surveillance parlance, however, the role of Level 1 screening is to first identify children who are at risk for any developmental disability, which may include ASD as well as other types. Another term for this type of screener is "broadband." In the case of autism-specific screening, the intention is to identify those at risk for ASD specifically, but on a population level. Regardless, the intent to screen populations has implications for feasibility characteristics of screeners, for tolerance limits for levels of Se and Sp, and for research methods.

Feasibility refers to practical features related to cost, time, and ease of administration, scoring, and interpretation. Therefore, one expects a Level 1 screener to be quick and low cost so that it can fit into well-child visits as easily as possible. In terms of performance, there is somewhat more of an emphasis on Se rather than Sp, so that as few as possible cases are missed. Thus, there is more latitude for lower Sp, as long as it is close to being acceptable (>.80).

There is a particular set of methodological hurdles to conducting research for screening instruments at a population level, which involves screening thousands to tens of thousands of children. The first hurdle is actually screening this large a number of children, but just as challenging is following up enough of the children to find out who did have ASD or did not. After the initial screening, researchers typically call the parents/caregivers to invite them to come in for an evaluation that will take time and effort on the family's part. Participation is voluntary, so there may be a bias for families who are motivated to come in for further evaluation.

Table 2: Level 1 ASD screening instruments reviewed.

(a)

Screener	Dates of paper(s)	Country developed	Ages (mos)	Strategy
Infant-Toddler Checklist (ITC)†	2004 2008 2011*	US	8–24	Caregiver checklist
First-Year Inventory (FYI)	2007 2013* 2014	US	12	Caregiver checklist

(b)

Excluded from in-depth review	Dates of paper(s)	Country developed	Ages (mos)	Reason for exclusion
Pervasive Developmental Disorders Screening Test (PDDST-II)		US		No peer-reviewed articles (ROC or otherwise)
Early Screen for Autism Traits (ESAT)		Netherlands	14-15	No prospective studies done in age range; two-stage screening
Checklist for Early Signs of Developmental Disorders (CESDD)	2010 2012	Netherlands	3–40	Two-stage screening
Infant-Toddler Checklist (ITC) (2 of 3 studies)	2004 2008	US	8–24	Studies involved two-stage screening

†The ITC was evaluated for ASD prediction and the authors concluded that it functions best as a broadband screener, identifying children at risk for disabilities, a proportion of whom will be diagnosed with ASD.
*This paper was reviewed in detail for research methods because it was an ROC study.

Usually quite a bit of attrition occurs at this step that lowers the percentage of the population sample examined with the "gold standard" compared to those who were screened. If the investigators have basic demographic information on those who did not come in for the next phase, the best they can do is test if there are any significant differences between those who consented to move on to a full evaluation and those who did not on some baseline or demographic variables.

Most investigators focus first on getting positive screens (families/participants) to come back for fuller evaluation, since at least PPV can be calculated. But the final hurdle is that children who screened negative may be in the tens of thousands, and thus it is virtually impossible to examine them all directly. Even taking a proportional sample is difficult because of the lack of motivation for parents to come in for a longer evaluation if they do not believe their child is at risk. Of families that do consent, there may be a bias for families with more financial resources, or where one parent does not work, and/or higher education on the part of these volunteer participants. The overall result is that "true" Se and Sp can rarely be estimated because of these attrition and sampling problems.

Level 1 screening instruments, therefore, are often *developed* by using smaller samples and involving relatively high numbers of children who do have ASD. This is necessary to determine which items discriminate among children with ASD, DD, and TD. Yet, the screener's validity as a Level 1 instrument cannot be known unless it is then tested on a large, low-risk, unselected sample. Obviously, such studies are expensive and labor-intensive, and even focused resources and efforts often cannot overcome the barrier of uneven participation.

One important discovery from this review was the extent that studies attempting to describe the predictive value of a given screener were actually describing a screening program with multiple phases and instruments rather than a more pure test of efficacy of one screener. Ideally, the screener is given, and as many children as possible are followed through to the diagnostic testing phase, and thus there is a relatively direct route between the screener and the diagnostic outcome. In the case of three fairly well-known instruments—the Early Screen for Autistic Traits (ESAT) [64, 65], the Checklist for Early Signs of Developmental Disorders (CESDD) [66], and certain studies with the Infant-Toddler Checklist (ITC) [59, 67]—the children were filtered through prescreens or two-stage screening without explication of the effect on potential true and false positives and negatives on the targeted screener. Based on the probe questions under the "Index Test" and "Timing and Flow" domains, these flaws were considered sufficiently problematic to exclude as studies of the ROC of the instruments. On the other hand, the studies are often able to provide PPV estimates, have other merits, and provide results that are informative about many features of the screening process. Thus, some are reviewed in the preliminary narrative for the instrument.

Table 2 presents first-level ASD screening instruments that have peer-reviewed papers reporting Se and Sp or PPV and NPV, as well as the studies that have been excluded once reviewed in depth.

3.1.2. Level 1 Instruments Excluded from Detailed Review. The *Pervasive Developmental Disorders Screening Test (PDDST-II)* [68] is a parent-report instrument for children ages 12 to 48 months. It is the only instrument that has three screening levels to it. However, the only ROC presented are in the manual, and there is no paper describing such a validity study published in peer-reviewed journals.

The *Early Screen for Autistic Traits (ESAT)* [64, 65], which targets 14-15-month-olds, is often reviewed as an early ASD screener, but it does not yet have peer-reviewed articles that report prospectively obtained Se and Sp for its intended age group. Dietz and colleagues [64] reported on its development and utilized retrospective parent reports to discover which items discriminate ASD from non-ASD. Swinkels and colleagues [65] further described validity testing and did apply the ESAT prospectively, giving results in terms of percentages and odds ratios, but not ROC.

As important, interpretation of the studies for this screener is limited by the two-phase protocol used for the ESAT. Specifically, first a four-item screening test was given to parents of children being screened, and it was only those who failed this prescreen (by failing any one or more of the four items) who were then given the ESAT. Although the ESAT's predictive value was tested in reference to children diagnosed with ASD, we do not know its performance if given as a first-level screener; it cannot be known who was left behind when the 4-item prescreening was given in terms of true and false positives and negatives. The study is really describing a screening program that the ESAT is part of, not the predictive value of the ESAT.

Oosterling and colleagues [69] compared ESAT to prediction with the Social-Communication Questionnaire (SCQ) [70] and Infant-Toddler Checklist [71], but the sample was older (primarily 18–24 months) than what the screener was originally developed for. Finally, Dereu and colleagues [72] included the ESAT in a screening study where children were first identified to be at risk through childcare staff rating the Checklist of Early Signs of Developmental Disorders [66]. Because the ESAT was given in a second phase along with several other screeners and many of the children were not in its intended age range, this report was not considered to reflect the predictive ability of the ESAT.

There are also feasibility concerns about the measure in that it is actually administered by a trained psychologist through parent interview. In the validity study, the psychologist was evaluating the child through play and a cognitive assessment at the same visit and making judgments on each item, overriding the parent if he or she expressed no concern about a given behavior when the psychologist did have concern. This is a protracted process for a screening instrument, one that approaches an abbreviated evaluation, and thus would not seem practical for most settings.

The studies of the ESAT do yield important information about the screening process (e.g., they found that the caregiver/parents had a very low rate of agreement with the psychologist about their child's symptoms when the child actually was shown to have ASD later). Further studies addressing these methodological issues would be required to substantiate the ESAT's use as an ASD screening instrument. It would also require a translation if not used in Dutch-speaking countries.

The *Checklist for Early Signs of Developmental Disorders (CESDD)* [66] is a daycare staff-rated checklist for children 3 to 36 months. There are at least two promising innovations embodied in this instrument, the first being its use of childcare staff as informants, given their familiarity with the children they care for and their presumed knowledge about child development. For the study, the staff were given training sessions about early symptoms of ASD as well. The second is that the checklist included slightly different sets of items depending on the age of the child, which helped in accommodating developmental changes over the age range.

The CESDD studies share interpretive challenges with the ESAT in that the tool was part of a two-phase screening process, with the CESDD as the first-phase screener. After a child was flagged as at-risk based on the CESDD, then parents filled out several more screeners and only advanced to the evaluation phase if their child then failed one of these additional screeners, a set of language items, or the MacArthur-Bates Communication Inventory [73]. Finally, a child could also go on to the full evaluation if parents requested it out of concern. Also, the attrition was high at this phase—only 31% of the families went on to Phase 2. By the time the children were evaluated for ASD, they no longer represented a group that had been determined to be at risk only by the CESDD. Therefore, although the Se (.80) and Sp (.94) were good to excellent, it is not clear how much these statistics represent the CESDD alone. Finally, the CESDD has only been used in the Dutch language.

3.1.3. Level 1 Instruments Included for Detailed Review

(A) Infant-Toddler Checklist (ITC)

(1) Background. The ITC is a 24-item caregiver-report checklist for children ages 8–24 months. It is part of the Communication and Symbolic Behavior Scales Developmental Profile [71]. The CSBS-DP was developed out of an earlier, longer version—the CSBS [74]. This instrument, which is for children 6–24 months of age, was originally developed for detection of early language delays, not ASD specifically. However, with its emphasis on prelinguistic communication, including social components such as eye gaze and emotion, it became clear that the instrument targeted key early features of ASD and was addressing younger children than many other instruments. There are three parts to both the original and the Developmental Profile version: a short, parent-rated ITC; a longer parent-rated Caregiver Questionnaire (CQ), which is an elaborated version of the ITC and includes some of the same questions; and the Behavior Sample (BS)—a semistructured clinician observation and rating procedure—that was shortened considerably (to 20–30 minutes) for the Developmental Profile version so that it could in fact function as a screener. At this point only the ITC has sufficient published research as an ASD screener.

The first published research on the ITC focused on its function as a language screener and in the context of using all three of the CSBS components as a child progressed through first- and then second-phase screening and then diagnostic evaluation [75]. In 2004 and 2008 the ITC, combined with other components of the CSBS-DP, was investigated as an autism spectrum disorder screener. The Wetherby and colleagues study [76] is not described here because most of the children were 18–24 months when screened, making the study more similar to those for ages 18+ months.

Wetherby et al.'s study [67] also was not reviewed using the probe questions because the study children went through a three-stage screening procedure wherein the CSBS-DP Behavior Sample and then the Systematic Observation of Red Flags (for autism) (SORF) further narrowed the group who were eventually diagnosed with ASD. This study is nonetheless reported on in the Research Summary section because parts of the study are very informative (see below).

More recently, the instrument was reported on in terms of its utility when used with children with a mean age of 12 months [59], again as a broadband screener.

(2) Instrument Development. The original choice of items for the CSBS and therefore for the CSBS-DP is noteworthy because they were informed by important foundational research on normal development of prelinguistic social communication [77, 78]; this essential knowledge about when and how children develop a range of communication strategies within an interactive caregiving context helps us understand how typically developing children bring their own capacities to engage the caregiver. It is through this engaged relationship, ongoing interaction, and the resulting perpetual feedback loops that children develop social-linguistic competence [79].

(3) Measurement Strategy, Constructs Measured, and Scoring. The ITC is a 24-item checklist that can be filled out by a very familiar caregiver in about 5 minutes. The ITC has been normed so that it can be used with cutoff scores (both the checklist and its normative tables for cutoff scores are free downloads) and, with the use of the purchased manual, will yield standard scores as well.

Because the ITC was originally developed as a language screening measure, it focuses almost exclusively on social and communication behaviors. It does include four items on object use or play. There are no items about repetitive behaviors, unusual sensory reactions, or temperament issues. (It was conceived as a screener that would lead to further evaluation, most specifically by the CSBS Behavior Sample, and it is from the Behavior Sample that repetitive behaviors are scored, using the SORF.)

In contrast to many other such checklists, the ITC yields a number of subscale scores in addition to a total score. The Social Composite consists of three subscales: *Emotion and Eye Gaze* (3 items), *Communication* (4 items), and *Gestures* (5 items). The Speech Composite includes *Sounds* (3 items) and *Words* (2 items), and the Symbolic Composite contains *Understanding* (2 items) and *Object Use* (4 items).

Given these subscales, failing the screen can be done in more than one way: if the child is below the cutoff on either the total score, or the Social Composite, or the Symbolic Composite. The category denoting a positive screen is "Of Concern." Scoring the ITC relies on a normative table with cutoff scores to classify as follows: (1) typical skills: readminister in 3 months; (2) elevated risk: monitor and readminister in 3 months; and (3) at-risk: refer immediately for further evaluation. Standard scores are also obtainable using the purchased manual.

In addition to these scores used as cutoff points, it appears that a "fail" also occurs when the parent checks off the single item "have a concern about your child."

(4) Research Summary. Wetherby and colleagues [67] went to great lengths to locate every child from the original ITC screening sample ($N = 5{,}385$) who was diagnosed with ASD at age of three years or older, finding them either through their own research program, through follow-up mailings to families, or through autism treatment programs in the catchment area. Sixty children with confirmed diagnoses were then compared to children with other DDs and TD children. Of the 60, 56 had at-risk ITC scores at some point before 24 months. At 6–8 months, only 20% of the children scored at-risk, but 77% did so at 9–11 months. However, for the 12–14-, 15–17-, 18–20-, and 23–24-month age groups, the percentages of at-risk scores ranged from 91% to 100%.

The study by Pierce and colleagues [59] is the only study reviewed in depth here because it met the criteria of including ROC analyses and did not involve two-stage screening (see Table 3). The authors tested the ITC as an autism screener when given to parents through pediatric practices at the one-year well-child checkup. The mean age the ITC was filled out by parents was 12 months, with a range of 10 to 15 months. Screening 10,479 children, they did have 1318 "fails," with an at-risk rate of 12.5%. For practical reasons, the researchers were only able to follow up and examine directly 184 (14%) of those children who screened positive for ASD. Of those failing the ITC between the ages of 10–15 months, 75% were found to have ASD, DDs, or LD (language disorder) at age of 3 years (i.e., PPV = .75). Twenty percent were diagnosed with ASD (PPV = .20). Therefore, ITC was again found to function best as a broadband screener.

(5) Conclusions. The ITC has the advantage of being a short parent checklist that can be applied in community settings and can identify children as young as 12 months as being at risk for developmental delays including ASD, language delay, and other delays, but it does not successfully distinguish ASD from other DDs. The authors have recommended it as a broadband screener, therefore, and suggest its use more as a continuous monitoring device over the second year of life. There is obvious utility in detecting other disabilities that require follow-up and attention. For the children with ASD, outcome developmental quotients demonstrated the presence of children with a range of functioning, including some children with average intellectual functioning.

The main methodological issues of this study were as follows: (1) it is not known if the evaluators were blind to the participants' screening status; and (2) the attrition from their original set of over a thousand children scoring at-risk was very high. Other studies on the ITC, including those with Se and Sp reported, were excluded because their methods did not allow for straightforward interpretation of the ITC's predictive power given that children were moved through to definitive evaluations for reasons unrelated to the ITC. This instrument has only reported PPV, which

TABLE 3: Research summaries for the Infant-Toddler Checklist (ITC) and First-Year Inventory (FYI).

Probe questions	ITC [59]	FYI [60]
Sample/participants		
Was the sample appropriate in size and scope?	Low-risk community sample; large to start with (10,479), but attrition was high for the reference standard evaluation phase; 184 at the end; 14% of high-risk sample.	Yes, population study; mailed to almost 6,000 and got a 25% return rate. 699 filled out developmental and ASD screening questionnaires after child's third birthday.
How representative was the sample?	These parameters were not reported.	Although the sample was diverse, there were a disproportionate number of Caucasian and highly educated families responding to later phases of the screening study.
Were there exclusion criteria based on other disabilities?	They specified that no exclusion criteria were exercised for either the population sample or the follow-up.	It was specified that children born preterm were excluded.
Screening instrument		
Was there anything about how the screener was administered that would be different from its intended use in a nonresearch, community setting?	No.	No.
Were there any issues regarding the way it is scored in the study?	Note that the ITC can be failed in four different ways—low score on either or both of two subscales, total score; there may be differences in true and false positives given the source of fail criterion.	The authors explored predictive validity based on several different ways of using subscales scores and total score.
Reference standard		
Did all children receive a BED from in-person evaluations? How extensive was the information available to the clinician making the Best Estimate Diagnosis?	Cognitive, ADOS-T, and ADI-R; children seen every 6 months up to three years of age. They evaluated children every 6 months and gave "at-risk" dx's of ASD from 12 to 18 months, "provisional" dx's from 19 to 31 months, and established dx's from 32 to 36 months with ADI-R. Five children with provisional dx's no longer had dx at the last evaluation.	Mixed—some children brought in for Best Estimate Diagnosis including all information, ADOS, and occupational therapy evaluation ($n = 9$). Three others were determined to have ASD based on diagnostic evaluations submitted by parents. Those evaluations all used the ADOS.
Were the reference standard evaluators blind to the screener risk status of the children?	Not reported.	Yes.
What diagnostic outcome categories were used to test prediction from screener to reference standard?	ASD, LD, DD, and no diagnosis. LD and DD defined by Mullen Scores, "other" by parameters such as motor delay.	ASD, other DDs' diagnosis, or treated through EI services, developmental concerns (no diagnosis but concerns), and no concerns.
Timing and flow		
Was there excessive attrition through any phase of screening and evaluation?	Out of 10,479, there were 1316 fails. Out of those, only 346 were referred for testing by the researchers, with a list of practical reasons why the others might have been missed. Out of 346 they lost another 232 for a variety of reasons, so in the end they worked with 184 high-risk children plus 41 TD children referred as a comparison group.	No.
Were there conditions besides attrition that filtered the negative and positive screens from the original screening to the reference standard diagnostic testing phase?	No.	No issues—they were able to make some assessment of developmental status of all 699.
Evaluation		
How were performance/predictive values calculated?	They combined ASD with other DDs to calculate PPV because they were considering the ITC a broadband screener.	They were not able to see the FYI negatives in person but did have parents report diagnoses, EI services, developmental concerns, and two parent-rated screening questionnaires for DD and ASD symptoms.

Table 3: Continued.

Probe questions	ITC [59]	FYI [60]	
Was performance/prediction for younger versus older children explored?	Screened at 12–15 months. But their breakdown showed that diagnosis was less stable at 12–18 months and became more stable towards 24 months.	N/A—all screened at 12 months.	
Performance			
What were the performance/predictive values?	PPV = .75 for all disabilities. PPV = .20 ASD alone.	*Total score* PPV = .14. NPV = .99. Se = .44. Sp = .97.	*Two-domain cutoff* PPV = .31. NPV = .99. Se = .44. Sp = .99.
What was the developmental level of children detected?	IQs ranged widely but did include higher functioning children: MSEL Composite (M = 100; SD = 15). M = 78.6. SD = 17.5. Range = 49–106.	Sample size includes higher-functioning children but difficult to characterize because 9 children had ASD and only 6 had Mullen Composite scores; four were average or higher and two were very low. M = 94.7. Range = 62–127.	
Of the false positives for ASD, what proportion had other developmental or learning disabilities?	69.7%.	65% (who met total score cutoff). 85% (who met two-domain cutoff).	

ITC = Infant-Toddler Checklist; ASD = autism spectrum disorder; FYI = First-Year Inventory; BED = Best Estimate Diagnosis; ADOS-T = Autism Diagnostic Observation Schedule-Toddler Module; ADI-R = Autism Diagnostic Interview-Revised; dx = diagnosis; LD = language disorder; DD = developmental disability; EI = early intervention; TD = typically developing; PPV = positive predictive value; NPV = negative predictive value; Se = sensitivity; Sp = specificity; MSEL = Mullen scales of early learning; M = mean; SD = standard deviation.

is appropriate because all children from screening sample could not be followed up to know the proportion of true and false negatives. The ITC would need further studies that reported Se and Sp using more conventional screening validity methods in order for more conclusive judgments to be made about its utility.

(B) First-Year Inventory (FYI)

(1) Background. The FYI is a 62-item caregiver-rated checklist meant for screening 12-month-olds. It was first produced in 2003 and remains an unpublished instrument. Its development and first applications were described in Reznick et al. [80] and Watson and colleagues [81]; a recent study focused on an analysis of what combinations of items were most predictive [82]. Turner-Brown et al. [60] reported Se and Sp on a community, low-risk sample. A shortened version (the FYI-Lite) has been reported upon [83], but no specificity and sensitivity estimates were produced. The development of the instrument is currently ongoing (Baranek, pers. comm.).

(2) Instrument Development. The authors chose target behaviors for items based on an extensive review of the literature that included retrospective studies, case studies, studies of home movies, and prospective studies from the Baby Sibling laboratories as well as from community programs and from videotapes of infants from the authors own laboratory. They obtained feedback from experts and parents on the item wording and eventually piloted the instrument with a community sample of parents. The final version of 63 questions is obtainable from the authors.

Reznick and colleagues [80] reported on a normative community sample that was gathered by a mass mailing to families who had an infant child based on birth records. Of the 5,941 sent out, there was a return rate of 25%. Parents filled out the questionnaire when their child was within a month of 12 months old. This paper described how the subscales of the FYI were developed based on the parent responses from this sample (see section below).

Watson and colleagues [81] used the population sample to test the ability of the FYI to discriminate among children who had been diagnosed with ASD, typically developing children, and children with non-ASD developmental disabilities by having parents of older children (but under 5 years of age) *retrospectively* rate their children at 12 months. They examined both the total risk scores and the risks scores for each of the eight constructs. Analyses of variance and post hoc analyses showed highly significant differences across the three groups, with the total score and most of the constructs showing an ability to discriminate among children with ASD, DD, and TD.

(3) Measurement Strategy, Constructs Measured, and Scoring. This is a parent-rated questionnaire with 63 items; the items have several different response types. The authors considered their items covering the broad categories of "social-communication" and "sensory-regulatory functions" and purposely included some items indicating "generalized

developmental delay" because of their increased association with autism.

Forty-six of the items are rated on a four-point scale from "never" to "often." Fourteen of the items revisit key questions but have the parent choose a frequency rating (e.g., "some of the time" to "all of the time"). There is one item asking the parent to circle the consonant sounds their child makes. The final two items are open-ended questions about concerns about development and other medical issues the child may have.

The authors then conducted a construct shaping procedure that yielded eight constructs under the two following domains: (1) social-communication domain—Social Orienting and Receptive Communication, Social-Affective Engagement, Imitation, and Expressive Communication; and (2) sensory-regulatory domain—Sensory Processing, Regulatory Patterns, Reactivity, and Repetitive Behavior.

Risk scores were developed by examining frequency distributions of items to find those of low endorsement but high atypicality; these were identified across the eight constructs, standardized to account for the different number of items within constructs, and a cutoff score determined for a combined or total risk score (cutoff = 17).

(4) Research Summary. Turner-Brown and colleagues [60] followed up the normative sample of 1,192 nonselected families who had filled out the FYI when their child was approximately 12 months old and agreed to be contacted after their child was three years old. A letter was sent out that included the Social Responsiveness Scale (Preschool) and a developmental questionnaire that inquire about developmental status, any early intervention, and any diagnoses. A total of 699 families returned the questionnaire.

Children whose parents' responses on these measures indicated, based on a set of score cutoff criteria, a high risk and/or possibility of ASD were invited to come for an in-person evaluation. Twenty-eight children were seen for a clinical evaluation. Between in-person assessment and parent report of community diagnoses, 9 or 1.3% of the 699 children were found to have ASD at age of 3.

Using a cutoff total score of 19.2, the PPV was .14. Investigators report that 4 out of 9 children identified with ASD met the total score cutoff (or 44% sensitivity) and that the majority of children (665/690) who did not have ASD at age of 3 screened negative (or 97% specificity). They also examined ROC using a two-domain cutoff. This yielded an improved PPV (.31) with very similar Se (.44) and Sp (.99).

(5) Conclusions. It would appear that the FYI is still in its formative stages. It has shown some ability to predict ASD from the early age of 12 months, but the sensitivity is unacceptably low for an ASD clinical instrument; thus further research is needed to increase its utility. This is one of the only studies of its kind that made an effort to ascertain the developmental status of the entire sample (who sent back questionnaires at age of three, $n = 699$). Over half of the ASD false positives had other developmental problems, which increases its utility as a developmental screener. Although their developmental outcome information was not extensive, there appeared to be a range of abilities including some very low and some high.

Its authors suggest that the 62-item length may be too long for routine office screening and an FYI-Lite version has been used in two papers (without Se and Sp information reported). They report on their research website that they are continuing to work with this screening tool.

3.1.4. Level 1 Conclusions and Recommendations. For this young age range, two screening instruments were examined after the criteria of published performance information and interpretable "timing and flow" filtered several others from consideration. Both instruments have demonstrated some success at detecting ASD under 18 months but actually function better as broadband screeners that detect other disabilities as well as ASD. The ITC identifies itself as such a screener, while the FYI endeavors to be autism-specific. Both were able to detect children under age of 18 months who had a range of developmental levels at age of three years, but both are also in need of continued research to demonstrate efficacy. The FYI appears to be in process of revision, as well.

3.2. Level 2 Early Screening Instruments for Autism Spectrum Disorder

3.2.1. Features of Autism-Specific Level 2 Screening. Level 2 screeners are intended to distinguish ASD *per se* among children already identified as being at high risk for a number of developmental disabilities and delays. In the field of autism screening, there are added nuances in that high risk is conferred in three major ways. The first involves children that have already been identified as being at risk, but this is operationalized in a variety of ways as well: children who have been referred to evaluation clinics and have appointments to be evaluated thoroughly, children who have failed an autism-specific screening instrument through parent report or clinician administration in a primary care or research setting, and children for whom their caregivers or primary care providers have expressed concerns. The second way is risk status unique to a relatively recently developed research paradigm: they are younger siblings of children that have been diagnosed with ASD, since the "Baby Siblings" research has shown the prevalence to be significantly increased among them [27]. A third way, not addressed in this review, is by a child having a congenital (preterm status) [84, 85] or genetic condition (e.g., Fragile X, Down syndrome, or Angelman syndrome) that is associated with increased risk of an ASD diagnosis [86, 87].

As with Level 1 screeners, the goals for Level 2 have implications for research and feasibility. Validity research designs typically compare identified groups of children with ASD and other DDs and frequently a TD group. Ideally the comparison groups are matched on gender, age, and developmental level. In terms of sensitivity and specificity, the latter becomes important because of the explicit effort to distinguish ASD from other DDs. In terms of feasibility, the length of administration may be longer, and need for

Table 4: Level 2 ASD screening instruments reviewed.

(a)

Screener	Dates of paper(s)	Country developed	Ages (mos)	Strategy
Screening Test for Autism in Two-Year-Olds (STAT)	2000 2004 2008*	US	12–24	Interactive clinician observation
Parent Observation of Early Markers (POEMS)	2012*	Canada	3–24	Caregiver checklist
Autism Detection in Early Childhood (ADEC)	2014 (2)* 2015	Australia US	12–36	Interactive clinician observation

(b)

Excluded from in-depth review	Country developed	Ages (mos)	Reason for exclusion
Autism Observation Scale for Infants (AOSI)	Canada	6–18	Studies eventually showed inadequate Se and Sp.

*This paper was reviewed in detail for research methods because it was an ROC study.

training may be present because of this more advanced phase of identification.

Table 4 presents second-level ASD screening instruments that have peer-reviewed papers reporting Se and Sp or PPV. They are presented in order of most recent publication (which reported Se and Sp) date.

3.2.2. Level 2 Instruments Excluded from Detailed Review. The *Autism Observation Scale for Infants (AOSI)* [88], a clinician observation instrument, was developed by a group of Canadian researchers who are part of the prospective infant sibling studies consortium. They were interested in developing a standardized measure for early autism symptoms for children as young as 6, 12, and 18 months. They developed the protocol in the early 2000s in response to this need and began to generate published reports in 2005. However, by 2014 the authors did not recommend it for clinical use based on inadequate sensitivity and specificity [89].

The AOSI is a semistructured interactive measure of 19 items that takes about 20 minutes to be administered by a clinical professional. The clinician must be trained in the AOSI and, in addition, needs to be quite familiar with infant behavior as well as young children with ASD.

The items reflect many of the social-communication behaviors identified through both basic studies of the development of ASD and the development of other infant screening instruments. Its creators also included early information-processing behaviors, such as the child's ability to shift visual attention away from one stimulus to another. The AOSI also includes some items reflecting temperamental features, such as atypical reactivity (under- and overreactive to environmental input).

The AOSI represents an intensive effort to take advantage of the infant sibling research protocol to reveal very early emerging behaviors of ASD and to create a manageable semistructured observation protocol to use in both research and clinical settings. At this point more work is needed to refine procedures to stabilize reliability coefficients and to realize adequate sensitivity and specificity.

3.2.3. Level 2 Instruments Included for Detailed Review

(A) Screening Test for Autism in Two-Year-Olds (STAT)

(1) Background. The STAT is a clinician-administered instrument for children 12–36 months and takes about 20 minutes to administer. It was developed in the late 1990s, with reports on development, reliability, validity, ROC, and community applications and feasibility from 2000 to the present. Although it was created for children from 24 through 35 months, there is one study that investigated its utility for children 12–24 months [61], and the authors are continuing to examine scoring strategies that address earlier detection (Stone, pers. comm.).

(2) Instrument Development. The development sample was described in a brief report by Stone and colleagues [20], and the results were considered preliminary evidence for the instrument's utility. They had a very small sample: 7 children with autism and 33 with DDs and/or language impairment (LI), all between 24 and 36 months. The participants were given the STAT while attending a clinic for a full evaluation because of developmental concerns. The authors developed the scoring and the cutoff scores and then applied it to another set of high-risk children to achieve Se of .83 and Sp of .86 for Autistic Disorder (AD) only.

Further development of the STAT was described in Stone and colleagues [21]. Groups of children referred for evaluation were given the STAT at the same time as their comprehensive evaluations at a university clinic. In Study 1, 26 children who were diagnosed with AD were compared to 26 children who were diagnosed with developmental delay and/or language disorder in order to establish cutoff scores for adequate sensitivity and specificity. They determined that a cutoff score of 2 resulted in Se of .92 and Sp of .85. In Study 2 of this paper, a similar procedure was used to look at other features of validity and reliability, but no ROC coefficients were reported. This time 50 children had AD and 39 had DDs and/or LI. All three of the above studies specified that the screening was intended to detect AD and not the milder presentation of Pervasive Developmental Disorder-Not Otherwise Specified (PDD-NOS), as referenced to the DSM-IV [58].

Chiang and colleagues [90] adapted the STAT to a Taiwanese version. These authors made some item substitutions, so their instrument would be considered an adaptation. They conducted the study in the same way that the Stone articles described and obtained an Se of .93 and Sp of .74, predicting to AD only and excluding PDD-NOS.

(3) Measurement Strategy, Constructs Measured, and Scoring. The STAT is a semistructured play-based interactive tool that takes about 20 minutes to complete. It can be given in less time if the child fails sufficient items to reach the at-risk cutoff score before all items are given. The clinician does have to be trained in order to administer it, and this involves an investment of time and cost. There is an online tutorial that takes several hours to complete and includes a reliability scoring test that must be passed in order to obtain the training certification. Vanderbilt University does conduct training workshops, including specialized ones for MDs. The information is available at http://vkc.mc.vanderbilt.edu/vkc/triad/training/stat/physicians.

There are four domains of two-to-four items each: Play, Requesting, Directing Attention, and Motor Imitation. In fact, the items are probing for social communication, joint attention, pretend play and functional object use, and motor/gestural imitation. There is an emphasis on social communication in this scale and there does not seem to be an opportunity to directly account for highly atypical behaviors (although this is reflected to some degree through *lack* of pretend and functional use with objects in this tool).

For each item, the child receives a Pass, Fail, or Refuse, using the child's best performance for up to three trials. Only the total score is used for determining at-risk status.

(4) Research Summary. The only study to be considered here is the one that looked at children 12–24 months [61], since it falls within our age inclusion criterion. Participants were younger siblings of children diagnosed with ASD ($n = 59$) and children referred for developmental concerns ($n = 12$). They had the STAT administered from 12 to 24 months and were evaluated for ASD at 24 months (see Table 5). Although for studies using high-risk children between 24 and 36 months the cutoff score was 2, it was adjusted for the study using children between 12 and 24 months. Performance measures were generated for a higher more optimal cutoff score, 2.75, as follows: Se = .95, Sp = .73, PPV = .56, and NPV = .97. The authors noted that prediction improved at 14 months and thus recalculated the measures after excluding the 12-13-month-olds, with the following results: Se = .93, Sp = .83, PPV = .68, and NPV = .97.

(5) Conclusions. The STAT is a clinician-administered, semistructured interactive screener that shows adequate to strong prediction up to this point. It requires an investment of time and money to train front-line providers; however, once this is accomplished, presumably the administrator has a skill set that facilitates identification and referral for ASD and DDs independent of the actual screener application. Although it was originally developed for children between age of two and three years of age, this one paper has shown in a preliminary way its utility for children between one and two years. One weakness in this study was that the sample size was relatively small (group with ASD ended up being 19, and typically developing group was 12). Another issue is that the children were evaluated for ASD at 24 months of age. A minority of children will change their diagnosis between 24 and 36 months, and thus it would be important to have a study that also evaluated the children at 3 years of age for more precise prediction coefficients. The original papers restricted the STAT to AD, but the study about younger children extended the prediction to ASD with good ROC. One important contribution was that prediction to later diagnosis was examined in for the youngest versus older children. Across a 12-month age range, starting at age of 12 months, prediction improved starting at 14 months. Fifty percent of false positives had developmental problems warranting evaluation and intervention. Based on the relatively high developmental quotients at outcome diagnosis, this instrument is detecting a group of children that includes those with milder levels of disability. The authors continue to refine its structure and scoring for future reports (Stone, pers. comm.).

(B) Parent Observation of Early Milestones Scale (POEMS)

(1) Background. The POEMS, a 61-item caregiver-rated checklist, was developed relatively recently by researchers in Canada who recruited, through an Internet site, families with infant siblings of children diagnosed with autism spectrum disorder. They were interested in tracking the emergence of ASD features to facilitate earlier identification in these high-risk children. Papers in 2012 and 2015 described development, reliability, and validity of the measure [62, 91]. The 2012 paper had ROC reported.

(2) Instrument Development. The researchers developed items based on established measures of symptoms of ASD in young children, such as the ADI-R [92] and the CARS [93].

(3) Measurement Strategy, Constructs Measured, and Scoring. This is a caregiver-report checklist, but in the one published study parents filled out the POEMS online and on paper and then sent it through the mail or reported it over the telephone (the parent and examiner both had a copy and the examiner recorded the parent responses).

The items represent a broad range of behaviors that are known to characterize young children with ASD, including those outside of the core behaviors. For example, the items addressed mood regulation, sensory responses, visual tracking, and motor skills. More specifically, the authors describe the items addressing the following types of behaviors: early social and communication skills or deficits, restricted interests, ritualistic, repetitive, nonfunctional behaviors, intolerance to transitions and waiting, difficulties with new foods, loud noises, sleeping, and toileting, problems with attention

Table 5: Research summaries for the Screening Test for Autism in Two-Year-Olds (STAT), Parent Observation of Early Milestones Scale (POEMS), and Autism Detection in Early Childhood (ADEC).

Probe questions	STAT [61]	POEMS [62]	ADEC [63]
Participants			
Was the sample appropriate in size and scope?	Small: 19 had ASD. All participants were of high risk because of diagnosed older sibling.	All participants were of high risk because of diagnosed older sibling.	All participants were of high risk based on being scheduled for an evaluation at a specialty clinic.
Did investigators use a sample matched for developmental level?	No.	No.	Yes.
Screening instrument			
Was there anything about how the screener was administered that would be different from its intended use in a nonresearch, community setting?	No.	The POEMS was filled out by families every three months. Giving the POEMS many times could sensitize parents to ASD behaviors, especially since they would already be so because of their older child with ASD. However, this is consistent with its intended use within this study.	The team administering the screener received some training.
Were there any issues regarding the way it is scored in the study?	No.	No.	See evaluation domain below.
Reference standard			
Did all children receive a BED from in-person evaluations? How extensive was the information available to the clinician making the Best Estimate Diagnosis?	Yes; the information available included ADOS and Mullen.	No direct examination for diagnostic status. They relied on parent report of community diagnosis. They were able to give ADI-R to 3 out of the 9 children with ASD to confirm.	BED with cognitive assessment, ADOS, and ADI-R if AD or PDD-NOS diagnosis considered. "77.5% had an independent confirmatory diagnosis from either two other independent professionals who were recognized by the state's autism association or other medical professionals such as pediatricians and psychologists."
Were the reference standard evaluators blind to the screener risk status of the children?	Not reported.	Most likely, considering they were clinicians in the community who were independent of the study.	Yes.
What diagnostic outcome categories were used to test prediction from screener to reference standard?	Autism, PDD-NOS, DD, LI (language impairment), BAP (Broader Autism Phenotype), and no diagnosis.	Only categories were ASD versus no-ASD. This is a departure from most studies, which also include other DDs. This appeared to be a function of the study methods, which involved using reports the parents obtained from the community.	For initial analyses, ASD (AD + PDD-NOS), other DDs, and TD. However, authors indicated that the ADEC is intended to detect Autistic Disorder, so PDD-NOS was left out for ROC analysis and this suggests that it will detect more severe children on the spectrum.
Timing and flow			
Was there excessive attrition through any phase of screening and evaluation?	No.	No, sample size was adequate.	N/A.

Table 5: Continued.

Probe questions	STAT [61]	POEMS [62]	ADEC [63]
Were there conditions besides attrition that filtered the negative and positive screens from the original screening to the reference standard diagnostic testing phase?	No.	No, sample size was adequate.	N/A.
Evaluation			
How were performance/predictive values calculated?	The groups were combined as follows: autism and PDD-NOS were all ASD; the others were non-ASD. With this categorization, the most false positives were found for 12-13-month-olds, so Se and Sp were calculated both with and without them. They achieved acceptable Se and Sp levels by raising the cutoff score compared to that for the 24–36-month-olds.	Predictive validity was first explored by forming two groups: infant siblings who were confirmed to have ASD at age of 36 months (n = 9) and those who were not (n = 63). They then compared how the POEMS score diverged over the different age levels.	Investigators left the PDD-NOS group out and compared AD to Other Developmental Disabilities (ODD) with and without the TD group. This can inflate performance compared to studies that include milder children.
Was performance/prediction for younger versus older children explored?	Yes—reported false positives for three different groups between 12 and 24 months. More false positives for the 12-13-month group than older children.	Yes—see below. The sensitivity got higher as age progressed over 3, 6, 9, 12, 18, and 24 months. Sensitivity reached the acceptable level at 18 months.	Yes, for 12–24 versus 24–36 with no differences found. Did not look at the youngest children (under 18 months).
Performance			
What were the performance/predictive values?	Using a cutoff of 2.75: Se = .95, Sp = .73, PPV = .56, NPV = .97. Excluding the 12-13-month-olds: Se = .93, Sp = .83, PPV = .68, NPV = .97.	A cutoff score of 70 resulted in a mean sensitivity (across all age groups) of .74 and specificity of .87; PPV overall was .21. At 12 months, Se = .71 and Sp = .68. At 18 months, Se = .89 and Sp = .65.	Using a cutoff score of 11. *Unmatched* AD versus ODD: Se = 1.0; Sp = .77. AD versus ODD + TD: Se = 1.0; Sp = .89. *Matched* AD versus ODD: Se = 1.0; Sp = .74. AD versus ODD + TD: Se = 1.0; Sp = .90.
What was the developmental level of children detected?	The sample included higher functioning children; at mean of 24 months, MSEL Early Learning Composite: M = 93.5; SD = 23.3.	Not reported.	Not reported.
Of the false positives for ASD, what proportion had other developmental or learning disabilities?	50% of false positives had other DD diagnoses.	Not reported.	10/70.

STAT = Screening Test for Autism in Two-Year-Olds; POEMS = Parent Observation of Early Milestones Scale; ADEC = Autism Detection in Early Childhood; ASD = autism spectrum disorder; BED = Best Estimate Diagnosis; ADOS = Autism Diagnostic Observation Schedule; ADI-R = Autism Diagnostic Interview-Revised; AD = Autistic Disorder; PDD-NOS = Pervasive Developmental Disorder-Not Otherwise Specified; DD = developmental delay; LI = language impairment; BAP = Broader Autism Phenotype; TD = typically developing; ROC = receiver operator characteristics; Se = sensitivity; Sp = specificity; ODD = Other Developmental Disabilities; PPV = positive predictive value; NPV = negative predictive value; MSEL = Mullen scales of early learning; M = mean; SD = standard deviation.

and visual tracking, and problems with motor agility and movement. Each item was scored on a 1–4 scale, with 1 representing typical and nonproblematic behavior and 4 representing extreme difficulty. Each item has its specific description for the low and high behavioral anchors. Only a total score is obtained; no subscales scores have been developed.

(4) Research Summary. Feldman and colleagues [62] recruited families with an older sibling diagnosed with autism and

then followed up younger, infant siblings with parents filling out the POEMS multiple times, at least a month apart. They followed up 108 children. Data analyses focused on scores they had for groups of both HR/ASD and HR/No ASD at 3, 6, 9, 12, 18, and 24 months. To get the high-risk siblings diagnosis by 36 months, they relied on parent report of community diagnoses. They were able to complete the ADI-R on ~70% of the HR/No ASD sibs (n = 99) and to confirm they did not have ASD. They were only able to give the ADI-R on 3 out of the 9 HR/ASD children (see Table 5). At 12 months, Se was .71 and Sp was .68; at 18 months, Se was .89 and Sp was .65. The overall PPV was .21.

(5) Conclusions. The POEMS is a medium-length parent checklist (61 items) for very early ASD detection. Although Se and Sp did not both reach ideal levels (>.80) at any age, it was the best at 18 months, with Se at .89 and Sp at .65. Given that Se was under acceptable levels until 18 months, the checklist does not offer an advantage for children below 18 months of age. It is noteworthy that the Se and Sp were around .70 at 12 months of age, given the difficulty of detecting ASD specifically at this early an age through a parent checklist.

For the sake of developing the measurement tool, the authors gave the checklist every three months, but presumably a choice would be made as to the ideal time to use the instrument for screening. However, the repeated parent reporting used in the instrument's development also may have served to heighten parents' observational skills, thus increasing veridicality of their reporting, and this would not be the case for one-time administration. The POEMS is a recently developed measure with one published study and future work may serve to increase the Se and Sp levels.

(C) Autism Detection in Early Childhood (ADEC)

(1) Background. The ADEC is a clinician-administered play interaction tool with 16 items for children 12–36 months. It was developed by a researcher in southern Australia. The development and initial examination is reported in a 2007 in-house publication [94]. In 2010, Hedley et al. [95] translated the instructions to Spanish and showed good Se (.94) and Sp (.92–100) for a sample of 19–36-month-old children. Subsequent papers were published in 2014 [63, 96], the latter reporting ROC. In 2015, a paper with ROC was published that used a sample from the US [97], but it focused on children from 18 months on. Importantly, the intent as specified in the first of these studies was to distinguish AD only. In the 2015 paper the authors changed the outcome category to ASD.

(2) Instrument Development. Behaviors were identified from retrospective parental reports [98] and video analysis [99].

(3) Measurement Strategy, Constructs Measured, and Scoring. The ADEC is a clinician interaction/observation instrument with 16 items that takes 10–15 minutes to administer.

The specific behaviors that are observed during the administration of the ADEC are response to name, imitation, ritualistic play, joint attention and social referencing, eye contact, functional play, pretend play, reciprocity of smile, reaction to common sounds, gaze monitoring, following verbal commands, delayed language, anticipation of social advances, nestling, use of gestures, and task switching.

As an example of scoring, *social response* has been operationalized as whether a child responds to his or her name when called by the examiner over five trials. If the child responds in the first or second attempt, he or she is scored a 0; in three to five attempts, he or she is scored a 1; and a 2 is given if the child does not respond to his or her name in any of the five attempts.

Response scores for each item range from 0 (*appropriate*) to 2 (*inappropriate*), with a possible maximum score of 32. Based on Se and Sp data provided in the manual, a score of 0–10 indicates a low risk for AD, 11–13 a moderate risk, 14–19 a high risk, and >19 a very high risk.

The training for ADEC is not formal. A video is supplied with purchase of the manual, and the clinician is expected to view it, study the manual, and practice until proficient. The ADEC website (https://shop.acer.edu.au/autism-detection-in-early-childhood-adec) specifies that the individuals qualified to administer the ADEC are "Master degree in a health profession (e.g., speech pathology, occupational therapy, special education, or social work) OR Bachelor degree in a health profession, PLUS evidence of training in assessment, OR ACER Specialist Certification."

(4) Research Summary. Nah and colleagues [63] recruited families with children 12–36 months from a variety of sources over a several-year period in order to accumulate a varied group of 70 children diagnosed with AD, PDD-NOS, and other DDs and as TD. They first had research assistants administer the ADEC, and then the children and parents returned for a full evaluation, using Best Estimate Diagnosis, including the ADOS. This study calculated performance measures using both matched and unmatched samples. For the matched sample, they selected children from two groups (AD and other DDs) that matched on NVIQ and Vineland Adaptive Behavior Scales Adaptive Behavior Quotient (VABS ABC). The unmatched group retained all the children that ended up in their diagnostic groups (AD and other DDs) but the groups had significantly different mean NVIQs and Vineland ABCs. The authors predicted from ADEC failure (cutoff score of 11) to outcome, but only to AD versus other DDs, leaving out the PDD-NOS group; this strategy will increase the Se and Sp. They also calculated measures with and without combining the other DDs and TD group (see Table 5). For all the comparisons, Se was 1.0, and Sp ranged from .74 to .90. In the unmatched sample PPV was .84 and NPV was 1.0.

(5) Conclusions. The ADEC is a clinician-administered structured play interaction tool. Se reached 1.0; however, investigators specifically removed milder children and this can inflate performance measures compared to studies that include the continuum of severity. Its outcomes need to be considered in the context that the measure was intended to detect Autistic Disorder and not milder presentations. Another issue was that it appeared that concurrent diagnoses were made to validate some very early screening ages. Therefore, if some of

the children were diagnosed at 24 months or less, then there is a chance that some would change diagnosis by age of three. Sp was in the high 70s (.74 unmatched sample and .77 matched sample) and was thus just under the acceptable level (>.80). Discriminating ASD from DDs was accommodated through a matched sample and performance remained essentially the same.

Although the authors intend for the instrument to be used by clinicians with limited training, the description of the instrument suggests that to score the items correctly the administrator would have to study the directions, including examples of passing and nonpassing behaviors, and practice with this tool to some extent before being able to administer it quickly. In the most recent paper, a more protracted training period was described.

3.2.4. Level 2 Conclusions and Recommendations. Three second-level screening instruments were reviewed that have a beginning research base. Two are clinician-administered tools. The STAT shows promise but needs continued study with larger subject samples. It has feasibility considerations in that there is time and cost for initial training; the training itself does confer the added value of a nonspecialized clinician understanding early ASD symptoms in greater depth. The ADEC is building a research base with adequate Se but Sp that is less so, and the research on the younger age continuum of its targeted population is just beginning. The ADEC requires study and practice on the part of the clinician but this training is less formal and resource-intensive than the STAT. One parent-report checklist, the POEMS, has a very beginning research foundation. Its current length may preclude widespread community use except in the case of children who are at higher risk for ASD and thus for whom the expenditure of extra time is warranted.

4. Discussion

4.1. Interpretation Challenges: Methodological Themes Associated with Study Design. After comparing these early screener studies, several essential method issues emerged that need to be addressed in order to create more consistent and comparable future screening studies for very young children.

4.1.1. Inclusion Criteria. The first is that important features of participant inclusion/exclusion are either not specified or inconsistent. Two of the five studies do not describe any neurodevelopmental features of either those initially included or those evaluated apart from developmental levels at the point of reference standard evaluation. The STAT authors [61] did specify that significant sensory, motor, genetic, and metabolic disorders were conditions for exclusion. Preterm status is another relevant participant characteristic; the FYI study excluded children born preterm because the researchers wanted the child to be 12 months of age and not have adjusted age complicating that goal. However, preterm children have been shown to be at higher risk for ASD [84, 85] so it is also relevant to the degree of risk present in the sample.

4.1.2. Outcome Categories. A second issue is inconsistency in the outcome categories when the reference standard diagnostic testing is performed. Both the STAT and the ADEC originally stated that the intent was to detect more severely affected children (AD and not PDD-NOS) but in the most recent articles changed that designation to ASD. The studies in general are variable in their designation of non-ASD disability detected. Some have clear criteria based on standardized tests for language disorder and developmental disorder, whereas others use more vague terms such as "broad autism phenotype" and "developmental concerns" [59]. While it is important to accommodate different levels of possible developmental delays and differences in the outcomes, consistency in definition will be important.

4.1.3. Developmental Level of Children at the Outcome Stage. This is also an important piece of information because it gives insight into whom the screener detected—higher versus lower functioning individuals, for example. There is considerable inconsistency across studies regarding this information. There is the complication that some children will not be able to respond to standardized tasks in order to achieve a score so that there will usually be children not represented by such scores.

4.2. Constructs Encompassed in Very Early Screening Instruments. Clearly, different approaches have been taken to construct measurement in the screeners. The ITC, for example, was developed as a social-communication measure and does not include repetitive behaviors (although play items function to some extent when typical milestones are not endorsed). Table 6 shows the different symptom domains that were derived from comparing the screeners and the items that represented them. The most common differences are the extent to which regulatory/temperament items (difficult to soothe, cannot tolerate waiting, and gets upset easily) and developmental items (language, motor, and play milestones) are included apart from the core social-communication and repetitive, restricted behavior symptom domains. Brian and colleagues [100] found that items related to temperament (difficulty with transitions and reactivity) at 18 months did discriminate well between high-risk infant siblings children diagnosed with ASD or not at age of three years and that these features added independent prediction from social-communication items.

A similar result was reported by the authors of the POEMS. When items were analyzed that were most predictive from early months to ASD diagnosis at age of three years among high-risk biologic younger siblings, "problems with waiting" was as strong as any of the social and communication items [91]. These results suggest that temperament and reactivity items may be important to include along with core symptom items, but the extent to which developmental items add predictive value has yet to be examined.

The AOSI authors attempted to add a very early neuropsychological feature to prediction. Although the screener has not been shown to be predictive at a level for clinical use at

Table 6: Behaviors examined by very early ASD screeners.

(a) Level 1 ASD screening instruments

Social communication: Communication	Social communication: Social	Repetitive behaviors	Sensory	Developmental	Reactivity/temperament	Atypical information processing
Early Screen for Autism Traits (ESAT)						
Eye contact		Has interest in different toys	Reaction to sensory stimuli			
Reacts when spoken to	Emotions understandable	Varied play	Likes cuddling			
	Facial expression	Stereotyped movements				
	Attracts attention					
	Brings/shows objects					
	Interest in people					
	Smiles directly					
Checklist for Early Signs of Developmental Disorder (CSEDD)						
Lack of eye contact		Shows stereotyped behavior	Dislikes touching and cuddling	Does not explore, passive		
Turns to name	Social smile	Lack of variable play*	Unusual sensory behavior	Lack of functional play*		
Seems to be deaf	Shares enjoyment	Lack of functional play*		Babbling at 12 months	Overreaction to change or other events*	
Gestures	Imitation	Unusual postures		Single words at 16 months		
Follows point	Prefers aloneness	Overreaction to change or other events*		Spontaneous two-word phrases at 24 months		
Points	Shows object for social bid			Loss of language		
Instrumental communication/hand-leading	Flat affect					
Infant-Toddler Checklist (ITC)						
Responds to name	Emotions readable	Interest in a variety of objects		Strings sounds together		
Follows point to object	Eye contact while playing	Uses objects appropriately*		Variety of consonant sounds		
Requests object	Shared affect	Repeats simple activity over and over		Comprehension vocabulary		

(a) Continued.

Social communication: Communication	Social communication: Social	Repetitive behaviors	Sensory	Developmental	Reactivity/temperament	Atypical information processing
Words for attention or help	Seeks attention			Block or ring stacking		
Points to objects	Gets you to laugh					
Waves to greet	Shows object for social attention					
	Initiating through handing object					
	Initiates joint attention					
First-Year Inventory (FYI)						
Looks when name is called		Upset when switching activities	Overly sensitive to touch	Babbles	Sleeping and waking patterns are regular	
Trouble hearing	Avoids looking at you	Enjoys staring at bright lights	Ignores loud or startling sounds	Uses pincer grip	Regular feeding patterns	
Looks at people when they talk	Looks at your face for comfort	Gets stuck on playing with a part of a toy	Spits out certain textures of foods	Eyes line up when looking at object		
Uses communicative gestures	Plays alone for an hour or more	Body gets stuck in positions or postures	Presses against things			
Responds to "Where's —?"	Looks up from play when shown new toy	Enjoys making objects spin over and over	Enjoys rubbing or scratching objects			
Uses finger to point at things	Easy to understand baby's expressions	Stares at fingers while wiggling them	Enjoys kicking feet over and over			
Plays or communicates less than in the past	Tries to get your attention to show things, or for interactive or physical games					
	Imitates mouth sounds, body movements, or movements, with objects					

(a) Continued.

Social communication: Communication	Social communication: Social	Repetitive behaviors	Sensory	Developmental	Reactivity/temperament	Atypical information processing
	Tries to get attention by sound and gaze Seems interested in other babies					

(b) Level 2 ASD screening instruments

Social communication: Communication	Social communication: Social	Repetitive behaviors	Sensory	Developmental	Reactivity/temperament	Atypical information processing	Adaptive skills
Autism Observation Scale for Infants (AOSI)							
Eye contact		Atypical motor behavior	Atypical sensory behavior	Motor control	Behavioral reactivity	Visual tracking	
Orientation to name	Differential response to facial emotion	Insistence on specific objects/activities				Engagement of attention	
Social babbling	Anticipatory social response					Disengagement of attention	
Shared interest	Imitation					Transitions	
	Reciprocal social smile						
Coordination of eye gaze and action	Social interest and shared affect						
Screening Test for Autism in Two-Year-Olds (STAT) (applied to children under 24 months)							
Requests when presented with communication challenge (2 items)	Takes turns	(Lack of) functional object use*		Functional object use*			
Directs attention and interacts socially (4 items)	Imitates motor acts (4 items)						
Parent Observation of Early Milestones Scale (POEMS)							
Eye contact		Shifts (does not shift) attention from one event to another	Cuddling	Object permanence	Demands attention	Visual tracking (2 items)*	Sleep (3 items)
Imitates sounds or words	Social smiling	Explores (does not explore) new toys and environments	Reaction to pain	Muscle tone	Stability of mood		Feeding (4 items)

(b) Continued.

Social communication		Repetitive behaviors	Sensory	Developmental	Reactivity/temperament	Atypical information processing	Adaptive skills
Communication	Social						
Points to request	Laughs appropriately	Diverse toy play	Reaction to noise	Agility in movement	Comforted when hurt		
Points to share interests	Attachment to parents	Repetitive body movements	Fearful of objects that move or make noise	Attention span	Unpredictable reactions		
Coordinates gaze and point	Recognizes parents voice	Atypical use of words	Tolerance to transitions	Stacks blocks	Activity level		
Points in response to question	Emotions appropriate			Pretend play	Cries to express needs		
Follows adult point	Anticipation to being picked up			Communicates with words*	Waiting tolerance		
Follows simple direction	Response to name			Visual tracking (2 items)*			
Brings toys to request	Attention to faces						
Greets	Shifts attention from object to person						
Coordinates gestures and communication	Imitating						
Communicates with words*	Social games						
	Interest in birthday present and cake						
	Interest in peers						
	Plays with peers						
Autism Diagnostic Evaluation for Children (ADEC)							
Responds to verbal command	Imitation	Functional play (lack of)	Responds to every day sounds	Demonstrates use of words			
Demonstrates use of words	Gaze switching from toy to person	Pretend play (lack of)					
Use of gestures (waves good-bye)	Eye contact						
Response to name	Reciprocity of smile						
	Following point						
	Anticipatory posture for being picked up						
	Nesting into caregiver						

* Item placed in two categories.

this time, it is noteworthy that they included items that are related to certain early differences that are pursued in more laboratory-based studies.

4.3. Challenges to Early Detection of ASD before 18 Months of Age. By sampling children from below 12 months up to 18–24 months, some of these very early screening studies were able to demonstrate that prediction was less stable the younger children were. Wetherby and colleagues [67] showed that of children diagnosed with ASD at 36 months fewer attained at-risk scores on the Infant-Toddler Checklist below 12 months (6–8 and 9–11 months), but from 12 to 24 months the percentages identified as being at risk (after serial screening) ranged from 91% to 100%. Wetherby and Prizant [71] examined concurrent validity by correlating ITC scores with clinician ratings on a structured play procedure tapping social-communication competence and found the correlations increased with age as follows: 6–11 months, .57; 12–17 months, .78; 18–24 months, .87. Stone and colleagues [61], testing the STAT as a screening tool for children 12–24 months, found that the number of false positives was much higher for the 12-13-month groups (38%) compared to 14–17 months (13%) and 18–23 months (11%) [61]. For the POEMS, Feldman and colleagues [62] reported that sensitivity improved and only received acceptable levels for the instrument as children were 18 and 24 months, compared to 3, 6, 9, and 12 months of age.

There are a number of reasons why these youngest children are more challenging to identify. They range from measurement challenges to features intrinsic to very young children who develop symptoms in different patterns in terms of timing and clinical presentation. These issues are considered as follows.

4.3.1. Difficulty with Parent Report for Early, Subtle Behaviors. Starting with the measurement methods themselves, many rely on caregiver report, asking them to make judgments on behaviors that are undoubtedly subtle at the ages up to 18 months. While parents and other consistent caregivers have the advantage of the greatest familiarity with and interest in their children, under certain circumstances parent report is not as reliable as direct observations [61, 101]. In a study comparing parent observation to detailed behavior counts from home videos, Ozonoff and colleagues [102] found that, while some aspects of the parent reporting were accurate, their reports regarding slowing of their child's development and gradual loss of skills were not consistent with video observations. The authors speculated that skill loss during this earliest period—between 12 and 18 months—may have been too gradual for parents to notice. During administration of the ESAT, wherein a trained psychologist was observing the child at the same time the parent was reporting on symptoms, it was common for the psychologist to override the parent judgment in the direction of more autism symptoms for the child [65]. Wetherby and colleagues' study [67] found that while parents were reporting a number of atypical symptoms, they often indicated that they did not have any concern, that is, regard them as problematic. Since several studies have found 18 months to be the average age of first parent concern for children diagnosed with ASD [103], it is possible that lack of language, underdeveloped social skills, and any unusual play patterns are more evident to them by the middle of the second year compared to earlier.

4.3.2. Timing Patterns of Symptom Emergence. Different timing patterns of symptom emergence among children with ASD make the ages before 12 months to 18 months particularly ambiguous. Retrospective parent-report, systematic observations from home movies and Baby Siblings consortium prospective studies have all been used to characterize the timing and nature of symptom development in ASD. Initially, mainly two trajectories had been described: early onset, wherein slow development is noted from about six months onward with gradual unfolding of more frank ASD symptoms after the one-year mark and throughout the second year, and later onset, often thought of as regressive autism [25]. In the latter pattern, parents reported that their child developed normally in all areas for the first year and then lost language and social skills in the second year, with this often becoming noticeable to them between 18 and 24 months. In contrast, more recent studies have endorsed three general patterns—(1) early onset, (2) relatively intact first-year development with loss of skills in the second year, but generally earlier than parents report [102], and (3) a "plateau" pattern, wherein first-year development is normal but soon after 12 months the child stops making progress and eventually manifests a full ASD profile by 24–36 months [22, 104]. It is likely, therefore, that for patterns (2) and (3) the first half of the second year may be a time of transition and ambiguous behavior.

One of the most important timing distinctions gleaned from prospective studies is that reported by Landa and colleagues [36]. Using a Baby Siblings prospective sample, approximately half the infants who would eventually be diagnosed with ASD showed symptoms at 12 months of age, but the other half was not detectable until after 14 months. Clearly, this distinction has important implications for attempts at very early screening. The differential prediction patterns of the STAT [61] and the ITC [67] reflect this symptom emergence timing.

The symptom domain of repetitive and restricted behaviors appears to present specific challenges in terms of timing and thus detection under 18 months. Although several studies have shown that certain types and rates of repetitive behaviors will distinguish groups of children with ASD versus DDs versus TD by 12 months [105–107], there is also evidence that repetitive behaviors as a whole may emerge or become more evident as the child approaches 3 years of age and older. For example, Moore and Goodson [108] reported the increase in repetitive behaviors from 2 years, 10 months to 4 to 5 years of age. The type of repetitive behavior plays a role; this effect was attributable in part to emergence of circumscribed interests and unusual preoccupations, symptoms that may not be observable at much younger ages. Guthrie et al. [109], using the ADOS-T, demonstrated this pattern but starting at early ages: restricted and repetitive behaviors became more prevalent in the second half of the second year, continuing through 30–46 months.

4.3.3. Phenotypic Variability. Phenotypic variability also complicates very early detection at these youngest ages. Children and individuals with ASD are known to vary widely in their presentation, and there are a number of sources of this variability. First, there is a difference in degree of variability between the two core symptom domains. Whereas social communication is always delayed and different in children with ASD, the RRB symptom domain has been observed to be more variable in children under three years [110], in addition to its tendency to increase in evidence over the second and third years of life.

Variability in degree of overall severity is also a known feature of ASD, and since young children with milder symptoms are more difficult to diagnose definitively under 24 months of age, it stands to reason that the less precise screening measures also are not as effective for early detection. With a Baby Siblings sample, Ozonoff and colleagues [111] reported that of those who were diagnosable at 36 months less than half (47%) were diagnosed at 18 months, and only 60% could be diagnosed at 24 months. These results represent a subgroup of the population of children with ASD, however (high-risk younger siblings). Guthrie and colleagues [109], using a community sample, showed that only a small proportion of their community sample had an unclear diagnostic presentation before 24 months and thus required follow-up for diagnostic clarification at three years of age.

The new designation of "specifiers" for the DSM-5 diagnostic criteria [112] encourages distinction between children with different cognitive levels, severity levels of the two symptom domains, and degree of language impairment. The earliest presentation of children with ASD and also with what will be enduring cognitive and language disability may be particularly difficult to differentiate from children with global delays. On the other hand, children with ASD but who are not inherently intellectually delayed and whose language is relatively intact may represent the more mildly affected children, who tend to be missed by ASD screeners in general and thus most likely by the very early screeners as well [3, 19]. In fact, all reviewed studies used DSM-IV criteria and thus it will be important to observe what impact the somewhat more conservative DSM-5 criteria will have on the predictive power of early screeners.

In addition to differences in the timing of symptom emergence, recent studies have begun to include other developmental domains, such as fine and gross motor, language, and nonverbal cognitive skills, when characterizing patterns of developmental disturbances. This approach generally yields more classes or models of trajectories [33, 113].

All told, these results suggest that prediction from behaviorally based screening instruments before 12 months to 14 months will be inherently unstable. From about 14 months on, more accurate prediction to later diagnosis is achievable. One important methodological recommendation that can be made with confidence is that when this age group is included in screening studies with older children, separate calculations must be made for the younger participants. If the participant sample includes children up to 24 months and even older, resulting ROC may overestimate prediction from the youngest group.

5. Conclusion

5.1. General Recommendations for Autism and Disability Screening Studies. Table 7 summarizes methodological recommendations for future early screening studies gleaned from all phases of this review, ranging from summaries from the general literature on disability screening as well as autism-specific screening to those generated from the probe questions adapted from the QUADAS system for evidence-based analysis of diagnostic tests, to conclusions gleaned from these specific studies.

5.2. Recommendations for Clinical Use of Very Early ASD Screening Instruments. It is important to consider what clinical practice recommendations can be made from the current evidence. In fact, the evidence base for these early screeners is just being developed and therefore cannot be considered strong. Most of the instruments focused on in this review do have more than one paper that describes development and establishes different features of reliability and validity; all of them have one paper with ROC coefficients for children less than 18 months, as well. Most of these studies have some shortcomings in terms of research quality or else can be viewed as one of several needed to build a case for efficacy.

Given the current strong interest in the earliest identification of ASD, it is likely that more studies will soon add to the evidence base, and there remains a strong rationale for their continued development and conservative use. The growing body of studies around early neurological and information-processing disturbances and their possible link to early emerging behavioral disturbances offer much promise for interventions that interrupt the "developmental cascade" that leads from a prodromal autism pattern to a fully developed ASD presentation [42, 45]. The early screeners reviewed are a starting point for this endeavor and offer the opportunity to monitor children at risk for ASD; in addition, all were shown to detect other developmental delays at about a 50% rate of their false positives. These advantages can be seen to outweigh concerns about overidentification. Another reasonable concern by practitioners may be whether intervention services are available for such early-identified children. Importantly, any child with a significant developmental delay can be referred, evaluated, and possibly provided services by the state-administered public early intervention program. However, for autism-specific services, there is recent emerging documentation for some success with children who are symptomatic at 9–15 months [3, 46], and this will likely continue to be a focus of practice and research.

Recommendations for their use first need to be put in the context of the larger effort of early developmental surveillance for all types of disabilities including ASD.

Table 7: Methodological recommendations for future early autism screening studies.

Domain	Essential study features for interpretability: general for disability and autism screening	Additional criteria for interpretability for screening that targets children under 18 months	Recommended for consistency across studies
Sample/participants	Level 1: large population studies needed; track at least a subset of representative screen negatives to determine true and false negatives so that accurate Se and Sp can be calculated. Report demographic characteristics.		Report inclusion/exclusion criteria related to other risks or other disabilities; consider % of preterm/low birthweight; suggest to exclude significant sensory, motor, and known genetic diagnoses.
	Level 2: smaller (not population level) high-risk samples acceptable. Level 2: include samples matched on cognitive level or compare DD to ASD at outcome. Report demographic characteristics.	Level 2: include samples matched on cognitive level and/or compare DD to ASD on outcomes.	Report inclusion/exclusion criteria related to other risks or other disabilities; see above.
Screening instrument	Make administration of instrument as close as possible to how it would be used in a community setting.		
Reference standard	Evaluations based on DSM criteria; in-person BED preferable. Evaluators must be blind to screening status of participants.		
	24-month-old diagnoses may be unstable in a minority of children; 36-month diagnosis is more reliable.	24-month-old diagnoses may be unstable in a minority of children; 36-month diagnosis is more reliable.	
	Include and define other disability outcomes.		Define other disability outcomes consistently; consider global delay, language delay, typical development, and other disabilities.
Timing and flow	Demonstrate a "clear path" between screening outcomes and scores and reference standard diagnosis. Describe attrition. No study to date has followed children up for diagnosis after the concurrent study age or at age of 3 years. It will be important for future studies to confirm longer-term diagnostic status.		
Evaluation and performance	Important to examine age groups separately; preferably in 6-month groupings up to 3 years of age.	Very important to examine young age groups separately, especially below 12 months versus 12–18 months versus 18–24 months.	Very important to examine young age groups separately, especially below 12 months versus 12–18 months versus 18–24 months.
	Very important to describe developmental level of children detected with screener. Account for different levels of ASD severity. Describe other disability outcomes for false positives.		Very important to describe developmental level of children detected with screener.

This should always be conducted via checking progress on developmental milestones and/or using an evidence-based broadband developmental screener, for example, Ages & Stages Questionnaire, knowing the red flags for developmental delay and early autism behaviors and being responsive any time a caregiver brings up a developmental concern. The recommendations regarding formal screening instruments are necessarily slightly more conservative, given the current practice climate calling for efficient, evidence-based instruments. The recommendation, therefore, is to use one of these instruments at these early ages only if a child falls into one of the risk categories: an older biologic sibling who has been diagnosed with ASD; a child who has already failed a developmental screening, one who has shown behaviors or whose parents have reported behaviors of concern to the health professional; or a child whose parent has expressed a concern over general development or ASD *per se*. The following are also considerations for use. First, each agency or practice may have its own priorities for resource expenditure and instrument administration in light of their capability and clinical flow. Second, the strengths and limitations of the screener should be understood and shared with caregivers. Third, rescreening and monitoring for developmental delays and autism symptoms should take place if results are equivocal and in fact are built into the intended administration strategy of some of the tools. Finally, ideally data can be collected using a sound prospective design or program evaluation approach to add to our knowledge base for the instruments.

Clearly the value of such early detection is to support the family to obtain early intervention as soon as possible, and there is a growing base of evidence for the effectiveness of early intervention. Very relevant to this review, there are now reports about intervention efforts for high-risk children detected with ASD symptoms early in the second year [3, 16, 105]. Given the potential consequences of not acting to build early skills and remediate barriers to more effective cognitive and social learning (more costs to society, less independence and access to full community participation by individuals), acting early with what is available seems prudent.

Acknowledgments

The authors are grateful for the assistance of graduate students participating in the first author's research team while completing their Leadership Education in Neurodevelopmental Disabilities (LEND) fellowship at the Westchester Institute for Human Development. This work was supported, in part, through Grant no. T73MC29073 from the Health Resources and Services Administration and through a subcontract from the Far Fund.

References

[1] M. L. Ganz, "The lifetime distribution of the incremental societal costs of autism," *Archives of Pediatrics and Adolescent Medicine*, vol. 161, no. 4, pp. 343–349, 2007.

[2] D. L. Sharpe and D. L. Baker, "Financial issues associated with having a child with autism," *Journal of Family and Economic Issues*, vol. 28, no. 2, pp. 247–264, 2007.

[3] J. Bradshaw, A. M. Steiner, G. Gengoux, and L. K. Koegel, "Feasibility and effectiveness of very early intervention for infants at-risk for autism spectrum disorder: a systematic review," *Journal of Autism and Developmental Disorders*, vol. 45, no. 3, pp. 778–794, 2015.

[4] V. Eapen, R. Črnčec, and A. Walter, "Clinical outcomes of an early intervention program for preschool children with Autism Spectrum Disorder in a community group setting," *BioMed Central Pediatrics*, vol. 13, no. 1, article 3, 2013.

[5] B. Reichow, "Overview of meta-analyses on early intensive behavioral intervention for young children with autism spectrum disorders," *Journal of Autism and Developmental Disorders*, vol. 42, no. 4, pp. 512–520, 2012.

[6] Centers for Disease Control and Prevention, "Autism and developmental disabilities monitoring network surveillance year 2010. Prevalence of autism spectrum disorders—Autism and Developmental Disabilities Monitoring Network, 11 sites, United States, 2010," *MMWR Surveillance Summary*, vol. 63, no. SS02, pp. 1–21, 2014.

[7] S. J. Spence, P. Sharifi, and M. Wiznitzer, "Autism spectrum disorder: screening, diagnosis, and medical evaluation," *Seminars in Pediatric Neurology*, vol. 11, no. 3, pp. 186–195, 2004.

[8] Centers for Disease Control and Prevention, Learn the Signs. Act Early, 2015, http://www.cdc.gov/ncbddd/actearly.

[9] D. L. Coury, "Babies, bathwater, and screening for autism spectrum disorder: comments on the USPSTF recommendations for autism spectrum disorder screening," *Journal of Developmental and Behavioral Pediatrics*, vol. 36, no. 9, pp. 661–663, 2015.

[10] G. Dawson, "Why it's important to continue universal autism screening while research fully examines its impact," *Journal of the American Medical Association*, vol. 170, no. 6, pp. 527–528, 2016.

[11] L. Zwaigenbaum, M. L. Bauman, D. Fein et al., "Early screening of autism spectrum disorder: recommendations for practice and research," *Pediatrics*, vol. 136, supplement 1, pp. S41–S59, 2015.

[12] American Academy of Pediatrics, Council on Children with Disabilities, Section on Developmental and Behavioral Pediatrics, Bright Futures Steering Committee, and Medical Home Initiatives for Children with Special Needs Project Advisory Committee, "Identifying infants and young children with developmental disorders in the medical home: an algorithm for developmental surveillance and screening," *Pediatrics*, vol. 118, no. 1, pp. 405–420, 2006.

[13] S. Porter, R. Qureshi, B. A. Caldwell, M. Echevarria, W. B. Dubbs, and M. W. Sullivan, "Developmental surveillance and screening practices by pediatric primary care providers: implications for early intervention professionals," *Infants & Young Children*, vol. 29, no. 2, pp. 91–101, 2016.

[14] C. P. Johnson and S. M. Myers, "Identification and evaluation of children with autism spectrum disorders," *Pediatrics*, vol. 120, no. 5, pp. 1183–1215, 2007.

[15] S. Baron-Cohen, S. Wheelwright, A. Cox et al., "Early identification of autism by the Checklist for Autism in Toddlers (CHAT)," *Journal of the Royal Society of Medicine*, vol. 93, no. 10, pp. 521–525, 2000.

[16] F. Soleimani, A. Khakshour, Z. Abasi, S. Khayat, S. Z. Ghaemi, and N. A. H. Golchin, "Review of autism screening tests," *International Journal of Pediatrics*, vol. 2, no. 4, pp. 319–329, 2014.

[17] P. García-Primo, A. Hellendoorn, T. Charman et al., "Screening for autism spectrum disorders: state of the art in Europe," *European Child and Adolescent Psychiatry*, vol. 23, no. 11, pp. 1005–1021, 2014.

[18] D. L. Robins, D. Fein, M. L. Barton, and J. A. Green, "The Modified Checklist for Autism in Toddlers: an initial study investigating the early detection of autism and pervasive developmental disorders," *Journal of Autism and Developmental Disorders*, vol. 31, no. 2, pp. 131–144, 2001.

[19] D. L. Robins, K. Casagrande, M. Barton, C.-M. A. Chen, T. Dumont-Mathieu, and D. Fein, "Validation of the modified checklist for autism in toddlers, revised with follow-up (M-CHAT-R/F)," *Pediatrics*, vol. 133, no. 1, pp. 37–45, 2014.

[20] W. L. Stone, E. E. Coonrod, and O. Y. Ousley, "Brief report: screening tool for autism in two-year-olds (STAT): development and preliminary data," *Journal of Autism and Developmental Disorders*, vol. 30, no. 6, pp. 607–612, 2000.

[21] W. L. Stone, E. E. Coonrod, L. M. Turner, and S. L. Pozdol, "Psychometric properties of the STAT for early autism screening," *Journal of Autism and Developmental Disorders*, vol. 34, no. 6, pp. 691–701, 2004.

[22] L. Zwaigenbaum, S. Bryson, and N. Garon, "Early identification of autism spectrum disorders," *Behavioural Brain Research*, vol. 251, pp. 133–146, 2013.

[23] G. T. Baranek, "Autism during infancy: a retrospective video analysis of sensory-motor and social behaviors at 9–12 months of age," *Journal of Autism and Developmental Disorders*, vol. 29, no. 3, pp. 213–224, 1999.

[24] J. A. Osterling, G. Dawson, and J. A. Munson, "Early recognition of 1-year-old infants with autism spectrum disorder versus mental retardation," *Development and Psychopathology*, vol. 14, no. 2, pp. 239–251, 2002.

[25] E. Werner and G. Dawson, "Validation of the phenomenon of autistic regression using home videotapes," *Archives of General Psychiatry*, vol. 62, no. 8, pp. 889–895, 2005.

[26] C. Saint-Georges, R. S. Cassel, D. Cohen et al., "What studies of family home movies can teach us about autistic infants: a literature review," *Research in Autism Spectrum Disorders*, vol. 4, no. 3, pp. 355–366, 2010.

[27] S. Ozonoff, G. S. Young, A. Carter et al., "Recurrence risk for autism spectrum disorders: a baby siblings research consortium study," *Pediatrics*, vol. 128, no. 3, pp. e488–e495, 2011.

[28] Autism Speaks, Research by the Autism Speaks Baby Siblings Research Consortium, 2013, https://www.autismspeaks.org/science/research-initiatives/high-risk-baby-sibs.

[29] S. J. Rogers, "What are infant siblings teaching us about autism in infancy?" *Autism Research*, vol. 2, no. 3, pp. 125–137, 2009.

[30] S. Ozonoff, A.-M. Iosif, F. Baguio et al., "A prospective study of the emergence of early behavioral signs of autism," *Journal of the American Academy of Child & Adolescent Psychiatry*, vol. 49, no. 3, pp. 256–266, 2010.

[31] H. Tager-Flusberg, "The origins of social impairments in autism spectrum disorder: studies of infants at risk," *Neural Networks*, vol. 23, no. 8-9, pp. 1072–1076, 2010.

[32] P. Szatmari, K. Chawarska, G. Dawson et al., "Prospective longitudinal studies of infant siblings of children with autism: lessons learned and future directions," *Journal of the American Academy of Child & Adolescent Psychiatry*, vol. 55, no. 3, pp. 179–187, 2016.

[33] R. J. Landa, A. L. Gross, E. A. Stuart, and M. Bauman, "Latent class analysis of early developmental trajectory in baby siblings of children with autism," *Journal of Child Psychology and Psychiatry and Allied Disciplines*, vol. 53, no. 9, pp. 986–996, 2012.

[34] A. Estes, L. Zwaigenbaum, H. Gu et al., "Behavioral, cognitive, and adaptive development in infants with autism spectrum disorder in the first 2 years of life," *Journal of Neurodevelopmental Disorders*, vol. 7, no. 1, article 9117, 2015.

[35] M. W. Wan, J. Green, M. Elsabbagh, M. Johnson, T. Charman, and F. Plummer, "Quality of interaction between at-risk infants and caregiver at 12–15 months is associated with 3-year autism outcome," *Journal of Child Psychology and Psychiatry and Allied Disciplines*, vol. 54, no. 7, pp. 763–771, 2013.

[36] R. J. Landa, K. C. Holman, and E. Garrett-Mayer, "Social and communication development in toddlers with early and later diagnosis of autism spectrum disorders," *Archives of General Psychiatry*, vol. 64, no. 7, pp. 853–864, 2007.

[37] J. D. Lewis, A. C. Evans, J. R. Pruett et al., "Inefficiencies in autism spectrum disorder at 24 months," *Translational Psychiatry*, vol. 4, article e388, 2014.

[38] A. S. Masten and D. Cicchetti, "Developmental cascades," *Development and Psychopathology*, vol. 22, no. 3, pp. 491–495, 2010.

[39] A. K. Ami Klin and W. J. Warren Jones, "Measurement and mismeasurement of social development in infants later diagnosed with autism spectrum disorder," *International Journal of Statistics in Medical Research*, vol. 4, no. 2, pp. 180–187, 2015.

[40] K. Chawarska, S. Macari, and F. Shic, "Decreased spontaneous attention to social scenes in 6-month-old infants later diagnosed with autism spectrum disorders," *Biological Psychiatry*, vol. 74, no. 3, pp. 195–203, 2013.

[41] J. J. LeBlanc and M. Fagiolini, "Autism: a 'critical period' disorder?" *Neural Plasticity*, vol. 2011, Article ID 921680, 17 pages, 2011.

[42] G. Dawson, "Early behavioral intervention, brain plasticity, and the prevention of autism spectrum disorder," *Development and Psychopathology*, vol. 20, no. 3, pp. 775–803, 2008.

[43] M. H. Johnson, T. Grossmann, and K. C. Kadosh, "Mapping functional brain development: building a social brain through interactive specialization," *Developmental Psychology*, vol. 45, no. 1, pp. 151–159, 2009.

[44] C. A. Nelson, M. de Haan, and K. M. Thomas, *Neuroscience of Cognitive Development: The Role of Experience and the Developing Brain*, John Wiley & Sons, Inc, Hoboken, NJ, USA, 2015.

[45] J. A. Brian, S. E. Bryson, and L. Zwaigenbaum, "Autism spectrum disorder in infancy: developmental considerations in treatment targets," *Current Opinion in Neurology*, vol. 28, no. 2, pp. 117–123, 2015.

[46] S. J. Rogers, L. Vismara, A. L. Wagner, C. McCormick, G. Young, and S. Ozonoff, "Autism treatment in the first year of life: a pilot study of infant start, a parent-implemented intervention for symptomatic infants," *Journal of Autism and Developmental Disorders*, vol. 44, no. 12, pp. 2981–2995, 2014.

[47] L. R. Watson, E. R. Crais, G. T. Baranek, J. R. Dykstra, and K. P. Wilson, "Communicative gesture use in infants with and without autism: A Retrospective Home Video Study," *American Journal of Speech-Language Pathology*, vol. 22, no. 1, pp. 25–39, 2013.

[48] F. P. Glascoe, "Developmental screening: rationale, methods, and application," *Infants and Young Children*, vol. 4, no. 1, pp. 1–10, 1991.

[49] E. Plante and R. Vance, "Selection of preschool language tests: a data based approach," *Language, Speech, and Hearing Services in Schools*, vol. 25, no. 1, pp. 15–24, 1994.

[50] J. K. Squires, "Identifying social/emotional and behavioral problems in infants and toddlers," *Infant-Toddler Intervention*, vol. 10, no. 2, pp. 107–119, 2000.

[51] P. F. Whiting, A. W. S. Rutjes, M. E. Westwood et al., "Quadas-2: a revised tool for the quality assessment of diagnostic accuracy studies," *Annals of Internal Medicine*, vol. 155, no. 8, pp. 529–536, 2011.

[52] S. Gates, L. A. Smith, J. D. Fisher, and S. E. Lamb, "Systematic review of accuracy of screening instruments for predicting fall risk among independently living older adults," *Journal of Rehabilitation Research and Development*, vol. 45, no. 8, pp. 1105–1116, 2008.

[53] S. D. McDonald, W. L. Brown, J. P. Benesek, and P. S. Calhoun, "A systematic review of the PTSD Checklist's diagnostic accuracy studies using QUADAS," *Psychological Trauma: Theory, Research, Practice, and Policy*, vol. 7, no. 5, pp. 413–421, 2015.

[54] A. McGovern, S. T. Pendlebury, N. K. Mishra, Y. Fan, and T. J. Quinn, "Test accuracy of informant-based cognitive screening tests for diagnosis of dementia and multidomain cognitive impairment in stroke," *Stroke*, vol. 47, no. 2, pp. 329–335, 2016.

[55] M. J. Stout, S. N. Conner, G. A. Colditz, G. A. Macones, and M. G. Tuuli, "The utility of 12-hour urine collection for the diagnosis of preeclampsia: a systematic review and meta-analysis," *Obstetrics & Gynecology*, vol. 126, no. 4, pp. 731–736, 2015.

[56] M. N. Plana, J. Zamora, G. Suresh, L. Fernandez-Pineda, S. Thangaratinam, and A. K. Ewer, "Diagnostic accuracy of pulse oximetry screening for critical congenital heart defects (protocol)," in *The Cochrane Library*, vol. 10, John Wiley & Sons, Chichester, UK, 2015.

[57] P. S. Fontela, N. P. Pai, I. Schiller, N. Dendukuri, A. Ramsay, and M. Pai, "Quality and reporting of diagnostic accuracy studies in TB, HIV and malaria: evaluation using QUADAS and STARD standards," *PLoS ONE*, vol. 4, no. 11, Article ID e7753, 2009.

[58] American Psychiatric Association, *Diagnostic and Statistical Manual of Mental Disorders*, American Psychiatric Association,, American Psychiatric, Washington, DC, USA, 4th edition, 2000.

[59] K. Pierce, C. Carter, M. Weinfeld et al., "Detecting, studying, and treating autism early: the one-year well-baby check-up approach," *Journal of Pediatrics*, vol. 159, no. 3, pp. 458–465, 2011.

[60] L. M. Turner-Brown, G. T. Baranek, J. S. Reznick, L. R. Watson, and E. R. Crais, "The first year inventory: a longitudinal follow-up of 12-month-old to 3-year-old children," *Autism*, vol. 17, no. 5, pp. 527–540, 2013.

[61] W. L. Stone, C. R. Mcmahon, and L. M. Henderson, "Use of the screening tool for autism in two-year-olds (stat) for children under 24 months: An Exploratory Study," *Autism*, vol. 12, no. 5, pp. 557–573, 2008.

[62] M. A. Feldman, R. A. Ward, D. Savona et al., "Development and initial validation of a parent report measure of the behavioral development of infants at risk for autism spectrum disorders," *Journal of Autism and Developmental Disorders*, vol. 42, no. 1, pp. 13–22, 2012.

[63] Y.-H. Nah, R. L. Young, N. Brewer, and G. Berlingeri, "Autism detection in early childhood (ADEC): reliability and validity data for a level 2 screening tool for autistic disorder," *Psychological Assessment*, vol. 26, no. 1, pp. 215–226, 2014.

[64] C. Dietz, S. Swinkels, E. van Daalen, H. van Engeland, and J. K. Buitelaar, "Screening for autistic spectrum disorder in children aged 14-15 months. II: population screening with the Early Screening of Autistic Traits Questionnaire (ESAT). Design and general findings," *Journal of Autism and Developmental Disorders*, vol. 36, no. 6, pp. 713–722, 2006.

[65] S. H. N. Swinkels, C. Dietz, E. Van Daalen, I. H. G. M. Kerkhof, H. Van Engeland, and J. K. Buitelaar, "Screening for autistic spectrum in children aged 14 to 15 months. I: the development of the Early Screening of Autistic Traits Questionnaire (ESAT)," *Journal of Autism and Developmental Disorders*, vol. 36, no. 6, pp. 723–732, 2006.

[66] M. Dereu, P. Warreyn, R. Raymaekers et al., "Screening for autism spectrum disorders in Flemish day-care centres with the checklist for early signs of developmental disorders," *Journal of Autism and Developmental Disorders*, vol. 40, no. 10, pp. 1247–1258, 2010.

[67] A. M. Wetherby, S. Brosnan-Maddox, V. Peace, and L. Newton, "Validation of the Infant-Toddler Checklist as a broadband screener for autism spectrum disorders from 9 to 24 months of age," *Autism*, vol. 12, no. 5, pp. 487–511, 2008.

[68] B. Siegel, *Pervasive Developmental Disorders Screening Test—II (PDDST-II): Early Childhood Screeners for Autistic Spectrum Disorders*, Harcourt Assessment, San Antonio, Tex, USA, 2004.

[69] I. J. Oosterling, S. H. Swinkels, R. J. van der Gaag, J. C. Visser, C. Dietz, and J. K. Buitelaar, "Comparative analysis of three screening instruments for autism spectrum disorder in toddlers at high risk," *Journal of Autism and Developmental Disorders*, vol. 39, no. 6, pp. 897–909, 2009.

[70] M. Rutter, A. Bailey, and C. Lord, *The Social Communication Questionnaire*, Western Psychological Services, Los Angeles, Calif, USA, 2003.

[71] A. M. Wetherby and B. M. Prizant, *Communication and Symbolic Behavior Scales-Developmental Profile*, Brookes Publishing, Baltimore, Md, USA, 1st edition, 2002.

[72] M. Dereu, R. Raymaekers, P. Warreyn, I. Schietecatte, M. Meirsschaut, and H. Roeyers, "Can child care workers contribute to the early detection of autism spectrum disorders? A comparison between screening instruments with child care workers versus parents as informants," *Journal of Autism and Developmental Disorders*, vol. 42, no. 5, pp. 781–796, 2012.

[73] L. Fenson, V. A. Marchman, D. Thal, P. S. Dale, J. S. Reznick, and E. Bates, *MacArthur-Bates Communicative Development Inventories: User's Guide and Technical Manual*, Brookes Publishing, Baltimore, Md, USA, 2006.

[74] A. M. Wetherby and B. M. Prizant, *Communication and Symbolic Behavior Scales*, Brookes Publishing Co, Baltimore, Md, USA, 1993.

[75] A. M. Wetherby, H. Goldstein, J. Cleary, L. Allen, and K. Kublin, "Early identification of children with communication disorders: concurrent and predictive validity of the CSBS developmental profile," *Infants and Young Children*, vol. 16, no. 2, pp. 161–174, 2003.

[76] A. M. Wetherby, J. Woods, L. Allen, J. Cleary, H. Dickinson, and C. Lord, "Early indicators of autism spectrum disorders in the second year of life," *Journal of Autism and Developmental Disorders*, vol. 34, no. 5, pp. 473–493, 2004.

[77] M. Tomasello and M. J. Farrar, "Joint attention and early language," *Child Development*, vol. 57, no. 6, pp. 1454–1463, 1986.

[78] E. Bates, B. O'Connell, and C. Shore, "Language and communication in infancy," in *Handbook of Infant Development*, J. Osofsky, Ed., John Wiley & Sons, New York, NY, USA, 1987.

[79] E. Z. Tronick, "Emotions and emotional communication in infants," *American Psychologist*, vol. 44, no. 2, pp. 112–119, 1989.

[80] J. S. Reznick, G. T. Baranek, S. Reavis, L. R. Watson, and E. R. Crais, "A parent-report instrument for identifying one-year-olds at risk for an eventual diagnosis of autism: the first year inventory," *Journal of Autism and Developmental Disorders*, vol. 37, no. 9, pp. 1691–1710, 2007.

[81] L. R. Watson, G. T. Baranek, E. R. Crais, J. S. Reznick, J. Dykstra, and T. Perryman, "The First Year Inventory: retrospective parent responses to a questionnaire designed to identify one-year-olds at risk for autism," *Journal of Autism and Developmental Disorders*, vol. 37, no. 1, pp. 49–61, 2007.

[82] J. Rowberry, S. Macari, G. Chen et al., "Screening for autism spectrum disorders in 12-month-old high-risk siblings by parental report," *Journal of Autism and Developmental Disorders*, vol. 45, no. 1, pp. 221–229, 2014.

[83] A. Ben-Sasson, S. Habib, and E. Tirosh, "Feasibility and validity of early screening for identifying infants with poor social-communication development in a well-baby clinic system," *Journal of Pediatric Nursing*, vol. 29, no. 3, pp. 238–247, 2014.

[84] A. Guy, S. E. Seaton, E. M. Boyle et al., "Infants born late/moderately preterm are at increased risk for a positive autism screen at 2 years of age," *Journal of Pediatrics*, vol. 166, no. 2, pp. 269–275, 2015.

[85] S. Sandin, A. Kolevzon, S. Z. Levine, C. M. Hultman, and A. Reichenberg, "Parental and perinatal risk factors for autism: epidemiological findings and potential mechanisms," in *The Neuroscience of Autism Spectrum Disorders*, J. D. Buxbaum and P. R. Hof, Eds., Elsevier Academic Press, Waltham, Mass, USA, 2013.

[86] G. B. Schaefer and N. J. Mendelsohn, "Clinical genetics evaluation in identifying the etiology of autism spectrum disorders: 2013 guideline revisions," *Genetics in Medicine*, vol. 15, no. 5, pp. 399–407, 2013.

[87] J. Moss and P. Howlin, "Autism spectrum disorders in genetic syndromes: implications for diagnosis, intervention and understanding the wider autism spectrum disorder population," *Journal of Intellectual Disability Research*, vol. 53, no. 10, pp. 852–873, 2009.

[88] S. E. Bryson, L. Zwaigenbaum, C. McDermott, V. Rombough, and J. Brian, "The autism observation scale for infants: scale development and reliability data," *Journal of Autism and Developmental Disorders*, vol. 38, no. 4, pp. 731–738, 2008.

[89] S. E. Bryson and L. Zwaigenbaum, "Autism observation scale for infants," in *Comprehensive Guide to Autism*, V. B. Patel, V. R. Preedy, and C. R. Martin, Eds., pp. 299–310, Springer, New York, NY, USA, 2014.

[90] C.-H. Chiang, C.-C. Wu, Y.-M. Hou, C.-L. Chu, J.-H. Liu, and W.-T. Soong, "Development of T-STAT for early autism screening," *Journal of Autism and Developmental Disorders*, vol. 43, no. 5, pp. 1028–1037, 2013.

[91] M. A. Feldman, A. M. Hendry, R. A. Ward, M. Hudson, and X. Liu, "Behavioral development and sociodemographics of infants and young children at higher and lower risk for autism spectrum disorders," *Journal of Autism and Developmental Disorders*, vol. 45, no. 5, pp. 1167–1175, 2015.

[92] C. Lord, M. Rutter, and A. Le Couteur, "Autism Diagnostic Interview-Revised: a revised version of a diagnostic interview for caregivers of individuals with possible pervasive developmental disorders," *Journal of Autism and Developmental Disorders*, vol. 24, no. 5, pp. 659–685, 1994.

[93] E. Schopler, R. J. Reichler, and B. R. Renner, *The Childhood Autism Rating Scale*, Western Psychological Services, Los Angeles, Calif, USA, 1988.

[94] R. L. Young, *Autism Detection in Early Childhood: ADEC*, Australian Council for Educational Research, Camberwell, Australia, 2007.

[95] D. Hedley, R. Young, M. Angelica, J. Gallegos, and C. M. Salazar, "Cross-cultural evaluation of the Autism Detection in Early Childhood (ADEC) in Mexico," *Autism*, vol. 14, no. 2, pp. 93–112, 2010.

[96] Y.-H. Nah, R. L. Young, and N. Brewer, "Using the Autism Detection in Early Childhood (ADEC) and Childhood Autism Rating Scales (CARS) to predict long term outcomes in children with autism spectrum disorders," *Journal of Autism and Developmental Disorders*, vol. 44, no. 9, pp. 2301–2310, 2014.

[97] D. Hedley, R. E. Nevill, Y. Monroy-Moreno et al., "Efficacy of the ADEC in identifying autism spectrum disorder in clinically referred toddlers in the US," *Journal of Autism and Developmental Disorders*, vol. 45, no. 8, pp. 2337–2348, 2015.

[98] R. L. Young, N. Brewer, and C. Pattison, "Parental identification of early behavioural abnormalities in children with autistic disorder," *Autism*, vol. 7, no. 2, pp. 125–143, 2003.

[99] S. Clifford, R. Young, and P. Williamson, "Assessing the early characteristics of autistic disorder using video analysis," *Journal of Autism and Developmental Disorders*, vol. 37, no. 2, pp. 301–313, 2007.

[100] J. Brian, S. E. Bryson, N. Garon et al., "Clinical assessment of autism in high-risk 18-month-olds," *Autism*, vol. 12, no. 5, pp. 433–456, 2008.

[101] D. L. Robins and T. M. Dumont-Mathieu, "Early screening for autism spectrum disorders: update on the modified checklist for autism in toddlers and other measures," *Journal of Developmental and Behavioral Pediatrics*, vol. 27, no. 2, pp. S111–S119, 2006.

[102] S. Ozonoff, A.-M. Iosif, G. S. Young et al., "Onset patterns in autism: correspondence between home video and parent report," *Journal of the American Academy of Child and Adolescent Psychiatry*, vol. 50, no. 8, pp. 796–806, 2011.

[103] P. Howlin and A. Asgharian, "The diagnosis of autism and Asperger syndrome: findings from a survey of 770 families," *Developmental Medicine and Child Neurology*, vol. 41, no. 12, pp. 834–839, 1999.

[104] R. J. Landa, A. L. Gross, E. A. Stuart, and A. Faherty, "Developmental trajectories in children with and without autism spectrum disorders: the first 3 years," *Child Development*, vol. 84, no. 2, pp. 429–442, 2013.

[105] L. Zwaigenbaum, S. Bryson, T. Rogers, W. Roberts, J. Brian, and P. Szatmari, "Behavioral manifestations of autism in the first year of life," *International Journal of Developmental Neuroscience*, vol. 23, no. 2-3, pp. 143–152, 2005.

[106] S. Ozonoff, S. Macari, G. S. Young, S. Goldring, M. Thompson, and S. J. Rogers, "Atypical object exploration at 12 months of age is associated with autism in a prospective sample," *Autism*, vol. 12, no. 5, pp. 457–472, 2008.

[107] J. J. Wolff, K. N. Botteron, S. R. Dager et al., "Longitudinal patterns of repetitive behavior in toddlers with autism," *Journal of Child Psychology and Psychiatry*, vol. 55, no. 8, pp. 945–953, 2014.

[108] V. Moore and S. Goodson, "How well does early diagnosis of autism stand the test of time? Follow-up study of children assessed for autism at age 2 and development of an early diagnostic service," *Autism*, vol. 7, no. 1, pp. 47–63, 2003.

[109] W. Guthrie, L. B. Swineford, C. Nottke, and A. M. Wetherby, "Early diagnosis of autism spectrum disorder: stability and change in clinical diagnosis and symptom presentation," *Journal*

of Child Psychology and Psychiatry and Allied Disciplines, vol. 54, no. 5, pp. 582–590, 2013.

[110] W. L. Stone, E. B. Lee, L. Ashford et al., "Can autism be diagnosed accurately in children under 3 years?" *Journal of Child Psychology and Psychiatry*, vol. 40, no. 2, pp. 219–226, 1999.

[111] S. Ozonoff, G. S. Young, R. J. Landa et al., "Diagnostic stability in young children at risk for autism spectrum disorder: a baby siblings research consortium study," *Journal of Child Psychology and Psychiatry and Allied Disciplines*, vol. 56, no. 9, pp. 988–998, 2015.

[112] American Psychiatric Association, *Diagnostic and Statistical Manual of Mental Disorders*, American Psychiatric Association, Arlington, Va, USA, 5th edition, 2013.

[113] S. L. Macari, D. Campbell, G. W. Gengoux, C. A. Saulnier, A. J. Klin, and K. Chawarska, "Predicting developmental status from 12 to 24 months in infants at risk for autism spectrum disorder: a preliminary report," *Journal of Autism and Developmental Disorders*, vol. 42, no. 12, pp. 2636–2647, 2012.

18

Neuropsychological Characteristics of Children with Mixed Autism and ADHD

Costanza Colombi and Mohammad Ghaziuddin

University of Michigan, Ann Arbor, MI, USA

Correspondence should be addressed to Costanza Colombi; ccolombi@umich.edu

Academic Editor: Roberto Canitano

Clinical heterogeneity is a well-established characteristic of autism spectrum disorder (ASD). While the comorbidity of ASD and ADHD is well known in clinical practice, relatively little research has examined the neuropsychological profile of children with ASD + ADHD. Our study showed significant differences in the neuropsychological characteristics of children with ASD + ADHD compared to those with ASD only. Children with ASD + ADHD showed higher symptoms of anxiety, worse working memory, and less empathy, as measured by the "Reading the Mind in the Eyes." This suggests that having ADHD brings further challenges to individuals with ASD and may negatively impact their management and outcome. Our findings may have implications for clinical assessment as well as for intervention.

1. Introduction

Clinical heterogeneity is a well-established characteristic of autism spectrum disorder (ASD). In addition to the core features of social communication impairment and restricted/repetitive behaviors and interests, a large number of children with ASD present with the symptoms of hyperactivity, inattention, and impulsivity, which may be severe enough to merit an additional diagnosis of attention deficit hyperactivity disorder (ADHD) [1]. Although the DSM-IV-TR [2] did not allow for a diagnosis of ADHD in individuals with ASD, reports about the comorbidity between the two conditions started appearing soon after its publication [3]. Recent studies have confirmed the initial reports. Goldstein and Schwebach [4] found that 16 (59%) of 37 individuals with ASD met DSM-IV criteria for a diagnosis of ADHD. Ogino et al. [5] reported the presence of ADHD in 6 (37.5%) of a sample of 16 individuals with ASD. Keen and Ward [6] found comorbidity of ASD and ADHD in 27 (13.7%) of a sample of 196 individuals. Siminoff et al. (2008) in a community-based study conducted in the UK found that approximately a third of participants with ASD presented with additional ADHD. Miodovnik et al. [7] in an epidemiological study involving 1496 children with ASD found that 20% of the participants had received a diagnosis of ADHD prior to the diagnosis of ASD. Fewer studies have examined the occurrence of autistic symptoms in persons with ADHD because most studies of ADHD tend to exclude subjects with autism and/or intellectual disability. While exact figures are difficult to estimate, a large number of children with ADHD also present with symptoms of ASD [8, 9]. In addition to the comorbidity between the two conditions, reports have also suggested a possible overlap in their symptoms [7].

It is crucial to identify the comorbidity between ASD and ADHD because of its treatment implications. For example, compared with children with ADHD only, those with ADHD and ASD symptoms have a lower adaptive functioning and a poorer quality of life [10, 11]. In addition, children with ADHD and ASD symptoms, compared with those with ADHD only, tend to be prescribed more medications [12] and respond less to stimulants [13] and may respond better to alternative agents such as atomoxetine (Harterftkamp et al., 2014).

However, despite the group differences reported in the literature, it can be extremely difficult to differentiate between ASD and ADHD in individual cases. Historical data and presentation of symptoms may not be helpful. For example, social deficits occur in both the disorders. Although the social deficits of autism are typically described as being "reciprocal" in nature resulting from an inborn lack of "affective contact" [14] and those of ADHD are said to be the result of inattention and distractibility, the distinction is not always easy to make in clinical practice. Rating scales and observation schedules also are of limited value especially when hyperactivity and impulsivity are marked.

In such cases, a careful evaluation of the neuropsychological characteristics may be helpful in identifying the comorbidity of ASD and ADHD. Cognitive profiles of individuals with ASD and those with ADHD are well described. For example, in a rigorous study of high functioning individuals with ASD, Wilson et al. [15] found that, compared to typically developing individuals, subjects with autism showed deficits in social cognition, executive function, and motor performance. On the other hand, individuals with ADHD consistently showed deficits in their working memory (Merkt et al., 2014), while facial emotion and mental states recognition was impaired in persons with ASD. Thus, individuals with ASD consistently perform worse than control subjects on the "Reading the Mind in the Eyes" Test (Eyes Test) (Golan and Baron-Cohen, 2006; Lombardo et al., 2007; Baron-Cohen et al., 2011), which is an advanced task to assess Theory of Mind, an index of facial emotion recognition and mental states attribution. While the Eyes Test has not been used in ADHD, many accounts report difficulties in emotion recognition in individuals with ADHD [16, 17]. Some authors have suggested that affect processing impairments in ADHD are due to difficulties in emotion recognition rather than to deficits in attention and inhibition [18].

Limited research has been done on the neuropsychological characteristics of individuals with ASD + ADHD. Some authors have suggested that those with ASD + ADHD show an "additive profile" rather than a qualitatively different set of difficulties compared with those with ASD only (Antshel et al., 2015). For example, Andersen et al. [19] found that children with ASD + ADHD were more impaired on verbal working memory than children with ASD only and those with ADHD only. In an investigation of attention and inhibition, Tye and others [20] found that ASD + ADHD children had impairments in all domains evaluated, while ASD children presented difficulties in response preparation and conflict monitoring only and ADHD children presented abnormalities in omission errors and reaction time. The aim of our study was to extend the work on the neuropsychological profile of individuals with ASD + ADHD and to explore the hypothesis that subjects with ASD + ADHD show higher degrees of impairment in social cognition than those with ASD only.

2. Methods

2.1. Participants. The study was conducted at the Department of Psychiatry, University of Michigan, and approved by the Institutional Review Board (HUM00008815). The participants, drawn from referrals to the ASD Clinic, consisted of 22 children with ASD and 25 children with mixed ASD and ADHD. The demographics are presented in Table 1.

Table 1: Background information.

Variable	ASD Mean (SD)	ASD + ADHD Mean (ASD)	F	p
Age	10.9 (3.6)	9.8 (2.2)	6.08	0.21
FIQ	91.5 (18.8)	90.8 (15.6)	0.56	0.89
VIQ	96.2 (21.6)	95.7 (15.4)	2.21	0.92
PIQ	94.2 (18.7)	97.2 (16.6)	1.23	0.56

The diagnosis of ASD, based on the DSM-IV [2], was reached after a comprehensive evaluation by a multidisciplinary team consisting, among others, of a board-certified child/adolescent psychiatrist, a neuropsychologist, a speech pathologist, a social worker, and a fellow in child psychiatry. Both parents/caregivers and the participant were directly interviewed. In addition to the clinical interview, supplemental information was obtained from the case-notes, medical records, and school reports. Additional diagnostic information was obtained on the basis of the Autism Diagnostic Interview-Revised (ADI-R, [21]). The subtypes of DSM-IV PDD were collapsed together to form a single category. For the diagnosis of additional ADHD, the participant had to meet the DSM-IV criteria of ADHD [2]. As in the diagnosis of ASD, the subtypes of DSM-IV ADHD were collapsed into a single category. From both the groups, participants with known genetic conditions and/or marked sensory deficits were excluded. All children had to have a Full Scale IQ of at least 70 to be eligible to participate.

2.2. Procedure. Neuropsychological measures were administrated using standardized procedures. Measures, based on the main ASD deficits identified in the scientific literature, evaluated cognitive level of functioning, emotion recognition, Theory of Mind, executive functions, and motor abilities. The following measures were administered.

The Wechsler Intelligence Scale for Children, 4th Edition (WISC IV). It includes 10 subtests, yielding four index scores that combine into the Full Scale IQ (FSIQ). The Verbal Comprehension Index (VCI) consists of three subtests (Similarities, Comprehension, and Vocabulary). The Perceptual Reasoning Index (PRI) comprises Block Design, Matrix Reasoning, and Picture Concepts. The Working Memory Index (WMI) comprises Digit Span and Letter-Number Sequencing. The Processing Speed Index (PSI) comprises Coding and Symbol Search. Index standard scores have a mean of 100 and a standard deviation of 15.

Trail Making Test. The Trail Making Test (TMT) [22] is a visuomotor task used to measure sustained visual attention and psychomotor speed. TMT part A requires the participant to rapidly draw lines to connect consecutively numbered circles on one worksheet. TMT part B requires connecting the same number of consecutively numbered and lettered circles by alternating between the two sets, which involves frequent switching between two mental sets.

Tower of London. The Tower of London (TOL; Shallice 1982) measures planning and problem solving performance. The mechanical version of the TOL used in this study consists of two identical wooden game boards, one for the participants and one for the examiner. Each game board includes three different size pegs and three different colored balls. The participant needs to move the balls on the pegs to match the examiner's game board in the minimum number of moves.

The Strange Stories Task [23]. It consists of vignettes depicting social situations. The task requires the participant to explain a character's behavior with reference to his or her mental states. This is a measure of Theory of Mind.

Reading the Mind in the Eyes, Revised Version [24]. The revised version of the Eyes Test [24] consists of 36 black-and-white photographs of the eye region. Each trial requires the participant to choose among four descriptors related to the feelings of the person in the picture. This test is considered a measure of Theory of Mind.

The Child Behavior Checklist (CBCL) [25]. It is a measure assessing disruptive behavior and social competency in children. Caregivers of the participants completed the Child Behavior Checklist (CBCL). We used the CBCL to confirm ADHD symptoms.

2.3. Statistical Analysis. Statistical analyses were performed using the IBM SPSS Statistics software (Version 23). We first performed independent samples t-tests comparing the two groups in terms of age and IQ. We then performed univariate analyses of covariance (ANCOVAs), comparing the two groups while including IQ as a continuous covariate, for the following dependent variables: working memory, Children's Color Trail Test, Tower of London, Category Fluency Test, Happe's Stories, and Reading the Mind in the Eyes Test.

3. Results

Descriptive statistics for the two groups are reported in Table 1. Means and standard deviations for the experimental measures are reported in Table 2. The independent samples t-tests showed that the two groups did not differ in terms of mean age, mean Full Scale IQ, mean Verbal IQ, and mean Performance IQ. ADHD symptoms ($t = -2.19$; $p = 0.03$) and anxiety symptoms ($t = -1.95$; $p = 0.05$), as measured by the CBCL, were higher in the group of children with ASD + ADHD compared with the ASD only group. Based on the results of the ANCOVAs, there was a significant difference between the two groups in working memory ($F(1, 34) = 4.52$; $p = 0.041$), with the ASD only group having a significantly higher mean when holding FIQ fixed, indicating that children with ASD + ADHD present more impairment in working memory. Additionally, there was a marginally significant difference in the Reading the Mind in the Eyes Test ($F(1, 44) = 3.44$, $p = 0.07$), with the ASD only group having a marginally higher mean when controlling for FIQ, indicating that the ASD + ADHD group present slightly higher difficulties in the Eyes Test. The Trail Making Test, Tower of London, Category Fluency Test, and Happe's Stories did not show significant differences between the groups.

TABLE 2: Means and standard deviations for the experimental measures.

Variable	ASD Mean (SD)	ASD + ADHD Mean (SD)	F	p
Working memory	93.00 (13.66)	85.78 (13.09)	4.5	0.04
Trail A	40.00 (18.43)	42.68 (14.27)	0.80	0.37
Trail B	46.75 (20.76)	45.22 (11.54)	0.15	0.69
TOL	51.20 (18.25)	52.30 (9.63)	0.37	0.54
Categories	51.23 (11.86)	48.70 (10.51)	0.55	0.46
Stories	5.86 (4.07)	5.39 (3.66)	0.09	0.75
Eyes	15.95 (3.28)	14.00 (3.98)	3.43	0.07
Anxiety (CBCL)	59.87 (10.21)	65.57 (7.49)	3.74	0.05
Withdrawal (CBCL)	62.81 (10.28)	65.71 (9.93)	−0.86	0.39
Attention (CBCL)	64.50 (11.20)	72.09 (9.78)	−2.19	0.03
Social (CBCL)	63.75 (12.10)	67.42 (9.26)	−1.04	0.30

4. Discussion

In 1902, about 50 years before Leo Kanner described autism, George Still laid down the main characteristics of the condition that later came to be known as ADHD (see Goldstein, 2006). While Kanner did not describe the comorbid disorders his eleven patients suffered from, a close reading of his seminal paper suggests that at least a few of them seemed to show symptoms that would today be diagnosed as ADHD. Before the DSM-5 [26] was published, it was believed that the two diagnoses of ASD and ADHD were mutually exclusive. The diagnosis of ADHD could not be given in persons with ASD on the assumption that symptoms of inattention and hyperactivity were rather common in those with autism resulting in artefactual comorbidity. However, research in the last two decades has established that despite the seeming overlap between the symptoms of the two disorders and the challenges of diagnosing ADHD in some patients with ASD, such as those with severe intellectual disability (mental retardation), there does seem to exist a subgroup of patients who have both the disorders based on behavioral features. The results of this study provide preliminary neuropsychological evidence of the existence of this patient group.

The main finding of this study is that compared with children who have ASD only those who have ASD + ADHD are more impaired in their ability to read other people's emotions and feelings ("Reading the Mind in the Eyes Test") and to hold and manipulate critical periods of information ("working memory"). Thus, when we compared the neuropsychological profiles of 22 children with ASD only with those of 25 children with ASD + ADHD, we found significant differences between the two groups. Working memory was significantly more impaired in children with additional ADHD. Moreover, a marginally significant difference was identified in the Eyes Test, indicating that children with ASD + ADHD may have more difficulties in emotion recognition. Regarding behavioral symptoms, children with ASD + ADHD showed higher levels of anxiety in line with other studies [19, 20]; however, we did not identify qualitative differences in the profiles of the two groups. The worse performance in working memory and in emotion recognition, along with the higher levels of anxiety found in individuals with ASD + ADHD, supports the hypothesis that having additional ADHD increases the level of their impairment and negatively impacts their management and outcome.

It is to be noted that the sample consisted only of those with normal level of intelligence. Therefore, the findings may not apply to lower functioning children with ASD and ADHD. The risk of intellectual disability (ID) increases the risk of both ASD and ADHD, acting alone and in combination with other factors. Indeed, diagnosing the two conditions in those with severe and profound intellectual disability is extremely difficult. Since working memory is impaired in those with ID [27], it can be speculated that lower functioning children with ASD and ADHD are more impaired in measures of social cognition than those with normal intelligence. Future studies should examine the effect of decreasing IQ on ASD children with comorbid ADHD. Other limitations of the study also need to be considered when interpreting our results. Thus, it is possible that the performance was affected by tiredness in our participants due to the large test battery administered. Finally, the size of our sample may have failed to identify differences.

In summary, identifying symptoms of ADHD in children with ASD has important diagnostic and treatment implications. However, a reliable diagnosis based only on developmental history and clinical observation is not always possible. Examining the cognitive and neuropsychological deficits in children with both the conditions can facilitate their diagnosis and inform treatment. Our results also confirm the greater overall impairment in children with ASD plus ADHD as indexed by their performance on tests of social cognition. Further studies in subjects with a wider range of cognitive abilities, using larger sample sizes of different age groups, should be undertaken to better define the profiles of individuals with ASD + ADHD and identify effective pharmacological and behavioral interventions.

Disclosure

Portions of this study were presented at the 2016 International Meeting for Autism Research (IMFAR).

Acknowledgments

The authors thank the children who participated in the study.

References

[1] S. D. Mayes, S. L. Calhoun, R. D. Mayes, and S. Molitoris, "Autism and ADHD: Overlapping and discriminating symptoms," *Research in Autism Spectrum Disorders*, vol. 6, no. 1, pp. 277–285, 2012.

[2] American Psychiatric Association, *Diagnostic and Statistical Manual of Mental Disorders: DSM-IV-TR*, American Psychiatric Association, Washington, DC, USA, 4th edition, 2000.

[3] M. Ghaziuddin, E. Weidmer-Mikhail, and N. Ghaziuddin, "Comorbidity of Asperger syndrome: a preliminary report," *Journal of Intellectual Disability Research*, vol. 42, no. 4, pp. 279–283, 1998.

[4] S. Goldstein and A. J. Schwebach, "The comorbidity of pervasive developmental disorder and attention deficit hyperactivity disorder: Results of a retrospective chart review," *Journal of Autism and Developmental Disorders*, vol. 34, no. 3, pp. 329–339, 2004.

[5] T. Ogino, J. Hattori, K. Abiru, K. Nakano, E. Oka, and Y. Ohtsuka, "Symptoms related to ADHD observed in patients with pervasive developmental disorder," *Brain & Development*, vol. 27, no. 5, pp. 345–348, 2005.

[6] D. Keen and S. Ward, "Autistic spectrum disorder: a child population profile," *Autism*, vol. 8, no. 1, pp. 39–48, 2004.

[7] A. Miodovnik, E. Harstad, G. Sideridis, and N. Huntington, "Timing of the diagnosis of attention-deficit/hyperactivity disorder and autism spectrum disorder," *Pediatrics*, vol. 136, no. 4, pp. e830–e837, 2015.

[8] A. Mulligan, R. J. L. Anney, M. O'Regan et al., "Autism symptoms in Attention-Deficit/Hyperactivity Disorder: a familial trait which correlates with conduct, oppositional defiant, language and motor disorders," *Journal of Autism and Developmental Disorders*, vol. 39, no. 2, pp. 197–209, 2009.

[9] E. Staikova, H. Gomes, V. Tartter, A. McCabe, and J. M. Halperin, "Pragmatic deficits and social impairment in children with ADHD," *Journal of Child Psychology and Psychiatry and Allied Disciplines*, vol. 54, no. 12, pp. 1275–1283, 2013.

[10] K. D. Gadow, C. J. Devincent, and J. Schneider, "Comparative study of children with ADHD only, autism spectrum disorder + ADHD, and chronic multiple tic disorder + ADHD," *Journal of Attention Disorders*, vol. 12, no. 5, pp. 474–485, 2009.

[11] S. Guttmann-Steinmetz, K. D. Gadow, and C. J. Devincent, "Oppositional defiant and conduct disorder behaviors in boys with autism spectrum disorder with and without attention-deficit hyperactivity disorder versus several comparison samples," *Journal of Autism and Developmental Disorders*, vol. 39, no. 7, pp. 976–985, 2009.

[12] T. W. Frazier, P. T. Shattuck, S. C. Narendorf, B. P. Cooper, M. Wagner, and E. L. Spitznagel, "Prevalence and Correlates of Psychotropic Medication Use in Adolescents with an Autism Spectrum Disorder with and without Caregiver-Reported Attention-Deficit/Hyperactivity Disorder," *Journal of Child and Adolescent Psychopharmacology*, vol. 21, no. 6, pp. 571–579, 2011.

[13] K. M. Antshel, Y. Zhang-James, K. E. Wagner, A. Ledesma, and S. V. Faraone, "An update on the comorbidity of ADHD and ASD: A focus on clinical management," *Expert Review of Neurotherapeutics*, vol. 16, no. 3, pp. 279–293, 2016.

[14] L. Kanner, "Autistic disturbances of affective contact," *Nervous Child*, vol. 2, pp. 217–250, 1943.

[15] C. E. Wilson, F. Happé, and S. J. Wheelwright, "The neuropsychology of male adults with high-functioning autism or asperger syndrome," *Autism Research*, vol. 7, no. 5, pp. 568–581, 2014.

[16] J. Sinzig, D. Morsch, and G. Lehmkuhl, "Do hyperactivity, impulsivity and inattention have an impact on the ability of facial affect recognition in children with autism and ADHD?" *European Child & Adolescent Psychiatry*, vol. 17, no. 2, pp. 63–72, 2008.

[17] A. Downs and T. Smith, "Emotional understanding, cooperation, and social behavior in high-functioning children with autism," *Journal of Autism and Developmental Disorders*, vol. 34, no. 6, pp. 625–635, 2004.

[18] N. Yuill and J. Lyon, "Selective difficulty in recognising facial expressions of emotion in boys with ADHD. General performance impairments or specific problems in social cognition?" *European Child & Adolescent Psychiatry*, vol. 16, no. 6, pp. 398–404, 2007.

[19] P. N. Andersen, K. T. Hovik, E. W. Skogli, J. Egeland, and M. Øie, "Symptoms of ADHD in Children with High-Functioning Autism Are Related to Impaired Verbal Working Memory and Verbal Delayed Recall," *PLoS ONE*, vol. 8, no. 5, Article ID e64842, 2013.

[20] C. Tye, P. Asherson, K. L. Ashwood, B. Azadi, P. Bolton, and G. McLoughlin, "Attention and inhibition in children with ASD, ADHD and co-morbid ASD + ADHD: An event-related potential study," *Psychological Medicine*, vol. 44, no. 5, pp. 1101–1116, 2014.

[21] C. Lord, M. Rutter, and A. Le Couteur, "Autism diagnostic interview-revised: a revised version of a diagnostic interview for caregivers of individuals with possible pervasive developmental disorders," *Journal of Autism and Developmental Disorders*, vol. 24, no. 5, pp. 659–685, 1994.

[22] M. D. Lezak, D. B. Howieson, and D. W. Loring, *Neuropsychological Assessment*, Oxford University Press, New York, USA, 2004.

[23] F. G. E. Happe, "An advanced test of theory of mind: understanding of story characters' thoughts and feelings by able autistic, mentally handicapped, and normal children and adults," *Journal of Autism and Developmental Disorders*, vol. 24, no. 2, pp. 129–154, 1994.

[24] S. Baron-Cohen, S. Wheelwright, J. Hill, Y. Raste, and I. Plumb, "The "Reading the Mind in the Eyes" Test revised version: A study with normal adults, and adults with Asperger syndrome or high-functioning autism," *Journal of Child Psychology and Psychiatry and Allied Disciplines*, vol. 42, no. 2, pp. 241–251, 2001.

[25] T. Achenbach, C. Howell, H. Quay, C. Conners, and J. Bates, "National Survey of Problems and Competencies among Four- to Sixteen-Year-Olds: Parents' Reports for Normative and Clinical Samples," *Monographs of the Society for Research in Child Development*, vol. 56, no. 3, pp. 1–130, 1991.

[26] American Psychiatric Association, *American Psychiatric Association Diagnostic and Statistical Manual of Mental Disorders (DSM-5)*, American Psychiatric Association, Washington, DC, USA, 5th edition, 2013.

[27] K. Schuchardt, M. Gebhardt, and C. Mäehler, "Working memory functions in children with different degrees of intellectual disability," *Journal of Intellectual Disability Research*, vol. 54, no. 4, pp. 346–353, 2010.

19

Social Skills Intervention Participation and Associated Improvements in Executive Function Performance

Shawn E. Christ,[1,2] Janine P. Stichter,[2,3] Karen V. O'Connor,[3] Kimberly Bodner,[1] Amanda J. Moffitt,[1] and Melissa J. Herzog[3]

[1] *Department of Psychological Sciences, University of Missouri, Columbia, MO, USA*
[2] *Thompson Center for Autism & Neurodevelopmental Disorders, University of Missouri, Columbia, MO, USA*
[3] *Department of Special Education, University of Missouri, Columbia, MO, USA*

Correspondence should be addressed to Shawn E. Christ; christse@missouri.edu

Academic Editor: Herbert Roeyers

Autism spectrum disorder (ASD) is a neurodevelopmental disorder characterized by impairments in social communication. It has been postulated that such difficulties are related to disruptions in underlying cognitive processes such as executive function. The present study examined potential changes in executive function performance associated with participation in the Social Competence Intervention (SCI) program, a short-term intervention designed to improve social competence in adolescents with ASD. Laboratory behavioral performance measures were used to separately evaluate potential intervention-related changes in individual executive function component processes (i.e., working memory, inhibitory control, and cognitive flexibility) in a sample of 22 adolescents with ASD both before and after intervention. For comparison purposes, a demographically matched sample of 14 individuals without ASD was assessed at identical time intervals. Intervention-related improvements were observed on the working memory task, with gains evident in spatial working memory and, to a slightly lesser degree, verbal working memory. Significant improvements were also found for a working memory-related aspect of the task switching test (i.e., mixing costs). Taken together, these findings provide preliminary support for the hypothesis that participation in the SCI program is accompanied by changes in underlying neurocognitive processes such as working memory.

1. Introduction

Autism Spectrum Disorder (ASD) is a neurodevelopmental disorder characterized by persistent impairments in social communication and social interactions as well as the presence of restricted/repetitive patterns of behavior [1]. The core impairments of ASD often manifest as difficulties in basic social and communicative behavior (e.g., eye contact, intonation, and facial expressions) as well as rigidity relating to routines and pervasive preoccupations [2]. Difficulties in social interaction skills often include a lack of social reciprocity, lack of nonverbal behaviors/gestures, and difficulty maintaining peer relationships [1, 3]. Although the onset and diagnosis of ASD most often occur in early childhood, the impairments are present across the lifespan [4] and may be particularly challenging during the adolescent period.

Research has suggested that the significant social-communicative impairments in individuals with ASD are directly related to negative long-term outcomes [5, 6]. Social communication impairments may manifest differently based on an individual's overall level of intellectual functioning. For example, social-communicative difficulties observed in individuals with high functioning autism (HFA; i.e., individuals average to above average cognitive abilities) often include the failure to recognize social cues and contexts, and therefore students struggle with appropriate conversational skills and interpreting nonverbal behaviors of others [7]. Specifically, the social impairments for individuals with HFA include impairments in the use of nonverbal behaviors, developmentally inappropriate peer relationships, failure to seek out others for enjoyment, and poor social-emotional reciprocity [1, 8]. These impairments can manifest both from a lack of knowledge of social skills and from difficulties in demonstrating these skills in the required contexts [9].

1.1. Social Challenges and Social Competence Intervention. Social difficulties experienced by individuals with ASD appear to be related to disruptions in various social cognitive processes. Prominently discussed constructs underlying the social challenges for individuals with autism include emotion recognition [10, 11], theory of mind [12, 13], and executive functioning [14, 15]. Other contributing constructs include social motivation [16, 17], social reciprocity [18], and social problem solving [19, 20]. Importantly, these constructs are not orthogonal; rather, they appear to be interrelated components to an integrated whole (for brief review, see [21]).

The Social Competence Intervention-Adolescent (SCI-A; [22, 23]) is based on cognitive behavioral intervention and applied behavior analytic principles and targets EF, theory of mind, and emotion recognition as key constructs in addressing social competence impairments. Although other researchers have investigated the potential role of EF, theory of mind, and emotion recognition in existing intervention programs [21], SCI-A was developed specifically with these target constructs in mind. The SCI curriculum is designed to challenge thinking patterns related to these underlying constructs and includes the following key components: use of metacognitive strategies, self-monitoring and self-regulation, and exposure and response situations [21, 24]. The curricular units (recognizing facial expressions, sharing ideas, turn taking in conversations, recognizing feelings and emotions of self and others, and problem solving) are presented in a scaffolded fashion, with each new unit building upon the content and skills of the previous ones (for additional description of the SCI program, see [22, 23]). Maintenance of learned skills is reinforced throughout the curriculum by the use of repetition, integration, and feedback as new skills are added. The curricular units utilize a combination of didactic instruction, behavior modeling, rehearsal, and in vivo practice with other intervention participants as a means to teach and/or modify social behavior specific to a student's needs.

1.2. Executive Function and Its Role in Social Competence. Although a precise definition of EF remains elusive, EF can be generally conceptualized as referring to a set of higher-order cognitive processes that allow for the flexible modification of thought and behavior in response to changing cognitive or environmental contexts [25]. It encompasses abilities such as planning, strategy use, organization, working memory, inhibitory control, and cognitive flexibility. These abilities are considered "executive" in that they require the integration and processing of information from a wide range of internal and external sources. Empirical evidence [26] suggests that at least three core component processes may comprise EF: updating (working memory), inhibition (inhibitory control), and shifting (cognitive flexibility).

Working memory is broadly defined as the active maintenance and manipulation of a limited amount of information over a short period of time [27, 28]. Inhibitory control refers to the ability to suppress the activation, processing, or expression of information that would otherwise interfere with efficient attainment of a cognitive or behavioral goal [29, 30]. Shifting, also called cognitive flexibility or rule shifting, refers to switching between tasks or mental sets in response to changing task demands [31]. While distinguishable, these three component processes are not necessarily orthogonal and, in fact, the interplay among them provides the foundation for more complex executive abilities such as planning, strategy use, and organization.

Previous research indicates that EF represents an area of particular weakness for individuals with ASD even after accounting for comorbid conditions such as ADHD [32, 33]. Meta-analytical reviews of the existing literature point to cognitive flexibility and working memory as areas of consistent weakness in individuals with ASD as compared to healthy individuals without ASD (for reviews, see [34, 35]). Findings on inhibitory control in ASD, however, have been much more mixed. Whereas a number of studies have reported significant impairments on measures of inhibitory control in individuals with ASD [36–39], others have failed to find a difference between individuals with ASD and their control counterparts [40–42]. Literature reviews on ASD and inhibitory control have also come to differing conclusions [35, 43].

Each of the aforementioned EF component processes can be hypothesized to play an important role in proficient social competence. For example, working memory allows one to follow the flow of a conversation/interaction while at the same time preparing his/her own contribution to the conversation [44]. Cognitive flexibility is critical in that moment-to-moment changes in conversational topic or context may necessitate a shift in which social cues are relevant and the appropriate response to such cues [45]. Lastly, inhibitory control allows one to ignore irrelevant cues/stimuli so that socially relevant information may be processed more efficiently [37].

Although a number of studies have examined potential group-related differences in EF and social competence within the same study (e.g., ASD group has both poorer EF and poorer social communication abilities compared to non-ASD group), few studies have reported analysis of within-group covariability of the two factors (i.e., the correlation between EF and social competence within a given ASD sample). For the handful of studies that have done so, the results have been mixed. Some studies have found significant correlations between measures of EF and social competence [46–49], but others have failed to find any such evidence [50, 51]. In a recent randomized clinical trial, Kenworthy et al. [52] found similar gains in social competence for individuals with ASD who participated in an executive function-focused intervention compared to those who participated in a more general social skills-focused intervention.

Developmental research with younger children provides additional support for the interrelationship between EF and social competence. Findings from several studies suggest that early EF abilities are correlated with later theory of mind ability [53–56]. Also, in a more recent study, Pellicano [57] found that individual differences in early EF performance

Table 1: Sample characteristics.

Variable	ASD intervention group (n = 22)		Non-ASD group (n = 14)	
	M (SD)	Range	M (SD)	Range
Age (years)	12.3 (1.1)	10.8–14.7	12.8 (0.9)	11.0–14.5
Gender (M/F)	22/0		22/0	
FSIQ	100.5 (13.1)	78–130	103.4 (7.2)	81–111
Parent-report SRS (at baseline)				
Raw score	106.1 (18.8)	71–144	—	—
T score	84.6 (9.0)	68–103	—	—
ADI-R (n = 18)*				
A (social interaction)	15.2 (6.9)	3–29	—	—
B (communication)	13.4 (5.4)	5–21	—	—
C (restricted/repetitive behavior)	4.7 (2.4)	1–10	—	—
ADOS-original algorithm (n = 7)*				
Communication	1.9 (0.7)	1–3	—	—
Social interaction	6.6 (3.3)	0–10	—	—
ADOS-revised algorithm (n = 8)*				
Social effect	7.4 (2.5)	4–11	—	—
Restricted, repetitive behavior	2.6 (1.7)	0–5	—	—

*Note that a subset of children (n = 10) received both the ADI-R and ADOS.

at age 5–7 years predicted social communication ability (as well as extent of repetitive behaviors/restricted interest) in children three years later.

Previous research [22, 23] supports the effectiveness of the SCI-A program in improvements in parent reports of social competence behaviors and characteristics of adolescents with HFA. In addition, pre- to postintervention improvements in EF as assessed by measures such as the Behavior Rating Inventory of Executive Function (BRIEF; [58]) and the Test of Problem Solving-3 (TOPS-3; [59]) were also found in these studies. The BRIEF is a parent- or teacher-report measure designed to assess behavioral manifestations of EF problems in daily life. The TOPS-3 is a performance-based measure in which participants are shown photographic or written scenarios and asked questions designed to assess the participants' interpretation of what factors may have contributed to the scenario and potential ways to solve the situation. Both the BRIEF and TOPS-3 focus primarily on complex manifestations of EF (e.g., everyday problem solving), which rely on a confluence of working memory, inhibitory control, and cognitive flexibility. Little is currently known regarding the relationship between Social Competence Intervention and potential changes in individual EF component processes.

1.3. The Current Study. As noted above, there is growing evidence [22, 23] of potential improvements in EF for adolescents who participated in the SCI-A intervention. To date, however, these studies have relied primarily on measures (e.g., the BRIEF and TOPS) that capture EF in broad-brush strokes. The current study builds on these results by examining the nature of such improvements via laboratory behavioral performance measures to evaluate potential intervention-related changes in individual EF component processes in a sample of adolescents with HFA who participated in SCI-A. A demographically matched sample of adolescents without ASD was assessed at identical time intervals for comparison purposes.

Digit span and spatial span tests were used to assess verbal and nonverbal working memory, respectively. Cognitive flexibility was assessed using a computerized switching task in which participants performed a visual matching task in which the response rule (i.e., whether to match the stimuli based on shape or color) was pseudo-randomly switched from trial to trial. In terms of inhibitory control, we focused on the ability to filter and resist interference from visual distractors, an aspect of inhibitory control that is known to be particularly affected in ASD [36, 37].

Based on previous research, we hypothesize that the ASD group will perform more poorly than the non-ASD group at baseline on all of the EF tests. However, we also hypothesize that improvements in EF performance will be observed in the ASD group with participation in the SCI intervention, thus decreasing the magnitude of group differences observed at follow-up.

2. Methods

2.1. Participants and Setting. Data is presented for a sample of 22 individuals (all male) with HFA ranging in age from 10.8 to 14.7 years (M = 12.3, SD = 1.14) who completed the SCI-A program. Additional demographic information on the sample is included in Table 1.

The program was delivered at a university-affiliated interdisciplinary diagnostic and outpatient treatment center for ASD and neurodevelopmental disorders in the Midwest. In total, SCI-A included 20 hours of group intervention delivered in 1-hour lessons twice weekly for 10 weeks. The groups met during academic semesters after school hours

Table 2: Association of SCI-A curricular units and executive functions.

SCI-A unit	Curricular content	Executive function*
(1) Recognizing facial expressions	Visual recognition of key facial features Displaying facial expressions Strategies for scanning facial features to read emotions	
(2) Sharing ideas	Speaker skills: gaining attention, staying on topic, sharing the main idea, appropriate eye contact/body proximity/volume Listener skills: appropriate eye contact/body proximity	*Working Memory:* staying on topic *Inhibitory Control:* sharing only the main idea/not sharing irrelevant information; avoiding interrupting others
(3) Turn taking in conversation	Conversational reciprocity Using questions and comments Transitioning in/out of conversations	*Inhibitory Control:* avoid interrupting others *Working Memory:* staying on topic, building off another person's comments *Cognitive Flexibility:* switching/transitioning topics
(4) Feelings and emotions	Understand emotional range/variance/intensity Self-control and emotion regulation Using context to understand others' emotions/perspective taking	
(5) Problem solving	Identify components of problems (who, what) Generate and evaluate possible solutions Collaborate with others to solve problems	*Inhibitory Control:* use appropriate conversational skills to collaborate *Working Memory:* holding the ideas of others to collaborative problem solving *Cognitive Flexibility:* generate alternate solutions

*Consistent with EF being only one of several interrelated constructs that contribute to social competence, the content in any given unit involves a combination of EF and other processes (e.g., social reciprocity, and pragmatic language).

in a classroom setting within the autism center. Master's level implementers with specific training in special education with ASD specializations led all current sessions. Cohorts were restricted to no more than seven participants each (range = 4–7 participants). As noted earlier, both content and instruction were scaffolded over time with new skills and practice opportunities layered upon each other as the curriculum progressed. Table 2 provides a description of how the SCI-A curricular units are conceptually linked to different EF component processes.

As noted previously, the SCI-A program designed for adolescents with HFA with a specific, predetermined set of characteristics (phenotype) related to their age, level of functioning, and general education placement. To be enrolled in the SCI-A program, participants had to meet the following criteria [22]: (a) age 11–14 years; (b) a clinical or medical diagnosis of an ASD; (c) a full scale IQ score above 75; (d) scores on the Autism Diagnostic Observation Schedule (ADOS; [60]) and/or Autism Diagnostic Interview-Revised (ADI-R; [61]) that met or exceeded clinically designated cutoffs; and (e) access to typically developing peers without ASD for at least part of their day (e.g., via general education classrooms). These are similar to the criteria utilized by Solomon et al. [21].

The current participants represent a subset of individuals across four semesters that were concurrently enrolled in a larger efficacy study of the SCI-A program [22]. Within these targeted four semesters, some participants were excluded from the present analysis for various reasons. Five were excluded due to excessive absences from the SCI-A program (>20% of sessions missed; attendance for the remaining participants were very high, with an average of <5% of sessions missed). Three participants were excluded due to compliance issues at pre/posttesting.

For comparison purposes, data was also reported for an age- and gender-matched comparison sample of 14 neurologically uncompromised individuals (all male) without ASD. Participants in the non-ASD comparison group ranged in age from 11.0 to 14.5 years ($M = 12.8$; $SD = 0.91$). They were recruited from the Columbia, Missouri community. Prior to enrollment, the parents of potential participants were asked to complete an extensive questionnaire detailing past developmental and medical history. Individuals with significant medical and/or psychiatric history were excluded. Additional demographic information on the sample is included in Table 1.

The non-ASD comparison group was evaluated at an equivalent time interval (12–14 weeks) to the ASD intervention group; however, they did not receive the SCI intervention. The ASD and non-ASD groups did not differ significantly in terms of age [$t(34) = 1.43$, $p = .16$] or FSIQ [$M_{ASD} = 100.5$; $M_{TYP} = 103.4$; $t(34) < 1$, $p = .45$].

2.2. Procedure. The present study was approved by the University of Missouri-Columbia Internal Review Board and completed in accordance with the Helsinki Declaration. Informed consent and assent were obtained for all participants in the present study.

Baseline evaluations were conducted with intervention participants within a 2-week window prior to beginning the

SCI-A program. The SCI-A program was then delivered over a 10-week period twice a week for an hour within a clinic-based classroom setting. Participants completed postintervention evaluation within two weeks following completion of the program. The non-ASD comparison group did not receive the intervention but had baseline and postevaluation at an equivalent time interval (12–14 weeks) to the intervention group. All measures reported below were administered at both baseline and posttest.

All EF tasks were administered in a small, quiet room with sufficient overhead lighting. For the computerized tests, reaction time (RT) and error rate were recorded for each condition. Children used both hands to respond during the inhibitory control task (i.e., left hand to the left button; right hand to the right button). For the cognitive flexibility/switching task, participants used their dominant hand to respond. The order of task administration was varied randomly across participants.

As evidenced by the relatively low error rates observed, none of the children exhibited difficulties in understanding task instructions or feedback for any of the tasks. In addition, to further ensure that the children had time to become comfortable with the computer tasks, each task included a block of practice trials that was administered prior to data collection. [Note that the Digit Span and Spatial Span working memory tasks were administered as per their standardized instructions, which does not include "practice trials" per se.]

2.3. Measures

2.3.1. Working Memory. The Digit Span and Spatial Span subtests of the Wechsler Intelligence Scale for Children – Fourth Edition Integrated (WISC-IV Integrated; [62]) were administered to assess verbal and nonverbal working memory, respectively. The Digit Span subtest has two components: Digits Forward and Digits Backwards. In the Digits Forward component, the participant must repeat back a series of auditorily-presented digits in the same order as they were presented. In the Digits Backwards component, the participant again receives a series of auditorily presented digits, but he/she must now repeat them back in reverse order. In both components, the length of the sequence increases as the participant responds correctly.

The Spatial Span subtest was designed as a visual analogy to the Digit Span subtest and also includes forward and backwards span components. In the Forward Span component, the examiner points one-at-a-time to a series of spatial locations (demarked by blocks on a board). The participant must then point to the same spatial locations in the same order. In the backwards span component, the examiner again points to a series of spatial location, but the participant must now respond in the reverse order. As with the Digit Span subtest, the length of the sequence increases as the participant responds correctly.

2.3.2. Inhibitory Control. A flanker visual filtering task was used to assess inhibitory control. The stimuli and procedure are identical to those employed in another recent study of inhibitory control in ASD [37]. In brief, participants were seated in front of a computer monitor and two large response buttons. They were asked to respond as quickly as possible based on the orientation of a centrally presented stimulus (e.g., "press the left button if the fish is facing left, and press the right button if the fish is facing right"). At the time of presentation, the target stimulus was closely flanked ($<0.5^\circ$) to the left and right by distracting stimuli (i.e., additional fish). These stimuli were either compatible (i.e., facing the same direction) or incompatible (i.e., facing the opposite direction) with the target stimulus.

Together the stimuli subtended approximately 1° vertically and 10° horizontally (1.9° per fish). For each trial, stimuli were presented until a response was made or until more than 3000 ms elapsed. After an intertrial interval of 1500 ms, a new trial was presented.

If a child responded in less than 200 ms after presentation of the target (an anticipatory error), a brief tone followed by the message "early response" was presented. If a child failed to respond within 3000 ms (an inattentive error), a tone and "too slow" were presented. If a child responded by pressing the incorrect button (an accuracy error), a tone and "wrong response" were presented.

Children completed two practice blocks of 20 trials. In the first block, target stimuli were presented without flankers. In the second block, practice trials were identical to experimental trials (i.e., flankers were present). After practice, children completed 120 experimental trials, with 60 trials in each of the two conditions. Presentation was balanced such that all possible stimulus-flanker pairings were equally likely to occur. The conditions were mixed randomly. At intervals of 40 trials, children were offered a break.

Response time (RT) and error rates were recorded. Inhibitory control is assessed by comparing performance in the incompatible condition (in which participants must inhibit the conflicting flanker stimuli) and performance in the compatible condition.

2.3.3. Task Switching. The experimental apparatus and task conditions are illustrated in Figure 1. Children were seated in front of a computer monitor and three large response buttons. On each trial, participants were shown a target stimulus at the top of the display and a row of three response stimuli near the bottom of the display. The target stimulus could be any of four different shapes (square, circle, cross, and triangle) presented in any of four different colors (red, green, blue, and yellow). One of the response stimuli shared the same shape as the target stimulus but not the same color. Another of the response stimuli shared the same color as the target stimulus but not the same shape. And the last response stimulus was a different shape and color than the target stimulus. The horizontal location (left, center, or right) of the different response stimuli varied randomly from trial to trial. A large response button was located below each of the three horizontal locations.

Concurrent with presentation of the aforementioned stimuli, a cue stimulus was presented at the center of the display. Participants were instructed that when they saw

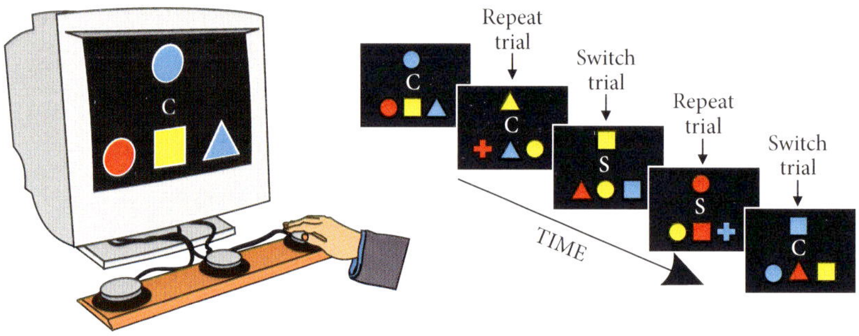

FIGURE 1: Illustration of the experimental apparatus and task conditions for the task switching test. Participants were instructed to match the top shape with one of the bottom three shapes. If the letter in the middle was a "C," then they were to match based on color. If it was an "S," then they were to match based on shape. [Note that the relative size of the stimuli has been enlarged for illustrative purposes.]

the "shape" cue (the letter "S" superimposed on a gray-colored hexagon shape), they should press the response button corresponding to the response stimulus that matched the target stimulus in shape. Similarly, when they saw the "color" cue (the letter "C" superimposed on a rainbow-colored diamond shape), they were to press the response button corresponding to the response stimulus that matched the target stimulus in color. RT and error rate were recorded. Following the participant's response and a short intertrial interval (50 ms), a new trial was presented.

Prior to beginning the task, participants were shown an illustration of both color and shape trials. Participants first completed a practice block of 24 trials of randomly intermixed color and shape trials. Next, 6 blocks of trials, each comprising 48 experimental trials, were administered. One experimental block included only color trials (the "pure color" block), and another block included only shape trials (the "pure shape" block). The remaining four blocks ("mixed" blocks) included an equal number of color and shape trials (24 of each) that were randomly intermixed. Prior to each block, the task instructions were reviewed, and participants were informed that the upcoming block would include color trials, shape trials, or a mix of both. The presentation order of the 6 experimental blocks varied randomly from participant to participant.

2.3.4. Social Communication Abilities. The Social Responsiveness Scale (SRS; [63]) is a standardized, parent report, 65-item rating scale that measures social impairments associated with ASD across five domains: social awareness, social cognition, social communication, social motivation, and autistic mannerisms. A four-point Likert scale was used to rate items and scores were summed to form five subscales. A higher score reflected greater social impairment in that domain. *T*-scores derived from large-scale norming were provided in the scoring manual; however in order to better represent variations among very high scores, raw scores served as the unit of analysis in this study (consistent with other intervention research).

As noted above, the ASD participants in the present study were also concurrently enrolled in a larger efficacy study of the SCI-A program and their SRS outcome data has been reported in the prior study [22]. For comparison purposes, however, data is represented here as the primary measure of social competence improvement to be associated with any concurrent EF gains. The SRS was administered only for ASD/intervention participants; the non-ASD group did not receive the SRS.

3. Results

EF task data were available for all participants with the following exceptions: Due to technical problems, complete pre/postintervention data on the task switching test was unavailable for five participants with ASD. Data on the task switching test was also unavailable for the non-ASD comparison group. [Note that the non-ASD group data were originally collected as part of another (unpublished) study effort. However, given that the sole difference in study battery between the two groups related to the absence of the task switching test, we felt that the value of including their data for comparison purposes on the working memory and inhibition tasks outweighed any potential concerns.]

For the inhibitory control and task switching tests, median response time (RT) for nonerror trials served as the primary dependent variable. Error rates were very low for both tasks (overall error rate for inhibitory and task switching tests = 2.9% and 5.7%, resp.) and thus were not considered further. For the current analyses, we employed mixed model analysis of variance (ANOVA) as the primary statistical model. ANOVA has been generally found to be robust to the assumption violations (e.g., assumptions of normality and homoscedasticity) that frequently arise with the analysis of RT data [64]. However, so as to further validate the present results, the analyses of EF performance were repeated utilizing a nonparametric statistical model (i.e., Mann–Whitney *U* test) that does not rely on such assumptions. The resulting pattern of statistically significant and nonsignificant findings was identical to that found with ANOVA. When applicable, effect sizes are reported in terms of Hedge's *g*, which provides a better estimate (in comparison to Cohen's *d*) when dealing with relatively smaller sample sizes. Descriptive statistics (mean, standard deviation, and range) for performance on each task are included in Table 3.

TABLE 3: Descriptive statistics for performance on each task.

Variable	ASD intervention group				Non-ASD group			
	Timepoint 1		Timepoint 2		Timepoint 1		Timepoint 2	
	M (SD)	Range	*M* (SD)	Range	*M* (SD)	Range	*M* (SD)	Range
Working memory measure								
Spatial subtest	12.8 (3.3)*	6–19	14.6 (3.7)*	7–22	16.4 (3.1)	12–21	16.1 (2.0)	12–20
Verbal (digit) subtest	13.6 (2.4)	9–18	14.6 (3.3)	7–22	16.1 (2.5)	13–23	15.6 (2.5)	12–21
Combined (spatial + verbal)	26.4 (4.7)*	17–33	29.2 (5.8)*	14–40	32.6 (4.3)	27–40	31.7 (3.8)	26–40
Inhibitory control measure								
Inhibitory effect	.09 (.06)	−.03–.23	.07 (.04)	−.01–.12	.08 (.05)	.00–.18	.09 (.05)	.00–.16
Task switching measure								
Switching costs	.18 (.17)	−.02–.72	.15 (.13)	−.01–.42	—	—	—	—
Mixing costs	.54 (.24)	.26–1.21	.40 (.20)	.08–.82	—	—	—	—

*Effect of Timepoint, $p < .05$.

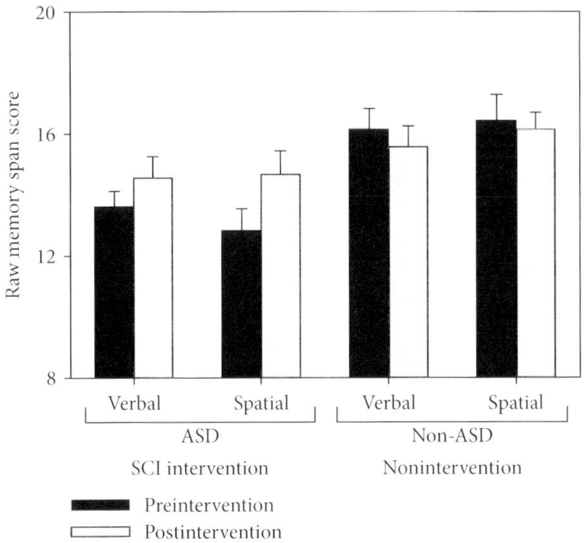

FIGURE 2: Mean raw scores for the working memory span tests, shown separately for each group (ASD and non-ASD), modality (verbal/digit and spatial), and timepoint (before and after intervention). Error bars represent standard error of the mean.

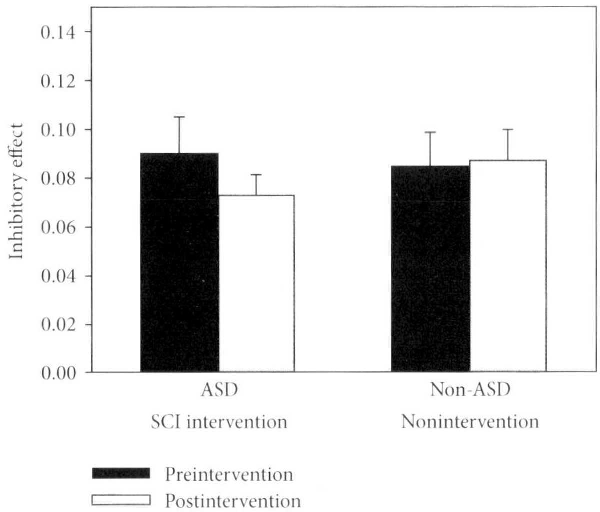

FIGURE 3: Mean inhibitory control effect $[(RT_{INCOMPATIBLE} - RT_{COMPATIBLE})/RT_{COMPATIBLE}]$ for the inhibitory control test, shown separately for each group (ASD and non-ASD) and timepoint (before and after intervention). Error bars represent standard error of the mean.

3.1. Working Memory. Mean raw scores for each working memory span test are shown in Figure 2. Data were entered into a 2 × 2 × 2 mixed model ANOVA with group (ASD and non-ASD) as a between-subjects factor, and modality (verbal and spatial) and timepoint (pre- and postintervention) as within-subject factors. There was no main effect of modality or timepoint [$F(1,34) < 2.6$, $p > .12$, $\eta_p^2 < .07$ in both instances]. However, a main effect of group was found, with the non-ASD group performing better overall than the ASD group [$F(1,34) = 7.89$, $p = .008$, $\eta_p^2 = .19$]. There was also a significant interaction between group and timepoint [$F(1,34) = 9.05$, $p = .005$, $\eta_p^2 = .21$]. No other interactions approached significance [$F(1,34) < 1$, $p > .39$, $\eta_p^2 < .03$ in all instances].

As can be seen in Figure 2, then interaction between group and timepoint was driven by the fact that the ASD intervention group showed improvements on the spatial subtest [$M_{PRE} = 12.8$; $M_{POST} = 14.6$; $t(21) = 2.55$, $p = .02$, $g = .51$] and the verbal (digit) subtest albeit to a slightly lesser degree [$M_{PRE} = 13.6$; $M_{POST} = 14.6$; $t(21) = 1.70$, $p = .10$, $g = 0.33$]. In contrast, the non-ASD group showed effectively no change in spatial or verbal working memory task performance over the same period of time [$t(13) < 1$, $p > .41$, $g < .23$ in both instances].

3.2. Inhibitory Control. Inhibitory control data are shown in Figure 3. Potential intervention-related changes in the *inhibitory effect* or the additional time needed to respond on incompatible trial (i.e., a trial with flanking stimuli that are mapped to a competing response) as compared to a compatible trial (i.e., a trial with flanking stimuli that are mapped to the same response) were examined. Note that, in order to account for individual differences in general response speed, inhibitory effect was calculated as a proportion of the

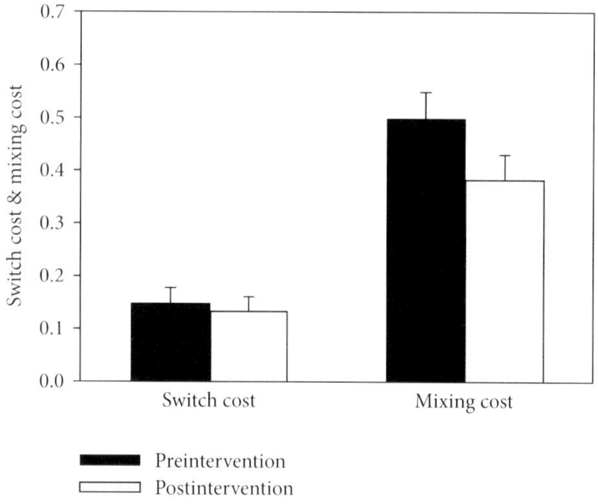

FIGURE 4: Mean switch cost [$(RT_{Switch} - RT_{Repeat})/RT_{Repeat}$] and mixing cost [$(RT_{Mixed} - RT_{Pure})/RT_{Pure}$] for the ASD intervention group on the task switching test, shown separately for each trial type (switch and repetition), block type (pure and mixed), and timepoint (before and after intervention). Error bars represent standard error of the mean.

RT in the baseline compatible condition [$(RT_{INCOMPATIBLE} - RT_{COMPATIBLE})/RT_{COMPATIBLE}$]. Resulting data were entered into a 2 × 2 mixed model ANOVA with group (ASD and non-ASD) as a between-subjects factor and timepoint (before and after intervention) as a within-subject factor.

No main effect of group or timepoint was found [$F(1, 33) < 1$, $p > .55$, $\eta_p^2 < .02$ in both instances]. The interaction between group and timepoint also did not approach significance [$F(1, 33) < 1$, $p = .46$, $\eta_p^2 = .02$]. No significant changes in inhibitory effect were observed for either the ASD intervention group [$M_{PRE} = .090$; $M_{POST} = .073$; $t(20) = 1.08$, $p = .30$, $g = 0.31$] or non-ASD group [$M_{PRE} = .085$; $M_{POST} = .087$; $t(20) < 1$, $p = .92$, $g = .04$].

3.3. Task Switching

3.3.1. Switch Costs. Data for the task switching test are shown in Figure 4. Potential intervention-related changes in the *switch cost* or the additional time needed to respond on a switch trial (i.e., a trial in which the matching rule is different from that required on the previous trial) as compared to nonswitch/repetition trial (i.e., a trial in which the matching rule is the same as that required on the previous trial) within the mixed blocks were examined. In order to account for individual differences in general response speed, the switch cost effect was calculated as a proportion of the RT in the repetition trial condition [$(RT_{Switch} - RT_{Repeat})/RT_{Repeat}$]. No significant pre/postintervention differences in switch cost were observed for the ASD group [$M_{PRE} = .149$; $M_{POST} = .134$; $t(16) < 1$, $p = .62$, $g = .13$]. [Note that, as explained earlier, comparison data from the non-ASD group were unfortunately unavailable for the task switching test.]

3.3.2. Mixing Costs. Inclusion of pure blocks of trials (i.e., blocks of trials where the matching rule remained the same throughout the block) in the experimental design allowed for evaluation of another task-related phenomenon, namely, the *mixing cost*. The mixing cost reflects the observation that RT for repetition trials within mixed blocks (i.e., blocks also containing switch trials) tends to be slower than RT for repetition trials within pure trial blocks. It is generally believed that whereas switch costs (see above) reflect task switching ability, mixing costs may be better conceptualized as reflecting the added working memory demands associated with maintenance of two sets of task rules for the mixed blocks as compared to only one set for the pure blocks [31].

In order to account for individual differences in general response speed, the mixing cost effect was calculated as a proportion of the RT in the pure block condition [$(RT_{Mixed} - RT_{Pure})/RT_{Pure}$]. A clear trend towards decreased mixing cost from pre- to postintervention was found [$M_{PRE} = .50$; $M_{POST} = .38$; $t(16) = 1.97$, $p = .07$, $g = .57$].

3.4. Relationship between Improvements in Executive Function and SRS Scores. As anticipated, participation in the SCI-A program was associated with improved social competence as reflected by significantly lower SRS raw scores at postintervention ($M_{POST} = 87.6$; Range: 59–118) as compared to preintervention ($M_{PRE} = 106.1$; Range: 71–144) [$t(21) = 6.81$, $p < .001$, $g = 0.99$]. No direct relationship was found between the observed intervention-related improvements in overall SRS scores and performance changes in the working memory ($r_s = .09$, $p = .68$), inhibitory control ($r_s = .32$, $p = .16$), or switching task (switch costs: $r_s = .14$, $p = .54$; mixing costs: $r_s = .34$, $p = .13$). Analysis of changes in SRS subscales (i.e., Social Awareness, Social Cognition, Social Communication, Social Motivation, and autistic mannerisms) and task performance yielded similar findings ($r_s < .36$, $p > .09$ in all instances).

4. Discussion

Whereas previous research on the SCI-A program has found significant improvements in measures of social competence and EF [22, 23], the measures utilized in these past studies have been largely limited to parent report questionnaires (e.g., BRIEF) and broad nonspecific measures of EF (e.g., TOPS). Consequently little is known regarding potential changes in specific EF component processes. By separately assessing working memory, inhibitory control, and cognitive flexibility at both pre- and postintervention, the current study was designed to further elucidate the nature of changes in EF functioning associated with participation in the SCI-A program.

Consistent with the aforementioned previous research, the present study found significant improvements in EF as measured by the present behavioral tasks. Specifically, intervention participants' performance on the working memory task improved significantly before to after intervention, with clear gains evident in spatial (nonverbal) working memory ($g = 0.51$). A nonsignificant trend towards improvement was also observed for verbal working memory performance (g = 0.33). At the same time, no such improvements were observed for the nonintervention comparison group suggesting that the performance gains of the intervention group are likely not attributable to practice and/or maturational factors. The finding of improved working memory performance for the intervention group is consistent with research with other clinical populations suggesting that working memory represents an aspect of cognition that may be malleable and responsive to intervention [65–67].

We also examined potential intervention-related changes in inhibitory control, specifically the ability to resist interference from visual distractors. As noted earlier, research has found that children with ASD are particularly impaired in this aspect of inhibitory control [36, 37]. Interestingly, we found no evidence of inhibitory control impairment in the present sample of ASD participants when compared to their non-ASD counterparts. It is important to note, however, that, in the aforementioned study by Christ et al. [37], they found a significant group by age interaction such that inhibitory control impairments were much more evident in their younger as compared to older participants. Within this context, it is possible that the age of the current participants was prohibitive (i.e., they were relatively too old) in terms of the manifestation of inhibitory difficulties.

With no impairment evident for the ASD group at baseline, it is not completely surprising that we also failed to find significant pre-to-post changes in inhibitory control ability for this group. It remains possible, had we targeted a younger cohort (whom would have presumably shown inhibitory impairment at baseline), that intervention-related improvements in inhibitory ability may have been observed as well. Indeed, even with no impairment at baseline in the present ASD sample, there was a nonsignificant trend (g = 0.31) towards improved inhibitory performance in this group following the intervention. Additional research is needed to further examine these possibilities and whether inhibitory ability may be responsive to intervention as well.

With regard to the switching task, we failed to observe intervention-related changes in our primary measure of cognitive flexibility/switching ability, namely, *switching costs* or the additional time needed to respond on a switch trial (i.e., a trial in which the matching rule is different from that required on the previous trial) as compared to nonswitch/repetition trial (i.e., a trial in which the matching rule is the same as that required on the previous trial). We did, however, find evidence of a nonsignificant trend (g = 0.57) towards intervention-related improvements in a secondary measure, namely, *mixing costs* or the additional time taken to respond when trials are presented within mixed blocks (i.e., blocks containing both "shape" and "color" matching trials) as compared to pure blocks (i.e., blocks containing "shape" or "color" matching trials but not both). Importantly, mixing costs are believed to not reflect switching ability per se but rather to reflect the added working memory demands associated with maintenance of two sets of task rules for the mixed blocks as compared to only one set for the pure blocks [31]. Within this context, the observed pre- to postintervention change in mixing cost may better conceptualized as an improvement in working memory performance rather than switching ability. Although speculative, the same neurocognitive processes underlying the improvements observed on the working memory span tests may also be responsible for this improvement as well.

As noted earlier, switching task data was unavailable for the nonintervention group. As such, even though there was no evidence of practice effects for either of the other two tasks, we cannot fully rule out the possibility that practice and/or maturational factors may have contributed to the *mixing costs* improvement observed on the switching task. Additional research is needed to rule out this possibility and to further explore the relationship between the improvements observed on the working memory span tasks and those on the switching task.

The present findings add to the growing evidence of improvements in EF in children with ASD participating in social skills training that emphasizes the use of EF skills such as problem solving in conversation [22, 23]. This line of research further supports the use of curricula such as SCI-A that integrates EF skills and application within its delivery. Furthermore, whereas these earlier studies relied almost exclusively on parent report measures (e.g., the BRIEF), the current study utilized performance-based behavioral measures, which are generally accepted to be less susceptible to informant bias. The present methodology also allowed for more precise characterization of the observed improvements such that we found that EF improvements associated with participation in the SCI program were most apparent on working memory-related measures (as compared to inhibitory control or switching). Future research utilizing a similarly approach may prove useful in also refining our understanding intervention-related changes in non-EF processes as well (e.g., emotion recognition, pragmatic language). In addition, by identifying those contributing processes which are most malleable, research such as this may inform future intervention design and planning.

4.1. Additional Limitations and Future Directions. Although both social competence and executive function performance improved with SCI-A participation, we failed to find a direct correlation between the measures of the two constructs within the current study. A number of factors may have contributed to this finding (or lack thereof). For example, whereas the present sample size was comparable to that utilized in several past social competence- and EF-focused ASD intervention studies [10, 21, 22, 68, 69] and appeared sufficient to detect group-related changes in the aforementioned constructs, it was likely undersized/underpowered to fully elucidate the relationship among individual differences in these constructs. Additional research with a larger sample size is also needed to confirm the generalizability of the present findings to the broader population as well as evaluate the extent to which the observed differences may be "clinically meaningful."

Another potential factor relates to differences in the nature of the measures used to assess EF and social competence. Executive function was assessed using performance-based behavioral measures administered within a laboratory setting. In contrast, social competence was assessed using a report-based measure (i.e., the SRS) which focused on the manifestation of social competence ability within the participants' everyday environment. In light of previous research demonstrating only a modest correlation between performance-based and report-based measures even when assessing the same construct (e.g., EF: [70, 71]), the present lack of correlation between performance- and report-based measures of EF and social competence, respectively, is not all too surprising and is not necessarily indicative of a lack of relationship between the two underlying constructs.

The aforementioned methodological mismatch reflects a larger issue within the field, namely, a paucity of performance-based measures of social competence that are well-established and have been demonstrated to be psychometrically sound. The continued development and validation of such measures are essential for future efforts to fully elucidate the nature of the relationship between social competence and other cognitive constructs such as EF.

On a related note, the present tasks were designed to assess core EF component processes in relative isolation while placing minimal demand on other social-related cognitive processes such as language and affect processing. This approach may be viewed as a double-edged sword. On one hand, it allows for isolation of individual component processes. On the other, implementation of executive function in everyday life typically involves placing concurrent demands on multiple EF and non-EF processes. It is possible that a more robust effect would have been observed on more complex multidemand tasks, for example, one aimed at assessing EF in a social context (i.e., the focus of the present intervention).

Lastly, it is worth considering whether or not undiagnosed secondary symptoms related to ADHD or another comorbid condition may have contributed to the present findings. This is particularly relevant given the relatively high prevalence rate of children with comorbid ASD and ADHD [72–74]. Research suggests that these two disorders are each associated with distinct profiles of executive dysfunction [32, 47]. For example, whereas ADHD is associated with significant impairments in inhibitory control [75], findings on inhibitory control in ASD (in absence of ADHD) are much less clear [35]. In addition, while both ASD and ADHD are associated with working memory impairment, the severity of impairment appears exacerbated in individuals with comorbid ASD and ADHD [33]. In terms of the present study, the lack of a significant inhibitory impairment at baseline runs contrary to expectations if there had been extensive ADHD comorbidity among the study's ASD participants. Regardless, additional research is necessary to examine whether the presence/absence of comorbid ADHD symptomatology may influence the effectiveness of the SCI-A program for improving not only social competence ability but also underlying core EF processes such as working memory.

In the present study, intervention targeting social competence and the application of EF skills within a social context appeared to result in generalized benefits for performance on more basic nonsocial EF tasks. This finding is admittedly unusual. Research in this area typically centers on the somewhat reverse of this phenomenon, namely, how focused training (on EF or another particular area of cognition) leads to improvements in a more general area such as social competence. As such, if taken in isolation, the present results might be dismissed as spurious – particularly given the relatively modest effect sizes observed ($g = 0.33–0.57$). However, the current findings are only the latest in a growing body of evidence [22, 23] supporting the possibility of generalized EF improvements in SCI-A intervention participants. Taken together with these past studies, the present results raise a number of interesting questions about the dynamic relationship between social competence ability and underlying cognitive processes such as EF, questions that necessitate additional research.

As detailed earlier, the SCI-A program is designed for children who fit a specific phenotype (i.e., adolescent with HFA) and specifically targets EF as a critical factor in social competence impairments. Within this context, additional research is needed to evaluate to what extent the presently observed gains in EF performance may translate to other age ranges, levels of symptom severity, and variations of the SCI program (e.g., SCI-School: [23]; SCI-Elementary: [68]) as well as other social skills interventions.

4.2. Conclusions and Summary. The present results are consistent with previous reports [22, 23, 68] of generalized improvements in EF associated with participation in the SCI program. By using behavioral tests to separately evaluate core components of EF, we were able to more precisely characterize the nature of the changes in these cognitive processes. Specifically, the findings suggest that participation in the SCI program is associated with improvements in working memory performance, particularly spatial working memory. Working memory (both spatial and verbal) would seem to play a critical role in several aspects of proficient social communication such as turn taking in conversations (i.e., the ability to follow the flow of a conversation while concurrently preparing one's own contribution to the conversation), and identification of social cues and subsequent implementation and maintenance of appropriate metacognitive strategies to enhance a given social interaction. Additional research is needed to fully understand how EF improvements such as those observed in the present study may relate to improved social competence.

Acknowledgments

This work was supported by the University of Missouri Alumni Association (Shawn E. Christ); University of Missouri Research Board (Shawn E. Christ); and Autism Speaks (Shawn E. Christ). The authors would like to thank Tia Schultz and Kourtney Christopher for their assistance with data collection.

References

[1] American Psychiatric Association, *Diagnostic and Statistical Manual of Mental Disorders*, DSM-5, American Psychiatric Association, Arlington, Va, USA, 5th edition, 2013.

[2] C. Lord, "Epidemiology: How common is autism?" *Nature*, vol. 474, no. 7350, pp. 166–168, 2011.

[3] P. Howlin, "Outcomes in autism spectrum disorders," in *Handbook of Autism and Pervasive Developmental Disorders: Diagnosis, Development, Neurobiology and Behavior*, F. R. Volkmar, R. Paul, A. Klin, and D. Cohen, Eds., vol. 1, pp. 201–220, John Wiley & Sons, Inc, Hoboken, NJ, USA, 2005.

[4] M. M. Seltzer, P. Shattuck, L. Abbeduto, and J. S. Greenberg, "Trajectory of development in adolescents and adults with autism," *Mental Retardation and Developmental Disabilities Research Reviews*, vol. 10, no. 4, pp. 234–247, 2004.

[5] L. C. Eaves and H. H. Ho, "Young adult outcome of autism spectrum disorders," *Journal of Autism and Developmental Disorders*, vol. 38, no. 4, pp. 739–747, 2008.

[6] P. Howlin, "Outcome in high-functioning adults with autism with and without early language delays: implications for the differentiation between autism and asperger syndrome," *Journal of Autism and Developmental Disorders*, vol. 33, no. 1, pp. 3–13, 2003.

[7] S. W. White, K. Koenig, and L. Scahill, "Group social skills instruction for adolescents with high-functioning autism spectrum disorders," *Focus on Autism and Other Developmental Disabilities*, vol. 25, no. 4, pp. 209–219, 2010.

[8] T. Atwood, *The Complete Guide to Asperger's Syndrome*, Jessica Kingsley, London, UK, 2007.

[9] K. D. Cummings, R. A. Kaminski, and K. W. Merrell, "Advances in the assessment of social competence: Findings from a preliminary investigation of a general outcome measure for social behavior," *Psychology in the Schools*, vol. 45, no. 10, pp. 930–946, 2008.

[10] N. Bauminger, "The facilitation of social-emotional understanding and social interaction in high-functioning children with autism: intervention outcomes," *Journal of Autism and Developmental Disorders*, vol. 32, no. 4, pp. 283–298, 2002.

[11] K. A. Loveland, B. Tunali-Kotoski, Y. R. Chen et al., "Emotion recognition in autism: Verbal and nonverbal information," *Development and Psychopathology*, vol. 9, no. 3, pp. 579–593, 1997.

[12] S. Baron-Cohen, A. M. Leslie, and U. Frith, "Does the autistic child have a "theory of mind"?" *Cognition*, vol. 21, no. 1, pp. 37–46, 1985.

[13] C. M. Hale and H. Tager-Flusberg, "Social communication in children with autism: the relationship between theory of mind and discourse development," *Autism: The International Journal of Research and Practice*, vol. 9, no. 2, pp. 157–178, 2005.

[14] B. A. Corbett, L. J. Constantine, R. Hendren, D. Rocke, and S. Ozonoff, "Examining executive functioning in children with autism spectrum disorder, attention deficit hyperactivity disorder and typical development," *Psychiatry Research*, vol. 166, no. 2-3, pp. 210–222, 2009.

[15] S. Ozonoff, M. South, and S. Provencal, "Executive functions," in *Handbook of Autism and Pervasive Developmental Disorders: Diagnosis, Development, Neurobiology and Behavior*, F. R. Volkmar, R. Paul, A. Klin, and D. Cohen, Eds., vol. 1, pp. 606–627, John Wiley & Sons, Inc, Hoboken, NJ, USA, 2005.

[16] H. D. Garman, C. J. Spaulding, S. J. Webb, A. Y. Mikami, J. P. Morris, and M. D. Lerner, "Wanting it too much: an inverse relation between social motivation and facial emotion recognition in autism spectrum disorder," *Child Psychiatry and Human Development*, vol. 47, no. 6, pp. 890–902, 2016.

[17] A. M. Scheeren, R. Banerjee, H. M. Koot, and S. Begeer, "Self-Presentation and the Role of Perspective Taking and Social Motivation in Autism Spectrum Disorder," *Journal of Autism and Developmental Disorders*, vol. 46, no. 2, pp. 649–657, 2016.

[18] L. R. Qualls and B. A. Corbett, "Examining the relationship between social communication on the ADOS and real-world reciprocal social communication in children with ASD," *Research in Autism Spectrum Disorders*, vol. 33, pp. 1–9, 2017.

[19] S. Channon, S. Crawford, D. Orlowska, N. Parikh, and P. Thoma, "Mentalising and social problem solving in adults with Asperger's syndrome," *Cognitive Neuropsychiatry*, vol. 19, no. 2, Article ID 809659, pp. 149–163, 2014.

[20] S. L. J. Jackson and B. Dritschel, "Modeling the impact of social problem-solving deficits on depressive vulnerability in the broader autism phenotype," *Research in Autism Spectrum Disorders*, vol. 21, pp. 128–138, 2016.

[21] M. Solomon, B. L. Goodlin-Jones, and T. F. Anders, "A social adjustment enhancement intervention for high functioning autism, Asperger's syndrome, and pervasive developmental disorder NOS," *Journal of Autism and Developmental Disorders*, vol. 34, no. 6, pp. 649–668, 2004.

[22] J. P. Stichter, M. J. Herzog, K. Visovsky et al., "Social competence intervention for youth with Asperger Syndrome and high-functioning autism: An initial investigation," *Journal of Autism and Developmental Disorders*, vol. 40, no. 9, pp. 1067–1079, 2010.

[23] J. P. Stichter, M. J. Herzog, S. A. Owens, and E. Malugen, "Manualization, Feasibility, and Effectiveness of the School-Based Social Competence Intervention for Adolescents (sci-A)," *Psychology in the Schools*, vol. 53, no. 6, pp. 583–600, 2016.

[24] B. J. Webb, S. P. Miller, T. B. Pierce, S. Strawser, and W. P. Jones, "Effects of social skill instruction for high functioning adolescents with autism spectrum disorders," *Focus on Autism and Other Developmental Disabilities*, vol. 19, no. 1, pp. 53–62, 2004.

[25] D. T. Stuss, "Biological and psychological development of executive functions," *Brain and Cognition*, vol. 20, no. 1, pp. 8–23, 1992.

[26] A. Miyake, N. P. Friedman, M. J. Emerson, A. H. Witzki, A. Howerter, and T. D. Wager, "The unity and diversity of executive functions and their contributions to complex "frontal lobe" tasks: a latent variable analysis," *Cognitive Psychology*, vol. 41, no. 1, pp. 49–100, 2000.

[27] A. Baddeley and G. Hitch, "Working memory," in *The Psychology of Learning and Motivation*, vol. 8, pp. 47–89, Academic Press, New York, USA, 1974.

[28] N. Cowan, *Attention and Memory: An Integrated Framework*, Oxford University Press, New York, USA, 1995.

[29] D. Dagenbach and T. Carr, *Inhibitory Processes in Attention, Memory, & Language*, Academic Press, San Diego, Calif, USA, 1994.

[30] F. N. Dempster, "The rise and fall of the inhibitory mechanism: Toward a unified theory of cognitive development and aging," *Developmental Review*, vol. 12, no. 1, pp. 45–75, 1992.

[31] S. Monsell, "Task switching," *Trends in Cognitive Sciences*, vol. 7, no. 3, pp. 134–140, 2003.

[32] P. N. Andersen, E. W. Skogli, K. T. Hovik, H. Geurts, J. Egeland, and M. Øie, "Working memory arrest in children with

high-functioning autism compared to children with attention-deficit/hyperactivity disorder: Results from a 2-year longitudinal study," *Autism*, vol. 19, no. 4, pp. 443–450, 2015.

[33] P. N. Andersen, K. T. Hovik, E. W. Skogli, J. Egeland, and M. Øie, "Symptoms of ADHD in Children with High-Functioning Autism Are Related to Impaired Verbal Working Memory and Verbal Delayed Recall," *PLoS ONE*, vol. 8, no. 5, Article ID e64842, 2013.

[34] E. L. Hill, "Evaluating the theory of executive dysfunction in autism," *Developmental Review*, vol. 24, no. 2, pp. 189–233, 2004.

[35] C. L. E. Lai, Z. Lau, S. S. Y. Lui et al., "Meta-analysis of neuropsychological measures of executive functioning in children and adolescents with high-functioning autism spectrum disorder," *Autism Research: Official Journal of the International Society for Autism Research*, vol. 10, no. 5, pp. 911–939, 2017.

[36] S. E. Christ, D. D. Holt, D. A. White, and L. Green, "Inhibitory control in children with autism spectrum disorder," *Journal of Autism and Developmental Disorders*, vol. 37, no. 6, pp. 1155–1165, 2007.

[37] S. E. Christ, L. E. Kester, K. E. Bodner, and J. H. Miles, "Evidence for selective inhibitory impairment in individuals with autism spectrum disorder," *Neuropsychology*, vol. 25, no. 6, Article ID a0024256, pp. 690–701, 2011.

[38] B. Luna, N. J. Minshew, K. E. Garver et al., "Neocortical system abnormalities in autism: An fMRI study of spatial working memory," *Neurology*, vol. 59, no. 6, pp. 834–840, 2002.

[39] M. W. Mosconi, M. Kay, A.-M. D'Cruz et al., "Impaired inhibitory control is associated with higher-order repetitive behaviors in autism spectrum disorders," *Psychological Medicine*, vol. 39, no. 9, pp. 1559–1566, 2009.

[40] M. C. Goldberg, S. H. Mostofsky, L. E. Cutting et al., "Subtle executive impairment in children with autism and children with ADHD," *Journal of Autism and Developmental Disorders*, vol. 35, no. 3, pp. 279–293, 2005.

[41] E. M. Griffith, B. F. Pennington, E. A. Wehner, and S. J. Rogers, "Executive functions in young children with autism," *Child Development*, vol. 70, no. 4, pp. 817–832, 1999.

[42] J. Russell, C. Jarrold, and B. Hood, "Two intact executive capacities in children with autism: Implications for the core executive dysfunctions in the disorder," *Journal of Autism and Developmental Disorders*, vol. 29, no. 2, pp. 103–112, 1999.

[43] H. M. Geurts, S. F. W. M. van den Bergh, and L. Ruzzano, "Prepotent response inhibition and interference control in autism spectrum disorders: two meta-analyses," *Autism Research: Official Journal of the International Society for Autism Research*, vol. 7, no. 4, pp. 407–420, 2014.

[44] S. E. Gathercole and A. D. Baddeley, *Working Memory and Language*, Psychology Press, 2014.

[45] H. M. Geurts, B. Corbett, and M. Solomon, "The paradox of cognitive flexibility in autism," *Trends in Cognitive Sciences*, vol. 13, no. 2, pp. 74–82, 2009.

[46] C. S. Ames and S. J. White, "Are ADHD traits dissociable from the autistic profile? Links between cognition and behaviour," *Journal of Autism and Developmental Disorders*, vol. 41, no. 3, pp. 357 363, 2011.

[47] S. E. Christ, S. M. Kanne, and A. M. Reiersen, "Executive function in individuals with subthreshold autism traits," *Neuropsychology*, vol. 24, no. 5, Article ID a0019176, pp. 590–598, 2010.

[48] R. E. McEvoy, S. J. Rogers, and B. F. Pennington, "Executive function and social communication deficits in young autistic children," *Journal of Child Psychology and Psychiatry and Allied Disciplines*, vol. 34, no. 4, pp. 563–578, 1993.

[49] S. Ozonoff, B. F. Pennington, and S. J. Rogers, "Executive function deficits in high-functioning autistic individuals: relationship to theory of mind," *Journal of Child Psychology and Psychiatry and Allied Disciplines*, vol. 32, no. 7, pp. 1081–1105, 1991.

[50] J. H. R. Maes, C. T. W. M. Vissers, J. I. M. Egger, and P. A. T. M. Eling, "On the relationship between autistic traits and executive functioning in a non-clinical Dutch student population," *Autism: The International Journal of Research and Practice*, vol. 17, no. 4, pp. 379–389, 2013.

[51] S. J. White, P. W. Burgess, and E. L. Hill, "Impairments on "open-ended" executive function tests in autism," *Autism Research: Official Journal of the International Society for Autism Research*, vol. 2, no. 3, pp. 138–147, 2009.

[52] L. Kenworthy, L. G. Anthony, D. Q. Naiman et al., "Randomized controlled effectiveness trial of executive function intervention for children on the autism spectrum," *Journal of Child Psychology and Psychiatry and Allied Disciplines*, vol. 55, no. 4, pp. 374–383, 2014.

[53] S. M. Carlson, D. J. Mandell, and L. Williams, "Executive function and theory of mind: stability and prediction from ages 2 to 3," *Developmental Psychology*, vol. 40, no. 6, pp. 1105–1122, 2004.

[54] C. Hughes, "Finding your marbles: does preschoolers' strategic behavior predict later understanding of mind?" *Developmental psychology*, vol. 34, no. 6, pp. 1326–1339, 1998.

[55] C. Hughes and R. Ensor, "Executive function and theory of mind: Predictive relations from ages 2 to 4," *Developmental Psychology*, vol. 43, no. 6, pp. 1447–1459, 2007.

[56] E. Pellicano, "Individual Differences in Executive Function and Central Coherence Predict Developmental Changes in Theory of Mind in Autism," *Developmental Psychology*, vol. 46, no. 2, pp. 530–544, 2010.

[57] E. Pellicano, "Testing the predictive power of cognitive atypicalities in autistic children: Evidence from a 3-year follow-up study," *Autism Research: Official Journal of the International Society for Autism Research*, vol. 6, no. 4, pp. 258–267, 2013.

[58] G. Gioia, P. Isquith, S. Guy, and L. Kenworthy, *Behavior Rating Inventory of Executive Function*, Psychological Assessment Resources, Odessa, Fla, USA, 2000.

[59] L. Bowers, R. Huisingh, and C. LoGiudice, *Test of Problem Solving 3: Elementary*, LinguiSystems, Inc., East Moline, Ill, USA, 2005.

[60] C. Lord, S. Risi, L. Lambrecht et al., "The Autism Diagnostic Observation Schedule—generic: a standard measure of social and communication deficits associated with the spectrum of autism," *Journal of Autism and Developmental Disorders*, vol. 30, no. 3, pp. 205–223, 2000.

[61] C. Lord, M. Rutter, and A. Le Couteur, "Autism diagnostic interview-revised: a revised version of a diagnostic interview for caregivers of individuals with possible pervasive developmental disorders," *Journal of Autism and Developmental Disorders*, vol. 24, no. 5, pp. 659–685, 1994.

[62] E. Kaplan, D. Fein, J. Kramer, D. Delis, and R. Morris, *Wechsler Intelligence Scale for Children: Fourth Edition Integrated (WISC-IV Integrated) [Assessment Instrument]*, Pearson, San Antonio, Tex, USA, 2004.

[63] J. N. Constantino, S. A. Davis, R. D. Todd et al., "Validation of a brief quantitative measure of autistic traits: comparison

of the social responsiveness scale with the Autism Diagnostic Interview-Revised," *Journal of Autism and Developmental Disorders*, vol. 33, no. 4, pp. 427–433, 2003.

[64] W. Hays, *Statistics*, Harcourt Brace, Fort Worth, Tex, USA, 1994.

[65] S. A. Gray, P. Chaban, R. Martinussen et al., "Effects of a computerized working memory training program on working memory, attention, and academics in adolescents with severe LD and comorbid ADHD: A randomized controlled trial," *Journal of Child Psychology and Psychiatry and Allied Disciplines*, vol. 53, no. 12, pp. 1277–1284, 2012.

[66] R. J. Gropper, H. Gotlieb, R. Kronitz, and R. Tannock, "Working memory training in college students with ADHD or LD," *Journal of Attention Disorders*, vol. 18, no. 4, pp. 331–345, 2014.

[67] T. Klingberg, H. Forssberg, and H. Westerberg, "Training of working memory in children with ADHD," *Journal of Clinical and Experimental Neuropsychology*, vol. 24, no. 6, pp. 781–791, 2002.

[68] J. P. Stichter, OK. V. Connor, M. J. Herzog, K. Lierheimer, and S. D. McGhee, "Social competence intervention for elementary students with Aspergers syndrome and high functioning autism," *Journal of Autism and Developmental Disorders*, vol. 42, no. 3, pp. 354–366, 2012.

[69] N. Fisher and F. Happé, "A training study of theory of mind and executive function in children with autistic spectrum disorders," *Journal of Autism and Developmental Disorders*, vol. 35, no. 6, pp. 757–771, 2005.

[70] S. McCandless and L. O'Laughlin, "The clinical utility of the Behavior Rating Inventory of Executive Function (BRIEF) in the diagnosis of ADHD," *Journal of Attention Disorders*, vol. 10, no. 4, pp. 381–389, 2007.

[71] M. E. Toplak, S. M. Bucciarelli, U. Jain, and R. Tannock, "Executive functions: Performance-based measures and the behavior rating inventory of executive function (BRIEF) in adolescents with attention deficit/hyperactivity disorder (ADHD)," *Child Neuropsychology*, vol. 15, no. 1, pp. 53–72, 2009.

[72] K. D. Gadow, C. J. DeVincent, and J. Pomeroy, "ADHD symptom subtypes in children with pervasive developmental disorder," *Journal of Autism and Developmental Disorders*, vol. 36, no. 2, pp. 271–283, 2006.

[73] S. Goldstein and A. J. Schwebach, "The comorbidity of pervasive developmental disorder and attention deficit hyperactivity disorder: Results of a retrospective chart review," *Journal of Autism and Developmental Disorders*, vol. 34, no. 3, pp. 329–339, 2004.

[74] H. Sturm, E. Fernell, and C. Gillberg, "Autism spectrum disorders in children with normal intellectual levels: associated impairments and subgroups," *Developmental Medicine & Child Neurology*, vol. 46, no. 7, pp. 444–447, 2004.

[75] E. G. Willcutt, A. E. Doyle, J. T. Nigg, S. V. Faraone, and B. F. Pennington, "Validity of the executive function theory of attention-deficit/hyperactivity disorder: a meta-analytic review," *Biological Psychiatry*, vol. 57, no. 11, pp. 1336–1346, 2005.

20

What Do Parents Think about Chromosomal Microarray Testing? A Qualitative Report from Parents of Children with Autism Spectrum Disorders

Lei Xu,[1] Linda Crane Mitchell,[2] Alice R. Richman,[1] and Kaitlyn Clawson[1]

[1] *Department of Health Education and Promotion, College of Health and Human Performance, Greenville, East Carolina University, Greenville, NC 27858, USA*
[2] *Department of Child Development and Family Relations, College of Health and Human Performance, East Carolina University, Greenville, NC 27858, USA*

Correspondence should be addressed to Lei Xu; xul14@ecu.edu

Academic Editor: Herbert Roeyers

Background. Chromosomal Microarray Analysis (CMA) is increasingly utilized to detect copy number variants among children and families affected with autism spectrum disorders (ASD). However, CMA is controversial due to possible ambiguous test findings, uncertain clinical implications, and other social and legal issues related to the test. *Methods.* Participants were parents of children with ASD residing in the North Eastern region of North Carolina, USA. We conducted individual, face-to-face interviews with 45 parents and inquired about their perceptions of CMA. *Results.* Three major themes dominated parents' perceptions of CMA. None of the parents had ever heard of the test before and the majority of the parents postulated positive attitudes toward the test. Parents' motivations in undergoing the test were attributed to finding a potential cause of ASD, to being better prepared for having another affected child, and to helping with future reproductive decisions. Perceived barriers included the cost of testing, risk/pain of CMA testing, and fear of test results. *Conclusion.* This study contributes to the understanding of psychosocial aspects and cultural influences towards adoption of genetic testing for ASD in clinical practice. Genetic education can aid informed decision-making related to CMA genetic testing among parents of children with ASD.

1. Introduction

Autism Spectrum Disorders (ASD) represent a group of highly inheritable disorders [1]. Although the practices, implementation, and availability of genetic testing for ASD vary in different countries, a growing trend is the embracing of more advanced genetic testing in clinical settings [2–6]. Based on the current clinical guidelines by the American College of Medical Genetics and Genomics (ACMG), an established technology known as Chromosomal Microarray Analysis (CMA) has been recommended as the first-tier test for all children with ASD [7]. CMA is also considered as part of routine care in the ASD diagnostic process and has been available in multiple clinical settings in the United States (USA) such as Duke University Health Systems (DUHS) Clinical Laboratories, Medical Genetics Laboratories at Baylor School of Medicine, and the Division of Genetics and Genomics at Boston Children's Hospital. Furthermore, next-generation prenatal screening for ASD is already under development, although still considerably debated [8].

Research on the clinical benefits/usage of CMA has shown that this test can potentially help ASD patients and their families to explain the causal link of genetics and autism, predict the recurrence risk, help develop timely treatment (medical, educational, and behavioral) plans, and guide parental decision on reproductive options [9–13]. Moreover, compared with traditional tests, CMA has the following features: (1) CMA offers the highest detection rate (approximately 12–19%, compared with G-banded Karyotyping at <3%) [14]; (2) CMA has the ability to detect extra or missing segments of genetic material; therefore, it can provide evidence for other neurological conditions associated with ASD [4]; and (3) CMA test results can influence the medical management among the test-taker who underwent CMA and received abnormal test results [15].

Although CMA has proven to be a more powerful technology in detecting genetic variations over conventional cytogenetic tests [14], this emerging test might raise potential ethical and social considerations, such as genetic discrimination, insurance concerns, confidentiality issues, ambiguous explanation of the test results, and psychological burdens related to the test [12, 13, 15–18]. For instance, in a recent study conducted by Reiff et al. [13] among parents of children with ASD who had CMA testing, parents expressed concerns about the limited usage of the test, the misunderstandings and ambiguities of the test results, and the negative emotions (e.g., "a lot of guilt") associated with the test results. It was also noted that clinicians and other providers who order the test might face challenges in sharing the extensive details from the tests with the test-takers. In addition, as Riggs and colleagues pinpointed [18], genetic health care professionals might have reservations to order CMA for their patients due to both practical and perceived barriers. The reasons included the difficulty of interpreting test results and other negative impacts on the test-takers, for instance, lack of "actionable" medical plans after the test and the denied coverage by insurance companies. Although reimbursement status for CMA genetic testing varied in the US, who would pay for the test remains a big concern among patients and families who intend to undergo CMA genetic testing.

Albeit CMA has both potential benefits and harms, parents' awareness and interest in taking their children with ASD to undergo CMA are still largely unknown. To ensure adequate access to genetic technologies and to reduce the potential negative impact of concerns regarding CMA, there is an immediate need to understand perspectives from parents of children with ASD regarding their awareness, motivations, and inhibitors regarding undergoing CMA testing, including testing themselves and their affected children.

This study focused on parents of children with ASD in Eastern North Carolina (ENC), which is rural area that serves a largely diverse, agricultural, and economically challenged area of the state. ASD identification in North Carolina (1 in 58) is higher than the national average (1 in 68) [19]. This geographical location has one of the highest rates of families who are Medicaid-eligible (Medicaid is a joint federal and state program in the US which helps people with limited income and resources), disadvantaged parents who have children diagnosed with ASD.

This study was part of a larger pilot research project investigating the genetic literacy, education needs, and decisions with regard to CMA genetic testing among parents of children with ASD in ENC. We sought to address three main questions in this particular study. (1) Are parents of children with ASD aware of the availability of CMA testing? (2) What are motivating factors for parents to participate in CMA testing? (3) What do parents identify as barriers that would keep them from participating in CMA testing? The questions we asked containing parents' motivations and barriers associated with both taking their children to undergo the test and test themselves. Our investigations specifically related to parents' perceptions on undergoing prenatal CMA were not reported in this paper. Parents were informed that their answers should be provided in a hypothetical scenario.

2. Materials and Methods

Based on the current literature and our previous published work [13, 20–23], we developed a multipart, semistructured interview guide with 14 questions examining parents' perceptions regarding CMA genetic testing. The questions covered general information regarding CMA genetic testing, inquiries about parental knowledge, perceptions, family planning, and communication related to CMA genetic testing. We used individual, face-to-to face interviews to elicit information about parents' perceptions and decision-making about CMA genetic testing. This study was conducted between December 2014 and February 2015.

The reasons we adopted this qualitative research method are threefold: (1) qualitative methods are more relevant for research areas that have not been adequately researched before, (2) qualitative methods are advantageous in procuring in-depth information about a largely unknown topic, and (3) qualitative methods are powerful in understanding a complex decision-making process [24] such as the one examined in this research.

2.1. Sample and Recruitment. A snowball sampling technique was used to recruit parents of children with ASD living in ENC [24]. In addition, we also reached our potential participants through verbal advertisement at a local autism research fair for parents of children with ASD and through flyers sent to parents through the Autism Society of North Carolina and other local autism education agencies. Our selection criteria included all parents of children with at least one child diagnosed with ASD residing in ENC. Interested parents contacted the researchers directly and scheduled an appointment for a face-to-face interview. Interviews were also scheduled for couples who were interested in study participation.

Our initial recruitment team was composed of three researchers who specialize in public health genomics, social behavioral sciences, and special education. We also used a train-the-trainer model and recruited one community member who was bilingual (English/Spanish) and worked with Hispanic families who have children with ASD due to the vast Hispanic population that is present in ENC. Prior to implementation, approval was acquired from the Institutional Review Board at East Carolina University.

2.2. Procedure. In order to protect confidentiality, participant information was coded using a numerical system. A master list of participants was kept in the office of the lead researcher (LX) in order to complete reality checks during data analysis.

Prior to the interview, the purpose of the study as well as the consent document for participation was reviewed with each participant. We also provided brief information regarding CMA genetic testing at the beginning of each interview session. Interviews lasted 45–60 minutes. Information was provided in Spanish for those who were non-English speaking. The community bilingual specialist conducted the interviews for Spanish-speaking participants. All interviews were audio recorded in order to provide a reliability check for information. Researchers also collected field notes during the interviews to ensure that all related information was collected. Each parent received $40 gift card for participation.

2.3. Data Analysis. Each interview was transcribed verbatim and analyzed using Nvivo 10 [25]. We used a thematic analysis approach, an inductive method, to analyze our qualitative data. The feature of this analytical approach was exploratory and theory-driven, rather than depending on preexisting coding themes. The research team members met weekly to define and redefine the thematic categories as well as resolve discrepancies when divergent opinions arose in the course of data analysis. This researchers' triangulation strengthened the reliability of our data [24].

3. Results and Discussion

3.1. Sample Characteristics. As illustrated by Table 1, the majority of the 45 participants were mothers (60%, $n = 27$). Parents had a mean age of 39.1 years. More than half of participants were spouses who were interviewed individually (57.8%, $n = 26$). Almost 56% of participants were White and the remaining were minorities. Slightly over half of the parents (57.8%, $n = 26$) had an annual income lower than $55K. Forty-four children (35 boys and 9 girls) with ASD were involved in this study and they represented diverse severity levels of ASD as reported by parents (Table 1). Guidelines provided by DSM-5 by American Psychiatry Association were used to assign severity levels of ASD with Level 1 representing mild characteristics of autism, Level 2 moderate, and Level 3 severe [26]. Among the 44 children involved in this study, 9% ($n = 4$) were in Level 1 (high functioning in social communication and less severe symptoms of repetitive behaviors), slightly more than half (52%) were in Level 2 (high functioning in social communication and moderate symptoms of repetitive behaviors), and a quarter of the sample (25%) were in Level 3 in the severe category (either with very low function in social interactions or with the need for very substantial support). Six parents were unable to define the severity level of their children's ASD which accounts for 14% of the children. When parents provided the information regarding severity level of ASD, three of them also mentioned that their children also had intellectual disability. According to the parents, none of them knew any identified etiology of their children's autistic conditions.

Table 1: Sample characteristics ($N = 45$).

Characteristics	n (%)
Participants' age: mean (range)	39.1 years (24–60)
Spouses' age: mean (range)	38.3 years (24–60)
Gender	
Females (mothers)	27 (60)
Males (fathers)	18 (40)
Number of children with ASD	
Boys	35 (79.5)
Girls	9 (20.5)
Race/ethnicity	
White	25 (55.5)
Hispanic/Latino	14 (31.1)
Black	4 (8.9)
American Indian/Alaskan native	1 (2.2)
Others	1 (2.2)
Education	
High school diploma or less	16 (35.6)
Some college	4 (8.9)
College graduate or above	25 (55.5)
Employment status	
Employed	32 (71.1)
Homemaker	11 (24.4)
Not employed	2 (4.4)
Annual household income	
<$15,000	7 (15.6)
$15,000–35,000	11 (24.4)
$35,001–$55,000	8 (17.8)
$55,001–$75,000	5 (11.1)
$75,001–$95,000	6 (13.3)
Over $95,001	8 (17.8)
Participants not born in USA	15 (33.3)
Child's age of diagnosis: mean (range)	4.3 years (1.5–13)
Severity level	
Level 1 (mild)	4 (9.1)
Level 2 (moderate)	23 (52.3)
Level 3 (severe)	11 (25)
Answer not provided	6 (13.6)

3.2. Interview Findings. Based on parents' perspectives on undergoing ASD genetic testing, three main themes emerged from the data: parental awareness of CMA genetic testing, test motivations, and perceived barriers to undergoing CMA genetic testing.

3.2.1. Parental Awareness of CMA Genetic Testing. Before we asked parents their attitudes toward CMA genetic testing, we asked parents "what is the first word that comes to your mind when you hear the word genetics." Then we provided brief information about CMA (e.g., what did CMA stand for, what was CMA, and what is the testing procedure). Regardless of the diverse socioeconomic status, none of the 45 parents reported that they were knowledgeable of CMA. One of the fathers with twin boys who was highly educated and had previous training in molecular genetics reported that he never knew that CMA was a genetic test that was available to his children (twins) with ASD. According to him,

> *This particular test I have not heard of. I've heard of general genetic testing, but not CMA.*

Another mother who also doubted that anyone in the local autism community had heard of the test before commented that

> *No, not in the group here, local – I don't know anybody that has (heard of CMA genetic testing).*

3.2.2. Test Motivations. Table 2 illustrates recurrent motivations for why parents reported that they would participate in CMA (including testing themselves and their children with ASD). The subthemes, percentages, and illustrative quotes are provided in Table 2.

Helping Identify a Potential Cause of Autism. The most recurrent motivation from participants was whether CMA genetic testing could help identify a potential cause of autism. Almost half of participants ($n = 21$, 46.7%) mentioned that the ability for CMA genetic testing to provide a link to the cause of their child's autism would motivate them to test themselves and their children. One participant noted that

> *Um... to see if there is a genetic link, to see if it's something that I've passed on versus something that I may have caused during my pregnancy. Because as a parent, when you find out your child has autism, your first reaction is- is it my fault? Did I do this? Is something wrong with me? Is something wrong with my child? So, I think a test like that would bring a little bit of peace to you to know whether or not it was in your bloodline, it was in your genetics, and you passed it down. (Male, White, Income: $15–$35K)*

Preparing for Having Another Child with ASD. Similarly, being prepared to have a child with autism was mentioned by the equal numbers of participants ($n = 21$, 46.7%). Participants particularly mentioned that CMA testing results would not change their decisions of giving birth to another child, but they still wanted to use CMA genetic testing as a tool to be more prepared for having another child with ASD. One mother specified that

> *I think it would be interesting. I would be open to be tested. I don't think that would sway my decisions of whether I would have another child or not, but it might prepare me for the eventually of possibly dealing with another child with autism. (Female, Hispanic, Income: <$15K)*

Family Planning. Less than half of the participants ($n = 18$, 40%) indicated that the CMA genetic testing would provide them with assistance in family planning. According to one participant,

> *For me, personally, yes, it [testing] would play a major role in family planning just because of my knowledge of a child with a disability, and the cost, stigma, and the opportunity for the child. (Male, American Indian/Alaskan native, Income: >$95K)*

Early Intervention. Nearly 40% ($n = 17$, 37.8%) of participants specified that early intervention for their child with ASD would be a motivation to participate in CMA genetic testing. For instance, one participant stated that

> *So that would be preparing the boys (autistic children), thinking about early intervention strategies to help the child learn how to communicate and develop. It would give us some more support when speaking with pediatricians and such about hey this is a real concern. What are the things we want to start working on early... so I think those would be some benefits of it. (Male, White, Income: $35–$55K)*

Research to Benefit Other Families with Autistic Children. One-third of participants ($n = 15$, 33.3%) indicated that the main motivation to undergo CMA genetic testing would be for research purposes to benefit other families. According to one interviewee,

> *I don't plan on having more family... and if it would help other people through my daughter, to know the motive why these things [autism spectrum disorders] happen, I would do it for that reason. (Male, Hispanic/Latino, Income: $15–35K)*

Benefit Their Own Child with Autism. A motivation for some participants was that the results of the CMA genetic testing would benefit their child with autism ($n = 14$, 31.1%). These benefits ranged from types of therapies to medical treatments to help their child with autism. One participant indicated that

> *Any type of testing that could help his ability to socialize more in the world. Whatever tests are out there or whatever that can help him... Let's do that [CMA testing]. (Female, African American, Income $35–$55K)*

Getting to Know the Recurrence Risk. A number of participants ($n = 8$, 17.7%) also demonstrated that a motivation to participate in the genetic testing was the ability to be informed about the recurrence risk, the risk that they may have another child with ASD. According to one participant,

> *This [CMA testing] also would benefit us though because it would give us, are we going to have a 90% chance that we will have another child with autism? That would be something that would be interesting to know. (Male, White, Income: $35–$55K)*

Confirming ASD Diagnosis. As indicated in Table 2, three participants (6.7%) specified that they would utilize genetic testing to confirm their child's diagnosis of ASD.

Table 2: Motivators for participants with at least one child with ASD to participate in CMA genetic testing (*N* = 45).

Theme	*n* (%)	Illustrative quote
Helping identify a potential cause of autism	21 (46.7)	*To know exactly where the origin of the problem of autism is that he has. (Female, Hispanic/Latino, Income: <$15K)* *The motivation would be to help the knowledge base better understand what causes autism... Having research like this can help the stigma of autism. (Male, American Indian/Alaskan native, Income: >$95K)*
Preparing for having another child with ASD	21 (46.7)	*I would like to know. I think it would be nice to know while you're pregnant with the child if the child is going to have autism... it would be a preparation tool. You know you would be able to prepare yourself, and to start preparing you and your family for what you're going to have to do when the child is growing up and prepare you for all the therapies and the cost of autism and the stress – that would be really helpful to know that information. (Male, White, Income: $15–35K)* *For me, if I wanted to have another child, I would be prepared if it was coming with autism.... (Female, Hispanic/Latino, Income: $15–35K)*
Family planning	18 (40)	*If I had done the test before I got pregnant, it would have been to make the decision if I would get pregnant or not or if I would have had this baby. (Female, Hispanic/Latino, Income: <$15K)*
Early intervention	17 (37.8)	*I can get help ahead of time... Instead of waiting until it is too late... so that he has to catch up. (Male, White, $75–95K)*
Research to benefit other families	15 (33.3)	*I think probably at this point in their [children with autism] lives the only reason why I would want to know is to help other people... but I think it would be especially at this point the testing would be more to help other people. (Female, White, Income: >$95K)*
Benefit their own child with autism	14 (31.1)	*I don't know that it will happen in my lifetime, but to help with drugs, chemicals, and could help even my son [with autism]. (Male, American Indian/Alaskan Native, Income: >$95K)*
Getting to know the recurrence risk	8 (17.7)	*I would personally do something like that, if I were to have another child I would want to know the risks, not that it would make a difference but it would be good to know. (Female, White, Income: $35–55K)*
Confirming autism diagnosis	3 (6.7)	*I would do it, [participate in CMA testing] not because I want to have more children, but to do away with doubts [that he has autism] and more than anything. (Male, Latino/Hispanic, Income: $35–55K)*

3.2.3. Barriers to Participating in CMA Testing. In addition to identifying participants' motivations to participate in CMA genetic testing, the research team also synthesized the barriers and reservations parents had before testing themselves and their children (Table 3).

Cost of Testing. The majority of participants ($n = 33$, 73.3%) were concerned with the cost of CMA testing. For example, one interviewee stated that

> *This is a common barrier a lot of times insurance does not pay for genetic testing, and we do not have Medicaid, we have private insurance... Genetic testing can be very expensive, and most families do not have access to that kind of money. (Female, White, Income: $55–75K)*

Risk/Pain Associated with CMA Testing. Over one-third ($n = 17$, 37.8%) of participants mentioned that either the risk or pain associated with CMA testing would be a barrier of participating in genetic testing. One parent expressed his concern:

> *My only concern would be he wouldn't want to take the blood out. You know he doesn't like doctors. He doesn't like needles, so that would be a challenge for him, to put him through that emotional rollercoaster.... (Male, White, $75–95K)*

Fear of Results. Fourteen participants ($n = 14$, 31.1%) mentioned that their fear of the results from the test would hinder them from participating in CMA testing. One of the participants has taken her son to undergo genetic testing for autism prior to our interview. She described her experience:

> *It took months for the test results to get back. It took a while to return and it was nerve racking. (Female, White, $55–75K)*

A portion of participants (15.6%, $n = 7$) expressed that they had *little to no motivation* to test themselves or their child. Moreover, six participants (13.3%) stated that *transportation and/or scheduling issues* would be a barrier for them to participate in genetic testing. In addition, five participants (11.1%) articulated that their *lack of knowledge and understanding about CMA genetic testing* would prohibit them from participating. The illustrative quotes are shown in Table 3.

3.3. Discussion. This exploratory study highlights important findings and applications associated with parents' before-testing perceptions of CMA. The unique value of this empirical research is fourfold: first, our study was among the first community-based studies that investigated the willingness/motivations related to CMA genetic testing among parents with at least once child diagnosed with ASD. Previous investigations on genetic testing for autism were primarily conducted in clinical settings [12, 13, 16], where participants probably were prone to genetic research and had better access to care. Our community-based approach allows us to elicit broad opinions from diverse members within autism communities, particularly in rural areas.

Second, half of our participants were spouses who participated in our study and were interviewed individually. Past studies had investigated couples' perceptions of undergoing genetic testing for other conditions, such as bipolar disorders and cystic fibrosis, and found that couples had different viewpoints on having themselves or spouses tested for the genetic conditions run in the families [27, 28]. Our study found that spouses might blame each other related to who has passed on an autistic condition to their affected children. Some of them might feel guilty or blame themselves for being the culprit for their children's autism. Our study suggests that future education interventions should have a component in helping parents to alleviate negative emotions related to the test, such as guilt and blame, and focus more on locating the therapeutic and educational approaches using the information obtained from the test.

Third, our study was one of the first studies that addressed the perceptions particularly from low-income parents with diverse ethnicities; for instance, over one-third of our participants were Hispanic/Latino and all were Medicaid eligible. The average age of these Hispanic participants was below 40 (they are still at the reproductive age) and they showed keen interest in undergoing the test if it is available. Before our interviews, we asked parents which language they would prefer, most of them (13 out of the 14 Latino parents) preferred to be interviewed in Spanish. All of these participants mentioned that the cost of testing was the biggest barrier that might hinder their actual behavior of taking their children to undergo the test. Future educational interventions need to be linguistically sensitive for ethnic minorities. This design can enhance both their willingness to participate in the genetic research projects and also the comfort level of sharing information with the researchers.

Fourth, another salient finding of our study was that the overwhelming majority of our participants (almost 85%) showed interest and indicated motivation to either take their children to undergo CMA genetic testing or participate in the testing themselves. We found that parents' favorable positon towards CMA was slightly higher than two prior published studies that explored parents' attitudes and interest towards genetic testing for autism [21, 22]. Specifically, parents' favorable attitudes in CMA in our study were potentially explained by parents' perceived benefits from the usage of the test, such as finding a potential cause of ASD, getting prepared for having a child with ASD, learning more guidance on family planning, and early intervention. In contrast, in another study assessing parents' intention related to undergoing genetic testing for autism, parents mentioned that one of the most deciding factors for testing was the intent to reduce the anxiety level [21]. Given that parents were not aware of the availability of CMA for their affected children and families before participating in our study, therefore, the willingness to test might be imposed by insufficient understanding about these yet-unknown tests.

Parents' lack of awareness of CMA testing might reflect parents' limited access to medical professionals, such as

Table 3: Barriers for participants with at least one child with ASD that would keep them from participating in CMA genetic testing ($N = 45$).

Theme	*n* (%)	Illustrative quote
Cost	33 (73.3)	*The cost for a child with autism is already so expensive just for the therapy and getting help for the child. You know, adding another cost would be difficult. (Male, White, Income: $75–95K)* *Cost would be something to consider. I know a lot of genetic testing can be expensive. Umm cost would be a factor. (Male, White, Income: $35–55K)* *Maybe the expense of it. If it wasn't covered by insurance that might be something that would sway me. (Female, White, Income: $75–95K)*
Risk and pain associated with testing	17 (37.8)	*The concerns would be... how invasive it is and then the potential psychological issues it may cause them. (Male, White, Income: $35–55K)* *Maybe the concern would be about him getting his blood taken. It would be difficult for him. He doesn't like it when they take blood samples. He's afraid of needles. It would be difficult. (Female, Hispanic/Latino, Income: $15–35K)*
Fear of result	14 (33.3)	*I think it probably would open up a big can of worms as far as pointing fingers at where those genes came from. (Female, White, Income: >$95K)* *My concerns would be it [test result] comes back positive. (Female, Hispanic/Latino, $35–55K)*
Lack of motivation for testing	7 (15.6)	*Me personally, I wouldn't want to do it [undergo CMA testing]. I don't think it would change anything. It sort of why we resisted the diagnosis from the very beginning... I don't want a preconceived notion of who they're going to be. (Female, Hispanic/Latino, Income: $33–55K)*
Transportation and/or scheduling Issues	6 (13.3)	*We really don't have a whole lot of time to be able to do things like this testing. I do not want them out of school; they need that kind of structure. (Female, White, Income: $15–35K)* *The procedure and the timing because of my job I can't get off, because there are only two people in the office, me and my boss.... (Female, White, Income: <$15K)*
Lack of knowledge about testing	5 (11.1)	*I would need more information for them [children with autism] if they are going to do a blood test. (Female, Hispanic/Latino, Income: $35–55K)* *It would all depend on what the test will give you. If the test says, 'Your son might have autism, your son might not,' I wouldn't want that because I wouldn't want to go looking for the problem without a cause. If you can give it to me definitively, 'yes your son has the markers. He's going to be expected by the autism spectrum in some way.' Then sure, I might want to know that up front. (Female, White, Income: >$95K)* *I don't know. I don't know enough about the test. (Male, White, Income: $75–95K)*

genetic counselors, medical geneticists, and pediatricians who can order the CMA testing for the children affected with ASD. Also, genetic testing/assessments were usually not provided before children complete/go through a long diagnostic process. Parents might be referred by primary care practitioners to speak to a medical geneticist or genetic counselor after the initial diagnosis; however, none of the parents in our study, as we discussed, had been referred to any genetic specialists about CMA testing. This might be contributed to the limited resources due to the fact that parents in our study live in relatively underserved areas. For instance, in the specific geographic location where this study was conducted, no genetic counselors are available who might provide the information regarding undergoing CMA for parents and children with ASD. During our research, participating parents queried who they could ask about CMA and who could provide any counseling or education sessions for them. Given the limited number of genetic counselors, health education specialists are in a better position of providing educational resources to parents pertaining to CMA testing. Providers need to be aware of parents' lack of understanding of CMA, particularly among low-income parents. Our study also suggests the necessity of providing pretest counseling strategies that can be incorporated into the educational materials.

Several limitations of this research deserve attention when interpreting the results. First, our recruitment strategy aimed to reach parents of children with at least one child diagnosed with ASD. However, although we recruited participants from various ASD communities in ENC, the diagnosis and the severity level were self-reported by the participants themselves. We were not able to confirm the information claimed by parents. Second, parents' attitudes toward CMA genetic testing involved a hypothetical scenario of undergoing the test. We realize that our findings might differ from the actual situations where parents decide to test themselves or take their children to undergo CMA.

Genetic education and counseling tailored to parents of children with ASD are needed. As one of the first studies that explored parents' attitudes toward CMA, our results indicate a clear need for supporting the genetic services/education interventions for people and families affected with ASD, particularly in economically disadvantaged regions. Future studies might consider using a quantitative method with a larger sample size, such as surveys in various forms, to better understand parents' attitudes toward CMA genetic testing. In order to maximize the quality of genetic services related to CMA genetic testing, educational efforts should be implemented among clinicians, genetic counselors, and other health professionals, particularly in the context of precounselling stage prior to offering CMA to parents and their children with ASD.

Acknowledgments

The authors want to give special acknowledgments to all parents of children who were willing to participate in this qualitative study.

References

[1] J. H. Miles, "Autism spectrum disorders—a genetics review," *Genetics in Medicine*, vol. 13, no. 4, pp. 278–294, 2011.

[2] S. G. McGrew, B. R. Peters, J. A. Crittendon, and J. Veenstra-VanderWeele, "Diagnostic yield of chromosomal microarray analysis in an autism primary care practice: which guidelines to implement?" *Journal of Autism and Developmental Disorders*, vol. 42, no. 8, pp. 1582–1591, 2012.

[3] I. Maya, B. Davidov, L. Gershovitz et al., "Diagnostic utility of array-based comparative genomic hybridization (aCGH) in a prenatal setting," *Prenatal Diagnosis*, vol. 30, no. 12-13, pp. 1131–1137, 2010.

[4] D. T. Miller, M. P. Adam, S. Aradhya et al., "Consensus statement: chromosomal microarray is a first-tier clinical diagnostic test for individuals with developmental disabilities or congenital anomalies," *The American Journal of Human Genetics*, vol. 86, no. 5, pp. 749–764, 2010.

[5] E. E. Palmer, G. B. Peters, and D. Mowat, "Chromosome microarray in Australia: a guide for paediatricians," *Journal of Paediatrics and Child Health*, vol. 48, no. 2, pp. E59–E67, 2012.

[6] H.-M. Liao, S. S.-F. Gau, W.-C. Tsai et al., "Chromosomal abnormalities in patients with autism spectrum disorders from Taiwan," *American Journal of Medical Genetics, Part B: Neuropsychiatric Genetics*, vol. 162, no. 7, pp. 734–741, 2013.

[7] G. B. Schaefer and N. J. Mendelsohn, "Clinical genetics evaluation in identifying the etiology of autism spectrum disorders: 2013 guideline revisions," *Genetics in Medicine*, vol. 15, no. 5, pp. 399–407, 2013.

[8] B. R. Jordan and D. F. C. Tsai, "Whole-genome association studies for multigenic diseases: ethical dilemmas arising from commercializationd the case of genetic testing for autism," *Journal of Medical Ethics*, vol. 36, no. 7, pp. 440–444, 2010.

[9] S. Darilek, P. Ward, A. Pursley et al., "Pre- and postnatal genetic testing by array-comparative genomic hybridization: genetic counseling perspectives," *Genetics in Medicine*, vol. 10, no. 1, pp. 13–18, 2008.

[10] M. A. Eriksson, J. Westerlund, Å. Hedvall, P. Åmark, C. Gillberg, and E. Fernell, "Medical conditions affect the outcome of early intervention in preschool children with autism spectrum disorders," *European Child and Adolescent Psychiatry*, vol. 22, no. 1, pp. 23–33, 2013.

[11] C. Lintas and A. M. Persico, "Autistic phenotypes and genetic testing: state-of-the-art for the clinical geneticist," *Journal of Medical Genetics*, vol. 46, no. 1, pp. 1–8, 2009.

[12] M. Reiff, K. Ross, S. Mulchandani et al., "Physicians' perspectives on the uncertainties and implications of chromosomal microarray testing of children and families," *Clinical Genetics*, vol. 83, no. 1, pp. 23–30, 2013.

[13] M. Reiff, E. Giarelli, B. A. Bernhardt et al., "Parents' perceptions of the usefulness of chromosomal microarray analysis for children with autism spectrum disorders," *Journal of Autism and Developmental Disorders*, vol. 45, no. 10, pp. 3262–3275, 2015.

[14] Y. Shen, K. A. Dies, I. A. Holm et al., "Clinical genetic testing for patients with autism spectrum disorders," *Pediatrics*, vol. 125, no. 4, pp. e727–e735, 2010.

[15] M. E. Coulter, D. T. Miller, D. J. Harris et al., "Chromosomal microarray testing influences medical management," *Genetics in Medicine*, vol. 13, no. 9, pp. 770–776, 2011.

[16] B. A. Bernhardt, D. Soucier, K. Hanson, M. S. Savage, L. Jackson, and R. J. Wapner, "Women's experiences receiving abnormal prenatal chromosomal microarray testing results," *Genetics in Medicine*, vol. 15, no. 2, pp. 139–145, 2013.

[17] G. Mcgillivray, J. A. Rosenfeld, R. J. Mckinlay Gardner, and L. H. Gillam, "Genetic counselling and ethical issues with chromosome microarray analysis in prenatal testing," *Prenatal Diagnosis*, vol. 32, no. 4, pp. 389–395, 2012.

[18] E. R. Riggs, K. E. Wain, D. Riethmaier et al., "Chromosomal microarray impacts clinical management," *Clinical Genetics*, vol. 85, no. 2, pp. 147–153, 2014.

[19] CDC, March 2015, http://www.cdc.gov/ncbddd/autism/states/addm-north-carolina-fact-sheet.pdf.

[20] M. Trottier, W. Roberts, I. Drmic et al., "Parents' perspectives on participating in genetic research in autism," *Journal of Autism and Developmental Disorders*, vol. 43, no. 3, pp. 556–568, 2013.

[21] V. Narcisa, M. Discenza, E. Vaccari, B. Rosen-Sheidley, A. Y. Hardan, and E. Couchon, "Parental interest in a genetic risk assessment test for autism spectrum disorders," *Clinical Pediatrics*, vol. 52, no. 2, pp. 139–146, 2013.

[22] L.-S. Chen, L. Xu, T.-Y. Huang, and S. U. Dhar, "Autism genetic testing: a qualitative study of awareness, attitudes, and experiences among parents of children with autism spectrum disorders," *Genetics in Medicine*, vol. 15, no. 4, pp. 274–281, 2013.

[23] L.-S. Chen, L. Xu, S. U. Dhar, M. Li, D. Talwar, and E. Jung, "Autism spectrum disorders: a qualitative study of attitudes toward prenatal genetic testing and termination decisions of affected pregnancies," *Clinical Genetics*, vol. 88, no. 2, pp. 122–128, 2015.

[24] Y. S. Linclon and E. G. Guba, *Naturalisitic Inquiry*, Sage, Newbury Park, Calif, USA, 1985.

[25] P. Bazeley, *Qualitative Analysis with Nvivo*, Sage, Thousand Oaks, Calif, USA, 2007.

[26] American Psychiatric Association, *Diagnostic and Statistical Manual of Mental Disorders: DSM-5*, American Psychiatric Association, Washington, Wash, USA, 2013.

[27] H. K. Tabor, T. Brazg, J. Crouch et al., "Parent perspectives on pediatric genetic research and implications for genotype-driven research recruitment," *Journal of Empirical Research on Human Research Ethics*, vol. 6, no. 4, pp. 41–52, 2011.

[28] C. L. Trippitelli, K. R. Jamison, M. F. Folstein, J. J. Bartko, and J. R. DePaulo, "Pilot study on patients' and spouses' attitudes toward potential genetic testing for bipolar disorder," *The American Journal of Psychiatry*, vol. 155, no. 7, pp. 899–904, 1998.

21

Factor Structure, Internal Consistency, and Screening Sensitivity of the GARS-2 in a Developmental Disabilities Sample

Martin A. Volker,[1] Elissa H. Dua,[2] Christopher Lopata,[3] Marcus L. Thomeer,[3] Jennifer A. Toomey,[4] Audrey M. Smerbeck,[5] Jonathan D. Rodgers,[3] Joshua R. Popkin,[2] Andrew T. Nelson,[4] and Gloria K. Lee[1]

[1] *Department of Counseling, Educational Psychology, and Special Education, College of Education, Michigan State University, East Lansing, MI 48824-1034, USA*
[2] *Department of Counseling, School and Educational Psychology, Graduate School of Education, University at Buffalo, The State University of New York, Buffalo, NY 14260-1000, USA*
[3] *Institute for Autism Research, Canisius College, 2001 Main Street, Buffalo, NY 14208, USA*
[4] *Summit Educational Resources, 150 Stahl Road, Getzville, NY 14068, USA*
[5] *Psychology Department, College of Liberal Arts, Rochester Institute of Technology, Rochester, NY 14230, USA*

Correspondence should be addressed to Martin A. Volker; volkerma@msu.edu

Academic Editor: Klaus-Peter Ossenkopp

The Gilliam Autism Rating Scale-Second Edition (GARS-2) is a widely used screening instrument that assists in the identification and diagnosis of autism. The purpose of this study was to examine the factor structure, internal consistency, and screening sensitivity of the GARS-2 using ratings from special education teaching staff for a sample of 240 individuals with autism or other significant developmental disabilities. Exploratory factor analysis yielded a correlated three-factor solution similar to that found in 2005 by Lecavalier for the original GARS. Though the three factors appeared to be reasonably consistent with the intended constructs of the three GARS-2 subscales, the analysis indicated that more than a third of the GARS-2 items were assigned to the wrong subscale. Internal consistency estimates met or exceeded standards for screening and were generally higher than those in previous studies. Screening sensitivity was .65 and specificity was .81 for the Autism Index using a cut score of 85. Based on these findings, recommendations are made for instrument revision.

1. Introduction

Autism spectrum disorder (ASD) is characterized by a complex profile of symptoms including social communication impairments and repetitive and restricted interests and behaviors [1]. Although core diagnostic features have been delineated, individuals with ASD exhibit significant variability in their presentation and severity of symptoms. Significant variability in symptom manifestation makes diagnosis complex [2]. Diagnosis is further complicated by the need to differentiate individuals with ASD from individuals with other developmental disabilities that may share some associated features (e.g., language impairment, intellectual disability). Klin et al. [3] noted that "the number of children being referred for developmental disabilities assessments with a differential diagnosis of autism continues to increase each year" (page 772). Given the multiple areas affected, variable symptoms, and challenges involving differential diagnosis, there is a significant need for assessment tools that contribute to accurate diagnosis. This is particularly urgent for individuals with ASD as early diagnosis is essential for access to intensive intervention which has been associated with better long-term outcomes [2].

Measures used in assessments for ASD have been categorized along different dimensions including purpose (i.e., screening versus diagnosis) and level of training needed for administration/scale completion (i.e., professional/trained raters versus untrained raters [4, 5]). At present, two measures recognized for their diagnostic accuracy are the Autism Diagnostic Interview-Revised (ADI-R [6]) and Autism Diagnostic Observation Schedule-Second Edition (ADOS-2 [7]). These measures are the most widely respected diagnostic measures; however they are lengthy to administer and require considerable skill and experience working with individuals with ASD [4, 8]. As a result, the ADOS-2 and ADI-R may be beyond the training of many practitioners and less feasible in some settings (e.g., schools [2, 9]).

Issues with the feasibility (training/expertise requirements, lengthy administration, etc.) of these measures have led to increased reliance on rating scales that can be completed by parents and teachers familiar with the functioning of the individual being assessed. A survey by Allen et al. [9] found rating scales were used far more frequently in ASD assessments by school psychologist than the original ADOS or ADI-R. Although informant rating scales may not be diagnostic on their own, they can contribute important information as part of screenings and/or comprehensive assessments [2, 10] and can assist with differential diagnosis [11]. This is especially useful when the measure assesses multiple constructs, is keyed to a diagnostic framework (e.g., *DSM-IV or DSM-5*), and provides a quantification of symptoms [3, 5, 8]. Informant rating scales may offer advantages over professionally administered scales (e.g., ADI-R) such as greater efficiency and reduced training. Rating scales also provide normative data, are standardized, and may assist with progress monitoring [4]. Despite their potential, rating scales may have limitations (e.g., lack of alignment between scale items and diagnostic criteria, inadequate psychometric properties) that reduce their validity [4]. These potential problems have led to recommendations for psychometric studies of commonly used rating scales [4, 5].

One of the most commonly used ratings scales is the Gilliam Autism Rating Scale-Second Edition (GARS-2 [12]). A survey published in 2008 found that 40% of school psychologists used the GARS-2 in the majority of their ASD-related assessments [9]. The GARS-2 (a revision of the original scale) is a 42-item informant rating scale designed to assist in the identification and diagnosis of autism and provide information on symptom severity. It can be completed by parents, teachers, and/or clinicians. The items are grouped to form three subscales (Stereotyped Behaviors, 14 items; Social Interaction, 14 items; and Communication, 14 items) and an overall Autism Index. Items were based on definitions of autism delineated at that time in the *DSM-IV-TR* [13] and by the Autism Society of America. For noncommunicative individuals, the Communication subscale is omitted and the Autism Index is calculated based on the other two subscales. While the GARS-2 item content is very similar to the original scale items [5], the test author reported improvements including the rewriting of some items to increase clarity, elimination of the Early Development scale (replaced by a parent interview not included in scoring), renorming based on the 2000 census, and modification of the guidelines for score interpretation [12].

Reliability data are presented in the GARS-2 manual for both internal consistency and stability. Internal consistency estimates were .88 for Social Interaction, .86 for Communication, .84 for Stereotyped Behaviors, and .94 for the Autism Index. Corrected test-retest coefficients (1-week interval) based on parent ratings of 37 children with autism were .88 for Social Interaction, .70 for Communication, .90 for Stereotyped Behavior, and .88 for the overall Autism Index. Validity data were presented based on correlations between subscale items and the subdomain total score. Median values were Social Interaction .55, Communication .53, and Stereotyped Behaviors .53, and the median coefficient for the sum of all items was .47. Sensitivity and specificity were assessed using matched samples of individuals with autism compared to individuals with intellectual disability, multiple disabilities, and typical controls. Using a cut score of 85 for the GARS-2 Autism Index, sensitivity for the autism group was 1.00 versus typical controls, .85 versus the group with intellectual disability, and .84 versus those with multiple disabilities. Specificity values for the same groups were .87, .85, and .84, respectively [12].

Despite the support reported in the manual, concerns have been noted regarding the need for additional details on the standardization sample characteristics, online recruitment, and lack of diagnostic confirmation [14, 15]. Norris and Lecavalier reviewed the GARS-2 and noted other potential problems including the large numbers of children rated by the same teachers (potential response bias) and the similarity between items on the previous version and the GARS-2 which may lead to problems similar to those of the original GARS involving poor sensitivity and specificity [15]. In a study examining the factor structure and reliability of the original GARS using parent ($n = 241$) and teacher ($n = 119$) ratings, Lecavalier found a three-factor solution consisting of Stereotyped Behaviors, Social Interaction impairments, and communication deficits [4], although these appeared generally consistent with the conceptually derived scales of the GARS, nearly half (i.e., 48%) of the items loaded on the stereotyped behavior scale. Most items had an acceptable factor loading on a single factor; however 26% of the items loaded on scales other than that proposed by the test author. Internal consistency (coefficient alpha) was .82 for Stereotyped Behavior, .85 for Social Interaction, and .84 for Communication. Despite all cases in the sample reportedly having ASD, the Autism Quotient score (using the original GARS probability categories) placed nearly two-thirds of the sample in the "below average" probability of autism category or lower, indicating low sensitivity. (Similar concerns regarding the GARS were raised by South and colleagues [16], who reported a screening sensitivity of .48 for the Autism Quotient in their study sample.) Interrater reliability was low (.31–.48) which may have been affected by the use of informants having different roles (parents versus teachers) or other factors. Overall, Lecavalier cautioned that the amount of explained variance in the factor solution was low (i.e., 38%) and recommended caution when using the GARS for screening or diagnosis as many facets of social and communicative impairment were not adequately assessed and several items may only be tapping related features [4].

While prior studies have provided useful psychometric information on the original GARS, the current review yielded only one published psychometric study of the GARS-2.

Pandolfi and colleagues conducted an exploratory factor analysis (EFA), as well as a follow-up confirmatory factor analysis (CFA; to determine if the model was replicated) using matched subgroups from the GARS-2 standardization sample [5]. The protocols were completed by parents, educators, and clinicians for individuals reported to have autism. EFA results yielded a four-factor model (accounting for 38.6% of the variance) which consisted of stereotyped/repetitive behaviors, stereotyped/idiosyncratic language, word use problems, and social impairment. Items from the GARS-2 Communication scale were found to be dispersed across the four factors identified in the EFA, with seven items splitting to help create two language/communication-related factors (stereotyped/idiosyncratic language and word use problems). Correlations were moderate between the stereotyped/repetitive behaviors, stereotyped/idiosyncratic language, and social impairment factors. In contrast, the word use problems factor had very weak correlations with the other factors suggesting that it was relatively independent and not autism-specific. The CFA replicated the results and the word use problems factor was again weakly associated with the other factors. Reliability for each scale was above .80 and median item-total correlations were ≥.45. The empirically derived four-factor model led Pandolfi and colleagues to question the clinical utility of the GARS-2 subscales and suggest that the three conceptually derived subscales put forth by the test developer are measuring more than one construct [5]. The researchers suggested that scale/item problems may be a function of some items only describing a correlate of the intended construct and/or the inclusion of complex or "double-barreled" items that assess multiple behaviors or characteristics. Additionally, some items appeared to assess non-autism-specific characteristics which may restrict discrimination between individuals with autism or other developmental disabilities [5].

Given the prominence of rating scales in the assessment of ASD, research is needed to determine their psychometric adequacy. Information in the GARS-2 technical manual details a number of positive attributes; however independent empirical evaluation is limited. Only one study has examined the GARS-2 factor structure and that study raised significant concerns about the validity of the subscales and the measure's clinical utility. Additionally, there have been no published studies evaluating the sensitivity and specificity of the GARS-2 utilizing samples with ASD and other developmental disabilities. Such studies will help establish "cut points that optimize diagnostic accuracy" [5, page 1128]. The prior study of the GARS-2 failed to independently confirm the diagnosis of those in the sample, relied on data from the standardization sample, and did not have data on functional level (e.g., IQ). The studies by Pandolfi and colleagues [5] and Gilliam [12], as well as Lecavalier [4], used ratings by various sources. Use of sources having different roles (e.g., teacher versus parent) may confound results [4]. The purpose of this study was to extend previous research by examining the factor structure, internal consistency, and screening characteristics of the GARS-2 using ratings provided by special education teaching staff for a sample of individuals with ASD and other significant developmental disabilities. Psychometric studies of GARS-2 teaching staff reports are warranted, as teachers and other educational staff members have been identified as being among the most likely individuals to complete the scale in actual practice [12].

2. Method

2.1. Participants

2.1.1. Developmental Disabilities Sample. Data for the present study were in the form of GARS-2 teacher and agency-staff ratings of 240 communicative individuals with an ASD diagnosis or a diagnosis of another significant developmental disorder. All students were attending a self-contained special education agency for students with ASDs and other significant developmental delays/disabilities in upstate New York. All participants were between the ages of thee and 21 years.

For the overall sample, the mean age was 9.50 (SD = 4.88). Prior test data regarding cognitive skills was extracted from the students' educational and psychological records indicating a mean IQ of 60.61 (SD = 19.61). (The cognitive data were based on a sample of 228 participants. Twelve were deemed untestable due to behavior issues but were considered clearly low functioning based on other available data.) Given the variability in ages, communicative skills, and functional levels, cognitive measures used varied considerably and were not consistent across cases. The gender ratio was approximately 4 : 1 male-to-female (i.e., male = 78.75%, female = 21.25%). The ethnic distribution was 79.58% Caucasian, 15.42% African American, 2.50% Hispanic, 0.4% Native American, and 2.08% unknown. Although socioeconomic status data were unavailable at the individual case level, the agency's records indicated that 31.1% of its students qualified for free and reduced lunch.

Comparisons across ASD and non-ASD subgroups were nonsignificant for all major demographic variables (i.e., IQ $t[226] = 0.627$, $p = .532$; age in years $t[238] = 0.369$, $p = .712$; gender $\chi^2(1, N = 240) = 1.373$, $p = .241$; and ethnicity: analyzed as a 2 × 2 majority versus minority status comparison $\chi^2(1, N = 235) = 1.874$, $p = .171$). (See Table 1 for additional demographic information.)

The ASD subsample consisted of 99 cases diagnosed with autistic disorder and 22 cases diagnosed with Pervasive Developmental Disorder-Not Otherwise Specified (PDD-NOS). ASD diagnoses were made by either a developmental pediatrician, child psychiatrist, or licensed psychologist using *DSM-IV-TR* criteria [13]. Diagnoses for the non-ASD subsample consisted of other developmental disorders and medical conditions (e.g., intellectual disability, severe developmental language disorder, and severe motor impairments). Though such conditions frequently cooccur with ASD, these cases did not meet comorbid ASD criteria.

Importantly, staff psychologists identified 38 cases from the non-ASD condition that had not yet completed an ASD evaluation (to confirm or rule out an ASD diagnosis) at the time of the study. These 38 cases were included in the factor analysis and reliability estimates, but given the diagnostic ambiguity, they were excluded from any discriminant validity comparisons and screening sensitivity/specificity estimates.

TABLE 1: Developmental disabilities sample demographic characteristics by subsample and overall.

Demographic characteristic	Autism spectrum disorders n = 121	Nonautism spectrum disorders n = 119	Overall sample N = 240
Age in years	M = 9.39 (SD = 4.58)	M = 9.63 (SD = 5.19)	M = 9.50 (SD = 4.88)
IQ	M = 59.82 (SD = 19.69)	M = 61.45 (SD = 19.57)	M = 60.61 (SD = 19.61)
Gender	Male 81.81% (n = 99) Female 18.18% (n = 22)	Male 75.63% (n = 90) Female 24.37% (n = 29)	Male 78.75% (n = 189) Female 21.25% (n = 51)
Ethnicity			
Caucasian	82.64% (n = 100)	76.47% (n = 91)	79.58% (n = 191)
African American	13.22% (n = 16)	17.65% (n = 21)	15.42% (n = 37)
Hispanic	1.65% (n = 2)	3.36% (n = 4)	2.50% (n = 6)
Native American	0.0% (n = 0)	0.84% (n = 1)	0.42% (n = 1)
Unknown	2.47% (n = 3)	1.68% (n = 2)	2.08% (n = 5)

2.1.2. Teaching Staff Raters. Ratings of behaviors associated with ASD were required as part of the pretesting for a large program evaluation project. Raters consisted of the primary and extended teaching staff of a large special education agency for students with developmental disabilities in upstate New York. Rating assignments were made by the staff psychologists in consultation with classroom team leaders. The goals of the assignment process were to have each student rated by the staff member who knows her/him best, while also maximizing statistical independence of the cases being rated. Rater familiarity with the student ranged from a minimum of six weeks to a maximum of 28 months (Mo = 4.5 months) of contact. In order to maintain statistical independence across cases, a different teaching staff rater was assigned to each student. This was possible for the majority of available cases, because most classes maintained a 6 : 1 : 1 ratio for instruction and included a substantial classroom team consisting of primary special education teacher, secondary teacher or teaching assistant, classroom aid(s), personal student aid(s), trained volunteer assistant(s), speech pathologist, occupational therapist, physical therapist, and so forth. Typically, if the student had a personal aid, then the personal aid was assigned to be the rater. All ratings were performed over a two-week period in the middle of the school year and were not a part of any diagnostic evaluations.

Though clearly all teaching staff members were aware that each student had a developmental disability, they were not typically aware of whether or not a particular student had a formal diagnosis of autistic disorder or PDD-NOS. However, most teaching staff members were familiar with the general characteristics of ASD, as a result of their special education training or work experience.

2.2. Measures

2.2.1. Gilliam Autism Rating Scale-Second Edition. The Gilliam Autism Rating Scale-Second Edition (GARS-2; [12]), a revision of the original GARS [19], is a screening instrument for assessing individuals ages from three to 22 years who exhibit significant clinical and adaptive behavior issues that may reflect symptoms of autism. It is a third-party rating scale intended to be completed by a primary caregiver or someone else who is very familiar with the day to day behavior of the person being rated. It consists of 42 items divided into three subscales with 14 items each. The subscales are named Stereotyped Behaviors, Communication, and Social Interaction. Items are rated on a four-point frequency scale from 0 (*Never Observed*) to 3 (*Frequently Observed*). Each subscale is scored by summing the individual item scores and converting the result into norm-referenced scaled scores with a mean of 10 and standard deviation of 3. The Communication subscale is not completed for cases that are not sufficiently communicative to allow for adequate ratings. Subscale scores are summed and converted to a deviation quotient metric (normative mean of 100 and standard deviation of 15) to form a composite called the Autism Index. This index can be calculated based on the sum of all three subscales for communicative cases or the sum of only the Stereotyped Behaviors and Social Interaction subscales for noncommunicative cases. According to the manual, Autism Index scores ≥85 suggest that autism is "very likely," scores from 70 to 84 suggest autism is "possibly" present and scores ≤69 suggest that autism is "unlikely" [12, page 31]. A parent interview assessing delays and abnormalities in development during the first three years of life is also included but does not contribute to the GARS-2 scores.

The standardization sample for the test consisted of ratings of 1,107 children and young adults with autism. Raters were recruited through a variety of methods. Sample proportions for geographic region and ethnicity were consistent with census estimates of the general school-age population, while the 4 : 1 male-to-female gender ratio was consistent with expectations based on autism samples in the research literature. Diagnostic confirmation and data regarding cognitive functioning for sample participants were not obtained. The ratio of ratings contributed by professionals versus parents was 8 : 3 for the normative sample. Separate norms are not available by rater type. The manual includes information concerning internal consistency, test-retest reliability, and concurrent validity for the test (see [12]). Pandolfi and colleagues [5] factor-analyzed the standardization sample for the GARS-2 and concluded the relationships among the item responses reflected a four-factor structure.

2.3. Procedures

2.3.1. Rating and Data Collection. All data were collected as part of a larger program evaluation project for a large special education agency serving students with ASD and other developmental disabilities. Students ranged in age from three to 21 years and were served in either 6 : 1 : 1 self-contained, 12 : 1 : 1 self-contained, or integrated classrooms. As part of the program evaluation pretesting, the GARS-2 was completed along with three other behavior rating scales. Each staff member completed the four instruments in counterbalanced order. (Results concerning these other instruments will be reported in other forthcoming articles.)

Every attempt was made to assign teaching staff raters who knew each student best, while also maximizing the independence of the ratings across cases. In order to achieve these simultaneous goals, rating responsibilities were distributed across the different types of teaching staff who worked within each classroom (i.e., lead special education teachers, teaching assistants, classroom aids, 1 : 1 personal aids, speech/language pathologists, occupational therapists, and physical therapists). All ratings were performed without access to student records.

A total of 336 students with autistic disorder, PDD-NOS, or other significant developmental disabilities were rated. All ratings took place over a two-week period in the middle of the school year. Completed rating scale packets were immediately reviewed by project research assistants who made sure that all items were completed on each rating scale. These research assistants returned any incomplete rating scales to staff members with instructions (consistent with test manual instructions [12]) for missed item completion.

Each completed rating scale was independently scored by at least two advanced research assistants with graduate level psychometric training, and data from all rating scales were independently double entered into the database by trained research assistants under the supervision of the doctoral level research coordinator.

Based on data supplied by speech/language pathologists who worked with the students, 72 cases were judged to be insufficiently communicative to allow for completion of the 14 Communication subscale items on the GARS-2. Given that complete data on all 42 GARS-2 items were required for inclusion in the factor analysis, these cases were removed. An additional 24 cases were removed due to a lack of rater independence. Thus, the final sample consisted of 240 sufficiently communicative students with ASDs or other developmental disabilities who were independently rated by teaching staff members with the GARS-2.

2.3.2. Data Analyses. Exploratory factor analysis (EFA) was chosen over confirmatory approaches due to the limited literature available concerning the factor structure of the original GARS and GARS-2. The GARS-2 item data were analyzed using principal axis common factor analysis. This particular factor extraction method was chosen because it is considered robust to violations of normality-related assumptions [20]—which were anticipated to be issues for an ASD sample (e.g., most items yielded considerable positive skew).

An additional issue was the ordinal nature of the item scaling. Each of the 42 GARS-2 items is rated on a four-point frequency scale. The discrete nature of the four ordered categories makes the polychoric correlation coefficient, as opposed to the Pearson correlation coefficient, the more appropriate correlation estimation procedure for the matrix of interitem relationships (see [17]). Thus, the 42 $\times$ 42 interitem polychoric correlation matrix was used for the EFA.

According to simulations performed by MacCallum and colleagues [21], the sample size required for factor analysis is dependent upon indicator communalities and level of factor saturation. Larger sample sizes are needed when communalities and factor saturation are lower, while smaller samples are likely to yield convergent solutions for the correct number of factors in the presence of high communalities and high factor saturation. Assuming an indicator to factor ratio of 20 : 3 and wide communality (ranging from .20 to .80), simulations demonstrated convergent solutions for the correct factors 100% of the time with samples as small as 60 subjects [21, page 93]. Squared multiple correlation prior communality estimates based on the Pearson correlation matrix ranged from .38 to .81, while maximum correlation prior communality estimates based on the polychoric correlation matrix ranged from .53 to .91. Assuming 42 indicators and three factors, based on the number of GARS-2 items and subscales, the sample size of 240 cases appears more than adequate for assessing the factor structure of the instrument.

The EFA followed the standard factor extraction, rotation, and interpretation phases. In the extraction phase, several strategies were used to determine the number of factors to retain. Parallel analysis [22, 23] was used in conjunction with the Guttman-Kaiser criterion (i.e., eigenvalue >1.00 [24–26]). Initially, a factor was retained if its obtained eigenvalue exceeded the 95th percentile of the random eigenvalue distribution [23] and met the Guttman-Kaiser criterion. Once the number of factors that met these criteria was established, factor solutions consisting of that number of factors ±1 were examined. The most interpretable solution of the three was retained.

Rotation of the factor solution is conducted to enhance the interpretability of the factors. An oblique (promax) rotation was attempted first. If the factors yielded correlations $\geq$.30, then the obliquely rotated solution was retained. Otherwise, an orthogonal (varimax) rotation was conducted and retained instead.

Each factor was interpreted and named based on what was conceptually common across the items with the highest loadings on it. Factor loadings <.30 were considered nonsubstantive, loadings $\geq$.30 and <.40 were considered questionable, and loadings $\geq$.40 were considered substantive. Three of the investigators independently interpreted the factor solutions.

Internal consistency estimates for the factor-based scales and the original GARS-2 subscales were generated using

Cronbach's alpha and ordinal alpha [18]. The internal consistency of the Autism Index was calculated using Mosier's 1943 formula for the reliability of a weighted composite [27]. Correlations between the factor-based scales and the original GARS-2 subscales were examined for evidence of convergent and divergent validity. Mean differences between the ASD and non-ASD subsamples were evaluated for all GARS-2 scores. A classification analysis was conducted to evaluate the sensitivity, specificity, positive predictive value, and negative predictive value of the GARS-2 Autism Index's ASD versus non-ASD classifications compared to the prior clinician-determined ASD and non-ASD diagnoses of the cases.

All analyses involving R programming language [28] software packages were run in SPSS 19.0 [29] using the SPSS R menu for ordinal factor analysis [17], which allows users to access and run analyses available through R packages via the SPSS R plugin [30]. The SPSS R menu was used to generate the polychoric correlation matrix, conduct the parallel analysis using the raw item data to generate polychoric correlation matrices, and calculate both Cronbach's alpha and ordinal alpha coefficients. The PAF was conducted in SAS 9.2 [31] using the polychoric correlation matrix exported from R. All other statistical calculations were performed through SAS.

3. Results

A principal axis factor analysis (PAF) was conducted in SAS version 9.2 using the polychoric correlation matrix for the 42 GARS-2 items generated by the SPSS R menu for ordinal factor analysis [17]. Prior item communalities were estimated using the maximum correlation method. The number of factors was determined by a combination of parallel analysis with the Guttman-Kaiser criterion and factor interpretability.

The parallel analysis, based on 100 samples, indicated that the obtained eigenvalues from the first three factors exceeded the 95th percentile of the randomly generated eigenvalue distributions. These first three eigenvalues also met the Guttman-Kaiser criterion (i.e., eigenvalue >1.0; first = 18.75, second = 2.59, and third = 2.42) and each accounted for substantial estimates of the common variance (i.e., first = 62.22%, second = 8.58%, and third = 8.03%). (Though an additional three factors also met the Guttman-Kaiser criterion, they did not meet the parallel analysis threshold.)

Based on these preliminary results, solutions consisting of two to four factors (i.e., 3±1) were examined for interpretability. For interpretive purposes, factor loadings <.30 were considered nonsubstantive, ≥.30 <.40 were questionable, and ≥.40 were deemed substantive. The three-factor solution was determined to be most interpretable and will be described in detail. (The two- and four-factor solutions will also be briefly discussed to explain why they were less suitable.)

An oblique (promax, Kappa = 3) rotation was attempted first, given the anticipated correlated structure of ASD symptoms and the conceptual structure of the GARS-2 (i.e., three subscales combined into an overall score). All three factor solutions examined yielded correlated solutions. In the case of the three-factor solution, Factor I correlated .62 with Factor II and .51 with Factor III, while Factor II correlated .47 with Factor III. Thus, the three-factor correlated solution was retained for interpretation.

Both the pattern and structure loading matrices were examined to help interpret the factors—with primary reliance on the pattern matrix. The pattern matrix for the three-factor solution compared to the GARS-2 conceptually derived subscales is given in Table 2. The matrices were examined and interpreted by three of the investigators independently. For the two- and three-factor solutions, factor names assigned across the three investigators were either identical or equivalent in meaning for all factors. Final factor names assigned within the two-, three-, and four-factor solutions were determined by discussion and consensus among the three investigators involved.

3.1. Three-Factor Solution

3.1.1. Factor I. Items which loaded highest on this factor were as follows: *whirls, turns in circles; makes rapid lunging, darting movements; flaps hands or fingers; and makes high-pitched sounds (e.g., eee-eee-eee-eee) or other vocalizations for self-stimulation; flicks fingers rapidly in front of eyes*; and so forth. This factor was named Stereotyped and Repetitive Behaviors. Based on the highest factor loading (≥.30 minimum) per item, this factor contained 18 items—including 12 of the 14 items originally located in the GARS-2 Stereotyped Behavior subscale. This factor also includes two items from the GARS-2 Communication subscale and four items from the Social Interaction subscale. In most cases, these additional items either make direct references to repetitive-type behavior (e.g., *repeats unintelligible sounds, does things repetitively*) or could be peripherally related to such behaviors (e.g., *uses toys inappropriately; laughs, giggles, cries inappropriately; uses gestures instead of speech; and responds negatively to commands*).

3.1.2. Factor II. Factor II was defined primarily by items such as the following: *is unaffectionate; avoids establishing eye contact; withdraws, remains aloof, or acts standoffish in group situations; looks away or avoids looking at speaker when name is called; resists physical contact with others.* This factor was named Social Avoidance and Withdrawal. Based on the highest factor loading (≥.30 minimum) per item, this factor contained 16 items—including 8 of the 14 items originally located in the GARS-2 Social Interaction subscale. However, it also includes six items from the GARS-2 Communication subscale and two items from the Stereotyped Behaviors subscale. The higher-loading items from these other GARS-2 subscales make conceptual sense as expressions of social avoidance or withdrawal (e.g., *avoids eye contact, looks away when name is called, avoids asking, and fails to initiate conversation*) or problems with the social use of language (e.g., *speaks with flat affect*) that may repel others involved in the social interaction.

3.1.3. Factor III. This factor was named Atypical Language and Communication. Items loading highest on Factor III were as follows: *uses pronouns inappropriately (e.g., refers to*

TABLE 2: Pattern matrix of factor loadings for GARS-2 three-factor solution.

GARS-2 *subscale*/item	Factor I	Factor II	Factor III
Stereotyped Behaviors			
(1) Avoids eye contact	.08	***.80***	−.03
(2) Stares	***.59***	.27	.07
(3) Flicks fingers	***.79***	.05	−.08
(4) Eat specific foods	.16	***.34***	.22
(5) Licks or eats inedible objects	***.75***	.15	−.23
(6) Smells or sniffs objects	***.63***	.12	.00
(7) Whirls, turns	***.88***	−.14	.06
(8) Spins objects	***.64***	−.04	.08
(9) Rocks back and forth	***.73***	.10	−.12
(10) Lunging Movements	***.82***	−.10	−.03
(11) Prances	***.73***	−.10	**.30**
(12) Flaps hands or fingers	***.80***	−.04	.00
(13) High-pitched sounds	***.81***	.10	.04
(14) Injures self	***.63***	.11	.09
Communication			
(15) Repeats (echoes) words	**.43**	−.10	***.58***
(16) Repeats words out of context	.14	−.03	***.82***
(17) Repeats over and over	.19	−.01	***.73***
(18) Speaks with flat affect	−.07	***.52***	**.39**
(19) Responds inappropriately	**.31**	***.34***	.21
(20) Looks away when name is called	.08	***.77***	.03
(21) Avoids asking	.05	***.70***	−.04
(22) Fails to initiate conversation	.10	***.58***	.14
(23) Uses "yes"/"no" inappropriately	.13	***.31***	**.30**
(24) Uses pronouns inappropriately	−.13	−.09	***.91***
(25) Uses "I" inappropriately	−.16	.03	***.83***
(26) Repeats unintelligible sounds	***.55***	.22	.07
(27) Uses gestures instead of speech	***.44***	**.33**	−.17
(28) Inappropriately answers questions	−.10	.12	***.70***
Social Interaction			
(29) Avoids eye contact	.15	***.71***	.02
(30) Stares or looks unhappy	.19	***.67***	−.02
(31) Resists physical contact	−.04	***.74***	−.09
(32) Nonimitative of others	.10	***.68***	−.04
(33) Withdrawn, aloof, standoffish	−.01	***.80***	.09
(34) Unreasonably fearful	.05	***.48***	.15
(35) Unaffectionate	−.24	***.82***	.03
(36) Looks through people	.21	***.70***	−.08
(37) Laughs, giggles, cries inappropriately	***.45***	**.31**	.11
(38) Uses toys/objects inappropriately	***.66***	.11	.09
(39) Does things repetitively	***.55***	.10	**.34**
(40) Upset when routines change	.24	.19	***.32***
(41) Responds negatively to commands	***.38***	.19	.18
(42) Lines up objects	**.30**	.07	***.31***

Note. All items are paraphrased to conserve space. Factor loadings ≥.30 are in bold, while the highest factor loading for each item is in italic font.

self as "he," "you," and "she"); uses the word I inappropriately (e.g., does not say "I" to refer to self); repeats words out of context (i.e., repeats words heard at an earlier time, e.g., repeats words heard more than one minute earlier); repeats words or phases over and over; inappropriately answers questions about a statement or brief story; and so forth. Based on the highest factor loading (≥.30 minimum) per item, this factor contained 8 items—including six of the 14 items originally located in the GARS-2 Communication subscale. Beyond these core six items, the weak loading item *upset when routines change* (originally from the GARS-2 Social Interaction subscale) may make some conceptual sense as being related to atypical language (e.g., as a result of failing to understand the change or not having sufficient expressive language to communicate displeasure appropriately), but it is not directly associated with language/communication. Any other items that loaded on this factor had loadings in the questionable range (>.30 <.40) and tended to yield such questionable loadings on multiple factors.

3.1.4. Problematic Items. Within the three-factor solution, several items yielded questionable loadings (≥.30 <.40). These items are as follows: 4: eat specific foods; 19: responds inappropriately; 23: uses "yes"/"no" inappropriately; 40: *upset when routines change*; 41: *responds negatively to commands*; and 42: *lines up objects*. In addition, items 19, 23, and 42 each yielded questionable loadings on more than one factor. As a result, all six of these items do not clearly and cleanly belong to any factor-based scale.

Most potentially mixed items showed a clear dominant loading on one factor, making item assignment clear (e.g., 11: *prances*). However, item 15 (*repeats [echoes] words*) and item 18 (*speaks with flat affect*) required more discussion and judgment, because in each case the primary loading was moderate and the secondary loading was not far from it and close to the .40 cut for a substantive loading. For both, each item's statistical overlap between the two factors made conceptual sense (i.e., repeating or echoing words is both a type of atypical language use/communication and a type of repetitive behavior; speaking with flat affect is both socially awkward and communicatively atypical). Though revising these items should be considered, there appear to be both statistical and conceptual reasons to retain them and assign each to its primary factor.

3.2. Two-Factor Solution. In the two-factor solution, high loading items for Factor I appeared to be predominantly about Social Avoidance and Withdrawal, while high loadings on Factor II primarily reflected language and communication abnormalities. The items from the GARS-2 Stereotyped Behaviors subscale were distributed across the two factors and tended to load in a mixed manner on both of them. (Overall, at least 16 items loaded on both factors.) These results were not clearly interpretable for a large number of items and suggested the need for at least one additional factor.

3.3. Four-Factor Solution. The first three factors of the four-factor solution were similar to those of the three-factor solution (Factor I = Social Avoidance and Withdrawal, Factor II = Stereotyped and Repetitive Behaviors, and Factor III = Atypical Language and Communication). The fourth factor consisted of six items: *uses gestures instead of speech*; *repeats unintelligible sounds*; *responds negatively to commands*; *licks*

Table 3: Internal consistency estimates for factor-based scales and GARS-2 subscales.

Factor/subscale	Cronbach's alpha	Ordinal alpha	Number of items
Factor I	.92	.95	18
Factor II	.92	.94	16
Factor III	.84	.89	8
Stereotyped Behavior	.90	.94	14
Communication	.89	.92	14
Social Interaction	.89	.92	14

Note. Cronbach's and ordinal alpha coefficients are estimated using the SPSS R menu [17]. Ordinal alpha is calculated using polychoric correlation coefficients in the alpha formula [18].

or eats inedible objects; *injures self*; and *laughs, giggles, cries inappropriately*. In general, the items of this factor appeared reflective of lower functioning behaviors, with the first two items suggesting lack of verbal expression, the third item perhaps a result of a lack of understanding spoken language, and the remaining three being tendencies toward pica, self-injurious behavior, and lack of emotional control (e.g., labile emotions/inappropriate affect).

This factor was not well defined and resulted in considerable discussion over how it could be interpreted. In addition, this overall solution included a greater number of items loading on more than one factor than the three-factor solution. Following discussion among those who independently interpreted the factor solutions, it was decided that the fourth factor was not well defined and included a majority of items that would fit reasonably well elsewhere and that the overall four-factor solution included too many items with mixed loadings and was less readily interpretable when compared to the three-factor solution. It was therefore rejected in favor of the three-factor model.

3.4. Internal Consistency Estimates. Internal consistency reliability estimates were calculated for each factor, original GARS-2 subscales, and the GARS-2 Autism Index. Estimates based on both Cronbach's alpha and ordinal alpha are reported in Table 3 for the factor-based scales and original GARS-2 subscales. Cronbach's alpha is the better known estimate but tends to be biased low for ordinal, skewed, and non-tau equivalent data [18, 32]. The ordinal alpha estimate is calculated by replacing the Pearson correlations with polychoric correlations in the alpha formula [18]. This estimation procedure corrects alpha for the ordinal and skewed nature of the data. (However, the assumption of tau equivalence is still necessary and, thus, the corrected estimate will still be considered a lower-bound estimate of reliability.) For the factors, Cronbach's alpha estimates ranged from .84 to .92 and ordinal alpha estimates ranged from .89 to .95. For the original three GARS 2 subscales, Cronbach's alpha estimates ranged from .89 to .90 and ordinal alpha estimates ranged from .92 to .94.

Given that the GARS-2 Autism Index is calculated as a linear transformation of the sum of subscale scores and not derived directly from the sum of the item scores, the composite reliability was calculated using the formula provided by Mosier [27]. This formula takes into account the subscale reliability estimates, subscale variances, and the correlations among the subscales. When calculated using Cronbach's alpha estimates for the subscales, the composite reliability was .96. When calculated using ordinal alpha estimates for the subscales, the composite reliability was .97.

3.5. Relationships between Factors and GARS-2 Subscales. By examining Table 4, within each row across columns, it is clear that each factor correlates highest, though imperfectly, with its target GARS-2 subscale and correlates relatively lower with the other GARS-2 subscales. This pattern of correlations suggests that the three-factor solution demonstrates some level of consistency with the intended construct pattern reflected in the three original GARS-2 subscales. However, the lack of near perfect convergence reflects important factor versus subscale disagreements over item placement (see Section 4). In addition, an examination of specific items suggests that Factor III likely reflects a more narrow atypical language/communication construct than originally intended for the GARS-2 Communication subscale.

3.6. Clinical Validity and Classification Accuracy. As mentioned under Method, 38 cases from the non-ASD group had not yet been evaluated for possible ASD at the time of the study. Because of the potential ambiguous diagnostic status of these cases, they were not included in the following discriminant validity comparisons or classification accuracy analyses. Thus, for the following analyses, the revised overall sample size was 202 cases (n = 121 ASD, n = 81 non-ASD).

The clinical or discriminant validity of the GARS-2 Autism Index and subscales was assessed via mean comparisons. As expected, the GARS-2 scores for the Autism Index and all the three subscales were significantly higher for the ASD group than the non-ASD group. (See Table 5 for details.)

A classification analysis of the GARS-2 Autism Index was conducted by comparing the known clinician-determined ASD status of cases with the predicted ASD status of cases based on the Autism Index cut score of ≥85 (indicative of a "very likely" probability of autism according to the test manual and the interpretive guide on the cover of the GARS-2 summary/response booklet [12]). For the study sample, the Autism Index classifications yielded a sensitivity of .6529 (indicating accurate test detection of 65.29% of the cases with known formal ASD diagnoses), a specificity of .8148 (indicating 81.48% accuracy in ruling out of ASD among those cases without an ASD diagnosis), positive predictive value of .8404 (indicating that a positive ASD classification by the GARS-2 suggests an 84.04% likelihood of the case actually having a formal ASD diagnosis), and negative predictive value of .6111 (indicating that a negative or non-ASD classification by the GARS-2 suggests a 61.11% likelihood of the case not having a formal ASD diagnosis).

4. Discussion

In the context of the study sample of 240 participants with ASDs and other conditions frequently confused with ASDs,

TABLE 4: Correlations between factor-based scales and GARS-2 subscales.

	GARS-2 Stereotyped Behaviors subscale	GARS-2 Social Interaction subscale	GARS-2 Communication subscale
Factor I: Stereotyped and Repetitive Behaviors	***.97***	.81	.73
Factor II: Social Avoidance and Withdrawal	.68	***.91***	.79
Factor III: Atypical Language and Communication	.51	.57	***.87***

Note. Raw sums of item scores were used to calculate the factor-based scales and GARS-2 subscale scores. In the case of the factor-based scales, only items with primary loadings ≥.40 were used in the composite. Correlations on the diagonal are convergent and correlations on the off diagonal are divergent.

TABLE 5: GARS-2 means and standard deviations for total sample, adjusted total sample, ASD cases, and non-ASD cases.

GARS-2 subscale/composite	Total sample $N = 240$	Total sample (adjusted) $N = 202^a$	ASD cases $n = 121$	Non-ASD cases $n = 81^a$	ASD versus non-ASD comparisons
Stereotyped Behavior	M = 6.71 (SD = 3.58)	M = 6.80 (SD = 3.57)	M = 8.05 (SD = 3.53)	M = 4.93 (SD = 2.74)	$t(200) = 6.722$, $p < .001^{***}$
Communication	M = 8.23 (SD = 3.80)	M = 8.32 (SD = 3.84)	M = 9.70 (SD = 3.48)	M = 6.26 (SD = 3.41)	$t(200) = 6.943$, $p < .001^{***}$
Social Interaction	M = 6.72 (SD = 3.45)	M = 6.76 (SD = 3.46)	M = 7.94 (SD = 3.10)	M = 4.99 (SD = 3.23)	$t(200) = 6.532$, $p < .001^{***}$
Autism Index	M = 82.14 (SD = 21.20)	M = 82.62 (SD = 21.33)	M = 90.81 (SD = 18.94)	M = 70.40 (SD = 18.78)	$t(200) = 7.533$, $p < .001^{***}$

Note. GARS-2 subscale scores are in standard score units (normative M = 10, SD = 3) and the Autism Index is standardized according to a deviation quotient metric (normative M = 100, SD = 15).

[a]Thirty-eight cases were removed from the non-ASD condition for this analysis, because they had not yet had an ASD evaluation to rule out the possibility of an ASD diagnosis. Without these cases, the adjusted total sample size is 202 cases and the non-ASD condition consists of 81 cases.

$^{***}p < .001$.

the three-factor correlated solution for the GARS-2 was most interpretable. The three factors named Stereotyped and Repetitive Behaviors (Factor I), Social Avoidance and Withdrawal (Factor II), and Atypical Language and Communication (Factor III) showed reasonable correspondence to the three GARS-2 conceptually derived subscales, respectively, named Stereotyped Behaviors, Social Interaction, and Communication. In terms of item overlap, 85.71% of the GARS-2 Stereotyped Behavior subscale items loaded primarily on Factor I (Stereotyped and Repetitive Behaviors), 57.14% of the Social Interaction subscale items loaded primarily on the Factor II (Social Avoidance and Withdrawal), and 42.86% of the Communication subscale items loaded on Factor III (Atypical Language and Communication). Though imperfect, convergent correlations ranged from .87 to .97 between each factor-based scale and its corresponding GARS-2 subscale, with all other factor-to-subscale relationships yielding the expected divergent pattern. Additionally, the correlated nature of the three factors is consistent with a possible higher-order factor reflecting the composite Autism Index. Thus, these data generally support a three-subscale and overall composite conceptualization of the GARS-2.

However, the factor analytic results also suggest a number of concerns that could inform the revision of the instrument. The lack of near perfect convergence between each factor-based scale and its corresponding GARS-2 subscale (see Table 4) reflects the presence of wrongly placed items on the GARS-2 subscales, which contribute construct irrelevant variance to the subscale scores and attenuate the correlation with the intended factor. The pattern matrix indicated that 16 (i.e., 38.10%) of the GARS-2 items did not load on the factor most reflective of the intended subscale but typically loaded on a different factor. Such results suggest that these discrepant items have been assigned to the wrong subscale. Though the GARS-2 was conceptualized with 14 items per subscale, the EFA suggested that a subscale based on Factor I contains 18 items, second subscale based on Factor II has 16 items, and a third subscale based on Factor III contains 8 items. In addition, six items (i.e., 4, 19, 23, 40, 41, and 42) yielded questionable or even low and mixed loadings, which suggested that they do not belong to any of the three factor-based subscales. This pattern of results gives clear direction for potential item-to-scale reassignment and item revisions.

A comparison of this three-factor correlated solution with that of Lecavalier [4] is very instructive. Lecavalier examined the factor structure of the original GARS using principal components analysis. (Differences in item wording between the GARS and GARS-2 for the core 42 items are negligible.) Lecavalier also found a correlated three-factor structure. An examination of the item overlap between the three-factor structures across the two studies indicated that 36 out of 42 items (i.e., 85.71%) loaded on the equivalent factor across both studies. In addition, five of the six items that loaded differently across the two studies (i.e., items 4, 19, 23, 40, and 42) were among the six items determined to be problematic (due to questionable or low and mixed loadings) in the current study.

Three of the six discrepant items (i.e., items 19, 40, and 42) also yielded primary loadings below .30 in the Lecavalier results, while still another (i.e., item 4) yielded a questionable range primary loading. (Though it should be noted that the factor analytic approach in the Lecavalier study likely yielded generally lower factor loadings due to the use of Pearson correlations, the level of relative agreement across the two studies on where items fit and which items are problematic is impressive.) The factor structures across the two studies are clearly convergent and virtually identical, even given different samples, different rater types, and different EFA approaches.

A comparison of the correlated three-factor model from the current study with the correlated four-factor solution found by Pandolfi and colleagues [5] using the GARS-2 standardization sample is also instructive. Pandolfi et al.'s Factor I, Stereotyped Behavior (17 items), and Factor IV, Social Impairment (14 items), both line up well with present study's Factor I, Stereotyped and Repetitive Behaviors (18 items), and Factor II, Social Avoidance and Withdrawal (16 items), respectively. The stereotyped behavior factor shares 16 items across the two studies (i.e., 88.88%–94.12% overlap), while the social impairment/avoidance factor shares 12 items across the two studies (i.e., 75%–85.71%). The high level of agreement between the corresponding factors across the two studies strongly indicates that they measure the same, conceptually consistent construct. In contrast, the items from the Atypical Language and Communication factor in the present study split up to form two separate language factors in the Pandolfi et al. study—one reflecting stereotyped/idiosyncratic language and the other assessing word use problems. When the four-factor EFA solution was assessed in the present study, it clearly did not lead to two separate and interpretable language factors. This difference between the factor solutions across the two studies may be a reflection of differences between the cases and/or raters between the present study and the GARS-2 standardization sample. However, the two studies agree on the presence of a factor reflecting stereotyped behavior, another reflecting social impairments, and at least one other language/communication factor. It is also noteworthy that five of the seven items (i.e., items 2, 4, 18, 19, 23, 40, and 41) that loaded differently across the two studies were among the six problematic items noted in the three-factor solution for the present study. Five of these seven items also yielded low to questionable loadings in the Pandolfi et al. four-factor EFA solution. Taken together with the Lecavalier [4] results, several of the same items were identified consistently as problematic across GARS and GARS-2 factor analytic studies.

4.1. Internal Consistency Estimates. Both Cronbach's alpha and ordinal alpha estimates were reported in the current study. It is noteworthy that these coefficients were generally higher than those reported in other sources (e.g., [4, 5, 12]), and this was the case regardless of the type of alpha coefficient. Though these estimates clearly meet or exceed reliability standards for screening purposes (see [33]), it is likely that the greater heterogeneity of the present study sample contributed to the relatively higher internal consistency numbers. For example, the Autism Index standard deviation for the total (i.e., combined ASD and non-ASD) sample was 21.20 in the present study, which is higher than that of the GARS-2 standardization sample (SD = 15) and the Autism Quotient standard deviation (SD = 15.4) for the original GARS reported by Lecavalier [4].

4.2. Clinical Comparisons. As expected mean comparisons between the ASD and non-ASD groups were statistically significant ($p < .001$) and substantive for all GARS-2 subscales and the Autism Index. The mean Autism Index for the ASD subsample (M = 90.81) indicated that the average ASD case fell within the "very likely" range for autism according to the GARS-2 manual, while the mean score for the non-ASD subsample (M = 70.40) placed the average non-ASD case at the lower end of the autism being "possibly" present range.

The classification accuracy of the GARS-2 Autism Index in classifying the known ASD and non-ASD cases yielded a sensitivity of .6529 and specificity of .8148. The sensitivity estimate is higher than that reported in prior studies with the GARS (e.g., [4, 16]). One factor likely critical to the higher sensitivity is that the original GARS manual recommended a cut score of ≥90 for the Autism Quotient [19], while the GARS-2 manual recommends a cut score of ≥85 for the Autism Index [12]. With a ≥90 cut score, the sensitivity for the present study sample would drop to .5289. This estimate is still higher than the .378 sensitivity reported in the Lecavalier [4] study with the GARS but similar to the .48 sensitivity reported in the South et al. [16] study with the GARS. Other factors to consider are that the teaching staff members who provided the ratings in the present study were very familiar with developmental disabilities, as a result of education and/or direct work experience. Thus, they may be unusually well suited to identify ASD relative to a more typical rater from the general population. However, it is also important to note that the non-ASD comparison cases in the setting for this study tend to share at least some associated features with ASD. Thus, the clinical discrimination context is maximally difficult. Regardless of these various factors, it is still critical to note that the ratings ended up misclassifying 34.71% of the ASD cases as non-ASD—even with the lower Autism Index cut score of ≥85. This suggests that even when completed by special education teaching staff, the GARS-2 would likely miss one-third of the cases with ASD. Thus, it should be used only with caution and clearly not in isolation.

4.3. Strengths of the Study. The study involved a number of strengths. First, instruments like the GARS-2 are intended to be used with those suspected of having an ASD. The mixed sample used in this study, including both those with formal ASD diagnoses and those with other significant developmental disabilities, matches well to the actual population and discriminant clinical situation intended for such a measure. Factor analyzing the GARS-2 with such a population is a useful preliminary assessment of the robustness of the factor structure—beyond just those with a known ASD diagnosis. Second, diagnostic and educational records were available for staff psychologists (who were not raters) to verify diagnoses.

Third, cognitive data were available for 95% of the sample—with clear indications of lower functional levels for the 12 cases without cognitive test data. Fourth, the use of special education teaching staff only as raters allowed for a more clearly defined rater population, in contrast to prior studies (including the standardization sample for the GARS-2) that combined ratings across professionals and parents. It is noteworthy that the GARS-2 manual suggests that professionals, and not parents, are likely to be the primary GARS-2 raters more often in actual practice [12]. Fifth, steps taken to assure rater independence, scale completeness, and data quality control were very thorough. Sixth, data were factor analyzed using methods appropriate for ordinal item data (i.e., polychoric correlations) and used a factoring method (i.e., PAF) robust to deviations in the item distributions. Finally, the availability of relatively large ASD and non-ASD subsamples allowed for a more comprehensive assessment of the sensitivity, specificity, positive predictive value, and negative predictive value than was possible in most prior studies.

4.4. Limitations. Most of the study limitations relate to the generalization of the results. First, though the formal ASD diagnoses likely generalize well to clinical practice, it would have been preferable to have diagnoses independently confirmed using a gold standard diagnostic instrument (e.g., ADI-R [6], ADOS-2 [7]). However, given the lack of a perfectly reliable and valid ASD diagnostic approach, understanding the relationships between a measure and a variety of different diagnostic outcome sources is helpful. Second, all study raters were special education teaching staff with experience working with those with ASD and other significant developmental disabilities. Thus, results may not generalize well to raters without such backgrounds. However, the similarity of the resulting factor structure to that found by Lecavalier [4] in the original GARS suggests at least some preliminary generality across rater types and sample contexts. Third, the 14 items of the Communication subscale can only be completed for cases that are sufficiently communicative. Given that the factor analysis examined the facture structure for all 42 items, results only generalize to communicative cases. Fourth, though also being a strength of the study, the use of the mixed developmental disabilities sample likely increased heterogeneity—which may restrict generalization of some results (e.g., alpha coefficients) to more homogenous populations.

4.5. Recommendations for Instrument Revision. Given a review of the GARS-2 manual, available research, and factor analytic findings, the following recommendations are made concerning the revision of the instrument. First, the manual needs a more clearly defined sampling plan and better sample characterization. It is most important that ASD diagnoses be verified and functional levels established. Second, clarify the ratio of raters to ASD cases rated. Ideally, each rater contributes one rating to the normative sample in order to maintain statistical independence. Third, thoroughly explore the development of separate normative tables for different rater types (e.g., parents versus teachers) and for different age groups. Though the manual notes that score correlations with age are low to negligible, this does not necessarily rule out nonlinear age changes or small but potentially important differences. Fourth, strongly consider the reassignment of items to scales based on factor analyses—paying particular attention to those item clusters that appear consistent across different factor analytic studies. Fifth, examine problematic GARS-2 items from the factor analyses. Consider revising or deleting and replacing items with low primary factor loadings, low and mixed loadings, or that including complex wording. Finally, it appears likely that some items yielding low loadings may include content considered important for diagnosing ASDs. In such cases, it is important to assess the wording of the item, whether item revision is reasonable, and to consider whether more items with similar content should be added as the basis for a new factor/subscale.

References

[1] American Psychiatric Association, *Diagnostic and Statistical Manual of Mental Disorders*, American Psychiatric Association (APA), Washington, DC, USA, 5th edition, 2013.

[2] National Research Council (NRC), *Educating Children with Autism*, edited by: Committee on Educational Interventions for Children with Autism, C. Lord, J. P. McGee, Division of Behavioral and Social Sciences and Education, National Academy Press, Washington, DC, USA, 2001.

[3] A. Klin, C. Saulnier, K. Tsatsanis, and F. R. Volkmar, "Clinical evaluation in autism spectrum disorders: psychological assessment within a transdisciplinary framework," in *Handbook of Autism and Pervasive Developmental Disorders: Vol. 2. Assessment, Interventions, and Policy*, F. R. Volkmar, R. Paul, A. Klin, and D. Cohen, Eds., pp. 772–798, John Wiley & Sons, Hoboken, NJ, USA, 3rd edition, 2005.

[4] L. Lecavalier, "An evaluation of the Gilliam autism rating scale," *Journal of Autism and Developmental Disorders*, vol. 35, no. 6, pp. 795–805, 2005.

[5] V. Pandolfi, C. I. Magyar, and C. A. Dill, "Constructs assessed by the GARS-2: factor analysis of data from the standardization sample," *Journal of Autism and Developmental Disorders*, vol. 40, no. 9, pp. 1118–1130, 2010.

[6] M. Rutter, A. LeCouteur, and C. Lord, *Autism Diagnostic Interview—Revised*, Western Psychological Services, Los Angeles, Calif, USA, 2003.

[7] C. Lord, M. Rutter, P. C. DiLavore, S. Risi, K. Gotham, and S. Bishop, *Autism Diagnostic Observation Schedule*, Western Psychological Services, Torrance, Calif, USA, 2nd edition, 2012.

[8] C. Lord and C. Corsello, "Diagnostic instruments in autistic spectrum disorders," in *Handbook of Autism and Pervasive Developmental Disorders: Vol. 2. Assessment, Interventions, and Policy*, F. R. Volkmar, R. Paul, A. Klin, and D. Cohen, Eds., pp. 730–771, John Wiley & Sons, Hoboken, NJ, USA, 3rd edition, 2005.

[9] R. A. Allen, D. L. Robins, and S. L. Decker, "Autism spectrum disorders: neurobiology and current assessment practices," *Psychology in the Schools*, vol. 45, no. 10, pp. 905–917, 2008.

[10] M. A. Volker and C. Lopata, "Autism: a review of biological bases, assessment, and intervention," *School Psychology Quarterly*, vol. 23, no. 2, pp. 258–270, 2008.

[11] E. E. Coonrod and W. L. Stone, "Screening for autism in young children," in *Handbook of Autism and Pervasive Developmental Disorders: Vol. 2. Assessment, Interventions, and Policy*, F. R. Volkmar, R. Paul, A. Klin, and D. Cohen, Eds., pp. 707–729, John Wiley & Sons, Hoboken, NJ, USA, 3rd edition, 2005.

[12] J. E. Gilliam, *Gilliam Autism Rating Scale*, PRO-ED, Austin, Tex, USA, 2nd edition, 2006.

[13] American Psychiatric Association, *Diagnostic and Statistical Manual of Mental Disorders*, Text Revision, American Psychiatric Association (APA), Washington, DC, USA, 4th edition, 2000.

[14] J. M. Montgomery, B. Newton, and C. Smith, "Test review: GARS-2: Gilliam Autism Rating Scale—Second Edition, Austin, TX: PRO-ED," *Journal of Psychoeducational Assessment*, vol. 26, no. 4, pp. 395–401, 2008.

[15] M. Norris and L. Lecavalier, "Screening accuracy of level 2 autism spectrum disorder rating scales: a review of selected instruments," *Autism*, vol. 14, no. 4, pp. 263–284, 2010.

[16] M. South, B. J. Williams, W. M. McMahon et al., "Utility of the Gilliam Autism Rating Scale in research and clinical populations," *Journal of Autism and Developmental Disorders*, vol. 32, no. 6, pp. 593–599, 2002.

[17] M. Basto and J. M. Pereira, "An SPSS R-menu for ordinal factor analysis," *Journal of Statistical Software*, vol. 46, no. 4, pp. 1–29, 2012.

[18] B. D. Zumbo, A. M. Gadermann, and C. Zeisser, "Ordinal versions of coefficients alpha and theta for likert rating scales," *Journal of Modern Applied Statistical Methods*, vol. 6, no. 1, pp. 21–29, 2007.

[19] J. E. Gilliam, *Gilliam Autism Rating Scale*, PRO-ED, Austin, Tex, USA, 1995.

[20] F. J. Floyd and K. F. Widaman, "Factor analysis in the development and refinement of clinical assessment instruments," *Psychological Assessment*, vol. 7, no. 3, pp. 286–299, 1995.

[21] R. C. MacCallum, K. F. Widaman, S. Zhang, and S. Hong, "Sample size in factor analysis," *Psychological Methods*, vol. 4, no. 1, pp. 84–99, 1999.

[22] J. L. Horn, "A rationale and test for the number of factors in factor analysis," *Psychometrika*, vol. 30, no. 2, pp. 179–185, 1965.

[23] L. W. Glorfeld, "An improvement on Horn's parallel analysis methodology for selecting the correct number of factors to retain," *Educational and Psychological Measurement*, vol. 55, no. 3, pp. 377–393, 1995.

[24] L. Guttman, "Some necessary conditions for common factor analysis," *Psychometrika*, vol. 19, pp. 149–161, 1954.

[25] H. F. Kaiser, "The application of electronic computers to factor analysis," *Educational and Psychological Measurement*, vol. 20, no. 1, pp. 141–151, 1960.

[26] H. F. Kaiser, "A note on Guttman's lower bound for the number of common factors," *British Journal of Statistical Psychology*, vol. 14, no. 1, pp. 1–2, 1961.

[27] C. I. Mosier, "On the reliability of a weighted composite," *Psychometrika*, vol. 8, no. 3, pp. 161–168, 1943.

[28] R Development Core Team, *R: A Language and Environment for Statistical Computing*, R Foundation for Statistical Computing, Vienna, Austria, 2011, http://www.R-project.org/.

[29] IBM Corporation, *IBM SPSS Statistics, Version 19*, IBM Corporation, Armonk, NY, USA, 2010, http://www-01.ibm.com/software/analytics/spss/.

[30] IBM Corporation, *SPSS R Plug-in 2.10*, IBM Corporation, Armonk, NY, USA, 2010, http://www.spss.com/devcentral/.

[31] SAS Institute, *The SAS System, Version 9.2*, SAS Institute, Cary, NC, USA, 2010, http://www.sas.com.

[32] T. Raykov, "Scale reliability, Cronbach's Coefficient Alpha, and violations of essential tau-equivalence with fixed congeneric components," *Multivariate Behavioral Research*, vol. 32, no. 4, pp. 329–353, 1997.

[33] J. Salvia and J. E. Ysseldyde, *Assessment in Special and Inclusive Education*, Houghton Mifflin, Boston, Mass, USA, 9th edition, 2004.

22

Defining Autism: Variability in State Education Agency Definitions of and Evaluations for Autism Spectrum Disorders

Malinda L. Pennington,[1] Douglas Cullinan,[2] and Louise B. Southern[2]

[1] *Special Education, Department of Curriculum, Instruction, and Counselor Education, NC State University, Poe Hall 602, Campus Box 7801, Raleigh, NC 27695-7801, USA*
[2] *North Carolina State University, Raleigh, NC 27607, USA*

Correspondence should be addressed to Malinda L. Pennington; mlpennin@ncsu.edu

Academic Editor: Geraldine Dawson

In light of the steady rise in the prevalence of students with autism, this study examined the definition of autism published by state education agencies (SEAs), as well as SEA-indicated evaluation procedures for determining student qualification for autism. We compared components of each SEA definition to aspects of autism from two authoritative sources: Diagnostic and Statistical Manual of Mental Disorders (DSM-IV-TR) and Individuals with Disabilities Education Improvement Act (IDEA-2004). We also compared SEA-indicated evaluation procedures across SEAs to evaluation procedures noted in IDEA-2004. Results indicated that many more SEA definitions incorporate IDEA-2004 features than DSM-IV-TR features. However, despite similar foundations, SEA definitions of autism displayed considerable variability. Evaluation procedures were found to vary even more across SEAs. Moreover, within any particular SEA there often was little concordance between the definition (what autism is) and evaluation procedures (how autism is recognized). Recommendations for state and federal policy changes are discussed.

1. Introduction

Autism spectrum disorder (ASD) refers to a group of pervasive neurodevelopmental disorders that involve moderately to severely disrupted functioning in regard to social skills and socialization, expressive and receptive communication, and repetitive or stereotyped behaviors and interests [1]. Only two decades ago ASD was considered rare, occurring or detected in about 1 in 1,000 children [2, 3]. Current estimates place the prevalence of ASD at 1 in 88 children [4], which suggests that roughly 800,000 US persons under age 20 have ASD.

In 1990, the US Congress amended the federal special education law (now called Individuals with Disabilities Education Improvement Act, or IDEA-2004) to make *autism* a category of education disability. Autism is defined for federal special education administrative purposes as stated below.

(i) Autism means a developmental disability significantly affecting verbal and nonverbal communication and social interaction, generally evident before the age of three that adversely affects a child's educational performance. Other characteristics often associated with autism are engagement in repetitive activities and stereotyped movements, resistance to environmental change or change in daily routines, and unusual responses to sensory experiences.

(ii) Autism does not apply if a child's educational performance is adversely affected primarily because the child has an emotional disturbance, as defined in paragraph (c) (4) of this section.

(iii) A child who manifests the characteristics of autism after the age of three could be identified as having autism if the criteria in paragraph (c) (1) (i) of this section are satisfied [5].

Autism is increasing in schools as well as in society. The US Department of Education (U.S. ED), which must monitor prevalence of autism and other educational disabilities, reported that US students with autism numbered 15,580 in 1992 [6]; by 2011 they numbered 406,957 [7].

The federal definition of autism preceded the fourth edition of the Diagnostic and Statistical Manual (DSM-IV) [8], and it is essentially unchanged since 1990. The federal definition is generally compatible with both the category of Pervasive Developmental Disorder (PDD) as described in DSM-IV and Autism Spectrum Disorder as described in DSM-5 [9], but it does not match any specific variety of PDD (see below). Within public school systems, students who have been clinically diagnosed with either a DSM-IV PDD or with DSM-5 Autism Spectrum Disorder are likely to be identified under the federal category of autism for the purpose of receiving special education services. Herein we use the term autism to include diagnoses of a DSM-IV PDD or DSM-5 Autism Spectrum Disorder.

In contrast to the IDEA-2004 definition, criteria for autism are more specific in the DSM-IV clinical diagnostic criteria. The *text revision* version [8] described four subcategories of PDD, including autistic disorder, Asperger's disorder, and a *not otherwise specified* subcategory (PDD-NOS) for presentations that clearly evidence autism but do not meet criteria for any named subcategory. In order to have qualified for DSM-IV autistic disorder, for example, a child must have exhibited a total of at least six listed characteristics, including at least two characteristics of "qualitative impairment in social interaction," one characteristic of "qualitative impairments in communication," and one characteristic of "restricted, repetitive and stereotyped patterns of behavior, interests, and activities" [8]. Additionally, DSM-IV autistic disorder has criteria that address age-of-onset and ruling out other conditions.

Recently, DSM-IV was superseded by DSM-5 [9]. The disorders comprising PDD in DSM-IV are largely addressed in DSM-5 by the Autism Spectrum Disorders category, which—unlike DSM-IV's PDD—has no subcategories. However, identification criteria still include substantial social problems (social initiations and responses, nonverbal social communication, and social relationships) and restricted, repetitive behaviors or interests (deviant speech or movements, rituals and resistance to change, preoccupations, and sensory reactivity). State education agencies (SEAs) have not yet incorporated DSM-5 information into their policies, procedures, and practices related to students with autism, and the DSM-5 definition was not involved in the present study. Implications of DSM-5 criteria for autism are presented in Section 4.

States also have administrative definitions of various categories of education disability, including autism. State education agency (SEA) definitions of a disability do not have to match the federal definition but must substantially address its elements or lose federal financial support for special education. Thus it is puzzling that the percentage of prevalence of autism varies greatly across different states. In 2012, for instance, when the mean rate of autism for all SEAs was 0.6% of the student-age population, Iowa reported the lowest prevalence at 0.1%, while Minnesota reported the highest rate at 1.2% [7]. No doubt the prevalence of ASD naturally varies somewhat with geography [4] but probably not by such a large factor, greater than tenfold in adjacent states. Conceivably, some state-by-state variation might be attributable to the content of SEA definitions of autism and perhaps the evaluation procedures required to accurately measure the concepts presented in definitions.

In a study of SEA definitions of autism, MacFarlane and Kanaya [10] found substantial variation in the eligibility criteria used by different states. By their analysis, 35% of SEAs based autism eligibility solely on the federal definition of autism, while 65% used diverse other criteria including symptoms of autism from the DSM-IV-TR. However, these researchers encountered difficulty obtaining eligibility information directly from SEAs through their websites and email requests to SEA administrators, so they based their findings on a review of special education definitions contained in state legal code documents (repositories of laws and supportive regulations). MacFarlane and Kanaya [10] noted that one limitation of this process is that state legal terminology may not accurately reflect SEA policies and practices.

MacFarlane and Kanaya [10] also considered SEA evaluation procedures for autism eligibility: they recorded the presence or absence of a requirement for clinical diagnosis of autism by a pediatrician or qualified clinician. However, this was the limit of their analysis of SEA evaluation procedures and their link to autism eligibility criteria. Because eligibility evaluation procedures can help operationalize a definition of autism, there clearly is a need to explore SEA evaluation information to a greater extent.

Federal special education law addresses, in a general way, evaluation procedures for determining whether a student is diagnosed as having a disability, including autism: "The child is assessed in all areas related to the suspected disability, including, if appropriate, health, vision, hearing, social and emotional status, general intelligence, academic performance, communicative status, and motor abilities" [11]. Based on this guidance, each state determines evaluation procedures, and these may be further modified by individual school districts. Obviously, this could lead to a wide variety of evaluation procedures implemented by diverse evaluators. It would be good to know what evaluation procedures different SEAs use for autism eligibility; however, we are aware of no compilation of them. To accurately determine eligibility, evaluation procedures should appropriately measure criteria established by SEAs. Similar criteria across states might be expected to call for similar evaluations. If evaluation procedures do not align with stated criteria or vary greatly across states, they throw into question the accuracy of autism identification by SEAs.

The purpose of the present study was to consider the current status of SEA definitions of autism and SEA evaluation procedures for autism eligibility. We wanted to analyze components found in the definitions in order to compare definitions to their probable sources and to each other. We also wished to analyze the evaluation procedures in order to compare them across SEAs and to consider the extent to which SEA evaluation procedures address concepts contained in the SEA definitions of autism.

2. Method

2.1. Data Collection. We looked for SEA definitions of autism for each of the states and the District of Columbia by accessing SEA websites and searching for "special education services" and as necessary, additional terms such as "rules and regulations" and "autism." Some SEAs had more than one apparently official definition of autism, presented on multiple SEA websites. In this instance, we coded the definition which included reference to state legal code. Some SEAs presented not only a statewide definition but additional definitions apparently reserved for particular school districts in the state. For this occurrence, we coded just the definition for the entire state.

For many SEAs, evaluation procedures for autism were located within the same website that stated the definition. If not, we searched the SEA website using "autism eligibility." All SEA definitions of and evaluation procedures for autism were collected between February and May, 2012.

2.2. Coding SEA Definition Components. To analyze and compare SEA definitions, we developed a list of ASD *components* based on consideration of three sources: (a) the definition of autism found in IDEA-2004, (b) the description of Autistic Disorder in DSM-IV-TR [8], and (c) the description of Childhood Autism in the tenth edition of *International statistical classification of diseases and related health problems* [12]. Our review of the descriptions of Asperger's Disorder and PDD-NOS in DSM-IV-TR showed that the criteria for these subcategories of PDD were subsumed by the criteria for Autistic Disorder (characteristics were the same, although not necessarily to the same degree). Therefore, our final list of definition components relied heavily on the main features of Autistic Disorder in DSM-IV-TR. We supplemented these with two components from the IDEA-2004 definition of autism that do not overlap with the DSM-IV-TR material: sensory processing problems and emotional disturbance exclusion (i.e., IDEA-2004 states that if the student qualifies for special education under the emotional disturbance disability, he or she cannot qualify under the autism disability). We judged that the characteristics of ICD-10 Childhood Autism are essentially similar to DSM-IV-TR Autistic Disorder, so the ICD-10 contributed no unique components to our list.

Our initial reading of the SEA definitions confirmed the suggestion of MacFarlane and Kanaya [10] that some SEAs appeared to rely heavily on either the DSM-IV-TR criteria or the IDEA-2004 statement for their definitions of autism. Therefore, we added two more components to the coding list: *Essentially DSM* and *Essentially IDEA*. We marked a SEA definition as Essentially DSM if it presented the three DSM-IV-TR set A criteria for autistic disorder (briefly stated as impaired social functioning, impaired communication, and stereotyped interests and activities), including the four specific subcriteria for each criterion, with no more than minor wording changes (e.g., "significant impairment" instead of "qualitative impairment"). We also coded Essentially DSM even if the DSM-IV-TR criterion B (onset before age 3) or criterion C (exclusion of Rett's disorder and childhood disintegrative disorder) was not included in the SEA definition. On the other hand, we marked an SEA definition as Essentially IDEA if it embodied either the entire IDEA-2004 definition or the major phrases in it verbatim.

2.3. Coding Evaluation Features. We developed a second coding list to analyze and compare SEA diagnostic evaluation procedures for autism. We began with the evaluation statement in IDEA-2004 regulations (which covers any educational disability, not just autism): "The child is assessed in all areas related to the suspected disability, including, if appropriate, health, vision, hearing, social and emotional functioning, general intelligence, academic performance, communicative status and motor abilities [11]."

Our evaluation coding list included each of the above statement's evaluation areas as *features*. In addition, our initial reading of the SEA evaluation statements revealed some other evaluation areas that we added to the list of features. These additions included the following: medical evaluation or information, observation, parent interview, social-developmental history, behavioral scale, adaptive behavior, sensory functioning, autism-specific diagnostic tool, and developmental assessment.

Following practice with coding, the authors clarified coding procedures through discussion. For example, SEA evaluation statements that included *psychological* assessment were coded as individual intelligence assessment and, if the statement indicated, additional psychological procedures. The first author coded the definition component list and the evaluation features list for all SEA definitions and all SEA evaluation statements. The second and third authors each coded definition components and evaluation features for an assigned half of the SEAs.

2.4. Coding Agreement. Intercoder agreement was calculated separately on each definition component and evaluation feature by dividing the number of coding agreements by the number of agreements plus disagreements. Disagreements between coders were resolved through discussion and review of material; if disagreements remained, the first author's coding was used.

3. Results

We obtained current SEA definitions of autism, as well as eligibility evaluation procedures for that category of special education for all states and the District of Columbia, from each SEA's website. We coded this information according to the definition and evaluation lists we created. Initial agreement (prior to discussion to achieve consensus) per coding item ranged from 0.88 to 1.0 with a mode of 0.96.

3.1. Basis of Definitions. A strong majority of SEA definitions of autism ($n = 35$, 69%) were coded as Essentially IDEA (IDEA-2004 definition entirely or in major part) as the sole basis of autism eligibility criteria for their state. Only 4 SEA definitions (8%) were considered Essentially DSM

Table 1: Components of state education agency autism definitions.

Definition component	Number of states	Percentage
Social interaction impairment—general statement	46	90
Impaired nonverbal social	15	29
Lack of peer relationships	21	41
Lack of spontaneous joint attention	14	27
Lack of social-emotional reciprocity	18	35
Communication impairment—general statement	46	90
Impaired development of spoken language	19	37
Impaired ability to initiate or sustain a conversation	17	33
Stereotyped and repetitive use of language	17	33
Lack of spontaneous make-believe or social imitative play	15	29
Restricted, repetitive, and stereotyped behaviors and interests—general statement	2	4
Preoccupation with stereotyped interests	49	96
Nonfunctional routines or rituals	50	98
Stereotyped and repetitive mannerisms	49	96
Preoccupation with parts of objects	17	33
Other components		
Onset prior to the age of three	47	92
Unusual sensory experiences	44	86
Exclusion conditions	45	88
Emotional disturbance	44	86
Intellectual/developmental delay	3	6
Pervasive developmental disorder	1	2
Rett's disorder or childhood disintegrative disorder	1	2
Schizophrenia	1	2
Visual or hearing impairments	1	2
Coexisting conditions allowed	3	6

(all three DSM-IV-TR criteria for Autistic Disorder (impaired social functioning, impaired communication, and stereotyped interests and activities), including the four specific subcriteria for each). Additionally, 10 SEA definitions (20%) used both the IDEA-2004 and the DSM-IV-TR criteria, incorporating essential elements from both sources either verbatim or with no more than minor wording changes. Two SEAs, California and Florida, presented unique state definitions that addressed some characteristics of autism such as those found in IDEA-2004 and DSM-IV-TR but did not contain enough similarity to be coded as either Essentially IDEA or Essentially DSM.

After definition basis was determined, we calculated a point-biserial correlation to investigate whether a relationship existed between source of definition (IDEA or DSM) and autism prevalence reported by states to the US Department of Education [7]. The analysis revealed no relationship based on this factor ($r_{37} = -0.11$, $P > .05$).

3.2. Autism Eligibility Criteria. The number of components in SEA autism definitions ranged from 5 to 17. The modal number of components was 8. Results of our examination of various components in each SEA definition are summarized in Table 1.

Social Interaction Impairment. Regardless of what source they appeared to be based on, 46 (90%) of the SEA definitions stated that impaired social interaction is required for the student to be qualified under the autism education disability. As Table 1 shows, considerable numbers of definitions included particular forms of social interaction impairment (impaired nonverbal social, lack of peer relationships, lack of spontaneous joint attention, lack of social-emotional reciprocity) as criteria for autism. In some definitions the particular forms were additions to a general statement about social interaction impairment, while in other definitions there was no general statement, just one or more of the particular forms of social interaction impairment.

Communication Impairment. Table 1 also shows that 46 (90%) of the SEA definitions contained a general statement to the effect that impairment in communication is a necessary characteristic to qualify for autism. Quite a few state definitions also presented particular forms of communication impairment as criteria for autism (impaired spoken language, impaired conversation ability, stereotyped language, impaired fantasy or social play). Again, in some but not all SEA definitions the particular forms were additions to a general statement.

Restricted, Repetitive, and Stereotyped Behaviors and Interests. Only 2 SEA definitions presented a general statement that to qualify for autism the student must show restricted or stereotyped behaviors or interests. However, all the definitions stated that one or more of the particular forms of restricted, repetitive, or stereotyped behaviors and interests had to be present for the student to qualify. Specifically, nearly all SEA definitions listed preoccupation with stereotyped interests, nonfunctional routines and rituals, and stereotyped mannerisms, while about one-third of definitions listed preoccupation with object parts.

Other Components. Among the other key features, 46 definitions (90%) stated that onset prior to three years of age was either generally evident or required. Of these, 41 stated that exceptions to the age of three onset guideline or requirement are permitted; 5 definitions did not state an age of onset.

An eligibility statement about unusual responses to sensory experiences was present in 44 SEA definitions (86%). The definitions contained six different exclusion conditions (see Table 1), most commonly identification under the emotional disturbance category of special education (86%). On the other hand, three states specified conditions that could coexist with autism eligibility.

3.3. Autism Evaluation Features. The number of SEA autism evaluation features ranged from 0 to 15 with 8 as the modal number of criteria. Only 10 SEAs used all, and only, features of the IDEA evaluation statement to indicate their evaluation criteria for autism eligibility. However, as Table 2 shows, the majority of SEAs used one or more features of the IDEA evaluation statement. Specifically, health evaluation was noted in 57% of SEA positions; vision evaluation in 57%; hearing evaluation in 57%; social and emotional evaluation in 59%; academic evaluation in 88%; speech-language evaluation in 88%; motor skills evaluation in 88%. In addition, the following other evaluation features were present in the majority of SEA evaluation statements: observation, 51%; parent interview, 53%; social-developmental history, 53%; psychological, 84%; adaptive behavior, 51%. Table 2 presents additional features that we found in less than 50 percent of SEA evaluation procedures. Among these less-recommended features is the requirement to administer an autism-specific evaluation as part of the eligibility process. Of the 15 SEAs (29%) that included an autism assessment in the evaluation process, none specified the use of a recognized instrument such as the Autism Diagnostic Observation Schedule (ADOS) [13] or the Childhood Autism Rating Scales (CARS) [14]. Although 3 of these SEAs did indicate the required use of a state-created autism checklist, none gave any reference to a source or psychometric characteristics of those checklists.

Table 2: Features of state education agency evaluation procedures for autism.

IDEA evaluation features	Number of states	Percentage
Academic	45	88
Speech-language	45	88
Intelligence (or psychological)	43	84
Social and emotional	30	59
Health	29	57
Vision	29	57
Hearing	29	57
Motor skills	29	57
Other evaluation features		
Parent interview	27	53
Social-developmental history	27	53
Observation	26	51
Adaptive behavior	26	51
Medical evaluations or information	18	35
Autism-specific	15	29
Behavioral scale	11	22
Sensory functioning	9	18
Developmental assessment	5	10

4. Discussion

The present study revealed that definitions of autism and the eligibility evaluation procedures for it are readily available on SEA websites. Most SEA definitions substantially resemble the federal definition of autism found in IDEA-2004, including its components about deviant responses to sensory experiences and exclusion of students with emotional disturbance. Many definitions have in addition some elements of DSM-IV-TR autistic disorder. On the other hand, only one-fifth of SEA evaluation procedures substantially reflect the IDEA-2004 statement on assessment for disability eligibility, although many SEAs incorporate a few aspects of that statement.

Study results suggest several points that call for criticism, but first we acknowledge that it is far easier to disapprove of existing definitions and evaluation statements about autism than to present demonstrably superior alternatives. That said, below we point to several drawbacks to the existing SEA information and offer a direction that could lead to their improvement.

Table 1 shows that most SEA definitions prohibit qualification under the category of autism for a student who has certain other conditions. This is a flaw because some of those other conditions are commonly found among children with autism. For example, children with autism often experience mood disorder, anxiety disorder, and other mental disorders [15–17] that might qualify the student for emotional disturbance. Yet in 44 SEA definitions, qualifying for emotional disturbance excludes qualifying for autism.

Moreover, despite the frequent definition emphasis on ruling out an emotional disturbance, only 11 SEAs (22%) require a behavioral evaluation that would document the presence or absence of emotional-behavioral problem characteristics. Given this disconnect, it is possible that students with characteristics of autism may either not be so identified due to rule-out criteria or may be identified under the autism category but not receive proper services for their unevaluated mental health issues.

The DSM-5 definition of autism spectrum disorder recognizes the comorbidity of autism with other mental disorders, such as anxiety and obsessive compulsive disorder, and allows for specification of these coexisting conditions within the clinical diagnosis. SEAs that undertake a revision of their autism special education category may wish to follow the lead of DSM-5 in this regard by recognizing that students whose emotional and behavior problems might qualify them for emotional disturbance may more appropriately be qualified for autism.

In addition to coexisting mental health conditions, many cases of ASD are characterized by abnormal brain development [18, 19] with documented seizures present in perhaps as much as 30% of this population [16]. Our study revealed that 29 SEAs called for health evaluations and 18 called for medical evaluations; however, what these evaluations entail was left unstated or vague. Although 3 SEAs called for a neurological examination as part of the health or medical evaluation, we recognize that such a universal requirement would represent an enormous cost to school districts. However, we do recommend that SEAs clarify the content and purpose of stated health and medical evaluations including whether they represent the same information. If SEAs were to incorporate elements of the DSM-5 autism criteria, they would see that recognition of coexisting medical or genetic conditions is part of the ASD in DSM-5. Developing a comprehensive description of the student beyond the basic categories of social functioning, communication skills, and repetitive behaviors will provide schools and families with a more complete picture of student needs and the services required to meet them by a variety of providers.

Of course, substantial communication impairments do characterize a large fraction of students with autism. These include failure to speak, echolalia, and other severe problems of receptive and expressive language [20]. While 45 SEAs called for speech and language evaluation to qualify for autism, none specified and few suggested language problem areas to evaluate. Only 6 SEAs prescribed evaluation of the student's needs regarding augmentative or assistive technology for language. SEA evaluation procedures for autism may be improved by the addition of more specifics on language evaluation.

Similarly, the present study noted that the majority of SEAs ($n = 44$, 86%) consider the presence of unusual responses to sensory stimuli to be a core feature of autism. However, as with other noted discrepancies, only 9 SEAs (18%) required an evaluation procedure to document the existence and nature of possible sensory functioning difficulties. The DSM-5 criteria for ASD recognize the pervasiveness and impact of sensory issues on students with autism and include this feature prominently.

The increasing prevalence of autism in recent years has been attributed, to some extent, to a broadening of the concept of autism [21, 22] to include children whose social problems, communication problems, stereotyped behaviors and interests, and other problems are less severe than most cases diagnosed two or three decades ago. Similarly, present results suggest that the large increase in students qualifying for special education under autism may have been caused, in part, by vague definitions together with ambiguous, variable, and irrelevant evaluation procedures. A particular example would be the underutilization of recognized autism diagnostic instruments. Improvements in SEA definitions of autism will be of limited use unless they are accompanied by better assessment procedures that will support better evaluation and other aspects of assessment (e.g., measurement of student progress per characteristic of autism).

Present results and their implications compel us to add a couple of qualitative judgments about most of the SEA definitions of and evaluation statements for autism. First, for many SEAs the definition and the evaluation procedures unfortunately did not correspond. Definition components often were not addressed by evaluation features, even in a cursory way. Second, many of the definitions and evaluation procedures as presently stated are too vague to be of much use. For example, one state's definition says that autism is a disorder "significantly affecting verbal communication," but its autism evaluation statement calls for evaluators to "assess all areas of need including… communicative status" [23]—hardly a specification of needed procedures or measurable criteria for verbal communication, suited for use in determining eligibility. Of course, that so many of SEA definitions and evaluation statements closely resemble those of the IDEA-2004 implies that the federal items are too vague as well. The federal and SEA definitions and evaluation procedures for autism must be improved.

There is no time like the present, literally, for making those improvements. As noted earlier, the number of students with autism continues to rise. This not only makes inferior definition and evaluation a disservice to more students but it also increases the number of parents and teachers who will probably support improved ones. With the publication of DSM-5, SEAs have the opportunity to expand and update their current definition of autism. The DSM-5 criteria encompass all of the elements stated by the current IDEA definition with the exception of allowing for the coexistence of potential emotional disorders rather than exempting autism eligibility based on those characteristics. Moreover, IDEA-2004 is overdue for Congressional reconsideration and possible amendment, so an opportunity window will open, but for a limited time, to also update and clarify the federal educational definition of autism.

Third, the DSM-5 concept of autism, like DSM-IV, emphasizes problems of social functioning and repetitive behaviors and interests, along with problems with social aspects of language. DSM-5 recognizes the salience of sensory processing problems and the possibility of coexisting mental health disorders. Officials of more SEAs should consider elements of DSM-5 autism spectrum disorders as they consider revisions to their state definition of autism and corresponding procedures by which assessors will provide data for eligibility determination.

The need is evident and the moment is favorable to make improvements to administrative definitions of and evaluation procedures for autism as an education disability on both the state and federal levels. Therefore, we propose that an appropriate national organization or agency seeks input and pursue consensus on this issue. Input should be obtained from representatives of special education and other professional groups, ASD advocacy organizations, state and federal education agencies, and other individuals and groups with significant interests in the appropriate education of students with autism.

An agenda might include addressing important questions, perhaps including some of the following: (a) what are the critical components that should be in an educational administrative definition of autism? (b) Are there other categories of educational disability that should be mutually exclusive with autism, and if so, how should this be presented? (c) Should the definition and evaluation procedures address the presence of autism overall, or its more specific components separately? (d) How is a balance established between evidence-based best assessment practices versus assessor professional judgment regarding individual student situations? (e) Are there critical validated or standardized evaluation procedures that should be specified, and if so, would SEA procedures that call for them incur large legal and financial obligations? As we see it, considering such fundamental questions will supplement other activities of participants to move toward the goal of this effort: to create ideal revisions to the IDEA definition of autism and its statement of evaluation procedures—in this case, procedures specific to autism eligibility.

If this goal is achieved, what might happen next? The model definition and evaluation procedures might be presented to federal authorities with the power to incorporate it into the next iteration of IDEA. They may be presented to SEAs for consideration in state-level revisions. Improved, more specific definitions and evaluation procedures will enable SEAs and school districts to better serve students with autism and better allocate resources. Ultimate outcomes such as school graduation, employment, and community involvement must begin with a correct first step. For autism, the first step is to accurately identify the disability and any accompanying individual conditions in a manner that students receive good services and opportunities regardless of where they live in our nation.

Disclosure

None of the authors received financial compensation to produce this study. This paper is the product of original research conducted by the primary author.

References

[1] S. E. Levy, D. S. Mandell, and R. T. Schultz, "Autism," *The Lancet*, vol. 374, no. 9701, pp. 1627–1638, 2009.

[2] C. Gillberg and L. Wing, "Autism: not an extremely rare disorder," *Acta Psychiatrica Scandinavica*, vol. 99, no. 6, pp. 399–406, 1999.

[3] J. K. Irwin, J. MacSween, and K. A. Kerns, "History and evolution of autism spectrum disorders," in *International Handbook of Autism and Pervasive Developmental Disorders*, J. L. Matson and P. Sturmey, Eds., pp. 3–16, Springer Science, Business Media, New York, NY, USA, 2011.

[4] Centers for Disease Control, "Prevalence of autism spectrum disorders: autism and developmental disabilities monitoring network, 14 sites, United States, 2008," *Morbidity and Mortality Weekly*, vol. 61, pp. 1–19, 2012, http://www.cdc.gov/mmwr/preview/mmwrhtml/ss6103a1.htm?s_cid=ss6103a1_w.

[5] Federal Register, vol. 71, no. 156, 2006, Rules and Regulations, p. 46756 a, 2006.

[6] U. S. Department of Education, "Number of children served under IDEA by disability and age group, during school years 1991-92 through 2000-01," Office of Special Education Programs, Data Analysis System (DANS), 2001, http://www.ideadata.org/tables24th%5Car_aa9.htm.

[7] U. S. Department of Education, "Children with disabilities receiving special education under Part B of the Individuals with Disabilities Education Act, 2011," Office of Special Education Programs, Data Analysis System (DANS), OMB #1820-0043, 2012, https://www.ideadata.org/arc_toc13.asp#partbCC.

[8] American Psychiatric Association, *Diagnostic and Statistical Manual of Mental Disorders*, American Psychiatric Association, Washington, DC, USA, 4th edition, 2000.

[9] American Psychiatric Association, *Diagnostic and Statistical Manual of Mental Disorders*, American Psychiatric Association, Washington, DC, USA, 5th edition, 2013.

[10] J. R. MacFarlane and T. Kanaya, "What does it mean to be autistic? inter-state variation in special education criteria for Autism services," *Journal of Child and Family Studies*, vol. 18, no. 6, pp. 662–669, 2009.

[11] Federal Register, vol 71, no. 156, 2006, p. 46785 b, 2006.

[12] WHO, *The ICD-10 Classification of Mental and Behavioural Disorders: Diagnostic Criteria for Research*, World Health Organization, Geneva, Switzerland, 1992, http://www.who.int/classifications/icd/en/GRNBOOK.pdf.

[13] C. Lord, M. Rutter, P. DiLavore, and S. Risi, *The ADOS-G (Autism Diagnostic Observation Schedule-Generic)*, Western Psychological Services, Los Angeles, Calif, USA, 1999.

[14] E. Schopler, J. Reichler, and B. Renner, *The Childhood Autism Rating Scale (C.A.R.S.)*, Western Psychological Services, Los Angeles, Calif, USA, 1988.

[15] A. B. Lewin, J. J. Wood, S. Gunderson, T. K. Murphy, and E. A. Storch, "Phenomenology of comorbid autism spectrum and obsessive-compulsive disorders among children," *Journal of Developmental and Physical Disabilities*, vol. 23, no. 6, pp. 543–553, 2011.

[16] S. Mohiuddin, S. Bobak, D. Gih, and M. Ghaziuddin, "Autism spectrum disorders: comorbid psychopathology and treatment," in *International Handbook of Autism and Developmental Disorders*, J. L. Matson and P. Sturmey, Eds., pp. 463–478, Spring Science, Business Media, New York, NY, USA, 2011.

[17] H. Tager-Flusberg and K. C. Dominick, "Comorbid disorders," in *Textbook of Autism Spectrum Disorders*, E. Hollander, A. Kolevzon, and J. T. Coyle, Eds., pp. 209–218, American Psychiatric, Washington, DC, USA, 2010.

[18] M. Bauman, "Neuroanatomy of the brain in autism spectrum disorders," in *Textbook of Autism Spectrum Disorders*, E. Hollander, A. Kolevzon, and J. T. Coyle, Eds., pp. 355–361, American Psychiatric, Washington, DC, USA, 2010.

[19] S. E. Levy, D. S. Mandell, and R. T. Schultz, "Autism," *The Lancet*, vol. 374, no. 9701, pp. 1627–1638, 2009.

[20] R. Paul and K. Gilbert, "Development of language and communication," in *Textbook of Autism Spectrum Disorders*, E. Hollander, A. Kolevzon, and J. T. Coyle, Eds., pp. 147–157, American Psychiatric, Washington, DC, USA, 2010.

[21] J. D. Bregman, "Pervasive developmental disorder not otherwise specified," in *Textbook of Autism Spectrum Disorders*, E. Hollander, A. Kolevzon, and J. T. Coyle, Eds., pp. 89–98, American Psychiatric, Washington, DC, USA, 2010.

[22] E. Fombonne, "Incidence and prevalence of pervasive developmental disorders," in *Textbook of Autism Spectrum Disorders*, E. Hollander, A. Kolevzon, and J. T. Coyle, Eds., pp. 117–136, American Psychiatric, Washington, DC, USA, 2010.

[23] Iowa Department of Education, "Administrative rules of special education," 2014, https://www.educateiowa.gov/pk-12/special-education/administrative-rules-special-education.

23

Characteristics of Two-Year College Students on the Autism Spectrum and their Support Services Experiences

Anne M. Roux,[1] Paul T. Shattuck,[1] Jessica E. Rast,[1] Julianna A. Rava,[1] Amy D. Edwards,[1] Xin Wei,[2] Mary McCracken,[2] and Jennifer W. Yu[2]

[1] *A.J. Drexel Autism Institute, Drexel University, 3020 Market Street, Suite 560, Philadelphia, PA 19104-3734, USA*
[2] *SRI International, 333 Ravenswood Avenue, BS 162, Menlo Park, CA 94025-3493, USA*

Correspondence should be addressed to Anne M. Roux; amr376@drexel.edu

Academic Editor: Hansen Wang

Approximately 80% of college-going youth with autism in the US attend a 2-year college at some point. These community-based, universally accessible institutions offer both academic and vocational courses and have experience in teaching diverse learners. This study used nationally representative survey data from the National Longitudinal Transition Study-2 to describe the characteristics and services experiences of adults with autism who attended postsecondary education after high school, focusing on those who attended a 2-year college. Over 60% of those who attended 2-year colleges had little to no trouble conversing or performing functional skills like counting change during high school, and extracurricular participation was common (93.8%). Most 2-year college attenders (85.7%) were able to navigate to places outside the home versus 43.9% of those with no postsecondary education. Over half took vocational courses at 2-year colleges, while one-quarter pursued academic study. Less than half (48.6%) of those who disclosed their disability to the school reported receiving services, accommodations, or other help. Most (87.3%) felt they received enough help, but fewer (68.0%) felt the services they received were useful. Future research should delineate specific needs of students with autism in 2-year college settings and identify what supports are needed to improve persistence and completion rates.

1. Introduction

The reported prevalence of autism has been increasing for over a decade. Most of the increasing prevalence is among children with average to above-average intelligence [1]. Approximately one-third of youth on the autism spectrum in the United States go to college within eight years of exiting high school [2, 3], and college attendance is projected to increase in this population [4]. Yet, very few population-based studies are available that describe the experiences of young adults on the autism spectrum who attend college.

Two-year colleges are a primary gateway to postsecondary education for youth on the autism spectrum in the US. The term "2-year colleges" primarily refers to over 1,100 locally funded community colleges throughout the US [5], which are attended by about 40% of undergraduate students [6]. These universally accessible, open-admission educational institutions offer both academic and vocational courses and are experienced in teaching diverse learners who may require developmental academic support.

Of youth on the autism spectrum in the US who attend college, the vast majority (81%) attend a 2-year college either solely or as a stepping stone to a 4-year college [7]. Approximately 70% of 2-year public institutions in the US report enrolling students with autism spectrum disorders [8]. However, little research has specifically examined the characteristics of 2-year college students on the autism spectrum as a whole, their educational experiences, and whether they receive the help they may need to complete a degree or certificate or to advance to a 4-year college. Understanding who these youth are and maximizing their potential for college attendance is important for those who advise them.

Like all colleges in the US, 2-year colleges are required to offer reasonable accommodations to students with self-disclosed disabilities. Some interpret these accommodations to include help aimed at organizational and social skills needed for academic success [9, 10]. Two-year college support programs for students on the autism spectrum vary widely: from noncredit college experience programs with a residential component and classroom-based supports, to center-based disability support services delivered to degree-seeking students, to off-campus supports provided by outside agencies or family members [9]. Dual-enrollment transition programs allow some high school students to take classes at the community college while continuing to receive academic and social skills supports through an Individualized Education Program until the age of 21. The prevalence and need for various types of support are currently unknown.

College students on the autism spectrum may require services and accommodations due to impairments in executive functioning (such as inattentiveness and poor organizational skills), communication (such as maintaining the topic of conversation and comprehending abstract language), social interactions, and social relationships [11–13]. Additionally, psychiatric comorbidities are known to affect about 70% of children and adolescents on the autism spectrum [14, 15]. Challenges associated with psychiatric comorbidities can impact a student's ability to succeed in college and navigate the dynamics of the social environment [13, 16–18]. Still other students may have significant functional skills deficits that necessitate more intensive services to support the student on campus. Such students might attend non-degree granting programs that focus on vocational preparation and opportunities for social inclusion. Yet, to date, there is almost no research that elucidates the characteristics of which students on the autism spectrum typically attend different types of college settings and what supports they might require.

Known factors of postsecondary outcomes for young adults with autism include conversational abilities and functional impairments in addition to socioeconomic position [19, 20]. Parental expectation that the student will attend postsecondary education is an identified predictor of participation in postsecondary education for students with autism [21].

Experiences during high school may also be relevant factors in predicting whether students will go on for further education. For typically developing youth, a connection exists between participation in high school extracurricular activities and college-going [22]. However, little research has explored the effect of participation in extracurricular activities on outcomes for youth on the autism spectrum. Over 70% of high school youth on the autism spectrum engage in some type of extracurricular activity, whether volunteering, taking classes outside of school, church activities, or postschool activities, including youth with a wide range of conversational abilities [23]. Extracurricular activities may provide opportunities to build self-advocacy and self-determination skills, which are important for success within postsecondary education.

Participation in Individualized Educational Program (IEP) meetings within school may be another example of self-advocacy. While 85% of students with ASD have a transition plan [24], students with autism are half as likely as their peers with learning disabilities to actively participate in their own transition planning (IEP) meetings [25], particularly for those with greater cognitive and social skill deficits. In general, however, we understand little regarding factors that predict participation in postsecondary education or at 2-year colleges specifically.

In this exploratory study we use nationally representative data to conduct one of the first examinations of 2-year college experiences in young adults on the autism spectrum in the US. We examine the following questions. First, of young adults with autism who attend postsecondary education, what are the characteristics and educational experiences of those who solely attend 2-year college? Second, what are the differences in characteristics and educational experiences between those who attend 2-year college and those who attend 4-year college, who attend vocational-technical education, or who never attended postsecondary education of any type? Last, what types of services and/or accommodations do students with autism receive at 2-year colleges compared to those who attend 4-year college or vocational-technical education? Findings will help colleges plan for the growing number of students on the autism spectrum and will provide useful anticipatory guidance for youth, their families, high school counselors, and special education staff who facilitate transition planning.

2. Methods

2.1. Participants. We analyzed data from Wave 5 of the National Longitudinal Transition Study-2 (NLTS2), collected in 2009 when participants were aged 21–25 years. The NLTS2 provides one of the largest sources of prospective, population based data on the postsecondary experiences of US students who received special education services during high school. Use of this data was approved by the US Department of Education (USDE) and deemed exempt by the Drexel University Institutional Review Board. Sample size reporting is rounded to the nearest 10 per agreement with the USDE.

The NLTS2 used a two-stage sampling plan. First, 500 local education agencies were randomly selected from across the US. Second, students who received special education services were sampled. This yielded 1,012 students who received special education services under the federal eligibility category of autism who were targeted for recruitment [26]. To ensure that results represented the target population, survey weighting was specifically calculated for each wave of data, and bias analysis was conducted at each wave as well [27, 28]. Results can be generalized to youth who were aged 13–17 and receiving special education services for autism at the start of the study in December 2000. More extensive discussion of NLTS2 methodology and questionnaire design is available [29].

Data analysis included students who received special education services under the special education categorical qualification of autism. At Wave 5, responses from 620 young adults who received special education services for autism during high school were available for analysis, yielding a retention rate of 67% at Wave 5 based on number of participants at Wave 1. For data presented in Table 1, rates of missing per covariate ranged from 0% to 17%. The highest rates of missing data were these variables: how well youth

TABLE 1: Demographic and disability characteristics of students on the autism spectrum across postsecondary education outcomes. Percentage (95% confidence interval), test for difference versus the 2-year college column.

	2-year college	4-year college	Vocational/technical school	No postsecondary education
Male	84.5 (76.7, 92.4)	88.1 (75.8, 100)	84.2 (68.5, 99.9)	85.8 (81.8, 89.7)
Hispanic ethnicity	2.4 (0, 5.2)	4.2 (3.4, 5.0)	5.2 (0, 11.1)	12.1** (4.3, 19.9)
Race				
White	85.3 (79.6, 90.9)	73.9 (63.0, 84.8)	69.3* (57.0, 81.5)	54.8*** (45.9, 63.7)
Black	8.3 (4.3, 12.2)	21.9** (11.4, 32.4)	15.8 (4.8, 26.8)	25.9*** (22.7, 29.2)
Other race	6.4 (2.0, 10.9)	4.2 (3.0, 4.5)	14.9 (4.9, 24.9)	19.3** (10.3, 28.2)
Either parent attended any postsecondary education	92.7 (87.2, 98.3)	100*** (100, 100)	78.5 (58.6, 98.3)	66.5*** (60.0, 73.0)
Parent or guardian household income				
Up to $25,000	12.1 (4.4, 19.7)	8.8 (2.3, 15.2)	11.0 (5.2, 16.8)	24.8* (19.1, 30.5)
$25,001–$50,000	19.4 (10.1, 28.7)	15.3 (2.6, 27.9)	32.1 (14.1, 49.7)	27.9 (22.3, 33.5)
$50,001–$75,000	47.1 (37.5, 56.8)	28.9 (15.2, 42.7)	28.5 (7.6, 49.3)	35.1 (28.9, 41.4)
More than $75,000	21.4 (14.8, 28.1)	47.0* (28.4, 65.6)	28.5 (11.2, 45.8)	12.1* (7.9, 16.3)
Characteristics of youth during high school				
How well youth converses				
Has a lot of trouble or not able to converse at all	38.5 (25.7, 51.4)	10.9 (7.3, 14.4)	39.3 (18.1, 60.5)	63.5** (54.7, 72.2)
Little trouble	52.1 (39.5, 64.7)	61.5 (48.7, 74.3)	35.4 (17.6, 53.1)	30.4** (22.4, 38.3)
No trouble	9.4 (4.6, 14.1)	27.7** (13.9, 41.4)	25.4* (4.8, 45.9)	6.2 (2.8, 9.5)
Counts change pretty or very well	64.6 (43.4, 85.7)	97.1** (90.4, 100)	64.2 (49.0, 79.4)	36.8* (30.0, 43.7)
Gets to places outside the home pretty or very well	85.7 (78.6, 92.8)	82.8 (74.2, 91.5)	61.5** (47.3, 75.8)	43.9*** (35.0, 52.9)
Parent expected youth to probably or definitely attend postsecondary school	60.9 (48.0, 73.7)	84.8 (80.6, 89.1)	53.5 (30.7, 76.2)	16.5*** (10.6, 22.4)
Any extracurricular activities	93.8 (89.8, 97.7)	90.3 (85.3, 95.3)	74.4*** (58.6, 90.1)	58.5*** (52.0, 65.0)
Participated in IEP or transition planning during high school (student provided some input or took leadership)	65.5 (55.6, 75.4)	82.7 (74.5, 90.9)	50.5 (31.0, 70.1)	33.4*** (27.6, 39.2)

Note: source: National Longitudinal Transition Study-2, Waves 1 and 5. Weighted to population levels. Variances adjusted for sampling method. Logistic regression analysis used 2-year college as the referent group; $^{*}p < .05$, $^{**}p < .01$, and $^{***}p < .001$.

gets to places outside the home (17.4%), role of youth in the IEP setting (16.3%), household income (6%), and how well youth converses (6%). Given the branching logic of questioning in the survey, the number of possible participants who were asked to respond to questions regarding services and accommodations was relatively small. Therefore, results for Table 2 should be treated as exploratory findings. Missing data were not imputed for this descriptive study.

Individual school districts determined whether students qualified for special education under the category of autism in accordance with federal law [30]. We could not clinically verify autism diagnosis because these are secondary data. However, virtually all students who meet eligibility criteria for special education under the category of autism also meet DSM-IV-TR criteria for autism, using the diagnostic guidelines in use during the period of NLTS2 administration [31, 32].

Table 2: Postsecondary education supports and services experiences of youth on the autism spectrum. Percentage (95% confidence interval), test for difference versus the 2-year college column.

	2-year college	4-year college	Vocational/technical school
Attendance and coursework at postsecondary institution			
Continuity of attendance			
Enrolled continuously	80.4 (67.8, 93.0)	93.6 (83.2, 100)	78.1 (66.8, 89.5)
Full- or part-time student as of most recent term			
Full time (≥12 hours' credit)	50.4 (36.5, 64.3)	86.2*** (77.7, 94.7)	78.4* (60.4, 96.3)
Universally available student supports			
Ever accessed help with school work available to all students at the postsecondary institution	43.2 (30.2, 56.2)	41.8 (35.0, 48.5)	20.3* (15.4, 25.3)
Received services or help on his/her own outside of school	17.6 (8.3, 26.9)	22.9 (7.5, 38.3)	17.5 (8.3, 26.6)
Disability-related services			
Young adult considers self to have a disability	70.2 (58.2, 82.1)	63.6 (39.9, 87.4)	80.6 (70.4, 90.0)
School was aware of disability either before or after enrollment	69.1 (57.9, 80.2)	62.7 (55.0, 70.4)	99.0** (96.6, 100)
Received any services, accommodations, or other help	48.6 (34.1, 63.1)	30.0 (18.5, 41.5)	65.5 (48.8, 82.3)
Type of accommodations or services received			
Human aides	62.5 (51.4, 73.7)	70.4 (39.3, 100)	44.9 (19.0, 70.9)
Testing accommodations	56.4 (40.9, 71.8)	84.2* (75.4, 92.9)	44.6 (16.2, 73.0)
Physical adaptation	34.3 (14.1, 54.4)	49.9 (25.5, 74.3)	13.1* (10.0, 16.1)
Out-of-classroom learning supports	19.8 (0, 41.3)	25.0 (19.6, 30.3)	19.5 (14.9, 24.1)
Materials/technology adaptations	16.0 (6.6, 25.4)	58.7** (24.3, 93.1)	—
Accommodations in assignments	14.4 (6.1, 22.6)	14.7 (2.1, 27.4)	27.2 (20.7, 33.6)
All supports and services			
Received enough help, services, or accommodations in and out of school	87.3 (78.5, 96.1)	91.2 (82.4, 100)	93.3 (—, —)
Help, services, and accommodations received in and out of school were somewhat or very useful	68.0 (52.8, 83.3)	55.5 (28.1, 82.8)	—

Note: source: National Longitudinal Transition Study-2, Wave 5. Weighted to population levels. Variances adjusted for sampling method. Cell sizes that are too small to report are denoted (—). Logistic regression analysis used 2-year college as the referent group; * $p < .05$, ** $p < .01$, and *** $p < .001$.

2.2. Procedures. Data for this study came from NLTS2 interviews primarily conducted by telephone. Responses were obtained directly from the young adult to the extent possible, if parents reported that the young adult was capable of answering survey items either through telephone interview or a mailed survey. A parent or guardian responded to the survey questions in cases where the young adult was not able to complete an interview. The role of the investigators was limited to analysis of previously collected NLTS2 survey data.

2.3. Materials. Variables that represent student and family demographics, impairment characteristics, high school experiences, and parent expectation of postsecondary school attendance are presented in Table 1. Variables representing characteristics of students during high school included how well youth conversed, ability to get to places outside the home, whether youth participated in any extracurricular activities, and participation in the IEP process.

We measured frequency of participation in postsecondary education experiences with the survey items, "Since leaving high school, have you ever taken any classes from a 2-year, junior, or community college?", from a "postsecondary vocational, business, or technical school," or from a "4-year college or university." Students were counted within only one

TABLE 3: Examples of services, accommodations, or other help received during postsecondary education by primary categories and subcategories.

Testing accommodations	More time to take tests Having tests read aloud Scribe to record answers Different tests Different grading standards Different setting to take tests
Assignment accommodations	Additional time to finish assignments Shortened length of assignments
Materials technology adaptations	Use of computer or spell checker in class or to take tests Special use of calculator, listening/recording devices, tape recorder Provision of written materials (e.g., copies of lectures, outlines, course notes) Books on tape Computer software designed for students with disabilities
Human aides	A reader or interpreter Note taker in class Personal aide or instructional assistant to help you in class Tutor Support person to monitor academic progress or help with managing workload
Out-of-classroom learning supports	Behavior management program Help with learning strategies or study skills Support group for students with disabilities Early registration
Physical adaptations in classroom	Physical changes to the classroom, special desks Changes to equipment, like different lab equipment in a science class

Note: source: National Longitudinal Transition Study-2, Wave 5. Youth Interview.

postsecondary outcome: 2-year college only, 4-year college only, vocational/technical education but no college, or no postsecondary education. If the respondent answered yes to both 2-year college and vocational/technical school, follow-up questions differentiated the most appropriate designation. Young adults were also asked whether they felt that they had a disability, a precursor to receiving disability-related accommodations in the postsecondary education setting.

Variables related to help and services experiences are presented in Table 2. A sequence of questions assessed student service and support experiences during their postsecondary education. The first question, posed to all young adults, concerned use of help that was available to all students, "Did you ever get help with school work from this school like going to a tutor, or a study center, or a writing center?" If young adults responded affirmatively to having a disability, a follow-up question asked whether the school was aware of the disability or special need either before or after enrollment. Students who disclosed the disability to the school, and were therefore potentially eligible to receive accommodations, were then asked whether they received "any services, accommodations, or other help from the school to help you do your best there, like a note taker or more time to take tests because of a learning problem, disability, or other special need." Those who responded affirmatively were asked, "What services, accommodations, or other help have you received there?" The NLTS2 interviewer coded the services, accommodations, and help that the student received.

Examples of categories and subcategories of services, accommodations, and help relevant to the needs of students on the autism spectrum are listed in Table 3. If the participant did not list any services, accommodations, or supports within the categories of human aides or out-of-classroom learning supports, follow-up prompts were asked: "Has there been any person assigned to help you, like a tutor, an interpreter, or someone who takes notes for you in class?" and/or "Have there been any supports for you outside of class, like a support group for students with disabilities or early registration?"

Students who received services, accommodations, or supports were next asked, "How useful have all the services, accommodations, and help with school work been in helping you stay in school and do your best there?" They were also asked whether they received enough services, accommodations, and help with schoolwork to do their best in school, as well as whether they had gotten any services or help on their own outside of the school.

2.4. Data Analysis. To understand the prevalence of postsecondary education experiences of youth with autism following high school, we estimated descriptive statistics for three groups of students to determine how many attended 2-year college only, 2-year and 4-year college, 4-year college only, vocational-technical education, or no postsecondary education. We examined postsecondary education attendance for these groups: (1) all youth with an autism spectrum disorder, (2) youth on the autism spectrum who ever attended postsecondary education of any type, and (3) youth on the autism spectrum who ever attended college. Those who attended both 2-year and 4-year colleges were excluded from further analysis due to inability to separate their experiences at each institution.

Our primary focus group for analysis was young adults on the autism spectrum who reported that they attended a 2-year college at some point since leaving high school but no other types of postsecondary schools. For purposes of contextualization and comparison, we also analyzed characteristics of young adults on the autism spectrum who experienced other postsecondary education outcomes: 4-year college, vocational/technical postsecondary education, and those who had never attended postsecondary education. We then compared postsecondary education and services experiences for those who attended a 2-year college to those who attended 4-year college, or vocational/technical education. Variables from Wave 1 were used to characterize students during high school (Table 1). Postsecondary outcomes and service experiences (Table 2) were measured using Wave 5 data. We used bivariate analyses and logistic regression to describe and test for group differences in characteristics of students during high school and in postsecondary education experiences, using young adults who attended 2-year college as the referent group for regression.

3. Results

Of all young adults on the autism spectrum represented in the NLTS2 at Wave 5, nearly one in five (17.7%) attended a 2-year college only, and an additional 9.2% attended both a 2-year and a 4-year college. Fewer students attended only a 4-year college (4.6%) or postsecondary vocational/technical education (7.4%). Most (61.1%) never attended any type of postsecondary education.

Of the 40% of young adults on the autism spectrum who attended postsecondary education of some type within the first eight years after high school, nearly 46% attended a 2-year college only; 11.7% attended a 4-year college only; 23.8% attended both 2- and 4-year colleges, and 19.1% attended a vocational/technical school. Of young adults on the autism spectrum who attended college, 85.6% ever attended a 2-year college, and 56.2% solely attended a 2-year college.

Students who reported that they attended a 2-year college only were primarily male (84.5%), White (85.3%), and non-Hispanic (97.6%) with a mean age of 23.2 years (range 21–25 years). Nearly 93% had at least one parent who attended any postsecondary education. Approximately half (47.1%) were from households with incomes in the $50,001–75,000 range. Significantly fewer 2-year college attendees were from households with incomes above $75,000 (21.4%) compared to those who attended 4-year colleges (47%, $p < .05$). Likewise, significantly fewer (12.1%) were from homes with incomes less than $25,000, compared to those who never attended postsecondary education (24.8%, $p < .05$).

Nearly 62% of students who attended 2-year college had little to no trouble conversing. Significantly more (63.5%, $p < .01$) of those who had no postsecondary education had a lot of difficulty or inability to hold a conversation. Most (64.6%) young adults who attended 2-year college reported doing "pretty well" to "very well" with functional skills like counting change, significantly more than students who never attended postsecondary education (36.8%, $p < .05$) but significantly fewer than those who attended 4-year college (97.1%, $p < .01$). Significantly more 2-year college students (85.7%) were able to navigate to places outside the home on their own than those who never attended postsecondary education (43.9%, $p < .001$) and those who attended vocational/technical school (61.5%, $p < .01$).

When asked at Wave 1, only 60.9% of parents of 2-year college students predicted that their youth would pursue postsecondary education, significantly higher than parents of those who never attended postsecondary education (16.5%, $p < .001$). Nearly all (93.8%) young adults who attended 2-year college participated in extracurricular activities during high school, significantly more than those who attended vocational education (74.4%, $p < .001$) or no postsecondary education (58.5%, $p < .001$). Nearly 66% provided some input in the IEP process or took leadership, significantly more than those who never attended postsecondary education (33.4%, $p < .001$).

Over half (56.1%) of students who attended only 2-year college took mostly vocational courses to train for a job, such as computer or business classes, as opposed to those who took mostly academic courses like English or science (26.1%), both vocational and academic (14.0%), or personal interest classes (3.8%). About 43% of 2-year college students utilized help with school work that was universally available to students, such as tutoring or writing lab. Other students used supports that were contingent upon disclosure of a disability.

Nearly half (48.6%) of those who attended 2-year college, and who disclosed their disability to the school, reported that they had received services, accommodations, or other help for their disability from the 2-year college. Further, 17.6% reported receiving services or help on their own outside of school. The most common accommodations for 2-year college students on the autism spectrum were human aides (62.5%), testing accommodations (56.4%), and physical adaptations in the classroom (34.3%) (Tables 2 and 3). Most students who attended 2-year college (87.3%) reported feeling that they had received enough services, accommodations, or help although only 68.0% reported that these services were somewhat or very useful.

4. Discussion

Continued education is an expectation for emerging adults in industrialized nations as a step along the pathway to a career [33]. In the US higher education is associated with higher incomes, better health, and improved quality of life [34]. Those with college degrees can expect to earn more and live longer lives [35, 36]. However, disparities in who attends college have persisted in the general population across the last half century, with nonattenders historically referred to as the "forgotten half" [37]. Public policy initiatives continue to attempt to close the gaps in college attendance and encourage college opportunities that include 2-year and community college programs.

The increase in youth with developmental disabilities, including autism spectrum disorder, who attend college is a relatively recent phenomenon, and there are few tracking mechanisms in place to tally the number of students who are accessing different postsecondary education options. This study found that over 85% of students on the autism spectrum who attend college in the US will enroll in a 2-year college at some point during the early years after high school. Well over half of these students solely attend a 2-year college.

It is critical for guidance counselors and transition planners to have useful predictors of which students might be candidates for 2-year college attendance. Overall, high school students who later attended a 2-year college could be characterized as having mid-range functional and communication abilities during high school relative to their peers on the autism spectrum with other types of postsecondary education outcomes. The conversational skills of young adults who attended 2-year college were generally of higher level than students who had no postsecondary education although students who attended 2-year college generally had greater levels of conversational impairment than their peers who had experiences at 4-year college. Similarly, they were able to navigate their community on their own and perform daily living skills more frequently than their peers in vocational/technical settings or those who had no postsecondary education but were not as adept as those who were able to attend 4-year college settings. This study also established that even students within the lowest conversational ability levels are accessing 2-year colleges.

Frequency of extracurricular participation and active participation in IEP transition planning activities was significantly higher in young adults who attended 2-year college compared to their peers in vocational education and those who did not attend postsecondary education. These indicators may be predictors of students who are candidates for 2-year college participation or may be viewed as transition experiences that could prepare a student for higher education settings.

Despite the finding that students with a wide range of abilities attended 2-year colleges, and the fact that all of these young adults required special education supports during high school, less than half of those who disclosed their disability to the 2-year college reported receiving any services, accommodations, or help. While the doors to 2-year colleges are open to students on the autism spectrum, gaps in supports may hinder their opportunities to succeed in this setting. Other studies have found lower rates of persistence and completion for students on the autism spectrum in 2-year settings [7], similar to students with other types of disabilities [38]. These issues must be addressed as more programs emerge that are designed to support these students in 2-year college programs.

While 2-year colleges are often touted as an avenue to success for students from disadvantaged backgrounds, students on the autism spectrum did not fit this characteristic. We found the majority of students on the autism spectrum who attended a 2-year college were from middle-to-upper income households with at least one parent who had some postsecondary education. The disadvantage these students experience appears to be primarily due to their disability, not their socioeconomic position.

Two-year college students on the autism spectrum in the US face significant gaps in access to supports for postsecondary education. Specialized college programs and supports offered for students with disabilities have increased in recent years due to federal support for comprehensive Transition and Postsecondary Programs for Students with Intellectual Disabilities (TPSIDs) authorized under the Higher Education Opportunity Act (HEOA) of 2008. However, these programs primarily serve students on the autism spectrum who have cooccurring intellectual disability, leaving students who are capable of accessing degree-seeking programs to pursue campus-based disability support services which are typically not tailored to the unique needs of students on the autism spectrum. Further, many TPSID programs are located on 4-year college campuses, not the 2-year/community college campuses which students on the autism spectrum frequently attend.

Issues of disability identity present another unique challenge in this population. College students must acknowledge and disclose a disability as a first step toward receiving disability support services in a college setting. Yet, one-third of college students on the autism spectrum who received special education during high school do not view themselves as having a disability or special need during young adulthood [39]. In cases where students are in need of help but are not receiving it, lack of identification of oneself as a student with a disability may signal an important barrier to receipt of disability support services. There is little research to explain lack of disability reporting among students on the autism spectrum. However, college students with other mental health disorders report feeling that they do not need services, lack time for services, or prefer to deal with issues on their own [40]. Nondisclosure may be related to stigma, limited student understanding of one's disability, or lack of resources [41]. Likewise, lack of service utilization by students with autism may be related to limited self-advocacy or self-determination skills, or not self-identifying a need for help [12, 42].

In summary, 2-year colleges are a frequent pathway in the transition to adulthood for many students in the U.S. and may offer a unique benefit for students on the autism spectrum. These settings serve as grounds for teaching and generalizing essential life skills including transportation navigation, employment, relationship-building, self-care, financial management, and sometimes residential living. Two-year colleges may function as a scaffold step between high school and independent living, offering a defined campus environment in which to develop life skills with potential support from fellow students who may be training to work with special needs populations. Yet, without adequate identification of students who may be candidates for 2-year programs, and corresponding improvements in access to the services they likely need for success in these institutions, this valuable option will be less than effective for helping young adults with autism to ultimately achieve higher quality lives.

5. Conclusions

Multiple opportunities exist for improving the success of students on 2-year college pathways beginning with enhancing planning for the transition to postsecondary education. Researchers note overall inadequate practices in transition planning [42], need for further research that explicitly connects transition planning interventions to intended outcomes [43], and a paucity of students with stated goals for transitioning into 2- or 4-year colleges [44]. Our findings of high rates of extracurricular activity participation during high school and active student participation in transition planning meetings indicate that many students who later go on to attend 2-year colleges do exhibit the seeds of self-determination skills that recent work has found to be related to positive postsecondary outcomes [45]. Further identification of which high school experiences and skills have the strongest relationship with positive postschool outcomes should be a primary research focus in the years ahead for informing transition practices.

Additional supports for parents of transition-age students may also be beneficial, as over one-fourth of families whose students attended 2-year colleges did not expect their child to attain this outcome. Parental expectations are contingent upon family awareness of available college options and support resources. A recent review of unmet needs of college students on the autism spectrum recommended further development of a student-in-training/parent-in-waiting model via dual-enrollment programs [46]. These programs would offer more explicit utilization of the student's IEP to develop supports in the college setting, gradual increase of ownership of academic and self-advocacy responsibilities to the student, and recognition that parents continue to play an important role in student support into the college years. Students and their families might also benefit from a focus on summer transition experiences between high school and 2-year college.

At the level of the postsecondary institution, few support programs are currently designed to address autism-specific needs of students. These needs may include highly specific guidance on understanding one's disability and related needs; navigating social situations and expectations; direct instruction in organizational systems; environmental accommodations for sensory integration dysfunction; and assistance for managing typical campus living skills including laundry, financial management, and sexual relationships [9].

This paper focused primarily on those who attended 2-year college to allow us to better examine student characteristics and support experiences in this setting alone. Findings from across our studies indicate differences in students who *only* attend a 2-year college versus those who *ever* attend a 2-year college. Although 9% of young adults with autism attended both 2-year and 4-year colleges, it was also not possible to accurately analyze their services experiences as these students may have had differing services, accommodations, or help across their 2-year and 4-year college settings. Wehman et al. (2014) [42] provide an extensive overview of the differences between 2- and 4-year settings and the needs of students who transfer from 2-year to 4-year programs.

5.1. Study Limitations. Study limitations were primarily related to the nature of the survey data. First, it was impossible to know whether students were enrolled in general or specialized postsecondary education programs such as TPSID-funded programs available on some college campuses. We were also unable to characterize important elements of educational quality identified by McEathron et al. (2013) including individualization of coursework, options for earning college credit, and degree of integration [47]. Third, while this study examined outcomes of those who were out of high school, we had no way to differentiate students who were able to access dual enrollment (in both high school special education and postsecondary education) during their transition-age years which may have provided some benefit to their postsecondary education outcomes. Finally, we were unable to accurately account for the potential effect of comorbid psychiatric diagnoses on postsecondary outcomes, as measures of medical diagnoses are limited in the NLTS2.

Despite these limitations, NLTS2 data offer an unprecedented glimpse into the postsecondary education outcomes and experiences of a large number of individuals on the autism spectrum in the US. Our findings indicate that students are accessing a variety of postsecondary education settings with a high prevalence of 2-year college experiences. Future research should delineate more specific needs of students in this setting and identify what supports are needed to improve persistence and completion rates as well as increase rates of transition into 4-year college programs.

Disclaimer

This information or content and conclusions are those of the authors and should not be construed as the official position or policy of, nor should any endorsements be inferred by, HRSA, HHS, or the US Government and they do not also represent the views of the National Institute of Mental Health or other funders.

Acknowledgments

This work was supported in part by funding from the Institute of Education Sciences, the National Science Foundation (HRD-1130088), and the National Institute of Mental Health (R01 MH086489). This work was also supported by the Health Resources and Services Administration (HRSA) of the US Department of Health and Human Services (HHS) under Grant no. UA6MC27364 and title Health Care Transitions Research Network for Youth and Young Adults with Autism Spectrum Disorders for the grant amount of $900,000.

References

[1] Centers for Disease Control and Prevention (CDC), "Prevalence of autism spectrum disorder among children aged 8 years—Autism and Developmental Disabilities Monitoring Network, 11 sites, United States, 2010," *Morbidity and Mortality Weekly Report. Surveillance Summaries*, vol. 63, no. 2, pp. 1–21, 2014.

[2] P. T. Shattuck, S. C. Narendorf, B. Cooper, P. R. Sterzing, M. Wagner, and J. L. Taylor, "Postsecondary education and employment among youth with an autism spectrum disorder," *Pediatrics*, vol. 129, no. 6, pp. 1042–1049, 2012.

[3] X. Wei, J. W. Yu, P. Shattuck, M. McCracken, and J. Blackorby, "Science, technology, engineering, and mathematics (STEM) participation among college students with an autism spectrum disorder," *Journal of Autism and Developmental Disorders*, vol. 43, no. 7, pp. 1539–1546, 2013.

[4] E. O. VanBergeijk and P. K. Cavanagh, "Brief report: new legislation supports students with intellectual disabilities in post-secondary funding," *Journal of Autism and Developmental Disorders*, vol. 42, no. 11, pp. 2471–2475, 2012.

[5] American Association of Community Colleges, "2014 fact sheet," 2014, http://www.aacc.nche.edu/.

[6] L. G. Knapp, J. E. Kelly-Reid, and S. A. Ginder, "Enrollment in postsecondary institutions, fall 2011: financial statistics, fiscal year 2011; and graduation rates, selected cohorts, 2003–2008: first look (provisional data) (NCES 2012-174rev)," http://nces.ed.gov/pubs2012/2012174rev.pdf.

[7] X. Wei, E. R. A. Christiano, J. W. Yu, J. Blackorby, P. Shattuck, and L. A. Newman, "Postsecondary pathways and persistence for STEM versus non-STEM majors: among college students with an autism spectrum disorder," *Journal of Autism and Developmental Disorders*, vol. 44, no. 5, pp. 1159–1167, 2014.

[8] K. Raue and L. Lewis, "Students with disabilities at degree-granting postsecondary institutions," NCES 2011-018, 2011, http://nces.ed.gov/pubsearch.

[9] E. VanBergeijk, A. Klin, and F. Volkmar, "Supporting more able students on the autism spectrum: college and beyond," *Journal of Autism and Developmental Disorders*, vol. 38, no. 7, pp. 1359–1370, 2008.

[10] D. Zager and C. S. Alpern, "College-based inclusion programming for transition-age students with autism," *Focus on Autism and Other Developmental Disabilities*, vol. 25, no. 3, pp. 151–157, 2010.

[11] B. McKeon, C. S. Alpern, and D. Zager, "Promoting academic engagement for college students with autism spectrum disorder," *Journal of Postsecondary Education and Disability*, vol. 26, no. 4, pp. 353–366, 2013.

[12] L. A. Sperry and G. B. Mesibov, "Perceptions of social challenges of adults with autism spectrum disorder," *Autism*, vol. 9, no. 4, pp. 362–376, 2005.

[13] S. W. White, T. H. Ollendick, and B. C. Bray, "College students on the autism spectrum: prevalence and associated problems," *Autism*, vol. 15, no. 6, pp. 683–701, 2011.

[14] M.-L. Mattila, T. Hurtig, H. Haapsamo et al., "Comorbid psychiatric disorders associated with asperger syndrome/high-functioning autism: a community- and clinic-based study," *Journal of Autism and Developmental Disorders*, vol. 40, no. 9, pp. 1080–1093, 2010.

[15] E. Simonoff, A. Pickles, T. Charman, S. Chandler, T. Loucas, and G. Baird, "Psychiatric disorders in children with autism spectrum disorders: prevalence, comorbidity, and associated factors in a population-derived sample," *Journal of the American Academy of Child & Adolescent Psychiatry*, vol. 47, no. 8, pp. 921–929, 2008.

[16] B. Hofvander, R. Delorme, P. Chaste et al., "Psychiatric and psychosocial problems in adults with normal-intelligence autism spectrum disorders," *BMC Psychiatry*, vol. 9, article 35, 2009.

[17] G. Joshi, C. Petty, J. Wozniak et al., "The heavy burden of psychiatric comorbidity in youth with autism spectrum disorders: a large comparative study of a psychiatrically referred population," *Journal of Autism and Developmental Disorders*, vol. 40, no. 11, pp. 1361–1370, 2010.

[18] G. Joshi, J. Wozniak, C. Petty et al., "Psychiatric comorbidity and functioning in a clinically referred population of adults with autism spectrum disorders: a comparative study," *Journal of Autism and Developmental Disorders*, vol. 43, no. 6, pp. 1314–1325, 2013.

[19] P. Howlin and P. Moss, "Adults with autism spectrum disorders," *Canadian Journal of Psychiatry*, vol. 57, no. 5, pp. 275–283, 2012.

[20] P. T. Shattuck, A. M. Roux, L. E. Hudson, J. L. Taylor, M. J. Maenner, and J.-F. Trani, "Services for adults with an autism spectrum disorder," *Canadian Journal of Psychiatry*, vol. 57, no. 5, pp. 284–291, 2012.

[21] H. M. Chiang, Y. K. Cheung, L. Hickson, R. Xiang, and L. Y. Tsai, "Predictive factors of participation in postsecondary education for high school leavers with autism," *Journal of Autism and Developmental Disorders*, vol. 42, no. 5, pp. 685–696, 2012.

[22] J. F. Zaff, K. A. Moore, A. R. Papillo, and S. Williams, "Implications of extracurricular activity participation during adolescence on positive outcomes," *Journal of Adolescent Research*, vol. 18, no. 6, pp. 599–630, 2003.

[23] P. T. Shattuck, G. I. Orsmond, M. Wagner, and B. P. Cooper, "Participation in social activities among adolescents with an autism spectrum disorder," *PLoS ONE*, vol. 6, no. 11, Article ID e27176, 2011.

[24] S. M. Zeedyk, L. A. Tipton, and J. Blacher, "Educational supports for high functioning youth with ASD: the postsecondary pathway to college," *Focus on Autism and Other Developmental Disabilities*, 2014.

[25] M. Wagner, L. Newman, R. Cameto, H. Javitz, and K. Valdes, "A national picture of parent and youth participation in IEP and transition planning meetings," *Journal of Disability Policy Studies*, vol. 23, no. 3, pp. 140–155, 2012.

[26] R. Cameto, M. Wagner, L. Newman, J. Blackorby, and H. Javitz, *National Longitudinal Transition Study II (NLTS2) Sampling Plan*, SRI International, Menlo Park, Calif, USA, 2000.

[27] H. Javitz and M. Wagner, *Analysis of Potential Bias in the Sample of Local Education Agencies (LEAs) in the National Longitudinal Transition Study-2 (NLTS2) Sample*, SRI International, Menlo Park, Calif, USA, 2002.

[28] H. Javitz and M. Wagner, *Analysis of Potential Bias in the Wave 1 and Wave 2, Respondents to the National Longitudinal Transition Study-2 (NLTS2) Sample*, SRI International, Menlo Park, Calif, USA, 2005.

[29] M. Wagner, K. Kutash, A. J. Duchnowski, and M. H. Epstein, "The special education elementary longitudinal study (SEELS) and the national longitudinal transition study (NLTS): study designs and implications for children and youth with emotional disturbances," *Journal of Emotional and Behavioral Disorders*, vol. 13, pp. 25–41, 2005.

[30] US Department of Education, *Individuals with Disabilities Education Act*, US Department of Education, Washington, DC, USA, 2004.

[31] J. Bertrand, C. Boyle, M. Yeargin-Allsopp, P. Decoufle, A. Mars, and F. Bove, "Prevalence of autism in a United States population: the Brick Township, New Jersey, investigation," *Pediatrics*, vol. 108, no. 5, pp. 1155–1161, 2001.

[32] M. Yeargin-Allsopp, C. Rice, T. Karapurkar, N. Doernberg, C. Boyle, and C. Murphy, "Prevalence of autism in a US metropolitan area," *The Journal of the American Medical Association*, vol. 289, no. 1, pp. 49–55, 2003.

[33] J. J. Arnett, *Debating Emerging Adulthood: Stage or Process?* Oxford University Press, Oxford, UK, 2011.

[34] J. Mirowsky, *Education, Social Status, and Health*, A. de Gruyter, New York, NY, USA, 2003.

[35] C. E. Ross and C.-L. Wu, "The links between education and health," *American Sociological Review*, vol. 60, no. 5, pp. 719–745, 1995.

[36] C. L. Ryan and J. Siebens, "Educational attainment in the United States, 2009," 2012, http://www.census.gov/prod/2012pubs/p20-566.pdf.

[37] The William T. Grant Foundation Commission on Work-Family and Citizenship, *The Forgotten Half: Pathways to Success for America's Youth and Young Families. Final Report, Youth and America's Future*, The William T. Grant Foundation Commission on Work, Family, and Citizenship, 1998.

[38] K. Mamiseishvili and L. C. Koch, "Students with disabilities at 2-year institutions in the United States: factors related to success," *Community College Review*, vol. 40, no. 4, pp. 320–339, 2012.

[39] P. T. Shattuck, J. Steinberg, J. Yu et al., "Disability identification and self-efficacy among college students on the autism spectrum," *Autism Research and Treatment*, vol. 2014, Article ID 924182, 7 pages, 2014.

[40] D. Eisenberg, J. Hunt, N. Speer, and K. Zivin, "Mental health service utilization among college students in the United States," *The Journal of Nervous and Mental Disease*, vol. 199, no. 5, pp. 301–308, 2011.

[41] D. Kranke, S. E. Jackson, D. A. Taylor, E. Anderson-Fye, and J. Floersch, "College student disclosure of non-apparent disabilities to receive classroom accommodations," *Journal of Postsecondary Education and Disability*, vol. 26, no. 1, pp. 35–51, 2013.

[42] P. Wehman, C. Schall, S. Carr, P. Targett, M. West, and G. Cifu, "Transition from school to adulthood for youth with autism spectrum disorder: what we know and what we need to know," *Journal of Disability Policy Studies*, vol. 25, no. 1, pp. 30–40, 2014.

[43] J. D. Westbrook, C. J. Fong, C. Nye, A. Williams, O. Wendt, and T. Cortopassi, "Transition services for youth With autism: a systematic review," *Research on Social Work Practice*, vol. 25, no. 1, pp. 10–20, 2015.

[44] K. A. Shogren and A. J. Plotner, "Transition planning for students with intellectual disability, autism, or other disabilities: data from the national longitudinal transition study-2," *Intellectual and Developmental Disabilities*, vol. 50, no. 1, pp. 16–30, 2012.

[45] K. A. Shogren, M. L. Wehmeyer, S. B. Palmer, G. G. Rifenbark, and T. D. Little, "Relationships between self-determination and postschool outcomes for youth with disabilities," *The Journal of Special Education*, vol. 48, no. 4, pp. 256–267, 2015.

[46] S. Pinder-Amaker, "Identifying the unmet needs of college students on the autism spectrum," *Harvard Review of Psychiatry*, vol. 22, no. 2, pp. 125–137, 2014.

[47] M. A. McEathron, T. Beuhring, A. Maynard, and A. Mavis, "Understanding the diversity: a taxonomy for postsecondary education programs and services for students with intellectual and developmental disabilities," *Journal of Postsecondary Education and Disability*, vol. 26, no. 4, pp. 303–320, 2013.

24

A Randomised Control Trial of the Impact of a Computer-Based Activity Programme upon the Fitness of Children with Autism

Kathleen Dickinson and Maurice Place

School of Health and Life Sciences, Northumbria University, Coach Lane Campus, Newcastle Upon Tyne NE7 7XA, UK

Correspondence should be addressed to Maurice Place; maurice.place@northumbria.ac.uk

Academic Editor: Manuel F. Casanova

The poor levels of fitness in children with autism are prompting concern for the children's future health. This study looked to assess if a computer-based activity programme could improve fitness levels (as reflected in cardiopulmonary function) of these children, and achieve a reduction in their body mass index. In a randomised controlled trial, 50 children with autism (of which 33 were under the age of 11 years and 39 were boys) were allocated to an intervention group which encouraged them to use the Nintendo Wii and the software package "Mario and Sonics at the Olympics" in addition to their routine physical education classes. 50 children with autism (34 under the age of 11 years and 40 being boys) acted as controls. At the end of one year, analysis of the changes in scores using analysis of covariance (ANCOVA) on the Eurofit fitness tests showed that the intervention group had made statistically significant improvement on all tests other than flexibility. These improvements were also significantly better than controls. This type of intervention appears to be an effective addition to standard fitness training in order to help children with autism improve their fitness levels.

1. Introduction

There is increasing concern about the decline in fitness among children generally and how this reduction increases the risk of ongoing health issues in these children. This fitness decline is associated with a dramatic rise of obesity among the young generally, and since many children and young people with autism have a relatively inactive lifestyle, it has been suggested that this decreased physical activity, together with other factors such as unusual dietary patterns, is the major factor in the relatively greater increased rate of obesity found in children with autism when compared to their typically developing peers [1–5].

Research has shown that increasing the physical activity of children with autism improves general fitness, has a positive impact upon cardiorespiratory function, and offers the potential to control weight gain [6]. Furthermore regular strenuous exercise is associated with decreases in other elements of difficult functioning, such as stereotypical behaviours, hyperactivity, aggression, self-injury, and destructiveness [6].

To achieve this change is however not easy, with the difficulty of encouraging exercise in children with special needs being well discussed in the literature [7, 8] and children with autism presenting a particular challenge in this regard. One method of encouraging physical activity which has been the focus of some interest is the use of computer-based activity programmes. In typically developing children such programmes have been shown to improve the general level of fitness of participants, particularly in those children who have a low level of initial fitness [9, 10]. Theoretically this type of intervention could be of advantage to children with autism because computers are often seen by them as nonthreatening, straight forward, and predictable, as well as demanding minimal social interaction.

In order to evaluate the potential value of computer-based activity programmes to children with autism, a study was undertaken to compare one such programme to standard school-based physical education in the children attending schools with classes specifically for children with autism in the North East of England.

2. Methods

The aim of the project was to assess whether additional physical activity in the form a computer-based activity game could improve the cardiopulmonary fitness of children with autism and have a positive impact upon their body mass index (BMI) which also is used as a proxy for fitness. The project was a parallel design with stratification to control for age and gender, and then block randomisation to the intervention and nonintervention groups.

2.1. Outcome Measures. One element of the assessment chosen was the multistage progressive shuttle run test (known as the bleep test), which has been shown to be a good measure of cardiopulmonary function because $VO_{2\ max}$ scores, a measure of the maximum capacity of an individual's body to transport and use oxygen during incremental exercise, can be calculated from it [11]. Power calculations indicated that a sample size of 34 in each group would allow the detection of a significant difference in $VO_{2\ max}$ with a power of 0.9 at a Type I error level of 0.05 for a two-tailed test and an effect size of 0.50 as measured by Cohen's *d*. It was decided to recruit 50 subjects for each group to allow for participant attrition. The secondary outcome assessment was the change in the children's BMI over the duration of the study.

2.2. Settings and Participants. Having obtained ethical approval from academic bodies, educational gatekeepers, and parents, the study was carried out over the period of one academic school year (September to June 2011-2012). Three schools in the locale that had classes specific for the teaching of children with autism agreed to take part in the study. The children in these settings ranged in age from 5 to 15 years of age and none had any physical disorder or illness that would reduce their ability to participate in the fitness programme. The families of all the children were approached to participate in the study. After the details of the study had been explained all agreed. The Statements of Special Educational Need for all of the children indicated that they all had an IQ in the moderate/severe range of ability. The children in this pooled sample were then randomly allocated to intervention or nonintervention groups, controlling for age and gender. Selection was completed when 50 families had been allocated to each group. Background information was collected from the family concerning make-up, medical conditions, employment of parents, and so forth.

2.3. Fitness Assessment. The physical fitness of the children was evaluated using elements of the Eurofit physical fitness test battery [12], which is a set of nine physical fitness tests covering flexibility, speed, endurance, and strength. These have been shown to have good reliability in typically developing children [13] and have adequate reliability in children with intellectual disability [14]. The five elements of the test that were chosen for this study are described in detail in Table 1. These items were chosen as the smallest number of the 9 tests that would assess the widest range of fitness aspects, while requiring little equipment and being easy to replicate. In fact this group of tests has become well established as the optimum programme for assessment [15].

As described in Table 1, the multistage progressive shuttle run test (known as the bleep test) has been shown to be a good measure of cardiopulmonary function and has been accepted as the standard measure by the British National Coaching Foundation [16]. This test also has the advantage of published norms for typically developing children and offers the opportunity to calculate the $VO_{2\ max}$ scores. This is seen as a reliable reflection of physical fitness and uses age as an influencing parameter [11].

2.4. Procedure. The testing was carried out in the schools' usual PE areas so the children would be familiar with the spaces. All the schools carried out the tests using the same set procedure, as described in the protocols which accompany each of the tests, and were fully explained to the participating staff. To help the children understand the test elements visual modelling was used together with simplified instructions. To ensure that the children gave their best effort they were instructed to go on until they could go on no longer. In addition, since the teaching staff leading the testing knew the children well they were allowed to explain this requirement in a way they felt the children would best understand.

To overcome the learning effect associated with field-based fitness tests, the children had two trial assessments, and then their scores were recorded at a further assessment, with one of the team (KD) in attendance. The study took place over three academic terms, with the same fitness level tests being repeated at the conclusion of the study period, again under supervision.

In addition to their standard school physical education programme, the children in the intervention group used a Nintendo Wii and the software package "Mario and Sonics at the Olympics." The participants and staff received an induction in relation to the Wii and associated software games package at the beginning of the intervention. The package was chosen because it had various levels of physical interaction, and each pupil played the game in groups of 2 to 4, under supervision, for a period of 15 minutes per day, three times per week. *Mario and Sonic at the Olympic Games* features authentic Olympic events for the single match and circuit modes. The events closely follow rules and regulations of the specific sports. The types of Wii events are classified as athletics, gymnastics, shooting, archery, rowing, aquatics, fencing, and table tennis. The children taking part in the intervention used the single match mode for up to 4 players. They took part in the athletics, aquatics, fencing, and table tennis. The most popular activities were the running events in the athletics and the swimming events in the aquatics activities. These allowed for four-player use at once. Table tennis allowed for two-player use and the other events were one-player use followed by the next player taking their turn as appropriate. The teachers had flexibility over the time of day the intervention would occur. Wherever possible, the school carried out their intervention at the same time each day so as not to significantly disrupt the children's routine. Random visits were made to the participating schools to monitor the intervention delivery.

TABLE 1: Fitness tests used in the study.

Test	Area of measurement/explanation	Equipment required
Body mass index	Body fat measurement	Height scale and weighing scales
National Coaching Foundation (NCF), multistage fitness test-progressive shuttle run test known as the bleep or beep test.	Cardiorespiratory fitness (aerobic) $VO_{2\ max}$. This is a maximal test. The bleep test is a maximal exercise test to measure aerobic fitness. It involves running up and down a 20 m track in time to increasingly faster beep signals.	Test CD and CD player or MP3 download, 20 m running space, marker cones.
Standing long jump test (broad jump)	Measurement of explosive leg strength. A starting line is marked on the floor and the participants have to take a standing two-footed jump from this line with the aim to jump as far as they can. The arms may be used to aid the jump.	2 m of space. Marker for starting line. Tape measure. Or Standing broad jump kit.
10 × 5 m shuttle test	Measurement of speed and agility and aerobic capacity. Subjects run between two markers of 5 m; there and back counts as 1 repeat and this is continued until 10 repeats have been carried out.	Cones, tape measure to mark out 5 m, stop watch.
Partial curl up test known as sit-ups	Measurement of abdominal strength and endurance. The child lies on the floor with knees flexed. The subject curls up his/her trunk then lowers back to the floor, repeating this as many times as they can. The test lasts for duration of 30 seconds.	Mat for the child to lie on. Stop watch. Additional person to hold legs or time test.
Sit and reach test	Test measures the flexibility of the lower back and hamstring muscles, that is, hip flexibility. The test involves sitting on the floor with legs out straight ahead and then reaching as far forward as possible.	Sit and reach board/equipment or tape measure.

Both groups received the standard physical education programme which, in England, is statutorily defined in the National Curriculum for Physical Education [17]. This consists of two PE lessons per week, of 30 or 45 minute duration. In accordance with the requirements of this curriculum these sessions cover sporting activities such as basketball, athletics, gymnastics, and swimming, as well as dance and other ball games, such as cricket.

2.5. Additional Assessment. To gain some measure of the dynamics of the families in each of the study groups, the general family functioning of the two groups was compared by asking the children's main care giver to complete the Family Adaptation and Cohesion Evaluation Scales (FACES IV) [18]. This is a self-report measure which gives two scales, one measuring family cohesion (the degree of emotional attachment between family members) and the other flexibility (the ability to change structure, roles, and relationships in response to situational and developmental stress). The scales have proven reliability [19], with moderate levels on each scale being assumed to be more functional than the extreme levels [20].

2.6. Sample Make-Up. As can be seen in Table 2, the purposive selection by age and gender resulted in there being 33/34 children under the age of eleven years in the intervention/control groups, and the groups contained 39/40 boys, respectively. All the children had moderate to severe intellectual difficulties, and 35/40 were living with both parents. There were some differences when identifying those that were the only children in the family (9/25), and in terms of parental employment 7/9 came from families where both parents were working, and 13/12 came from families where both parents were unemployed.

TABLE 2: The demographic information of the sample.

	Intervention group (n = 50)	Control group (n = 50)
Boys		
≤10 yrs	27	27
≥11 yrs	12	13
Girls		
≤10 yrs	6	7
≥11 yrs	5	3
Only child	9	25
Living with both parents	35	40
Both parents working	7	9
Both parents unemployed	13	12

All statistical analyses were conducted with IBM-SPSS version 21.0. Normalcy of the fitness and family data was assessed using the Shapiro-Wilk test [21], with the choice of statistical analysis being determined by the results and consideration of the Q-Q plots [22]. Student's t-tests were used for comparisons of parametric data and the impact of the intervention being assessed by analysis of covariance (ANCOVA).

3. Results

Testing of the family assessment data by the Shapiro-Wilk test confirmed it to be parametric, and the results from the FACES IV questionnaire showed no significant difference in family functioning between the two groups, with the control group mean for cohesion being 57.82 (std dev 12.77) and for the intervention group 60.54 (std dev 11.65, $t = 1.11$, 98 df). For flexibility of family functioning the mean score for the control group families was 51.3 (std dev 11.71) and the intervention group 50.16 (std dev 10.03, $t = 0.52$, 98 df).

3.1. Differences in Initial Parameters. The fitness results showed a wide variation, and the Shapiro-Wilk test confirmed that the results could not be considered to be normally distributed. As can be seen in Table 3, the initial physical fitness levels between the two groups showed some significant differences, with the intervention group being better at the broad jump, bleep test, and sit-up activities and the control group having better scores on the shuttle run test and flexibility.

3.2. Changes over Duration of Study. After the study period the children in the control group had shown minor improvements in flexibility, as assessed using the sit and reach test, over the time of the study, but the sit-up score showed little change, as did the broad jump score and bleep test. The control group actually showed a statistically significant increase in their body mass index (BMI), with only four children showing improvement. Also the group's shuttle run times showed an increase (deterioration) with only eight of the fifty improving their scores.

By contrast, the intervention group showed highly significant improvement in all of the fitness measures with, for instance, 46 showing improvement in their shuttle run times, (Table 3). The result that reflects cardiorespiratory fitness and the bleep test improved significantly, and the broad jump and the sit-up scores also showed significant increases. The flexibility median score had undergone a small increase after the intervention (reflecting a deterioration in function), but inspection of the individual scores showed that the majority showed a reduction, with four children whose poorer level of flexibility accounted for the change. The average body mass index (BMI) also showed a reduction in the intervention group, with 39 having a reduced (i.e., improved) score.

3.3. Differences between Control and Intervention Groups. When the degree of change seen in control and intervention groups over the time of the study is compared (Table 4), the children in the intervention group showed a significantly more positive level of change in all scores, except flexibility, when compared to the control group (Table 4). 43 had improved their bleep test scores, compared to 13 in the control group, and inspection of the results showed that the change in the control group's shuttle run scores achieved significance because eight children had improved their scores from a high baseline, while 46 of the children in the intervention group had shown improvement in their scores, but to a more modest degree. The broad jump and sit-up scores only improved in the intervention group, while the flexibility score only improved in the control group. With regard to the BMI, a reduction in BMI was taken to be a positive outcome.

To offer some insight as to whether out-of-school activity might bias the fitness results, the parents were asked about the index child's other activities. Only 10 children had any out-of-school activities, four in the intervention group and 6 in the controls.

4. Discussion

The potential benefits from using computer-based activity games has been demonstrated in adults [23], but to our knowledge this is the first report of its potential benefit for children with autism. In this study the intervention group showed highly significant improvement in certain aspects of physical activity, particularly in respect to cardiopulmonary fitness (as measured by the $VO_{2\ max}$ calculated from the bleep test score). Of perhaps equal note is that the anecdotal feedback from the school staff involved was that all of the children in the intervention group appeared to enjoy participation. One of the measures, the sit and reach activity, which was used to measure flexibility, was not an activity utilised in the computer programme chosen, though in various guises it is part of routine physical education activities. Although there has been some work to show that flexibility improves as general fitness improves [24], significant improvement in flexibility is generally only achieved when flexibility is specifically targeted.

The importance of improving physical fitness is well recognised given its strong association with physical health. Physically active children and adolescents have lower blood pressure levels, more favourable lipoprotein levels, higher bone density, and decreased adiposity compared to their sedentary counterparts [25]. Psychological health and general mental well-being are also improved by such a physically active lifestyle [26–28]. In addition, it has been shown that an active lifestyle has been shown to have a beneficial effect upon psychological health [29, 30], as well as being linked with higher academic achievement [31], especially if the activity improves aerobic capacity [32].

However in recent years there has been a growing concern about the reduction in physical exercise amongst children [33] and that this is increasing the risk of significant health problems for them in later life particularly if cardiorespiratory fitness is poor [34]. This is in part because active and energetic children tend to remain active throughout middle and late adulthood [35], whereas sedentary children are more likely to become sedentary adults [36].

Children with autism have greater difficulties than typically developing children with participating in physical activity because of the nature of their difficulties. Although the literature on physical activity levels in children with autism is sparse [37], several studies have found that children with autism are less active than children without disabilities [38, 39], and even when children with autism achieve recommended activity levels during physical activity lessons, they are significantly less active during break times [40–42] and when at home [37]. Also, when compared to young people

Table 3: Initial and follow-up fitness results as medians and interquartile range (IQR) scores (Z calculated using Wilcoxon signed rank test between time samples and Mann Whitney U for difference between initial scores of control and intervention groups).

	Control group			Intervention group			Difference between initial scores of control and intervention groups (Z)
	Median (IRQ)		Difference between initial and follow-up scores (Z)	Median (IRQ)		Difference between initial and follow-up scores (Z)	
	Initial score	Follow-up score		Initial score	Follow-up score		
Body mass index (BMI)	20.2 (5.6)	21.5 (5.5)	4.86^{***}	20.1 (6.1)	19.8 (5.6)	-5.37^{***}	0.72
Bleep test	2 (3)	2 (2)	1.61	3 (4)	4.5 (5)	5.92^{***}	2.52^{*}
Shuttle run	84.5 (49)	90 (42)	4.04^{***}	92 (27)	68 (43)	-4.89^{***}	2.33^{*}
Broad jump	54.5 (23)	52.5 (20)	−0.77	80 (41)	92.5 (50)	5.12^{***}	4.59^{***}
Sit-ups	7.5 (5)	7.5 (4)	1.94	10 (10)	13 (7)	5.08^{***}	2.27^{*}
Flexibility	10 (6)	10 (8)	2.48^{*}	8 (13)	9 (13)	0.09	2.05^{*}

$^{*}P < 0.05$, $^{**}P < 0.01$, and $^{***}P < 0.001$.

TABLE 4: Comparison of changes to fitness scores between the control and intervention groups (F calculated using ANCOVA with fixed factors of age and gender).

	Number of children showing improvement in score		Significance in difference of degree of change between control and intervention groups ($F(1,90)$)
	Control group ($n = 50$)	Intervention group ($n = 50$)	
$VO_{2\,max}$	13	43	16.13***
Body mass index (BMI)	4	39	30.06***
Bleep test	13	43	13.15***
Shuttle run	8	46	41.35***
Broad jump	18	39	40.30***
Sit-ups	9	38	25.72***
Flexibility	4	4	1.20

*$P < 0.05$, **$P < 0.01$, and ***$P < 0.001$.

without autism, young people with autism are more likely to have difficulties with balance, postural stability, gait, joint flexibility, and movement speed [43], all of which adds to their difficulty in participating in physical activity.

As with typically developing children, regular physical activity has been shown to reduce the BMI of children with autism [44] and reduce stereotypical and self-stimulating behaviour [45]. Physical activity has also been found to help improve other behavioural issues [24, 44, 46]. The impact however can be even wider, with improvements in social behaviour [47] and academic engagement also being reported [48]. Finally, at least one study has shown that physical exercise reduced stress levels, as measured by salivary cortisol and self-report measures, in children with autism; however, these improvements quickly faded when the exercise programme ceased [49].

These findings strengthen the conclusion that it is important for these children to have a continuous programme of exercise, with a method of delivery that maintains the child's engagement. There is evidence that children with autism have difficulty understanding the goals of physical exercise [50], increasing further the challenge of ongoing involvement with fitness programmes. The research that does exist on helping children with autism take more exercise and improve their physical fitness tends to be focussed upon jogging and swimming [45, 51], with modelling and physical guidance generally being the method of instruction [45]. However to achieve regular participation there must be some source of external regulation [52], and the activities of a nature that will engage them sufficiently such that they will wish to participate.

While there are an increasing number of computer-based programmes that offer guided fitness activities, programmes that are game-based have been viewed as being of little value to health and well-being. Indeed video games have often been blamed as contributing factors to the increasing obesity levels [53]; however, it is being increasingly shown that physical activity-focussed programmes increase the activity levels of participants [54]. This recognition has led to their use in various settings, with activity-based computer programmes making a positive impact upon physical rehabilitation after an accident [55], as well as reducing mild cognitive impairment in older adults [56]. There is also a growing evidence base in adults that computer- and web-based interventions are effective at promoting physical health more generally [23]. That such programmes would also be helpful in children would not be surprising [57] and perhaps particularly so in children with autism because computer-based interventions offer a visual and nonjudgemental opportunity for them to take part in games that make no social interaction demands.

In any such study there are limitations to the conclusions that can be drawn. In this case the sample was drawn from a small geographical area in the North of England which is urban in nature, making it difficult to be confident about how much the findings would represent the impact upon children with autism in other areas. Also, although efforts were made to match the two groups, the relatively small population from which to draw meant that the matching process could only use a limited number of parameters. By choosing age and gender the possibility of differences in initial fitness levels between the groups was accepted, and in the event this proved to be the case. However it was anticipated that the potential impact of this upon the results could be reduced by using nonparametric statistical analyses and the degree of change in scores as the main outcome measure. Using a pooled sample from three schools gave rise to a potential contamination between control and intervention children, but it was decided to proceed with this method because it gave a degree of control about wider school issues and reduced the extra sessions that the staff in each school had to undertake. The staff had been asked not to alter the standard PE lessons that all the children provided, but the project resources did not permit the content of these to be monitored. It was recognised that the ongoing research may have prompted some change in content of the routine PE sessions, but it was hoped that the fact that both control and intervention children were sharing these lessons would minimise the impact.

In addition, it is known that a child's level of physical activity is strongly influenced by family issues such as parental expectations and support, the modelling of siblings, and the opportunities that exist within their community to participate in physical exercise [58, 59]. In this study resources did not permit these specific issues to be explored in any detail, but the small number of children with out-of-school activities and the larger number being in the control group suggested this was unlikely to exert a negative effect upon the overall results.

5. Conclusion

The growing concern about deteriorating fitness levels and their impact upon children's health has a special significance for children with autism because of the way their patterns of functioning makes it difficult to encourage their participation in standard school physical education activities and how prone they are to become obese, further reducing their capacity to exercise. The results from this study indicate that an improvement in specific fitness measurements and BMI can be achieved by children with autism if they follow a computer-based activity programme (in this particular study the "Mario and Sonic at the Olympics" for the Nintendo Wii). Such an intervention is a practical option for schools, but the finding that some aspects of fitness did not improve emphasises the importance of offering such computer-based activities as part of a wider physical fitness regime so that physical functions that such programmes do not address can be tackled through other activities.

Acknowledgment

The authors gratefully thank all of the schools, staff, children and their parents who took part in this study. This research received no specific grant from any funding agency in the public, commercial, or not-for-profit sectors.

References

[1] J. E. Butcher and W. O. Eaton, "Gross and fine motor proficiency in preschoolers: relationships with free play behavior and activity level," *Journal of Human Movement Studies*, vol. 16, no. 1, pp. 27–36, 1989.

[2] A. D. Okely, M. L. Booth, and J. W. Patterson, "Relationship of physical activity to fundamental movement skills among adolescents," *Medicine and Science in Sports and Exercise*, vol. 33, no. 11, pp. 1899–1904, 2001.

[3] C. Curtin, S. E. Anderson, A. Must, and L. Bandini, "The prevalence of obesity in children with autism: A secondary data analysis using nationally representative data from the National Survey of Children's Health," *BMC Pediatrics*, vol. 10, article 11, 2010.

[4] N. B. Almandil, Y. Liu, M. L. Murray, F. M. C. Besag, K. J. Aitchison, and I. C. K. Wong, "Weight gain and other metabolic adverse effects associated with atypical antipsychotic treatment of children and adolescents: a systematic review and meta-analysis," *Pediatric Drugs*, vol. 15, no. 2, pp. 139–150, 2013.

[5] S. N. Grondhuis and M. G. Aman, "Overweight and obesity in youth with developmental disabilities: a call to action," *Journal of Intellectual Disability Research*, vol. 58, no. 9, pp. 787–799, 2014.

[6] K. N. Oriel, C. L. George, R. Peckus, and A. Semon, "The effects of aerobic exercise on academic engagement in young children with autism spectrum disorder," *Pediatric Physical Therapy*, vol. 23, no. 2, pp. 187–193, 2011.

[7] H. Oude Luttikhuis, L. Baur, H. Jansen et al., "Interventions for treating obesity in children," *Evidence-Based Child Health*, vol. 4, no. 4, pp. 1571–1729, 2009.

[8] B. Deforche, L. Haerens, and I. De Bourdeaudhuij, "How to make overweight children exercise and follow the recommendations," *International Journal of Pediatric Obesity*, vol. 6, no. 1, pp. 35–41, 2011.

[9] L. Lanningham-Foster, T. B. Jensen, R. C. Foster et al., "Energy expenditure of sedentary screen time compared with active screen time for children," *Pediatrics*, vol. 118, no. 6, pp. e1831–e1835, 2006.

[10] L. E. F. Graves, N. D. Ridgers, K. Williams, G. Stratton, G. Atkinson, and N. T. Cable, "The physiological cost and enjoyment of Wii fit in adolescents, young adults, and older adults," *Journal of Physical Activity and Health*, vol. 7, no. 3, pp. 393–401, 2010.

[11] L. A. Léger and J. Lambert, "A maximal multistage 20-m shuttle run test to predict $\dot{V}\ O_2$ max," *European Journal of Applied Physiology and Occupational Physiology*, vol. 49, no. 1, pp. 1–12, 1982.

[12] Council of Europe, *Eurofit Tests of Physical Fitness*, Council of Europe, Strasbourg, France, 2nd edition, 1993.

[13] N. Tsigilis, H. Douda, and S. P. Tokmakidis, "Test-retest reliability of the eurofit test battery administered to university students," *Perceptual and Motor Skills*, vol. 95, no. 3, pp. 1295–1300, 2002.

[14] C. M. Donncha, A. W. S. Watson, T. McSweeney, and D. J. O'Donovan, "Reliability of Eurofit physical fitness items for adolescent males with and without mental retardation," *Adapted Physical Activity Quarterly*, vol. 16, no. 1, pp. 86–95, 1999.

[15] M. Safrit and T. Wood, *Introduction to Measurement in Physical Education and Eexercise Science*, WBC McGraw-Hill, 3rd edition, 1995.

[16] British National Coaching Foundation, *Physiology and Performance (NCF Coaching Handbook)*, Coachwise, Chelsea, UK, 1998.

[17] Department of Education, 2013, https://www.gov.uk/government/publications/national-curriculum-in-england-physical-education-programmes-of-study.

[18] D. H. Olson, D. M. Gorall, and J. Tiesel, *FACES-IV Package: Administration*, Life Innovations, Minneapolis, Minn, USA, 2006.

[19] D. Olson, "FACES IV and the circumplex model: validation study," *Journal of Marital and Family Therapy*, vol. 37, no. 1, pp. 64–80, 2011.

[20] D. H. Olson and D. M. Gorall, "Circumplex model of marital and family systems," in *Normal Family Processes*, F. Walsh, Ed., pp. 514–547, Guilford Press, 3rd edition, 2003.

[21] S. S. Shapiro and M. B. Wilk, "An analysis of variance test for normality: complete samples," *Biometrika*, vol. 52, no. 3-4, pp. 591–611, 1965.

[22] J. J. Filliben, "Probability plot correlation coefficient test for normality," *Technometrics*, vol. 17, no. 1, pp. 111–117, 1975.

[23] C. Foster, J. Richards, M. Thorogood, and M. Hillsdon, "Remote and web 2.0 interventions for promoting physical activity," *The Cochrane Database of Systematic Reviews*, vol. 9, Article ID CD010395, 2013.

[24] I. Yilmaz, B. Birkan, F. Konukman, and M. Erkan, "Using a constant time delay procedure to teach aquatic play skills to children with autism," *Education and Training in Developmental Disabilities*, vol. 40, no. 2, pp. 171–182, 2005.

[25] E. Suter and M. R. Hawes, "Relationship of physical activity, body fat, diet, and blood lipid profile in youths 10–15 yr," *Medicine and Science in Sports and Exercise*, vol. 25, no. 6, pp. 748–754, 1993.

[26] S. Biddle, "Children, exercise, and mental health," *International Journal of Sport Psychology*, vol. 24, no. 2, pp. 200–216, 1993.

[27] B. M. Wipfli, C. D. Rethorst, and D. M. Landers, "The anxiolytic effects of exercise: a meta-analysis of randomized trials and dose-response analysis," *Journal of Sport and Exercise Psychology*, vol. 30, no. 4, pp. 392–410, 2008.

[28] M. A. I. Åberg, M. Waern, J. Nyberg et al., "Cardiovascular fitness in males at age 18 and risk of serious depression in adulthood: swedish prospective population-based study," *British Journal of Psychiatry*, vol. 201, no. 5, pp. 352–359, 2012.

[29] D. L. Schmalz, G. D. Deane, L. L. Birch, and K. K. Davison, "A longitudinal assessment of the links between physical activity and self-esteem in early adolescent non-Hispanic females," *Journal of Adolescent Health*, vol. 41, no. 6, pp. 559–565, 2007.

[30] I. Janssen and A. G. LeBlanc, "Systematic review of the health benefits of physical activity and fitness in school-aged children and youth," *International Journal of Behavioral Nutrition and Physical Activity*, vol. 7, article no. 40, 2010.

[31] T. A. Stevens, Y. To, S. J. Stevenson, and M. R. Lochbaum, "The importance of physical activity and physical education in the prediction of academic achievement," *Journal of Sport Behavior*, vol. 31, no. 4, pp. 368–388, 2008.

[32] D. M. Castelli, C. H. Hillman, S. M. Buck, and H. E. Erwin, "Physical fitness and academic achievement in third- and fifth-grade students," *Journal of Sport and Exercise Psychology*, vol. 29, no. 2, pp. 239–252, 2007.

[33] L. J. Griffiths, M. Cortina-Borja, F. Sera et al., "How active are our children? Findings from the millennium cohort study," *The British Medical Journal*, vol. 3, no. 8, Article ID e002893, 2013.

[34] A. Hurtig-Wennlöf, J. R. Ruiz, M. Harro, and M. Sjöström, "Cardiorespiratory fitness relates more strongly than physical activity to cardiovascular disease risk factors in healthy children and adolescents: the European Youth Heart Study," *European Journal of Cardiovascular Prevention & Rehabilitation*, vol. 14, no. 4, pp. 575–581, 2007.

[35] H. S. Friedman, L. R. Martin, J. S. Tucker, M. H. Criqui, M. L. Kern, and C. A. Reynolds, "Stability of physical activity across the lifespan," *Journal of Health Psychology*, vol. 13, no. 8, pp. 1092–1104, 2008.

[36] B. A. Spear, S. E. Barlow, C. Ervin et al., "Recommendations for treatment of child and adolescent overweight and obesity," *Pediatrics*, vol. 120, supplement 4, pp. 254–288, 2007.

[37] L. G. Bandini, J. Gleason, C. Curtin et al., "Comparison of physical activity between children with autism spectrum disorders and typically developing children," *Autism*, vol. 17, no. 1, pp. 44–54, 2013.

[38] C. Y. Pan and G. C. Frey, "Physical activity patterns in youth with autism spectrum disorders," *Journal of Autism and Developmental Disorders*, vol. 36, no. 5, pp. 597–606, 2006.

[39] C. L. Hilton, M. C. Crouch, and H. Israel, "Out-of-school participation patterns in children with high-functioning autism spectrum disorders," *The American Journal of Occupational Therapy*, vol. 62, no. 5, pp. 554–563, 2008.

[40] M. MacDonald, P. Esposito, and D. Ulrich, "The physical activity patterns of children with autism," *BMC Research Notes*, vol. 4, article 422, 2011.

[41] C.-Y. Pan, "Objectively measured physical activity between children with autism spectrum disorders and children without disabilities during inclusive recess settings in Taiwan," *Journal of Autism and Developmental Disorders*, vol. 38, no. 7, pp. 1292–1301, 2008.

[42] C. Y. Pan, C. L. Tsai, K. W. Hsieh, C. H. Chu, Y. L. Li, and S. T. Huang, "Accelerometer-determined physical activity among elementary school-aged children with autism spectrum disorders in Taiwan," *Research in Autism Spectrum Disorders*, vol. 5, no. 3, pp. 1042–1052, 2011.

[43] D. Green, T. Charman, A. Pickles et al., "Impairment in movement skills of children with autistic spectrum disorders," *Developmental Medicine and Child Neurology*, vol. 51, no. 4, pp. 311–316, 2009.

[44] K. H. Pitetti, A. D. Rendoff, T. Grover, and M. W. Beets, "The efficacy of a 9-month treadmill walking program on the exercise capacity and weight reduction for adolescents with severe autism," *Journal of Autism and Developmental Disorders*, vol. 37, no. 6, pp. 997–1006, 2007.

[45] R. Lang, L. K. Koegel, K. Ashbaugh, A. Regester, W. Ence, and W. Smith, "Physical exercise and individuals with autism spectrum disorders: a systematic review," *Research in Autism Spectrum Disorders*, vol. 4, no. 4, pp. 565–576, 2010.

[46] A. Prupas and G. Reid, "Effects of exercise frequency on stereotypic behaviors of children with developmental disabilities," *Education and Training in Mental Retardation and Developmental Disabilities*, vol. 36, no. 2, pp. 196–206, 2001.

[47] C.-Y. Pan, "Effects of water exercise swimming program on aquatic skills and social behaviors in children with autism spectrum disorders," *Autism*, vol. 14, no. 1, pp. 9–28, 2010.

[48] H. Nicholson, T. J. Kehle, M. A. Bray, and J. V. Heest, "The effects of antecedent physical activity on the academic engagement of children with autism spectrum disorder," *Psychology in the Schools*, vol. 48, no. 2, pp. 198–213, 2011.

[49] A. Hillier, D. Murphy, and C. Ferrara, "A pilot study: Short-term reduction in salivary cortisol following low level physical exercise and relaxation among adolescents and young adults on the autism spectrum," *Stress and Health*, vol. 27, no. 5, pp. 395–402, 2011.

[50] N. Ü. Yildirim, F. Erbahçeci, N. Ergun, K. H. Pitetti, and M. W. Beets, "The effect of physical fitness training on reaction time in youth with intellectual disabilities," *Perceptual and Motor Skills*, vol. 111, no. 1, pp. 178–186, 2010.

[51] C.-Y. Pan, "The efficacy of an aquatic program on physical fitness and aquatic skills in children with and without autism spectrum disorders," *Research in Autism Spectrum Disorders*, vol. 5, no. 1, pp. 657–665, 2011.

[52] C.-Y. Pan, C.-L. Tsai, C.-H. Chu, and K.-W. Hsieh, "Physical activity and self-determined motivation of adolescents with and without autism spectrum disorders in inclusive physical education," *Research in Autism Spectrum Disorders*, vol. 5, no. 2, pp. 733–741, 2011.

[53] S. Marsh, C. Ni Mhurchu, and R. Maddison, "The non-advertising effects of screen-based sedentary activities on acute

eating behaviours in children, adolescents, and young adults. A systematic review," *Appetite*, vol. 71, pp. 259–273, 2013.

[54] L. Graves, G. Stratton, N. D. Ridgers, and N. T. Cable, "Energy expenditure in adolescents playing new generation computer games," *British Medical Journal*, vol. 335, no. 7633, pp. 1282–1284, 2007.

[55] M. J. D. Taylor, D. McCormick, T. Shawis, R. Impson, and M. Griffin, "Activity-promoting gaming systems in exercise and rehabilitation," *Journal of Rehabilitation Research and Development*, vol. 48, no. 10, pp. 1171–1186, 2011.

[56] T. F. Hughes, J. D. Flatt, B. Fu, M. A. Butters, C. C. H. Chang, and M. Ganguli, "Interactive video gaming compared with health education in older adults with mild cognitive impairment: a feasibility study," *International Journal of Geriatric Psychiatry*, vol. 29, no. 9, pp. 890–898, 2014.

[57] A. G. LeBlanc, J.-P. Chaput, A. McFarlane et al., "Active video games and health indicators in children and youth: a systematic review," *PLoS ONE*, vol. 8, no. 6, Article ID e65351, 2013.

[58] S. G. Trost, J. F. Sallis, R. R. Pate, P. S. Freedson, W. C. Taylor, and M. Dowda, "Evaluating a model of parental influence on youth physical activity," *The American Journal of Preventive Medicine*, vol. 25, no. 4, pp. 277–282, 2003.

[59] A. F. Seabra, D. M. Mendonça, H. H. H. Göring, M. A. Thomis, and J. A. Maia, "Genetic and environmental factors in familial clustering in physical activity," *European Journal of Epidemiology*, vol. 23, no. 3, pp. 205–211, 2008.

25

Associations between Familial Rates of Psychiatric Disorders and De Novo Genetic Mutations in Autism

Kyleen Luhrs,[1] Tracey Ward,[2] Caitlin M. Hudac,[3] Jennifer Gerdts,[3] Holly A. F. Stessman,[4,5] Evan E. Eichler,[4,6] and Raphael A. Bernier[3]

[1] *University of Washington School of Medicine, Seattle, WA 91895, USA*
[2] *School of Psychology, Family, and Community, Seattle Pacific University, Seattle, WA 98119, USA*
[3] *Department of Psychiatry and Behavioral Sciences, University of Washington, Seattle, WA 91895, USA*
[4] *Department of Genome Sciences, University of Washington, Seattle, WA 91895, USA*
[5] *Department of Pharmacology, Creighton University Medical School, Omaha, NE 68178, USA*
[6] *Howard Hughes Medical Institute, Seattle, WA 91895, USA*

Correspondence should be addressed to Raphael A. Bernier; rab2@uw.edu

Academic Editor: Valsamma Eapen

The purpose of this study was to examine the confluence of genetic and familial risk factors in children with Autism Spectrum Disorder (ASD) with distinct de novo genetic events. We hypothesized that gene-disrupting mutations would be associated with reduced rates of familial psychiatric disorders relative to structural mutations. Participants included families of children with ASD in four groups: de novo duplication copy number variations (DUP, $n = 62$), de novo deletion copy number variations (DEL, $n = 74$), de novo likely gene-disrupting mutations (LGDM, $n = 267$), and children without a known genetic etiology (NON, $n = 2111$). Familial rates of psychiatric disorders were calculated from semistructured interviews. Results indicated overall increased rates of psychiatric disorders in DUP families compared to DEL and LGDM families, specific to paternal psychiatric histories, and particularly evident for depressive disorders. Higher rates of depressive disorders in maternal psychiatric histories were observed overall compared to paternal histories and higher rates of anxiety disorders were observed in paternal histories for LGDM families compared to DUP families. These findings support the notion of an additive contribution of genetic etiology and familial factors are associated with ASD risk and highlight critical need for continued work targeting these relationships.

1. Introduction

Autism Spectrum Disorder (ASD) is a neurodevelopmental disorder characterized by impairments in social communication and repetitive and restricted interests or behaviors [1]. The rate of diagnosis is estimated to affect as many as 2% of individuals in the US [2]. The etiology of ASD is likely a combination of genetic and environmental factors [2, 3]. Heritability of ASD is estimated to be as high as 90%, suggesting that genetics contribute significantly to ASD biology [4]. While no single event accounts for more than 1% of all cases of ASD, recent studies have identified putative causal genetic events in the form of de novo copy number variations (CNV) and likely gene-disrupting mutations (LGDM). Several hundred mutations have already been identified with estimates suggesting up to 1,000 ASD risk genes ([5], Sanders et al., 2012). As such, de novo mutations may account for 30% of all cases and up to 45% of female cases of ASD [5–7]. Recent evidence suggests increased maternal transmission rate of deleterious mutations and de novo CNV deletions that more often occur on the maternal haplotype [8]. However, exome studies indicate that de novo LGDMs are associated with the paternal line [9] and the transmission rate of ASD-associated paternal de novo point mutations increases with paternal age [5].

Elevated rates of psychiatric disorders have been consistently reported among the relatives of individuals with ASD, including schizophrenia, anxiety, depression, obsessive compulsive disorder, and bipolar disorder [10–18]. Long-standing evidence suggests that psychiatric disorders aggregate in family members affected by ASD [15, 16, 19, 20]. In addition, several studies indicate that the onset of familial psychiatric diagnoses originates before the proband's diagnosis, suggesting that vulnerability associated with psychiatric disorders may occur independently of psychosocial stressors related to the proband [11, 13]. Family members of individuals with ASD also exhibit elevated incidences of ASD-related traits known as the broader autism phenotype, underscoring the dimensional familial nature of ASD-related symptoms [15, 17, 21]. Maternal and paternal psychiatric histories vary considerably from an epidemiological standpoint as well as transmission rates of maternal and paternal de novo mutations [8, 9, 13], necessitating the separate examination of maternal and paternal factors.

Findings increasingly support the presence of common molecular and genetic features between ASD and other psychiatric disorders [22–29]. Shared genetic contributions between psychiatric disorders and ASD etiology indicate that unstable or deleterious underlying genetic architecture may lead to increased genetic vulnerability in ASD [11, 15, 16, 30]. For instance, recent work suggests that family history of psychiatric illness and de novo genetic events influence phenotypic ASD profiles [31].

Despite the confluence of genetic (e.g., de novo mutations) and familial (e.g., history of psychiatric illness) factors as major contributors to ASD risk, the extent by which these factors interact is less clear. Considering that familial psychiatric factors likely involve both genetic and environmental mechanisms, it is possible that these factors impact children with distinct genetic events in different ways. For instance, Girirajan and colleagues [32] proposed the multiple or "second hit" hypothesis for ASD, such that, in addition to a primary genetic event, a secondary insult is necessary to result in a more severe clinical presentation of ASD. This second hit could potentially be another unidentified ASD-associated genetic event or an environmental factor that influences development and confers ASD risk.

Here, in this exploratory study, we sought to test whether the presence of a psychiatric disorder in family members acts as a potential "second hit." Specifically, we targeted the potential additive risk for ASD from de novo genetic events and elevated familial psychiatric burden. We focused on families with a child with ASD and either a CNV deletion, CNV duplication, or LGDM who had completed a detailed interview regarding maternal and paternal family history of psychiatric illness. Building upon the "second hit" hypothesis for ASD, we hypothesized that less severe "first hit" mutations (CNV deletion or duplication) would be associated with higher rates of familial psychiatric disorders than more severe "first hit" mutations (truncating LGDM). In this way, we can evaluate whether an additional "second hit" insult (i.e., elevated familial psychiatric burden) is present with the less severe CNV duplication phenotype.

2. Materials and Methods

2.1. Participants. Participants ($N = 2514$) included families of 4- to 18-year-old children with ASD who had previously participated in genetic testing as part of the Simons Simplex Collection (SSC) with valid and complete medical history data. The objective of the SSC was to identify de novo genetic variants that contribute to the overall risk of ASD by focusing on simplex families (families with one child with ASD) without a family history of ASD [33]. Each family (i.e., biological parents, proband with ASD, and unaffected siblings) provided DNA via blood sample for sequencing and completed rigorous clinical and behavioral characterization of the proband. For all groups, ASD diagnosis was confirmed as part of inclusion criteria for the study using the Autism Diagnostic Interview-Revised [34], Autism Diagnostic Observation Schedule [35], and expert clinical judgment (APA, 2000). Families with complete family mental health history information were divided into groups based upon whether their child had an identified ASD-associated de novo genetic event as identified in [36]. The three genetic etiology groups included children with (1) a likely gene-disrupting mutation (LGDM group, $n = 267$, without any other relevant CNVs), (2) recurrent or rare CNV deletion event (DEL group, $n = 74$), and (3) recurrent or rare CNV duplication event (DUP group, $n = 62$). The remaining families whose child did not have an ASD-associated genetic event were included as a control group (NON group, $n = 2111$). Participant characteristics are provided in Table 1. The three supplementary tables in Supplementary Material available online at https://doi.org/10.1155/2017/9371964 list the participants' specific genetic events as identified by Sanders et al., 2015 (S1, DEL events; S2, DUP events; and S3, LGDM events). A series of one-way ANOVAs indicated no significant differences in age, verbal IQ, internalizing problems, or externalizing problems (Tukey HSD correction, all $p > .095$). There was a significant group difference of nonverbal IQ ($F(3, 2312) = 7.75$, $p < .01$) related to reduced nonverbal IQ for the DEL and LGDM groups relative to the NON group (p's $< .025$). The investigation was carried out in accordance with the most recent version of the Declaration of Helsinki and reviewed by the institutional review board. Written informed consent was obtained from participants including parents and children. Assent was obtained if developmental age was above 7 years in accordance with the ethical standards approved by the local institutional review board.

2.2. Familial Rate of Psychiatric Disorders Measure. Information regarding family history of psychiatric disorders was collected through semistructured caregiver interviews conducted as part of the SSC [33]. Caregivers identified the number of individuals that had been diagnosed with psychiatric disorders separately for maternal and paternal histories. Possible individuals included the proband's aunts, uncles, and grandparents. Due to exclusionary criteria, immediate family members with a history of schizophrenia were not eligible to participate in SSC or subsequently in this analysis. The following eight categories were created based on the type of psychiatric disorder endorsed. Diagnoses were categorized according to the Diagnostic and Statistical Manual of Mental Disorders, 5th edition [1]: (1) depressive disorders (depression disorder, dysthymic disorder, and other psychological disorders), (2) anxiety disorders (anxiety disorder and social phobia), (3) obsessive compulsive disorder,

Table 1: Genetic group demographic characterization.

Number of subjects	DEL		DUP		LGDM		NON	
	N	%	*N*	%	*N*	%	*N*	%
Total	74		62		267		2111	
Female	15	20.3%	10	16.1%	48	18.0%	286	13.5%
Male	14	18.9%	52	83.9%	219	82.0%	1825	86.5%
Race								
African-American	1	1.4%	0	0.0%	13	4.9%	89	4.2%
Asian	3	4.1%	1	1.6%	16	6.0%	86	4.1%
Native (American or Hawaiian)	0	0.0%	0	0.0%	0	0.0%	5	0.2%
More than one race	5	6.8%	3	4.8%	25	9.4%	155	7.3%
White	60	81.1%	54	87.1%	200	74.9%	1647	78.0%
Not specified/other	5	6.8%	4	6.5%	13	4.9%	129	6.1%
Household income								
<$20,000	1	1.4%	3	4.8%	4	1.5%	63	3.0%
$21,000–$35,000	2	2.7%	3	4.8%	13	4.9%	107	5.1%
$36,000–$50,000	8	10.8%	5	8.1%	23	8.6%	173	8.2%
$51,000–$65,000	7	9.5%	8	12.9%	27	10.1%	222	10.5%
$66,000–$80,000	8	10.8%	7	11.3%	37	13.9%	272	12.9%
$81,000–$100,000	11	14.9%	12	19.4%	50	18.7%	346	16.4%
$101,000–$130,000	11	14.9%	7	11.3%	29	10.9%	314	14.9%
$131,000–$160,000	9	12.2%	6	9.7%	27	10.1%	198	9.4%
>$161,000	14	18.9%	8	12.9%	47	17.6%	324	15.3%
Not specified	3	4.1%	3	4.8%	10	3.7%	92	4.4%
Measure	DEL		DUP		LGDM		NON	
	Mean	SD	Mean	SD	Mean	SD	Mean	SD
Age	113.67	45.23	103.03	43.52	113.98	44.12	107.34	43.17
Verbal IQ	67.08	34.40	76.83	30.90	74.44	30.12	77.14	31.36
Nonverbal IQ	70.45	32.26	78.39	27.94	78.39	25.10	83.34	26.25
Internalizing problems	59.68	9.88	59.86	9.62	60.39	9.15	60.02	9.66
Externalizing problems	54.67	11.69	58.20	11.58	56.65	11.13	56.48	10.68

(4) trauma and stress (adjustment disorder and posttraumatic stress disorder), (5) neurodevelopmental disorders (ADHD, behavior disorder, and Tourette's syndrome), (6) bipolar disorders, (7) feeding and eating disorders (eating disorder and pica), and (8) schizophrenia (schizophrenia and other psychotic disorders). Personality disorders were initially included; however, no indices of personality disorders were reported and, subsequently, this category was removed from analysis. Given the exclusion criteria for participation in the Simons Simplex Collection, none of the immediate or extended family members had been diagnosed with ASD.

To determine rates of psychiatric disorders, every family member that the respondent endorsed for a particular diagnostic category was given a value of 1. The overall sum was totaled for each participant separately for maternal and paternal family histories. To avoid false negatives related to the age-dependent nature of diagnosing many psychiatric disorders, siblings, half-siblings, and cousins were not included. The total score was then divided by the number of family members evaluated to produce a ratio that could be compared among families of different sizes, labeled as rate of psychiatric disorders separately for maternal and paternal rates. Only participants with complete quantitative family information were included.

2.3. Statistical Analysis. Rates of psychiatric disorder were analyzed using mixed modeling in SAS software version 9.4 (SAS Institute, Inc., Cary, NC, USA). The full-factorial model consisted of fixed effects and all possible interactions for kind of psychiatric disorder (8: depressive, anxiety, obsessive compulsive disorder, trauma/stress, neurodevelopmental, bipolar, feeding/eating, and schizophrenia), familial relation (2: maternal and paternal), and group (4: DEL, DUP, LGDM, and NON). The model was estimated using maximum likelihood, and fixed effects were tested by F-tests with Satterthwaite approximation of denominator degrees of freedom. Our primary hypothesis was to test group differences and potential familial relation interactions as main effects and also to consider secondary group differences related to specific kinds of psychiatric disorders. Thus, a priori pairwise comparisons were generated using least square means with Tukey correction for multiple comparisons [37].

Table 2: Mixed model fixed effects results.

Effect	F	df	p
Kind of disorder	62.280	7, 40000	<.0001
Familial relation	10.700	1, 40000	.001
Kind of disorder × familial relation	5.170	7, 40000	<.0001
Genetic group	2.700	3, 40000	.044
Genetic group × kind of disorder	1.230	21, 40000	.209
Genetic group × familial relation	1.160	3, 40000	.323
Genetic group × kind of disorder × familial relation	0.630	21, 40000	.903

Table 3: Rate of psychiatric disorders group comparisons by familial relation.

	DEL	DUP	LGDM	NON	A priori comparisons
Overall rates	0.015	0.022	0.017	0.020	*NON < DEL; DEL < DUP;* LGDM < DUP
Anxiety disorders	0.028	0.033	0.023	0.029	
Bipolar disorders	0.014	0.025	0.016	0.017	
Depressive disorders	0.046	0.077	0.067	0.077	*DEL < DUP; DEL < LGDM; DEL < NON; LGDM < NON*
Feeding/eating disorders	0.007	0.005	0.000	0.004	
Neurodevelopmental disorders	0.007	0.014	0.018	0.016	
Obsessive compulsive disorders	0.004	0.011	0.006	0.007	
Schizophrenia/psychotic disorders	0.005	0.006	0.002	0.004	
Trauma/stress disorders	0.005	0.005	0.004	0.003	
Maternal rates	0.018	0.022	0.022	0.024	DEL < NON
Anxiety disorders	0.028	0.028	0.032	0.037	
Bipolar disorders	0.003	0.018	0.015	0.018	
Depressive disorders	0.069	0.087	0.081	0.096	*DEL < NON; LGDM < NON*
Feeding/eating disorders	0.015	0.004	0.001	0.005	
Neurodevelopmental disorders	0.006	0.014	0.025	0.020	DEL < LGDM
Obsessive compulsive disorders	0.008	0.015	0.010	0.008	
Schizophrenia/psychotic disorders	0.006	0.003	0.003	0.004	
Trauma/stress disorders	0.005	0.006	0.007	0.005	
Paternal rates	0.012	0.022	0.012	0.015	*DEL < DUP; LDGM < DUP;* NON < DUP
Anxiety disorders	0.029	0.038	0.014	0.020	*LGDM < DUP;* NON < DUP
Bipolar disorders	0.025	0.032	0.018	0.015	
Depressive disorders	0.022	0.067	0.052	0.057	*DEL < DUP; DEL < LGDM; DEL < NON*
Feeding/eating disorders	0.000	0.005	0.000	0.002	
Neurodevelopmental disorders	0.008	0.014	0.011	0.013	
Obsessive compulsive disorders	0.000	0.006	0.001	0.005	
Schizophrenia/psychotic disorders	0.005	0.009	0.002	0.005	
Trauma/stress disorders	0.005	0.004	0.001	0.002	

3. Results

Mixed model fixed effects results are presented in Table 2, and least square means group comparisons are presented in Table 3. Results indicated an omnibus effect of genetic group ($F(3, 40000) = 2.70$, $p = .044$) such that DUP families exhibited increased rates of psychiatric disorders compared to DEL ($t(6400) = 2.21$, $p = .027$) and NON ($t(40000) = 2.01$, $p = .044$) and marginally significantly increased rates compared to LGDM ($t(40000) = 1.65$, $p = .098$) (Figure 1). This pattern of genetic group differences was evident for paternal rate [DEL < DUP, $t(40000) = 2.06$, $p = .039$; LGDM < DUP, $t(40000) = 2.32$, $p = .21$; and NON < DUP, $t(40000) = 1.87$, $p = .062$]. In contrast, there was only a marginal effect of maternal rate, such that DEL families had reduced rates of psychiatric disorders compared to NON families ($t(40000) = 1.88$, $p = .060$) (Figure 2). Overall, maternal rate was increased compared to paternal rate ($F(1, 40000) = 10.70$, $p = .001$), particularly within the LGDM ($t(40000) = 3.72$, $p = .0002$) and NON ($t(40000) = 10.39$, $p < .0001$) groups.

Genetic group differences were the most prominent for depressive disorders overall with the DEL group exhibiting reduced rates of psychiatric disorders compared to DUP, LGDM, and NON groups (t's > 2.73, p's < .006) (Figure 3(b)). Closer inspection indicated that this pattern was evident for paternal rates (t's > 2.76, p's < .006), but the DEL group

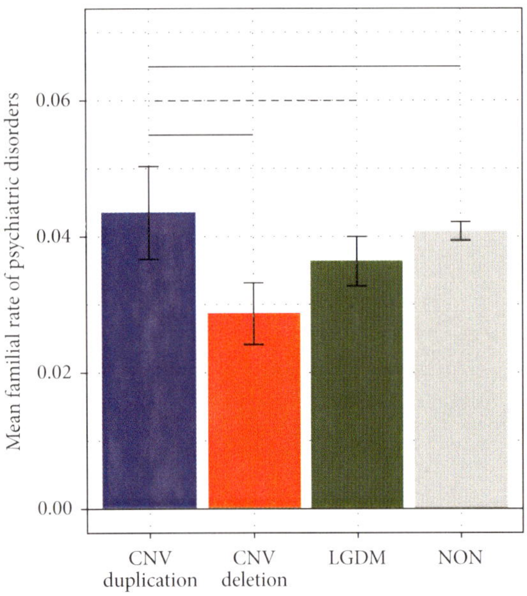

FIGURE 1: Group differences in familial rate of psychiatric disorders. Mean rate of psychiatric disorders is reported with standard error. Horizontal lines represent significance (solid line, $p < .05$; dashed line, $p < .1$).

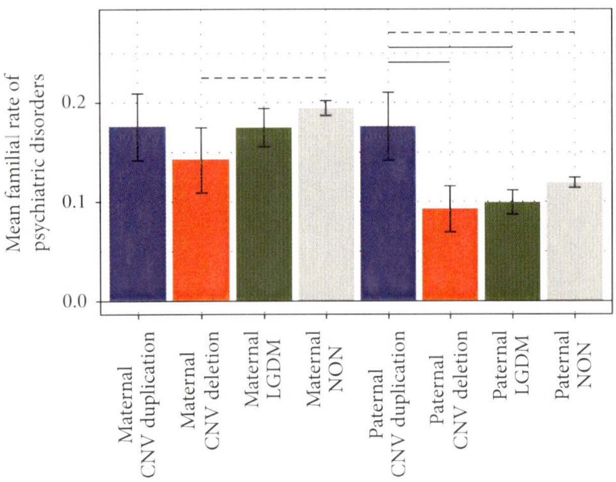

FIGURE 2: Group differences in familial rate of psychiatric disorders by familial relation. Mean rate of psychiatric disorders is reported with standard error. Horizontal lines represent significance (solid line, $p < .05$; dashed line, $p < .1$).

was only reduced relative to the NON group for maternal rates ($t(40000) = 2.72$, $p = .007$) (see Figure 3(a)). The LGDM group exhibited reduced rates of depressive disorders relative to the NON group for maternal rates ($t(40000) = 2.75$, $p = .006$) but not paternal rates ($t(40000) = .96$, $p = .34$), driving an overall effect between LGDM and NON ($t(40000) = 2.62$, $p = .009$) (Figure 3(b)). Of note, the rate of depressive disorders was greater overall for maternal compared to paternal families ($t = 4.84$, $p < .0001$) (Figure 3(c)). Lastly, LGDM families had a reduced rate of paternal anxiety disorders compared to DUP families [paternal, $t = 2.06$, $p = .04$; maternal, $t = 0.34$, $p = .74$]. There were no group differences in rates of obsessive compulsive disorder, trauma and stress, neurodevelopmental disorders, bipolar disorders, feeding and eating disorders, or schizophrenia.

4. Discussion

Our aim was to assess the familial rates of psychiatric disorders in relation to likely pathogenic genetic factors identified in children with ASD. We found that children with de novo CNV duplications have a significantly greater familial incidence of psychiatric disorders than children with de novo deletions and show a similar trend with likely gene-disrupting mutations. Critically, this increased rate in families with children with CNV duplication is similar to the rate of a control group of children without an ASD-associated genetic event. We also examined the contribution of psychiatric burden from maternal and paternal family histories separately and across genetic groups. Our results indicate that paternal rate of psychiatric disorders was greater in duplications than in deletions and LGDMs.

These results suggest that family psychiatric history may play a differential role in ASD depending on the type of genetic event contributing to ASD for a given individual. One explanation for the increased rate of psychiatric disorders for family members of children with duplications could be that duplications confer an overall psychiatric risk that necessitates an additional genetic disruption to result in a psychiatric presentation such as ASD [32]. In support of the "second hit" hypothesis, our results suggest that psychiatric burden (second hit) and the presence of a de novo CNV duplication (first hit) interrelate in a multiplicative manner, resulting in the development of the ASD phenotype. In other words, compared to deletion CNVs, duplication CNVs potentially may inflict a less severe impact on the ASD phenotype; however, the presence of both hits (CNV duplication and familial psychiatric burden) leads to the development of ASD. This "second hit" hypothesis is further strengthened by the fact that the de novo duplication group exhibited increased rates of familial psychiatric disorders to the idiopathic (NON) families whose children have no known genetic etiology.

While Girirajan and colleagues [32] show an inverse relationship between de novo cases and the prevalence of a "second hit," we limited our sample to only de novo CNV duplications/deletions and LGDMs without any additional CNVs. Therefore, our results extend the "second hit hypothesis" by proposing that individuals with de novo duplications have higher penetrance (relative to other de novo cases) due to a family history of psychiatric burden. As such, perhaps the presence of CNVs and LGDM confers independent risk factors for ASD and the "second hit" (psychiatric burden) uniquely exacerbates the ASD phenotype.

An alternative hypothesis is that family psychiatric history provides a vulnerable background upon which a CNV's deleterious effect can more easily be observed or propels an individual across a diagnostic threshold, such that the family psychiatric status can serve as either a protective or risk factor. This hypothesis is supported by evidence that individuals with a *16p11.2* locus CNV (i.e., duplication or deletion)

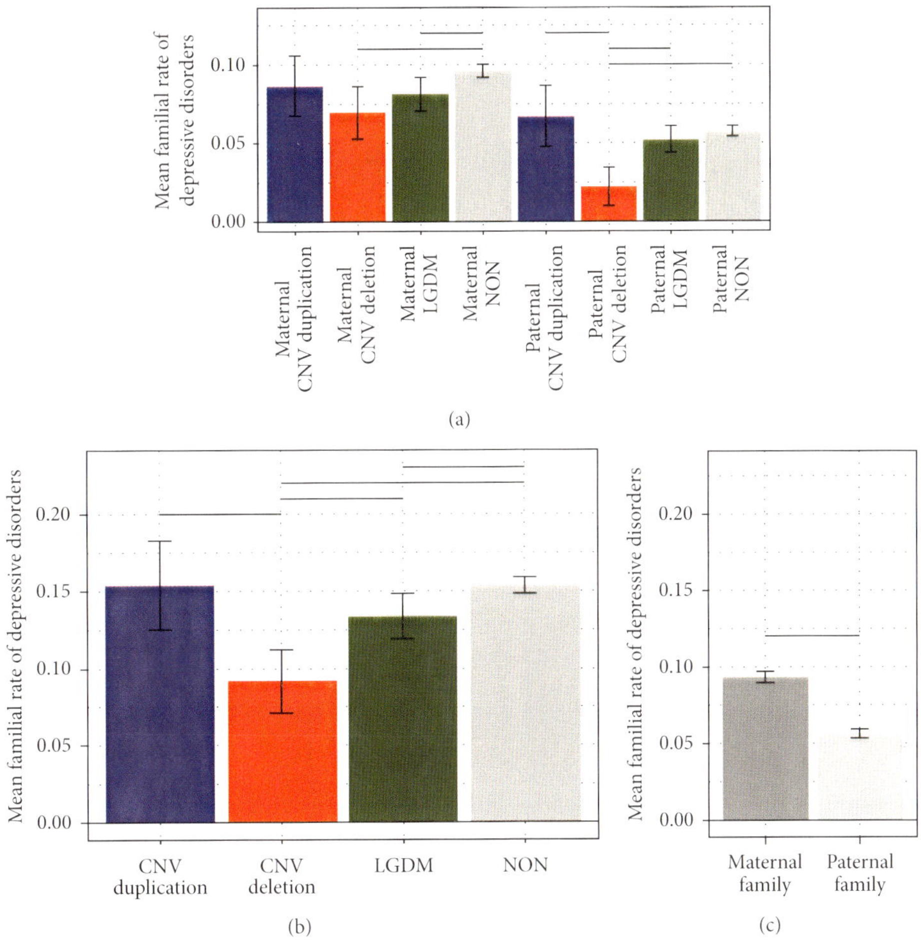

Figure 3: Familial rate of depression. Mean rate of depressive disorders is reported with standard error. Horizontal lines represent significance ($p < .05$). (a) Interaction between group and familial relation. (b) Main effect of group. (c) Main effect of familial relation.

show quantitative decrements in phenotypic domains that are reflective of the parental phenotype [38]. According to this perspective, a deleterious LGDM effect would prove more impactful such that family psychiatric history is less of a protective (or risk) factor. Given the heterogeneity in ASD-associated genetic events, it is likely that neither explanation is singularly sufficient and future work should continue investigating the impact of both psychiatric family burden and specific genetic events in the etiology of ASD.

The rate of depressive disorders was greater for paternal duplications than for maternal duplications, despite the fact that the rate of maternal depressive disorders was greater overall than paternal depressive disorders across genetic groups. These findings are particularly notable given the increased rates of maternal depression symptoms among the ASD population. Raising a child with ASD has been associated with increased parental stress and maternal depression compared to parents of children without ASD [39, 40]. Research suggests that mothers of children with ASD typically have greater parental strain than fathers associated with raising a child with ASD both in caregiving tasks and in expectations about family functioning. 79% of mothers report clinically significant depressive symptoms within one week of their child's ASD diagnosis and symptoms remain persistent for 37% of mothers one year later (Taylor and Warren, 2012). Approximately 29% of mothers report a delayed onset of depressive symptoms up to 16 months after the initial diagnosis. Factors such as child problem behaviors, ADHD symptoms [41], internalizing, externalizing, and behavior problems, access to services, financial barriers, family support, and parental adjustment [42] may interact in an additive or multiplicative way for mothers with children with ASD.

A relative strength of the current study is the ability to limit phenotypic and demographic confounders by closely matching participants in each group on a variety of domains. We focused only on individuals with clearly identified de novo ASD-associated events without additional inherited events. This study also expands the investigation of familial psychiatric history by including more family members (grandparents, aunts, and uncles), whereas most previous studies have focused on psychiatric history in only the parents [11, 13, 14, 18] and siblings [10, 16]. While previous studies have focused on parental psychiatric disorders in children with ASD compared to children without ASD [11, 13], this is the first study that compares the familial rate of psychiatric disorders between children with different types of genetic events associated with ASD.

Within this preliminary study, there are several limitations. First, we acknowledge that the population included in this study is limited by relatively small group sizes, particularly for the two de novo CNV groups (i.e., DUP, $n = 62$, and DEL, $n = 74$), and consists solely of children who participated in the Simons Simplex Collection (SSC). These children come from simplex families (i.e., only one known child or relative with ASD) and, subsequently, rates of familial psychiatric disorders may be lower than multiplex families. Considering the high functioning nature of the SSC cohort (i.e., large proportion of individuals with IQ > 70), future work should include increased sampling of children with ASD and intellectual disability. Second, although our structured interview was similar in scope to prior work (e.g., [17, 43]), our measurement consists of caregiver report of family mental health history information that could be influenced by possible reporting errors. Indeed, parents of a child with ASD report more psychiatric difficulties on self-report measures relative to clinical records [44], suggesting that the context of the interview (i.e., research versus clinical setting) may capture different aspects of the same outcome (i.e., subjective experiences versus clinical evaluation of functioning). Future work would benefit from a deeper understanding of the sensitivity of our measurement, as well as more detailed information such as the age of psychiatric disorder diagnosis. Lastly, although the groups were divided according to the specific type of structural mutation, it is possible that there remains a substantial amount of genetic heterogeneity within each group, which may be related to the extent by which familial factors contribute to ASD risk. Analysis of specific phenotypes tied to distinct genetic contributions and their relationship to family history may elucidate the relationship between ASD and other psychiatric disorders more clearly.

5. Conclusion

Our clarification of the differential association of family psychiatric history with distinct classes of genetic events in ASD provides a novel and informative step in elucidating the relationship between ASD and familial psychiatric burden. Our results support the proposal of the "second hit" hypothesis, such that elevated psychiatric burden (i.e., second hit) and the presence of a de novo copy number duplication (i.e., first hit) may generate an additive effect, subsequently resulting in the emergence of the ASD phenotype. In addition, our results suggest an elevated risk stemming from paternal family history of psychiatric burden, particularly related to depressive disorders. This is unusual in light of the fact that maternal rates of depressive disorders were greater across all genetic groups and highlights a critical avenue for future research. This work has important implications for diagnoses, pharmacological and psychological therapies, and strategies for investigating the etiology of neurodevelopmental disorders.

Disclosure

Kyleen Luhrs and Tracey Ward are co-first authors.

Acknowledgments

This work was supported by a grant from the National Institute of Mental Health (no. MH100047 to Raphael A. Bernier), by the Simons Foundation Autism Research Initiative (SFARI) (no. 137578 to Evan E. Eichler), and also by the Medical Student Research Training Program (MSRTP), University of Washington School of Medicine, Seattle, WA. The authors thank all of the families at the participating Simons Simplex Collection (SSC) sites, as well as the principal investigators (A. Beaudet, Raphael A. Bernier, J. Constantino, E. Cook, E. Fombonne, D. Geschwind, E. Hanson, D. Grice, A. Klin, R. Kochel, D. Ledbetter, C. Lord, C. Martin, D. Martin, R. Maxim, J. Miles, O. Ousley, K. Pelphrey, B. Peterson, J. Piggot, C. Saulnier, M. State, W. Stone, J. Sutcliffe, C. Walsh, Z. Warren, and E. Wijsman).

References

[1] American Psychiatric Association, *Diagnostic and statistical manual of mental disorders: DSM-5*, American Psychiatric Association, Ed., American Psychiatric Association, Washington, wash, USA, 5th edition, 2013.

[2] C. J. Newschaffer, L. A. Croen, J. Daniels et al., "The epidemiology of autism spectrum disorders," *Annual Review of Public Health*, vol. 28, pp. 235–258, 2007.

[3] I. Hertz-Picciotto, L. A. Croen, R. Hansen, C. R. Jones, J. van de Water, and I. N. Pessah, "The CHARGE study: An epidemiologic investigation of genetic and environmental factors contributing to autism," *Environmental Health Perspectives*, vol. 114, no. 7, pp. 1119–1125, 2006.

[4] A. Bailey, A. Le Couteur, I. Gottesman et al., "Autism as a strongly genetic disorder: evidence from a British twin study," *Psychological Medicine*, vol. 25, no. 1, pp. 63–77, 1995.

[5] B. J. O'Roak, L. Vives, S. Girirajan et al., "Sporadic autism exomes reveal a highly interconnected protein network of de novo mutations," *Nature*, vol. 484, no. 7397, pp. 246–250, 2012.

[6] I. Iossifov, B. J. O'Roak, S. J. Sanders et al., "The contribution of de novo coding mutations to autism spectrum disorder," *Nature*, vol. 515, no. 7526, pp. 216–221, 2014.

[7] N. Krumm, B. J. O'Roak, J. Shendure, and E. E. Eichler, "A de *novo* convergence of autism genetics and molecular neuroscience," *Trends in Neurosciences*, vol. 37, no. 2, pp. 95–105, 2014.

[8] S. Jacquemont, B. P. Coe, M. Hersch et al., "A higher mutational burden in females supports a 'female protective model' in neurodevelopmental disorders," *American Journal of Human Genetics*, vol. 94, no. 3, pp. 415–425, 2014.

[9] N. Krumm, T. N. Turner, C. Baker et al., "Excess of rare, inherited truncating mutations in autism," *Nature Genetics*, vol. 47, no. 6, pp. 582–588, 2015.

[10] P. F. Bolton, A. Pickles, M. Murphy, and M. Rutter, "Autism, affective and other psychiatric disorders: patterns of familial aggregation," *Psychological Medicine*, vol. 28, no. 2, pp. 385–395, 1998.

[11] J. L. Daniels, U. Forssen, C. M. Hultman et al., "Parental psychiatric disorders associated with autism spectrum disorders in the offspring," *Pediatrics*, vol. 121, no. 5, pp. e1357–e1362, 2008.

[12] M. Holtmann, S. Bölte, and F. Poustka, "Autism spectrum disorders: Sex differences in autistic behaviour domains and coexisting psychopathology," *Developmental Medicine & Child Neurology*, vol. 49, no. 5, pp. 361–366, 2007.

[13] H. J. Larsson, W. W. Eaton, K. M. Madsen et al., "Risk factors for autism: perinatal factors, parental psychiatric history, and socioeconomic status," *American Journal of Epidemiology*, vol. 161, no. 10, pp. 916–925, 2005.

[14] V. A. Morgan, M. L. Croft, G. M. Valuri et al., "Intellectual disability and other neuropsychiatric outcomes in high-risk children of mothers with schizophrenia, bipolar disorder and unipolar major depression," *The British Journal of Psychiatry*, vol. 200, no. 4, pp. 282–289, 2012.

[15] J. Piven, G. A. Chase, R. Landa, M. Wzorek, J. Gayle, and D. Cloud, "Psychiatric disorders in the parents of autistic individuals," *Journal of the American Academy of Child and Adolescent Psychiatry*, vol. 30, no. 3, pp. 471–478, 1991.

[16] J. Piven, J. Gayle, G. A. Chase et al., "A family history study of neuropsychiatric disorders in the adult siblings of autistic individuals," *Journal of the American Academy of Child and Adolescent Psychiatry*, vol. 29, no. 2, pp. 177–183, 1990.

[17] J. Piven and P. Palmer, "Psychiatric disorder and the broad autism phenotype: evidence from a family study of multiple-incidence autism families," *The American Journal of Psychiatry*, vol. 156, no. 4, pp. 557–563, 1999.

[18] P. F. Sullivan, C. Magnusson, A. Reichenberg et al., "Family history of schizophrenia and bipolar disorder as risk factors for autism," *Archives of General Psychiatry*, vol. 69, no. 11, pp. 1099–1103, 2012.

[19] M. E. Lobascher, P. E. Kingerlee, and S. S. Gubbay, "Childhood autism: an investigation of aetiological factors in twenty-five cases.," *The British Journal of Psychiatry*, vol. 117, no. 540, pp. 525–529, 1970.

[20] V. Lotter, "Epidemiology of autistic conditions in young children - 1. Prevalence," *International Journal of Social Psychiatry*, vol. 1, no. 3, pp. 124–135, 1966.

[21] J. Gerdts and R. Bernier, "The broader autism phenotype and its implications on the etiology and treatment of autism spectrum disorders," *Autism Research and Treatment*, vol. 2011, Article ID 545901, 19 pages, 2011.

[22] K. Kendler and L. Eaves, *Psychiatric genetics (review of psychiatry)*, American Psychiatric Press, Washington, wash, USA, 2005.

[23] B. Crespi, P. Stead, and M. Elliot, "Evolution in health and medicine Sackler colloquium: comparative genomics of autism and schizophrenia," *Proceedings of the National Acadamy of Sciences of the United States of America*, vol. 107, no. 1, pp. 1736–1741, 2010.

[24] A. Guilmatre, C. Dubourg, A.-L. Mosca et al., "Recurrent rearrangements in synaptic and neurodevelopmental genes and shared biologic pathways in schizophrenia, autism, and mental retardation," *Archives of General Psychiatry*, vol. 66, no. 9, pp. 947–956, 2009.

[25] P. Lichtenstein, E. Carlström, M. Råstam, C. Gillberg, and H. Anckarsäter, "The genetics of autism spectrum disorders and related neuropsychiatric disorders in childhood," *The American Journal of Psychiatry*, vol. 167, no. 11, pp. 1357–1363, 2010.

[26] A. Ronald, E. Simonoff, J. Kuntsi, P. Asherson, and R. Plomin, "Evidence for overlapping genetic influences on autistic and ADHD behaviours in a community twin sample," *Journal of Child Psychology and Psychiatry and Allied Disciplines*, vol. 49, no. 5, pp. 535–542, 2008.

[27] J. W. Smoller and C. T. Finn, "Family, twin, and adoption studies of bipolar disorder," *American Journal of Medical Genetics*, vol. 123C, no. 1, pp. 48–58, 2003.

[28] B. Xu, J. L. Roos, S. Levy, E. J. van Rensburg, J. A. Gogos, and M. Karayiorgou, "Strong association of de novo copy number mutations with sporadic schizophrenia," *Nature Genetics*, vol. 40, no. 7, pp. 880–885, 2008.

[29] N. M. Williams, B. Franke, E. Mick et al., "Genome-wide analysis of copy number variants in attention deficit hyperactivity disorder: The role of rare variants and duplications at 15q13.3," *The American Journal of Psychiatry*, vol. 169, no. 2, pp. 195–204, 2012.

[30] M. D. King, C. Fountain, D. Dakhlallah, and P. S. Bearman, "Estimated autism risk and older reproductive age," *American Journal of Public Health*, vol. 99, no. 9, pp. 1673–1679, 2009.

[31] E. B. Robinson, K. E. Samocha, J. A. Kosmicki et al., "Autism spectrum disorder severity reflects the average contribution of de novo and familial influences," *Proceedings of the National Acadamy of Sciences of the United States of America*, vol. 111, no. 42, pp. 15161–15165, 2014.

[32] S. Girirajan, J. A. Rosenfeld, G. M. Cooper et al., "A recurrent 16p12. 1 microdeletion supports a two-hit model for severe developmental delay," *Nature Genetics*, vol. 42, pp. 203–209, 2010.

[33] G. D. Fischbach and C. Lord, "The simons simplex collection: A resource for identification of autism genetic risk factors," *Neuron*, vol. 68, no. 2, pp. 192–195, 2010.

[34] C. Lord, M. Rutter, and A. Le Couteur, "Autism diagnostic interview-revised: a revised version of a diagnostic interview for caregivers of individuals with possible pervasive developmental disorders," *Journal of Autism and Developmental Disorders*, vol. 24, no. 5, pp. 659–685, 1994.

[35] C. Lord, M. Rutter, P. C. DiLavore, S. Risi, K. Gotham, and S. L. Bishop, *Autism diagnostic observation schedule*, ADOS: Manual. Western Psychological Services, Los Angeles, CA, 2002.

[36] S. J. Sanders, X. He, A. J. Willsey et al., "Insights into Autism Spectrum Disorder Genomic Architecture and Biology from 71 Risk Loci," *Neuron*, vol. 87, no. 6, pp. 1215–1233, 2015.

[37] J. W. Tukey, "Comparing individual means in the analysis of variance," *Biometrics - A Journal of the International Biometric Society*, vol. 5, pp. 99–114, 1949.

[38] D. Moreno-De-Luca, A. Moreno-De-Luca, J. F. Cubells, and S. J. Sanders, "Cross-Disorder Comparison of Four Neuropsychiatric CNV Loci," *Current Genetic Medicine Reports*, vol. 2, no. 3, pp. 151–161, 2014.

[39] R. McStay, D. Trembath, and C. Dissanayake, "Raising a child with autism: a developmental perspective on family adaptation," in *Current Developmental Disorders Reports*, vol. 2, pp. 65–83, URL https, //doi.org/10.1007/s40474-014-0037-z, 2015.

[40] B. Zablotsky, C. P. Bradshaw, and E. A. Stuart, "The association between mental health, stress, and coping supports in mothers of children with autism spectrum disorders," *Journal of Autism and Developmental Disorders*, vol. 43, no. 6, pp. 1380–1393, 2013.

[41] D. J. Steijn, A. M. van Oerlemans, M. A. G. Aken, J. K. van Buitelaar, and N. N. J. Rommelse, "The reciprocal relationship of ASD, ADHD, depressive symptoms and stress in parents of children with ASD and/or ADHD," *Journal of Autism and Developmental Disorders*, vol. 44, no. 5, pp. 1064–1076, 2013.

[42] J. L. Taylor and Z. E. Warren, "Maternal depressive symptoms following autism spectrum diagnosis," *Journal of Autism and Developmental Disorders*, vol. 42, no. 7, pp. 1411–1418, 2011.

26

Support Needs and Coping Strategies as Predictors of Stress Level among Mothers of Children with Autism Spectrum Disorder

Sheri R. Kiami[1] and Shelley Goodgold[2]

[1]*Department of Physical Therapy, Movement & Rehabilitation Sciences, Northeastern University, 301 Robinson Hall, 360 Huntington Avenue, Boston, MA 02115, USA*
[2]*Simmons College, Boston, MA, USA*

Correspondence should be addressed to Sheri R. Kiami; s.kiami@northeastern.edu

Academic Editor: Hansen Wang

This study examined maternal stress, coping strategies, and support needs among mothers of children with Autism Spectrum Disorder (ASD). A convenience sample of 70 mothers completed the Parent Stress Index Short Form (PSI-SF), Coping Health Inventory for Parents (CHIP), and Modified Family Needs Questionnaire (FNQ). PSI-SF scores reflected clinically significant levels of stress for 77% of mothers, and mothers identified 62.4% of important needs as unmet. The five most frequently reported important unmet needs were (1) financial support; (2) break from responsibilities; (3) understanding of other after-school program children; (4) rest/sleep; (5) help remaining hopeful about the future. Most coping strategies (81%) were identified as helpful. Additionally, both coping strategies and support needs served as predictors for maternal stress. Maternal stress scores decreased by .402 points for each percent increase in helpful coping strategy, and stress scores increased by .529 points with each percent increase in unmet needs. Given large variation in questionnaire responses across participants and studies, utilization of user-friendly questionnaires, such as the PSI-SF, CHIP, and FNQ, is advocated to determine the evolving important needs unique to each family over the child's lifetime as well as guide prioritization of care, compilation of resources, and referrals for additional services.

1. Introduction

With the ever-increasing number of children referred for developmental services, health professionals face larger caseloads and competing demands for direct care, caregiver education, provision of family resources, team meetings, and writing reports. These demands are especially challenging when treating children with Autism Spectrum Disorder (ASD) given its wide constellation of pervasive impairments and their impact on the whole family. ASD is a multidimensional, neurodevelopmental disability affecting social interactions and communication skills [1]. It is characterized by stereotyped repetitive strategies, interests and activities, and common comorbidities that vary in severity across the spectrum including aggression, impulsive behavior, anxiety, depression, sleep difficulties, and cognitive impairments. These impact the child's ability to attain developmental milestones and benefit from educational services.

Additionally, ASD impacts the well-being of the entire family. Parents of children with ASD experience a complex array of stressors that are both directly related to the child's characteristics, for example, difficult behaviors, and indirectly related to system stressors, such as barriers to accessing services for the child [2]. As stressors accumulate, families may experience financial strains, time pressures, marital conflicts, social isolation, increased time caregiving, decreased parenting self-efficacy, insufficient support services, ongoing child-advocacy, and uncertainty about their child's future [3].

Further, sources of caregiver strain change during the child's lifespan, especially during transitions [4]. For example, after the initial diagnosis, caregiver strain may arise from difficulty gathering information on ASD and obtaining early intervention services. During the school years, struggles may shift to accessing special education services and working with a different set of providers each academic year. With the child's transition to adulthood, key stressors may arise from barriers to community access, employment, and housing. Parents may also be faced with challenges related to estate planning, finances, and guardianship. When compared with parents of both typically developing children and children with other disabilities, parents of children with ASD experience greater parenting stress, fatigue, and health problems [5]. Additionally, lower family well-being creates a bidirectional, negative cycle that can exacerbate the child's problem behaviors as well as reducing the positive effects of therapeutic interventions [6–9]. Conversely, improved family functioning can positively impact child outcomes.

Utilization of effective coping strategies has been identified as an important mechanism of managing parental stress and promoting well-being [10, 11]. Hastings et al. [12] described four categories of coping strategies used by parents of children with ASD: (1) active-avoidance (e.g., substance use, self-blame, and venting of emotions); (2) problem-focused (e.g., planning, taking action to deal with problems, and seeking appropriate social supports); (3) positive coping (e.g., using humor, positive reframing, acceptance, and emotional social supports); and (4) religious/denial (e.g., using religion or spirituality, pretending problem does not exist). For mothers of children with ASD, active-avoidance and religious/denial coping strategies have been reported to be maladaptive and linked to decreased well-being and increased depression, anxiety, and stress [11]. In addition, Hastings and Brown [13] found that children's problematic behaviors were associated with the use of maladaptive coping strategies, which is then contributed to increased maternal stress. Furthermore, Hastings et al. [12] found that parents of children with ASD used maladaptive coping methods more often than both parents of typically developing children and parents of children with Down syndrome.

Additionally, assessing and addressing the self-perceived needs of parents of children with ASD not only may be linked to family outcomes but also may enhance the benefits of interventions the child receives [3]. However, there is a paucity of research in the United States on parents' perceptions of important support needs in spite of the potential benefits of family well-being and quality of life [3, 14, 15]. In addition, with the rapidly increasing number of children diagnosed with ASD, addressing family unmet needs may guide prioritization and allocation of limited resources, thereby reducing the burden on healthcare, school, and community services.

A few survey studies on parents' self-reported important needs have been conducted outside the United States. Siklos and Kerns [16] used a modified version of the Waaland et al. Family Needs Questionnaire [17] to compare the needs of parents of children with ASD with parents of children with Down syndrome in British Columbia. The questionnaire lists 54 potential support needs that the participant first self-reports as either "important" or "not important" and then as "met" or "unmet." Although both groups of parents in their study reported one-third of their important needs as being unmet, specific needs differed. For the parents of children with ASD, the five important needs most frequently rated as unmet were as follows: financial support, my child to have friends, help dealing with fears about my child's future, continuous services, and my other children's friends to feel comfortable around my child. Unmet parent needs were also examined in a more recent Canadian study of 101 parents of children with ASD aged 6–13 years [18]. Two of their most frequently identified unmet needs were similar to those reported by Siklos and Kerns [16], including social inclusion of their child and services provided continuously rather than only in times of crisis.

Examining the support needs of parents residing in a Midwestern US state, Hartley and Schultz [19] reported a higher proportion of important unmet needs for mothers than fathers. Mothers' unmet needs were most often related to the child's social development, family-wide impacts, emotional support, and planning for the future. The authors stated that understanding the important unmet support needs of parents of children with ASD is a critical first step towards improving parent well-being and family outcomes. This, in turn, is widely supported in the literature as a means of promoting better child outcomes [7].

The purpose of this study was, therefore, to better understand support needs and coping strategies among mothers of children with ASD, and how these factors may predict maternal stress. Specifically, we hypothesized that mothers would report high levels of stress as well as high levels of important unmet support needs. Further, we hypothesized that there would be an increase in maternal stress as important unmet needs increased, and a decrease in maternal stress as the utilization of helpful coping strategies increased. With greater understanding of the relationships among maternal stress, unmet needs, and coping strategies, healthcare professionals can better prioritize care within their scope of practice, compile key resources, and provide referrals for additional support services.

2. Methods

2.1. Participants. A convenience sample of mothers with children diagnosed with autism was recruited in-person during local parent meetings, educational events, and conferences hosted by four Boston-area organizations known to serve families of children with ASD, including the Asperger's Association of New England, Federation for Children with Special Needs, Boston Families for Autism/Towards Independent Living, and the Special Education Parent Advisory Council of the Boston Public Schools. Our rational reason for including only mothers was trifold: (1) mothers more frequently have the primary role of caregiver for children; (2) mothers experience higher level of stress; and (3) mothers have not only higher levels of unmet needs but types of needs which differ between mothers and fathers [2, 3, 15, 19, 20].

Data were collected via anonymous survey packets with stamped, self-addressed return envelopes. Each packet contained a cover letter explaining the purposes of the study, introducing the researchers, notifying mothers of their rights and that participation in the study was voluntary. All participants read and signed an informed consent to participate

Table 1: Demographic characteristics of the sample ($N = 70$).

Characteristics	n (%)
Race/ethnicity of mother	
Hispanic	4 (6)
White not Hispanic	55 (77)
Black not Hispanic	8 (11)
Others	3 (5)
Primary caregiver in home	
Mother	66 (94)
Other family/household members	3 (4)
Hired childcare provider	1 (1)
Income bracket	
Less than $15,000	6 (9)
$15,000– $24,999	3 (4)
$25,000–$49,999	10 (14)
$50,000–$74,999	10 (14)
$75,000–$99,999	15 (22)
$100,000 & over	26 (38)
Number of children in home: mean (SD)	2.1 (1.12)
Number of children in home with special needs: mean (SD)	1.34 (0.63)
Age of child with ASD (years): mean (SD)	9.7 (5.5)
Child with ASD BRIEF* score: mean (SD)	70 (12)
Child with ASD school placement	
Public school placement	57 (81)
Private School placement	8 (11)
Does not attend school or daycare	3 (4)
Residential placement	2 (3)

*BRIEF: Behavior Rating Inventory of Executive Function T score of 65 or above indicates clinically significant behavioral dysfunction.

in this research. To preserve anonymity, participants were instructed to exclude their names from the questionnaires, and completed questionnaires were immediately separated from the signed consent and raffle forms upon receipt.

Since recruitment of participants was in-person and anonymous, neither reminder letters nor a second survey packet could be mailed to enhance the return rate. Therefore, to incentivize participants, mothers could choose to enter a raffle for one of five $25.00 gift certificates. To maintain survey anonymity, raffle forms were immediately removed and kept separate from the returned survey packets. Study inclusion criteria were self-identification as a mother of a child with a diagnosis of ASD and the ability to read English.

Consistent with survey studies of this population published in the literature [16, 18, 21], the return rate of completed packets was 24% (70 packets out of 290 packets distributed).

2.2. Measures. Each packet included a demographic questionnaire developed by the researchers to identify participant characteristics (Table 1). To provide a measure of the child's everyday executive function, mothers also completed the Behavior Rating Inventory of Executive Function (BRIEF). T scores of 65 or above on the BRIEF indicate clinically significant behavioral dysfunction. For families with two or more children with ASD, mothers were instructed to choose one child and answer all questions with reference to that child only.

Packets also included the Parent Stress Index Short Form (PSI-SF) developed by Abidin [22] to measure maternal stress level, the Modified Family Needs Questionnaire (FNQ) developed by Siklos and Kerns [16] to identify parent self-reported important unmet needs, and the Coping Health Inventory for Parents (CHIP) by McCubbin et al. [23] to identify parent coping strategies and a self-addressed, stamped envelope.

2.2.1. Maternal Level of Stress. The PSI-SF, a derivative of the original tool used to measure parental stress levels [22], was developed to reduce the nearly prohibitive time required for typical assessment batteries. The short form is a 36-item questionnaire comprised of three subscales: parental distress, parent-child dysfunctional interaction, and difficult child. The parental distress (PD) subscale yields a score that indicates level of distress resulting from personal factors, such as depression or conflict with a partner and from life restrictions due to the demands of childrearing. The parent-child dysfunctional interaction (P-CDI) subscale provides an indication of the parent's dissatisfaction with interactions with their child and the degree to which the parent finds their child's strategies unacceptable. The difficult child (DC) subscale measures the parent's perceptions of their child's self-regulatory abilities. Each subscale consists of 12 items, and the entire short form takes about 10 minutes to complete. Validation of the short form was based on two samples of mostly white married mothers of young children, and the correlation coefficient on the short form was acceptably high at 87%.

2.2.2. Maternal Coping Strategies. The *Coping Health Inventory for Parents (CHIP)* is a 45-item questionnaire designed to identify coping strategies utilized by parents of children with serious or chronic health conditions [23]. Parents are instructed to circle the coping strategies they use and to rate its helpfulness on a 4-point scale: (3) extremely helpful, (2) moderately helpful, (1) minimally helpful, and (0) not helpful. In addition, for each coping behavior not used, the parent is asked to identify "chose not to use it" or "not possible" to use. The CHIP total score is the sum of points for all 45 items. The researchers reported that each of the subscales has shown adequate internal reliability (Cronbach's alphas = 0.79, 0.79, and 0.71, resp.) and validity. Rasch analysis, however, supported only two of the 3 subscales [24], and collapsing response categories was recommended.

2.2.3. Family Needs. The modified FNQ is a 54-item questionnaire modified by Siklos and Kerns [16] to examine the needs among parents of children with ASD and Down syndrome. It includes 23 "I need" statements from the original FNQ [17] and 31 new statements. In addition, in instances when the support benefit was clearly directed solely for the parent or for the child, need statements were also identified as parent-centered or child-centered. Cronbach's alpha coefficients ranging from 0.78 to 0.89 were reported as providing evidence of acceptable reliability. To investigate healthy lifestyle strategies, we added three self-care need statements related to the mother's health, participation in physical activity, and nutrition.

The FNQ utilizes a 4-point scale to indicate the degree that the need is important to the respondent: (1) not important, (2) slightly important, (3) important, or (4) very important. In addition, for each need statement, the respondent chooses "Yes," "Partly," or "No" to indicate if the need is currently being met. Responses are then classified as "Important" if respondents identify an "I need" statement as either "Important" or "Very Important" and "Unmet" if identified as either "Partly Met" or "Unmet."

2.3. Procedure and Data Analysis. The Institutional Research Board at the authors' academic institution reviewed and approved this study prior to participant recruitment. As survey packets were returned, the researchers scored individual surveys in accordance with each tool's administration manual, and scores were entered into Excel spreadsheets. To validate scoring and prevent data entry errors, a second researcher scored and checked data entry for 10% of participants via random sampling. Data were then exported to an IBM SPSS Statistics 23 software program for analyses.

2.3.1. Descriptive Statistics and Scoring. Descriptive statistics were used to analyze participants' demographics and questionnaire responses.

The PSI-SF utilizes a 5-point scale to indicate the degree to which the parent agrees with each of the 36 statements, from 5 (strongly agree) to 1 (strongly disagree.) Each subscale raw score was calculated by summing the points of the 12 items in that subscale. Higher raw scores reflect greater stress. The sum of the three subscales yields a total raw score, which was then converted into a percentile score based on a chart provided on the PSI-SF scoring sheet. PSI-SF percentile scores of 85% or above are identified as high, and scores of 90% or above reflect clinically significant levels of stress.

CHIP coping data for all analyses in this study were based on the sum of the three subscales and collapsed response categories of either helpful (extremely or moderately helpful) or not helpful (minimally or not helpful). Percentages of helpful coping strategies were then calculated by dividing the total score by the number of coping strategies identified as helpful (helpful coping strategy percentage = number of helpful coping strategies/total of coping strategies utilized).

FNQ support needs data used in our study were calculated in two ways. For need statements, we calculated the sums of participants identifying each statement as important or not important and as met or unmet. Percentages of important needs were calculated by dividing the sum of needs identified as important by the total number of need statements (important needs percentage = number of need statements identified as important/total number of need statements). In addition, need statements identified as both important and unmet were summed, and percentages were calculated by dividing the sum of important unmet needs by the sum of all important needs (important unmet needs percentage = number of important needs identified as unmet/total number of important needs). Similar calculations were also performed for individual participants.

2.3.2. Linear Regression. IBM SPSS Statistics 23 software program for linear regression was used to predict participants' stress levels based on percentages of helpful coping strategies and on percentages of important unmet needs and to predict the percentages of unmet support needs based on percentages of helpful coping strategies. In addition, after centering the data and creating an interaction term, SPSS linear regression was used to perform a moderator analysis to examine if the percent of helpful coping strategies altered the strength of the relationship between important unmet needs and maternal stress. Level of significance was set at 0.05 for all analyses.

3. Results

3.1. Descriptive Results

3.1.1. Demographics. A total of 70 mothers raising a child with ASD participated in this study. Two-thirds of the participants were white, non-Hispanic, and the majority of respondents identified an income bracket of $50,000 or higher per year (Table 1). These demographic characteristics are similar to those reported for the general population of children with a diagnosis of ASD [25].

3.1.2. Maternal Stress. PSI-SF mean raw scores for total stress (106.15; SD 22.57) and for mean raw scores of subscales P-CDI (29.52; SD 8.99) and DC (41.25; SD 9.72) when converted into percentile scores reached levels indicative of clinically significant levels of stress. The PD subscale raw mean (35.38, SD 8.74) when converted into a percentile score was considered high but missed the clinically significant level of stress by less than one point.

The total PSI-SF percentile scores reflected a clinically significant level of stress for 77% of the mothers participating in this study. For two of the subscales, clinically significant levels of stress were also found for the majority of participants, 63% of participants on the P-CDI Subscale, and 68% of participants on the DC Subscale. For the PD subscale, 48% of scores reflected a clinically significant level of distress.

3.1.3. Coping Strategies. A mean of 33 coping strategies were utilized by mothers, and 81% of these were reported to be helpful. The five most frequently reported coping strategies are presented in Table 2. "Believing that my child will get better" was reported as the most helpful coping strategy that our participants utilized. "Explaining our family situation to friends and neighbors so they will understand" and "eating" were the two coping strategies reported as least helpful. The least frequently utilized coping strategy was "Going out with my spouse on a regular basis."

3.1.4. Family Needs. FNQ data were analyzed for each mother and for each need statement. Table 3 presents percentages of self-reported "important needs" and "important unmet

Table 2: Most and least frequently reported coping strategies.

Coping strategy	n	%
Most frequently reported as extremely helpful.		
(1) Believing that my child will get better.	41	59.4
(2) Investing myself in my child.	37	53.6
(3) Having my child with special needs seen by professionals on a regular basis.	36	52.2
(4) Talking with other parents in the same situation and learning about their experiences.	33	47.8
(5) Doing things together as a family, including all members of the household.	32	46.4
Most frequently reported as *not* helpful.		
(1) Explaining our family situation to friends and neighbors so they will understand; eating. (Tied)	23	33.3
(2) Allowing myself to get angry.	21	30.4
(3) Encouraging my child with special needs to be more independent.	19	27.5
(4) Getting other members of the family to help with chores and tasks at home.	17	24.6
(5) Believing that things will always work out; telling myself that I should be thankful for. (Tied)	13	18.8
Least frequently reported as utilized		
(1) Going out with my spouse on a regular basis.	32	46.4
(2) Entertaining friends in my home.	31	44.9
(3) Concentrating on hobbies (art, jogging, etc.).	29	42.0
(4) Doing things with family relative; getting away by myself; and working outside employment; investing time & energy in my job (3-way tie).	25	36.2
(5) Purchasing gifts from myself/others.	24	34.8

needs" for each need statement. FNQ statement order is ranked by percentage from most to least frequently reported need identified as both important and unmet (far right column). Participants reported an average of 47.3 of the 57 (83%) need statements as "important." Percentages of important needs ranged from a high of 100% to a low of 49%, and all of the need statements except for two were rated as "important" by at least 65% of the participants.

On average, 62.4% of the need statements identified as important were also reported as unmet. Percentages of important unmet needs ranged from a high of 87% to a low of 25%, with a standard deviation of 23.7%. Important unmet needs that were reported by over 75% of mothers included (1) financial support for the child's therapies, treatment, and care; (2) a break from responsibilities; (3) having other after-school program children understand the child's special needs; (4) getting enough rest or sleep; (5) help remaining hopeful about the child's future; (6) counseling for the mother and her significant other; (7) family to understand the child's problems; and (8) time to care for the mother's own health needs. None of these items are categorized as child-centered.

Percentages of important needs that were identified as met ranged from a high of 75% to a low of 12%. The only important need reported as met by 75% of mothers was "to have professionals working with my child speak to me in terms I can understand."

3.2. Linear Regression Results

3.2.1. Helpful Coping Strategies as a Predictor of Maternal Stress. Linear regression using the PSI-SF total raw score as the dependent variable and the percent of helpful coping strategies as the predictor variable revealed an inverse relationship, with a β coefficient of -0.403 (se = .122; $t = -3.317$; $p = .001$). That is, maternal stress score decreased .403 points for each percent increase in helpful coping strategies.

3.2.2. Important Unmet Needs as a Predictor of Maternal Stress. Linear regression analysis using the PSI-SF total raw score as the dependent variable and the percent of important unmet needs as the predictor variable revealed a β coefficient of .529 (se = .099; $t = 5.138$; $p = .000$). That is, maternal stress score increased .529 percentage points for each percent increase in important unmet needs.

3.2.3. Helpful Coping Strategies as a Predictor of Important Unmet Needs. Linear regression analysis using the percent of important unmet needs as the dependent variable and the percent of helpful coping strategies as the predictor variable revealed and inverse relationship, with a β coefficient of $-.52$ (se = .176; $t = -2.950$; $p = .004$). That is, important unmet needs decreased .52 percentage points for each percent increase in helpful coping strategies. However, when a linear regression analysis was performed to examine helpful coping strategies as a moderator for the strength of the relationship between important unmet needs and maternal stress, the interaction failed to reach statistical significance.

4. Discussion

The purpose of this study was to better understand support needs and coping strategies among mothers of children with ASD and how these factors may predict maternal stress level. A convenience sample of 70 mothers completed the PSI-SF to

TABLE 3: Family needs questionnaire percentages ranked by important unmet needs.

"I need" statement[a]	% important unmet needs	% important needs
Financial support in order to provide my child with therapies, treatments, and care. (n/a)	87%	89%
To get a break from my responsibilities. (P)	86%	94%
To have the other children in my child's after-school program understand my child's special needs. (n/a)	79%	100%
To get enough rest or sleep. (P)	79%	96%
Help remaining hopeful about my child's future. (P)	79%	85%
To have counseling for myself and my spouse/partner/child's father. (P)	78%	69%
To have other family members understand my child's problems. (n/a)	77%	94%
To have time to care for my own health needs (Note: additional question added to Modified FNQ. (P)	76%	90%
Weekend and after-school activities for my child with special needs. (C)	74%	87%
To be told if I am making good decisions about my child. (P)	73%	82%
To be physical active or exercise. (P)	73%	96%
To be shown what to do when my child is acting unusually or is displaying difficult strategies. (P)	72%	93%
To have my child's therapies continue throughout the summer months and school breaks. (C)	72%	97%
Help dealing with my fears about my child's future. (P)	71%	81%
To have help in deciding how much to let my child do by himself/herself. (P)	71%	80%
To spend time with my friends. (P)	71%	84%
To have help from family members taking care of my child. (P)	70%	78%
Information about special programs and services available to my child and my family. (n/a)	70%	96%
For my child to have friends of his/her own. (C)	70%	94%
To have time to spend alone with a spouse/partner/companion. (P)	70%	90%
For my child with special needs to have social activities other than with his/her own parents and siblings. (C)	67%	93%
To have consistent behavioral therapy for my child. (C)	65%	96%
To have help with housework. (P)	65%	76%
To be encouraged to ask for help. (P)	65%	82%
To be reassured that it isn't uncommon to have negative feelings about my child's strategies. (P)	64%	65%
To be told why my child acts in ways that are different, difficult or unusual. (P)	64%	79%
Q To have my questions answered honestly. (P)	64%	97%
For my other children's friends to feel comfortable around my child. (n/a)	63%	88%
To have different professionals agrees on the best way to help my child. (n/a)	61%	93%
The children in my child's classroom to understand that my child cannot help his/her unusual strategies and difficulties. (n/a)	61%	80%
For professionals working with my child to understand my child's and family's needs. (n/a)	60%	94%
To have my child's teacher(s) understand his/her special needs. (P)	58%	93%
To have time to spend alone with my other children. (n/a)	57%	100%
My child's doctor and dentist to have experience working with children like my child. (n/a)	56%	97%
To eat nutritious meals. (P)	55%	96%
To have counseling for my other children. (n/a)	55%	73%
To take a family vacation each year. (n/a)	54%	88%
To work with professional with experience with child similar to my child. (C)	54%	93%
To have professional to turn to for advice or services when my child needs help. (P)	54%	96%
To have consistent speech therapy for my child. (C)	53%	85%
To take a vacation without my child with special needs each year. (n/a)	49%	65%
To be shown that my opinions are used in planning my child's treatment, therapies or education. (P)	49%	97%
To have information regarding my child's therapeutic or educational progress. (P)	47%	100%

Table 3: Continued.

"I need" statement[a]	% important unmet needs	% important needs
Q. Respite care for my child. (P)	46%	58%
Continuous services rather than only in times of crisis. (C)	46%	93%
To be actively involved in my child's treatment and therapies. (P)	44%	99%
For professionals to be discrete when talking about my child while he/she is in the room. (C)	43%	71%
My child to have a teacher's aide with him/her at school who has knowledge or experience working with children like my child. (C)	42%	83%
To go out to dinner with my family. (n/a)	41%	77%
To have my child's teacher(s) understand his/her special needs. (C)	40%	94%
To be well educated about my child's disorder so I can be an effective decision maker regarding the needs of my child. (P)	39%	100%
To have consistent occupational therapy for my child. (C)	38%	81%
To have my spouse/partner/child's father agree on decisions about our child with special needs. (P)	36%	89%
My child's school to set up a specialized education plan for my child. (C)	32%	100%
To have consistent physical therapy for my child. (C)	30%	49%
To be shown respect by the professional working with my child. (P)	28%	97%
To have professional working with my child to speak to me in terms I can understand. (P)	25%	97%

"I need" statement[a] (P) indicates parent-focused need; (C) indicates child-focused need; (n/a) indicates neither parent- nor child-focused need.

identify maternal stress level, the modified FNQ to identify important unmet support needs, and the CHIP to identify helpful coping strategies.

4.1. Maternal Stress. Consistent with previous studies [3, 15], the majority of mothers (77%) in our study presented with clinically significant levels of stress. Interventions for reducing high levels of maternal stress have often focused on training parents to better regulate the child's challenging strategies [3, 13, 15]. This approach, however, is narrow in scope and fails to address the social-emotional impact of parenting a child with ASD. In contrast, more recent models of stress for parents of children with ASD include family resources and support needs as intervening variables that may buffer or improve both family well-being and child outcomes [2, 3, 7, 15].

4.2. Maternal Important Unmet Needs. More than half of the needs identified as important by mothers in our study, 62.4%, were also reported as unmet. Hartley and Schultz [19] advocate that understanding parents' important unmet needs is a critical first step in prioritizing system-wide services. Our results highlight the prevalence of unmet needs among mothers of children with ASD and are consistent with previous research findings by Siklos and Kerns [16] and Brown et al. [18]. It is unclear whether our findings reflect the lack of available resources in the community or reflects knowledge, access, or utilization of support services. Nonetheless, these results reveal that, for many families, the service delivery system is failing to adequately address their needs.

Notably, the range of important unmet needs reported by mothers in this study varied widely, as evidenced by a large standard deviation of nearly 24%. Comparisons with other research studies are difficult since standard deviations were often not reported [16, 18, 19]. In addition, there is marked variation in the percentages of participants reporting each FNQ statement. For example, there are substantially lower percentages of maternal important unmet needs reported in the Hartley and Schultz study [19]. Their highest reported important unmet need, "my child to have friends of his/her own," was only 37% compared with our highest important unmet need, "financial support," at 87%. Financial support was not even among their five most frequently reported important unmet needs. Although financial support was the most frequently reported important unmet need in our study and the study by Siklos and Kerns [16], our other nine most frequently reported important unmet needs differed.

Variations in results among studies are not easily explained. Beyond the uniqueness of each child with ASD, family composition, and demographic characteristics, all of the studies employed convenience samples with inherent response bias. Further, differences across studies cannot be explained by the inclusion of fathers as participants. Hartley and Schultz's [19] data on fathers and mothers are presented separately, and over 90% of participants in the other two studies were mothers [16, 18]. Also, generalizability of the results to other jurisdictions is cautioned, since funding and school services were not reported. These variations across study participants underscore the importance of individual assessment of each unique family's important unmet needs. In addition, ongoing reassessment is advocated particularly during transitions as needs change, and the child and family face different demands and expectations.

4.3. Helpful Coping Strategies as a Predictor for Maternal Stress. As hypothesized, percent of helpful coping strategies was found to predict maternal stress level. Increases in helpful coping behavior were associated with decreases in maternal stress level. Similar to other study findings [26], participants in our sample utilized a wide variety of adaptive coping strategies that were problem-focused, for example, investing myself in my child, and that reflected positive thinking, for example, believing my child will get better.

The three coping strategies most frequently reported as not helpful were as follows: explaining the family situation to others, eating, and getting angry. None of these strategies tackle the challenges of raising a child with ASD directly and may therefore be categorized as maladaptive. Professionals are, therefore, encouraged to examine the strategies mothers are utilizing to help cope with high parenting demands and stress and to foster use of adaptive strategies.

4.4. Unmet Needs as a Predictor for Maternal Stress. As hypothesized, the percentage of important unmet needs was found to predict maternal stress level. Increases in important unmet needs were associated with increases in maternal stress level. This finding supports recommendations that healthcare practitioners seek opportunities to address family unmet needs. For mothers of children with ASD, however, other factors have also been associated with maternal stress level. For example, parental self-efficacy, belief in one's own ability to effectively assume the role of parenting, has been linked to the child's behavior problems and maternal anxiety and depression [3, 13, 15, 27].

4.5. Practice Implications. Pediatric healthcare practitioners widely endorse family-centered care (FCC) as a best practice [4, 15, 28]. This approach may be particularly critical when working with families raising children with ASD given the pervasive nature of the disability and bidirectional relationship between child outcomes and family well-being [3, 7, 15]. Although parental self-efficacy, coping strategies, and other parenting characteristics are important components for family well-being, the substantial demands associated with raising a child with ASD necessitate continued support from external sources [3]. Within the family-centered delivery model, pediatric services address both child and family needs and preferences, and professionals build family competency and capacity through interventions, resources, and supports [7]. One of the greatest challenges for pediatric service providers, however, is concurrently addressing the unique evolving needs of both the child and family.

Given the high prevalence and wide variation in identification of important unmet needs across participants in our study as well as across research studies, individual assessment of family support needs is advocated. Additionally, assessments should be ongoing as demands, responsibilities, and needs shift with transitions during the child's lifetime. Russa and colleagues [4] caution that even when professionals address needs in one developmental phase, caregivers' needs may shift from learning about the child's diagnosis to the child's special education rights, to resources for health insurance, recreation or respite, and then, with the child's transition to adulthood, to access for adult services.

Pediatric practitioners are well positioned to routinely screen mothers for high levels of stress, coping strategies, and important support needs using the PSI-SF, CHIP, and FNQ or other valid measures. These tools are low in cost, require little time to complete, and are self-administered. This avoids using therapist time that otherwise would have been available for direct child care and allows caregivers to complete the questionnaires at their convenience. Further, parents are often so overwhelmed or worried about their child's future that they cannot pinpoint specific desired child or family goals when asked verbally. In these instances, questionnaire items may help parents recognize problems their child and family are encountering, which in turn can facilitate their ability to identify specific child intervention goals that can enhance family functioning and well-being. As a result, positive child outcomes are believed to be more likely [3, 14, 18, 19].

Caregiver questionnaire responses can be used to prioritize and guide direct interventions that are within the clinician's scope of practice as well as compile resources. For example, depending on the parent's identified important unmet needs, pediatric practitioners can train parents to promote specific developmental skills or manage the child's difficult behaviors, help create family routines, plan outings to reduce social isolation, promote helpful coping strategies and parental self-efficacy, advise participation in healthy lifestyle strategies and other self-care activities that reduce stress and promote well-being, support teamwork, obtain access to therapies, and provide resources for support services, such as parent support groups, community recreation activities, or respite care. Practitioners are encouraged to refer to other healthcare professionals when parental stress and unmet needs are identified that are outside their scope of practice.

4.6. Study Strengths, Limitations, and Suggestions for Future Studies. One methodological strength in this study was the use of a support needs questionnaire that elucidates both whether the need is important to the respondent and whether each important need is met or unmet. Another strength is that the CHIP and FNQ-SF can be used readily by practitioners, are low in cost, require little time to complete, and are easy for family members to self-administer.

This study, however, has several methodological limitations. First, the small sample size and participation rate (24%) limit generalizability of our findings to parents of children with ASD in other geographical locations and with different demographics. Second, given the small sample size, we were unable to statistically account for differences related to the child's age or symptom severity. In addition, participants were mothers only, whose perceptions of unmet needs vary somewhat from those of fathers [19]. Further, this study examined only two variables related to maternal stress, and other factors, such as the child's problem behaviors, area resources, or parenting characteristics, may also produce reciprocal effects on child and family outcomes.

Future research is recommended to examine the underlying causes that produce such high percentages of important unmet needs and to examine the effectiveness of pediatric interventions on both child and caregiver outcomes. Studies on the feasibility of implementing family assessments that measure well-being are also needed. Even in organizations that endorse FCC, there are many barriers. Time is often reported as the greatest barriers, but other common barriers include a lack of training in FCC, lack of knowledge of resources within the community that might meet the family's needs, resistance to shifting to shared decision-making, meeting productivity levels, and lack of funding or insurance for services outside of direct care within the professional's scope of practice [14, 29–31].

5. Conclusions

Our findings further elucidate the relationships among maternal stress level, coping strategies, and support needs. Increases in helpful coping strategies utilized by mothers were associated with lower levels of maternal stress, but increases in important unmet needs were associated with increased levels of maternal stress. Given the high incidence of reported unmet needs and large variation across participants and studies, utilization of user-friendly questionnaires, such as the PSI-SF, CHIP, and FNQ, is advocated to determine the evolving important needs unique to each family over the child's lifetime. This may enhance the ability of pediatric healthcare practitioners to guide prioritization of direct care within the clinician's scope of practice, compile resources, and refer to other healthcare professionals when parent stress and unmet needs are identified that are outside their scope of practice.

Acknowledgments

This study was funded by a Simmons College President's Faculty Fund for Research Grant.

References

[1] American Psychiatric Association, *Diagnostic and Statistical Manual of Mental Disorders*, DSM-5, American Psychiatric Association, Arlington, Va, USA, 5th edition, 2013.

[2] K. Bluth, P. N. Roberson, R. M. Billen, and J. M. Sams, "A stress model for couples parenting children with autism spectrum disorders and the introduction of a mindfulness intervention," *Journal of Family Theory & Review*, vol. 5, no. 3, pp. 194–213, 2013.

[3] J. S. Karst and A. V. van Hecke, "Parent and family impact of autism spectrum disorders: a review and proposed model for intervention evaluation," *Clinical Child and Family Psychology Review*, vol. 15, no. 3, pp. 247–277, 2012.

[4] M. B. Russa, A. L. Matthews, and J. S. Owen-DeSchryver, "Expanding Supports to Improve the Lives of Families of Children With Autism Spectrum Disorder," *Journal of Positive Behavior Interventions*, vol. 17, no. 2, pp. 95–104, 2015.

[5] S. A. Hayes and S. L. Watson, "The impact of parenting stress: A meta-analysis of studies comparing the experience of parenting stress in parents of children with and without autism spectrum disorder," *Journal of Autism and Developmental Disorders*, vol. 43, no. 3, pp. 629–642, 2013.

[6] J. K. Baker, L. E. Smith, J. S. Greenberg, M. M. Seltzer, and J. L. Taylor, "Change in Maternal Criticism and Behavior Problems in Adolescents and Adults With Autism Across a 7-Year Period," *Journal of Abnormal Psychology*, vol. 120, no. 2, pp. 465–475, 2011.

[7] C. J. Dunst, C. M. Trivette, and D. W. Hamby, "Meta-analysis of family-centered helpgiving practices research," *Mental Retardation and Developmental Disabilities Research Reviews*, vol. 13, no. 4, pp. 370–378, 2007.

[8] D. S. Mandell, M. Xie, K. H. Morales, L. Lawer, M. McCarthy, and S. C. Marcus, "The interplay of outpatient services and psychiatric hospitalization among medicaid-enrolled children with autism spectrum disorders," *Archives of Pediatric and Adolescent Medicine*, vol. 166, no. 1, pp. 68–73, 2012.

[9] L. A. Osborne, L. McHugh, J. Saunders, and P. Reed, "Parenting stress reduces the effectiveness of early teaching interventions for autistic spectrum disorders," *Journal of Autism and Developmental Disorders*, vol. 38, no. 6, pp. 1092–1103, 2008.

[10] A. Ludlow, C. Skelly, and P. Rohleder, "Challenges faced by parents of children diagnosed with autism spectrum disorder," *Journal of Health Psychology*, vol. 17, no. 5, pp. 702–711, 2012.

[11] M. Seymour, C. Wood, R. Giallo, and R. Jellett, "Fatigue, stress and coping in mothers of children with an autism spectrum disorder," *Journal of Autism and Developmental Disorders*, vol. 43, no. 7, pp. 1547–1554, 2013.

[12] R. P. Hastings, H. Kovshoff, T. Brown, N. J. Ward, F. D. Espinosa, and B. Remington, "Coping strategies in mothers and fathers of preschool and school-age children with autism," *Autism*, vol. 9, no. 4, pp. 377–391, 2005.

[13] R. P. Hastinqs and T. Brown, "Behavior problems of children with autism, parental self-efficacy, and mental health," *American Journal on Intellectual and Developmental Disabilities*, vol. 107, no. 3, pp. 222–234, 2002.

[14] S. Hodgetts, L. Zwaigenbaum, and D. Nicholas, "Profile and predictors of service needs for families of children with autism spectrum disorders," *Autism*, vol. 19, no. 6, pp. 673–683, 2014.

[15] H. M. Kuhaneck, S. Madonna, A. Novak, and E. Pearson, "Effectiveness of interventions for children with autism spectrum disorder and their parents: A systematic review of family outcomes," *American Journal of Occupational Therapy*, vol. 69, no. 5, Article ID 2436569, pp. 1–14, 2015.

[16] S. Siklos and K. A. Kerns, "Assessing need for social support in parents of children with autism and Down syndrome," *Journal of Autism and Developmental Disorders*, vol. 36, no. 7, pp. 921–933, 2006.

[17] P. K. Waaland, C. Burns, and J. Cockrell, "Evaluation of needs of high- and low-income families following paediatric traumatic brain injury," *Brain Injury*, vol. 7, no. 2, pp. 135–146, 1993.

[18] H. K. Brown, H. Ouellette-Kuntz, D. Hunter, E. Kelley, and V. Cobigo, "Unmet Needs of Families of School-Aged Children with an Autism Spectrum Disorder," *Journal of Applied Research in Intellectual Disabilities*, vol. 25, no. 6, pp. 497–508, 2012.

[19] S. L. Hartley and H. M. Schultz, "Support Needs of Fathers and Mothers of Children and Adolescents with Autism Spectrum

Disorder," *Journal of Autism and Developmental Disorders*, vol. 45, no. 6, pp. 1636–1648, 2014.

[20] L. Abbeduto, M. M. Seltzer, P. Shattuck, M. W. Krauss, G. Orsmond, and M. M. Murphy, "Psychological Well-Being and Coping in Mothers of Youths with Autism, Down Syndrome, or Fragile X Syndrome," *American Journal on Intellectual and Developmental Disabilities*, vol. 109, no. 3, pp. 237–271, 2004.

[21] S. Hodgetts, D. Nicholas, L. Zwaigenbaum, and D. McConnell, "Parents' and professionals' perceptions of family-centered care for children with autism spectrum disorder across service sectors," *Social Science & Medicine*, vol. 96, pp. 138–146, 2013.

[22] R. R. Abidin, *Manual for the Parenting Stress Index*, Psychological Assessment Resources, Odessa, FL, USA, 1995.

[23] H. I. McCubbin, M. A. McCubbin, J. M. Patterson, A. E. Cauble, L. R. Wilson, and W. Warwick, "CHIP-Coping Health Inventory for parents: an assessment of parental coping patterns in the care of the chronically ill child," *Journal of Marriage and Family*, vol. 45, no. 2, pp. 359–370, 1983.

[24] V. K. Gothwal, S. Bharani, and S. P. Reddy, "Measuring coping in parents of children with disabilities: A Rasch model approach," *PLoS ONE*, vol. 10, no. 3, Article ID e0118189, 2015.

[25] M. Wingate, R. S. Kirby, S. Pettygrove et al. et al., "Prevalence of autism spectrum disorder among children aged 8 years-autism and developmental disabilities monitoring network, 11 sites, United States, 2010," *Morbidity and Mortality Weekly Report Surveillance Summaries*, vol. 63, no. 2, 2014.

[26] W. W. Lai and T. P. S. Oei, "Coping in Parents and Caregivers of Children with Autism Spectrum Disorders (ASD): a Review," *Review Journal of Autism and Developmental Disorders*, vol. 1, no. 3, pp. 207–224, 2014.

[27] D. L. Rezendes and A. Scarpa, "Associations between parental anxiety/depression and child behavior problems related to autism spectrum disorders: the roles of parenting stress and parenting self-efficacy," *Autism Research and Treatment*, vol. 2011, Article ID 395190, 10 pages, 2011.

[28] D. Z. Kuo, A. J. Houtrow, P. Arango, K. A. Kuhlthau, J. M. Simmons, and J. M. Neff, "Family-centered care: current applications and future directions in pediatric health care," *Maternal and Child Health Journal*, vol. 16, no. 2, pp. 297–305, 2012.

[29] M. E. O'Neil, R. J. Palisano, and S. L. Westcott, "Relationship of therapists' attitudes, children's motor ability, and parenting stress to mothers' perceptions of therapists' behaviors during early intervention," *Physical Therapy in Sport*, vol. 81, no. 8, pp. 1412–1424, 2001.

[30] L. M. Christon and B. J. Myers, "Family-centered care practices in a multidisciplinary sample of pediatric professionals providing autism spectrum disorder services in the United States," *Research in Autism Spectrum Disorders*, vol. 20, article no. 1072, pp. 47–57, 2015.

[31] P. E. Fingerhut, J. Piro, A. Sutton et al., "Family-centered principles implemented in home-based, clinic-based, and school-based pediatric settings," *American Journal of Occupational Therapy*, vol. 67, no. 2, pp. 228–235, 2013.

27

Experiences of Dental Care and Dental Anxiety in Adults with Autism Spectrum Disorder

My Blomqvist,[1] Göran Dahllöf,[1] and Susanne Bejerot[2]

[1] *Division of Paediatric Dentistry, Department of Dental Medicine, Karolinska Institutet, 141 04 Huddinge, Sweden*
[2] *Department of Clinical Neuroscience, Karolinska Institutet and Northern Stockholm Psychiatry, St. Göran Hospital, 112 81 Stockholm, Sweden*

Correspondence should be addressed to My Blomqvist; my.blomqvist@ki.se

Academic Editor: Manuel F. Casanova

Dental anxiety is associated with previous distressing dental experiences, such as lack of understanding of the dentist intentions, perceptions of uncontrollability and experiences of pain during dental treatment. People with autism spectrum disorder (ASD) are impaired in building flexible predictions and expectations, which is very much needed during a dental visit. The aims of the study were to investigate if people with ASD have more negative dental experiences and a higher level of dental anxiety compared to a matched control group. Forty-seven adults with ASD and of normal intellectual performance, and 69 age- and sex-matched typically developing controls completed questionnaires on previous dental experiences and dental anxiety, the Dental Anxiety Scale, and the Dental Beliefs Survey. The ASD group experienced pain during dental treatments more often than the controls and 22% had repeatedly experienced being forced to dental treatment they were not prepared for, compared to 3% of the controls. A higher level of dental anxiety was reported by the ASD group. Dental treatment and methods for supporting the communication with patients with ASD need to be developed, in order to reduce the negative dental experiences and dental anxiety in people with ASD.

1. Introduction

Dental anxiety, affecting approximately 20% of the adult population [1], is a feeling that something dreadful is going to happen in relation to dental treatment and is connected to a sense of losing control [2]. It is associated with dental caries and missed appointments [3, 4] and may extend to a total avoidance of dental care, reported by approximately 5% of the general population [1]. The development of dental anxiety is associated with previous distressing dental experiences, such as lack of understanding of the dentist intentions, or feeling of extreme helplessness or severe embarrassment during the treatment [5]. There is also a strong relationship between the number of previous experiences of pain during dental treatments and dental anxiety [6]. In children, both dental fear and pain connected to dental injections is more frequently reported in girls [7, 8]. Furthermore, medical treatments or conditions, other than dental, that might have caused pain, are associated with dental anxiety, at least in children [9]. However, Armfield [10] argued that it is the person's perception of the situation rather than the pain itself that is crucial for the development of dental anxiety. Perceptions of uncontrollability and feelings of danger have both showed strong associations with a high prevalence of dental anxiety [11].

Autism spectrum disorder (ASD) is considered to be a neurodevelopmental condition with early childhood onset [12]. It is characterised by persistent impairments in social interaction and communication and restricted, repetitive patterns of behaviour, interests, or activities and unusual sensory interests or sensitivities. In the recently revised American classification system for psychiatric disorders, the DSM-5 [12], ASD now includes previously separate diagnostic categories such as autistic disorder, Asperger disorder, and pervasive developmental disorder, not otherwise specified, specified (PDD-NOS) in the DSM-IV-TR [13] (American Psychiatric Association, 2000).

People with ASD commonly report abnormal responses to sensory stimuli [14]. Overreactivity to sound and under-reactivity to pain was stated by more than 40% of children with ASD. Sensory abnormalities affected to a greater extent those with more severe autistic traits compared to those with less autistic traits [14]. Sensory sensitivities in children with ASD are also related to behaviour difficulties in the dental office [15]. There are yet no studies on behaviour and experiences of dental care in adults with ASD.

People with ASD are impaired in building flexible predictions and expectations, which is very much needed in the highly unpredictable social world [16]. An inability to expect new sensory inputs and events leads to difficulties in perceptions and executive functions such as flexibility and planning [16] and this stress presumably causes anxiety. In addition, personality traits related to being more pessimistic and anxious is enhanced in ASD [17]. Thus, there are reasons to believe that dental anxiety could be common in adults with ASD but to our knowledge this has so far not been investigated.

The aims of the present study were twofold, first to investigate if people with ASD have more negative dental experiences compared to a matched control group composed of general dental patients. The second aim was to compare the level of dental anxiety between the two groups.

2. Material and Methods

2.1. Study Setting. The study is a double-cohort study, where a group of adults diagnosed with ASD is compared to a group of typically developing adults. It comprises part of a study on oral health and dental experience in adults with ASD living in the northern Stockholm area in 2008. All participants attended a dental examination appointment and completed questionnaires. Then, they were provided a written and verbal report on their dental status and necessary dental treatment. Written consent was obtained from the participants, and ethical approval was obtained from the regional ethical board in Stockholm, Sweden (2008/874-31/4).

2.2. Participants. Forty-seven adults with ASD and of normal intellectual performance, and 69 age and sex-matched typically developing controls were included in the study. Exclusion criteria for all participants were diagnosis of intellectual disability, a history of brain damage, current or past neurological disorder, epilepsy, alcohol abuse or dependence, past or present substance abuse, and psychosis. In addition, scores above cutoff for a probable ASD, according to a rating scale for assessing autistic traits (described below), were an exclusion criterion for the controls. Demographic characteristics and descriptive statistics are presented in Table 1.

2.3. Participants with ASD. The participants with ASD were recruited from tertiary units for diagnosing ASD in adulthood, the Neuropsychiatric unit, Northern Stockholm psychiatric clinic, and from a community-based unit for adults with ASD located in Stockholm. The diagnosis of ASD was based on a thorough examination, which took 12–18 hours to complete, during a time period of two weeks to three months. The diagnostic assessment included structured and semistructured clinical interviews following the DSM-IV-TR [13] criteria for autistic disorder, Asperger disorder, or PDD-NOS, rating scales and an interview with a parent. In addition, a licensed psychologist performed neuropsychological tests including the Wechsler Adult Intelligence Scale-Revised (WAIS-III-R). A senior psychiatrist and the psychologist, both trained in diagnosing ASD, performed all assessments and the diagnosis was established in consensus between the two, but the psychiatrist was ultimately responsible for setting the diagnosis.

An invitation letter was sent to patients diagnosed with ASD at the Northern Stockholm psychiatric clinic and to subjects with ASD who were registered at the community-based unit. Sixty-nine subjects with ASD agreed to participate by a letter of reply; fifty-nine of these completed a telephone interview. Seven patients were unavailable for the dental appointment and another five failed to attend, resulting in a final study group comprising 47 adults with ASD (25 males, 22 females).

2.4. Controls. Sixty-nine (34 males, 35 females) typically developing adults were recruited from six dental clinics in the Stockholm area, after being asked during their dental examinations. They were given the same invitation letter as the ASD group. The control group was matched to the clinical group with regard to age, gender, and area of residence.

2.5. Demographic and Background Information. Demographic and background information was collected from the participants in conjunction with the dental appointment, using a self-administered questionnaire comprising questions on medical diagnosis, medication, country of birth, education of parents, educational level, occupational status, and tobacco use.

2.6. Screening for ASD. In order to screen for behaviours related to ASD and thereby disclosing any subjects with symptoms of ASD from the control group, all participants completed the autism spectrum quotient, AQ [18]. The AQ is a self-rating scale that describes a variety of traits typically observed in individuals with ASD. It consists of 50 items, assessing personal preferences and habits. Subjects rate to what extent they agree or disagree with the statements on a 4-point Likert scale, ranging from definitely agree (0) to definitely disagree (3). Items are subsequently coded dichotomously into 0 and 1 to reflect the absence or presence of each symptom. Total AQ scores reflect the sum of all items; the lowest possible score (i.e., 0) indicates no autistic traits and the highest possible score (50) indicates severe autistic traits. A score above 32 has been proposed as a cutoff score for probable ASD [18], but people with a confirmed ASD diagnosis sometimes have lower scores [19].

2.7. Dental Experience. All participants completed a questionnaire on previous dental experiences included for the purpose of this study. If they had visited the dentist after 20 years of age (dental appointments are free of charge in Sweden until 20 years of age), the reasons for the appointment were

Table 1: Sociodemographic characteristics of adults with autism spectrum disorder (ASD) and controls.

	ASD group $n = 47$	Control group $n = 69$	P-value
Mean age (years)	33 ± 8	34 ± 7	0.466*
Male sex, n (%)	25 (53)	34 (49)	0.679#
Mother's country of birth n (%)			
Sweden	39 (83)	57 (83)	
Other Nordic countries	4 (9)	5 (7)	
Other European countries	1 (2)	2 (3)	
Rest of the world	3 (6)	5 (7)	0.985#
Father's country of birth, n (%)			
Sweden	36 (77)	59 (86)	
Other Nordic countries	5 (11)	3 (4)	
Other European countries	3 (6)	2 (3)	
Rest of the world	3 (6)	5 (7)	0.441#
Highest educational level, n (%)			
Elementary school	3 (6)	2 (3)	
High school	28 (60)	25 (36)	
University/college	16 (34)	41 (59)	0.021#
Working or studying, n (%)			
Full time	11 (23)	63 (91)	
Part time	7 (15)	5 (7)	
Unemployed/not studying	29 (62)	1 (1)	<0.001#
Smoking, n (%)	2/47 (4)	9/69 (13)	0.195a
Snuff, n (%)	4/47 (9)	8/69 (12)	0.759a
Medication, n (%)	31/47 (66)	7/69 (10)	<0.001#
Medication with reported side-effect xerostomia, n (%)	23/47 (47)	1/69 (1)	<0.001#
AQ (range)	133.8 ± 25.9 (66.0–182.8)	95.1 ± 11.1 (75.0–128.0)	$P < 0.001$*
AQ single count (range)	28.7 ± 10.4 (5.0–46.0)	11.4 ± 4.5 (4.0–28.0)	$P < 0.001$*

*t-test.
#χ^2 test.
aFisher's exact test.

requested (dental pain or for other reasons unrelated to pain). The four following items were (1) pain experience during dental treatment, (2) insufficient dental anaesthesia, (3) pain during other medical treatments, and (4) feelings of being forced into dental treatment that they were not prepared for. Each item could be answered by the alternatives "never," "once," or "more than once"; the items are shown in Table 2. The first three of these questions have previously been used in a Norwegian study on dental anxiety [4]. Responses reflecting "The answers never" and "once" were combined into one group versus "more than once" in the statistical analysis.

2.8. Dental Anxiety. The Dental Anxiety Scale (DAS) [20] is the most widely used test for measuring dental anxiety and is filled out by the patient. The primary focus of the scale is on the anticipation of dental treatment. The DAS comprises four multiple-choice questions addressing the individual's reactions and expectations of going to and being treated by a dentist (anticipation; waiting in a waiting room; waiting for the drill; waiting for the scraping; the items are shown in Table 2). Each question consists of five response alternatives ranging from 1 (no anxiety) to 5 (extreme anxiety) with a total score varying between 4 and 20. Average DAS scores of 8-9 for ordinary (nonfearful) patients and ≥13 among fearful dental patients have been reported [20–22]. The CDAS has shown good validity in Swedish studies on patients with dental fear [22, 23].

The Revised Dental Beliefs Survey, DBS-R [2] assesses the patient's subjective perceptions regarding the dentist's behaviour and the process of how the care is delivered and issues that are of primary concern to patients with general anxiety or who are distrustful [2]. The instrument consists of 28 items with a 5-point Likert scale and a sum of score ranging from 28 to 140. The DBS-R has been found to be a reliable and valid instrument for use in various Swedish patient and nonclinical population groups to assess attitudes to dentists and dental care [24]. DBS-R scores with a mean of 42 in ordinary patients and 88 among fearful dental patients have been reported [24].

2.9. Statistical Analysis. Mean scores were calculated for each rating scale. The scores for each rating scale were first summed to a total score and then divided by the number of items to which the patient had responded. Missing data

TABLE 2: Corah Dental Anxiety Scale.

Estimate the level of fear you would perceive in the situations described below.
(1) If you had to go to the dentist tomorrow, how would you feel about it?
(a) I would look forward to it as a reasonably enjoyable experience.
(b) I would not care one way or the other
(c) I would be a little uneasy about it.
(d) I would be afraid that it would be unpleasant and painful.
(e) I would be very frightened of what the dentist might do.
(2) When you are waiting in the dentist's office for your turn in the chair, how would you feel?
(a) Relaxed.
(b) A little uneasy.
(c) Tense.
(d) Anxious.
(e) So anxious that I sometimes break out in seat or almost feel physically sick.
(3) When you are in the dentist's chair waiting while he gets his drill ready to begin working on your teeth, how do you feel?
(a) Relaxed.
(b) A little uneasy.
(c) Tense.
(d) Anxious.
(e) So anxious that I sometimes break out in seat or almost feel physically sick.
(4) You are in the dentist's chair to have your teeth cleaned. While you are waiting and the dentist is getting out the instruments, which he will use to scrape your teeth around the gums, how do you feel?
(a) Relaxed.
(b) A little uneasy.
(c) Tense.
(d) Anxious.
(e) So anxious that I sometimes break out in seat or almost feel physically sick.

were analyzed by multiplying the mean item score for each response by the number of items in each scale, thus obtaining comparable scores. This method was chosen after it had been ascertained that no statistically significant differences occurred between the overall mean scores calculated in this way and the overall mean scores obtained using only complete questionnaires. A response rate above 80% was required in each questionnaire to be included.

Mann-Whitney U test was used to determine the significance of differences between continuous variables for the two groups, except for age and AQ, where Student's t-test was used. Categorical data were compared using the chi-square test. If the observed frequency was below five in one cell Fisher's exact test was used. The statistical software SPSS version 21.0 was used for statistical analyses.

3. Results

Results on questions regarding previous dental experiences are presented in Table 3. Significantly more patients with ASD had experienced pain during dental as well as other medical treatments compared to the typically developing adults (Table 3). Twenty-two percent (10/46) of the patients with ASD felt they had been forced into dental treatment they were not prepared for several times compared to only 3% (2/67) in the control group ($P = 0.003$).

All patients filled out the DAS and DBS-R. The ASD group reported more dental anxiety than the control group, according to the DAS and DBS-R (Table 4). DAS ≥ 13 was reported for 7/47 (15%) in the ASD group compared to 4/69 (6%) in the control group.

Participants with ASD who reported recurrent pain during dental treatment, insufficient local anesthesia or a feeling of being forced to dental treatment one was not prepared for, scored higher on DAS than those with ASD with one or no such experience (DAS pain dental treatment 9.8 ± 3.9 versus 7.0 ± 2.7 ($P = 0.022$); DAS insufficient anesthesia 11.1 ± 3.8 versus 7.2 ± 3.1 ($P = 0.045$); DAS being forced 11.6 ± 4.8 versus 8.2 ± 3.2 ($P = 0.030$)). However no association between DAS and pain during other medical treatments was found. In the controls no association between recurring negative dental or medical experience and higher DAS scores was found.

Table 5 shows separate item mean scores and ranking order of the DBS-R in the ASD and control groups. In both groups, the three highest ranked items were item number 8 "When a dentist seems in a hurry I worry that I am not getting good care," item number 23 "Once I am in the chair I feel helpless (things are out of my control)," and item number 21 "When I am in the chair I do not feel like I can stop the

Table 3: Dental experiences in autism spectrum disorder (ASD) and controls.

More than one experience of	ASD n (%)	Control n (%)	χ^2	P value
Pain during dental treatment[a]	33/46 (70)	30/67 (45)	6.8	0.009[#]
Insufficient local anaesthesia	20/47 (43)	14/67 (21)	14.7	0.001[#]
Pain during other medical treatment	27/47 (57)	11/67 (16)	20.9	<0.001[#]
A feeling of being forced to dental treatment one was not prepared for	10/46 (22)	2/67 (3)	10.1	0.003[a]

[#] χ^2 test and [a] Fischer's exact test.

Table 4: Dental anxiety and beliefs in autism spectrum disorder (ASD) and controls.

	ASD $n = 47$	Control $n = 69$	P-value
DAS, mean score (SD)	8.9 (3.8)	6.9 (2.8)	0.003
DAS, median score (range)	8 (4–19)	6 (4–18)	
DBS-R, mean score (SD)	50.1 (20.5)	34.3 (10.7)	<0.001
DBS-R, median score (range)	46 (28–108)	31 (28–89)	
DBS-R, mean item score (SD)	1.8 (0.7)	1.2 (0.4)	<0.001
DBS-R, median item score (range)	1.6 (1.0–3.9)	1.1 (1.0–3.2)	

DAS: Corah Dental Anxiety Scale.
DBS-R: Revised Dental Beliefs Survey.

appointment for a rest if I feel in the need." In the ASD group, this was followed by item number 26 "Dentists often seem in a hurry, so I feel rushed," item number 3 "I worry if the dentist is technically competent and is doing quality work," and item number 11 "I am concerned that dentists might not be skilled enough to deal with my fear or my dental problems," whereas the same items were ranked as numbers 16, 23, and 16 in the control group.

Only one subject in the ASD group had no dental contact, in addition another 7 had only booked an appointment when in dental pain, all others reported having a regular dental contact. When comparing the 7 patients with ASD that had only booked a dental appointment due to pain to the 39 with ASD that had regular dental contacts, there were no differences in mean values of DAS or DBS-R.

4. Discussion

This study shows that adults with ASD report more painful dental experiences and more often feel they have been forced to dental treatment that they were not prepared for, compared to typically developing people. The results also show that adults with ASD experience greater dental anxiety and emphasize different aspects of dental anxiety.

The great majority of the participants in the ASD group felt pain several times during dental treatment compared to less than half of the control group. Pain due to insufficient local anaesthesia was experienced several times by twice as many in the ASD group compared to the control group. The patients in the ASD group may have experienced more pain because of abnormal perception or other sensory sensitivities as both hyper- and hyposensitivity are frequently reported in ASD [16]. The patients in the ASD group might also have a lowered pain threshold for some qualities of pain. During dental treatment under general anaesthesia the need of anaesthetic medication (the propofol requirement) was found to be greater amongst patients with autism than intellectually impaired controls [25].

The presumably accompanied heightened stress level may have enhanced the experience of pain [26]. The sense of pain is also influenced by dental anxiety, as dental anxiety is a reinforcer of pain [8]. Participants with high dental anxiety and high pain sensitivity expect and experience more pain during dental treatment [27]. On the other hand, painful experiences during dental treatment increase the risk for future dental anxiety. A Norwegian study showed that 18-year-old participants who reported more than one previous experience of pain during dental treatment were ten times more likely to report high dental anxiety compared to those without this experience [6]. In the present study, those who had experienced recurrent pain or recurrent insufficient anaesthesia during dental treatment reported more dental anxiety in the ASD group, but not in the control group. This finding could be explained by sensory overresponsivity in the ASD group, which presumably can cause anxiety by mechanism of conditioning [28]. The characteristic smell of a dental office or the sound of the drill could become conditioned stimuli resulting in anxiety. However, in the present study there was no association between recurrent painful medical treatments and dental anxiety in either of the groups, suggesting that the association with dental anxiety does not extend to settings outside the dental office.

The ASD group reported that they more often felt they had been forced to dental treatment they were not prepared for than the control group. In the ASD group, but not

Table 5: Item mean scores and ranking of Dental Beliefs Survey (DBS-R) in autism spectrum disorder (ASD) and controls.

Items	ASD $n = 47$ Mean (SD)	Rank	Control $n = 69$ mean (SD)	Rank	P value[#]
(1) I am concerned that dentists recommend work that is not really needed	1.7 (1.0)	19	1.3 (0.7)	5	0.029
(2) I believe dentists say/do things to withhold information from me	1.3 (0.8)	28	1.1 (0.3)	27	0.022
(3) I worry if the dentist is technically competent and is doing quality work	2.0 (1.2)	5	1.1 (0.5)	23	<0.001
(4) I have had dentists say one thing and do another	1.5 (0.9)	24	1.3 (0.7)	10	n.s.
(5) I am concerned that dentists provide all the information I need to make good decisions	1.8 (1.3)	14	1.1 (0.3)	26	<0.001
(6) Dentists do not seem to care that patients sometime need a rest	1.9 (1.2)	11	1.2 (0.6)	10	0.001
(7) I have had dentists seem reluctant to correct work unsatisfactory to me	1.7 (1.3)	19	1.3 (0.6)	8	n.s.
(8) When a dentist seems in a hurry I worry that I am not getting good care	2.5 (1.4)	1	1.6 (1.0.)	1	<0.001
(9) I am concerned that the dentist is not really looking out for my best interests	1.9 (1.3)	9	1.1 (0.5)	16	<0.001
(10) Dentists focus too much on getting the job done and not enough on the patients comfort	1.9 (1.2)	8	1.3 (0.6)	9	0.001
(11) I am concerned that dentists might not be skilled enough to deal with my fear or my dental problems	2.0 (1.3)	6	1.1 (0.6)	16	<0.001
(12) I feel dentists do not provide clear explanations	1.8 (1.1)	14	1.2 (0.5)	13	0.001
(13) I am concerned that the dentists do not like to take the time to really talk to the patients	1.8 (1.1)	14	1.2 (0.5)	14	<0.001
(14) I feel uncomfortable asking questions	1.8 (1.2)	13	1.1 (0.5)	16	<0.001
(15) Dental professionals say things to make me feel guilty about the way I care for my teeth	1.7 (1.0)	19	1.4 (0.7)	4	n.s.
(16) I am concerned that the dentists will not take my worries (fears) about dentistry seriously	1.7 (1.2)	17	1.1 (0.5)	23	<0.001
(17) I am concerned that the dentists will put me down (make light of my fears)	1.3 (0.6)	27	1.1 (0.3)	27	0.003
(18) I am concerned that the dentists do not like it when a patient makes requests	1.9 (1.2)	9	1.2 (0.6)	14	<0.001
(19) I am concerned that the dental personnel will embarrass me over the condition of my teeth	1.4 (1.0)	26	1.1 (0.4)	22	n.s.
(20) I believe that dentists don't have enough empathy for what it is really like to be a patient	1.5 (0.8)	23	1.1 (0.3)	25	<0.001
(21) When I am in the chair I don't feel like I can stop the appointment for a rest if I feel in the need	2.3 (1.4)	3	1.4 (0.9)	3	<0.001
(22) Dentists don't seem to notice that patients sometime need a rest	1.9 (1.1)	7	1.3 (0.7)	6	<0.001
(23) Once I am in the chair I feel helpless (that things are out of my control)	2.4 (1.4)	2	1.6 (0.8)	2	0.004
(24) If I were to indicate that it hurts, I think that the dentist would be reluctant to stop and try to correct the problem	1.8 (1.2)	12	1.1 (0.5)	16	<0.001
(25) I have had dentists not believe me when I said I felt pain	1.6 (1.0)	22	1.2 (0.6)	12	0.021
(26) Dentists often seem in a hurry, so I feel rushed	2.1 (1.3)	4	1.1 (0.4)	16	<0.001
(27) I am concerned that the dentist will do what he wants and not really listen to me while I am in the chair	1.7 (1.1)	18	1.1 (0.4)	16	0.002
(28) Being overwhelmed by the amount of work needed (all the bad news) could be enough to keep me from beginning or completing treatment	1.5 (1.1)	25	1.3 (0.8)	7	n.s.

[#]Mann-Whitney U test, comparing the mean values.

among the controls, recurrent experiences of "being forced to dental treatment one was not prepared for," were associated with higher levels of dental anxiety. Across different cultures fearful patients put a strong emphasis on dentists' behaviour and performance of the dental treatment: emphatic behaviour and pain-free treatment are most important, while giving information and control are rated second [29]. Patients with ASD are impaired in predicting future events and have a low ability to build flexible predictions [16]. Thus the patient with ASD may feel completely un-prepared although others would think they were just as well prepared as any dental patient in a similar situation. Children with Asperger syndrome scored significantly lower on a language subtest on comprehension of instructions, while other subtests in the language tests showed no differences compared to typically developed controls [30] illustrating the risk of overestimating comprehension abilities in individuals with ASD.

The ASD group reported more dental anxiety compared to the control group. The control group scored lower than a comparative group of non-ASD Swedish patients, (mean DAS scores 8.0 and DBS-R scores 42.0) [24]. However, our ASD group reported higher scores, and the differences between the groups were marked when mean item scores were calculated: in the ASD group the mean DAS score was 1.8, in our control group 1.2 and in the Abrahamsson sample 1.5 [24]. The relatively low DAS scores in the control group could partly be due to the fact that they were familiar with their dentists, which may have reduced the anxiety level. On the other hand, high scores, reflecting dental anxiety, were also reported by some of the controls in the present study.

An intriguing finding was the different orders in ranking of items in the DBS-R between the groups. The group with ASD emphasized different aspects of dental anxiety than the control group. Although the three highest ranked items "When a dentist seems in a hurry I worry that I am not getting good care," "Once I am in the chair I feel helpless," and "When I am in the chair I do not feel like I can stop the appointment for a rest if I feel in the need" were identically ranked in the ASD and control groups, consistent with rankings in an earlier report [24], the items ranked as fourth, fifth, and sixth differed between the groups. These next three ranked items "Dentists often seem in a hurry, so I feel rushed," "I worry if the dentist is technically competent and is doing quality work," and "I am concerned that dentists might not be skilled enough to deal with my fear or my dental problems" were only ranked as numbers 16, 23, and 16 in the controls. Hence, the patients with ASD emphasized different aspects of dental fear compared to healthy controls (i.e., "dentist not technically competent, not skilled enough, I feel rushed"). Our findings suggest that people with ASD have a hard time trusting the professionals' ability to perform high-quality work, possibly related to deficits in mentalizing, a core symptom in ASD.

A sense of coherence (SOC) is defined by Antonovsky [31] as a pervasive feeling that (1) the stimuli deriving from one's internal and external environments are structured, predictable, and explicable; (2) resources are available to meet the demands posed by these stimuli; and (3) these demands are challenges, worthy of investment and engagement. According to a study on adolescents, those with higher dental fear have a weaker SOC than those with less dental fear [32]. In adult ASD extremely low SOC scores have been reported [33], but unfortunately SOC was not measured in our participants.

The DBS-R was constructed to assess to what degree patients perceive the interpersonal relationship with the dental professional as being the problem or possibly contributing to dental anxiety [2]. A change towards a more positive attitude in dentists' communication style early in the treatment has shown to predict a successful outcome in treatment of dental fear [34]. The communication impairment, critical for the diagnosis of ASD, suggests that specific communication skills are required from dental personnel, in order to meet the needs of the ASD population.

Dentists use a variety of techniques to meet the needs of fearful patients [35]. One of the most effective approaches to reducing dental anxiety is optimising controllability and predictability for the patient, by providing the patient with accurate explanations and information about what will happen and what type of experiences she/he might expect [36]. As ASD involves impairment in communication and sensory oversensitivity, this is particularly important. The latter is explained by the fact that people with ASD process visual and other stimuli differently presumably due to poor connections between parts of the brain that process these stimuli [37]. Thus the dentist should carefully inform the patient with ASD what she/he is about to do and what it may feel like, in addition to slowing down the pace of speech which facilitates comprehension. Another option is the use of visual pedagogy. Visual pedagogy is a way of introducing dentistry to children with ASD. When visual pedagogy was used to introduce dentistry to children with ASD, the capacity of children to cooperate during dental treatment one and a half year later was superior to that of children with ASD who had not been offered visual support [38]. In a recent study on adults with ASD and mild intellectual disability, the cooperation during a dental examination was significantly increased after a five-session training programme using a TEACCH-based approach [39]. Also, there is a growing interest in cognitive behavioural therapy for treating anxiety in adult ASD [33, 40]. The method is known to be helpful for treating dental anxiety in typically developing adults [1] but has not been studied for treating dental anxiety in people with ASD. Therefore, interventional studies on dental anxiety in ASD are warranted.

A limitation of the current study was the dropout in the ASD group due to patients not showing up at the dental appointment. The results regarding the ASD group might also not be representative of all persons with ASD, as the patients chose themselves to participate in the study. The present study assesses dental experiences and dental anxiety, known to be associated with dental avoidance [2]. Individuals who chose not to participate in the study or did not show up at the appointment probably included persons with high levels of dental anxiety. Dentally anxious persons, who believe they have bad oral health, tend to avoid going to the dentist [41]. Therefore, if persons with ASD and high dental anxiety chose not to participate in our study, this would have attenuated the differences in dental anxiety from the controls, which would further strengthen our findings. Another limitation was that as the control group consisted of regular dental patients recruited from dental practices, in this group we did not capture irregular attendees or the avoiders. Irregular attendees are more likely to be very afraid of visiting the dentist than regular attendees [42]. Levels of dental anxiety, general anxiety, and depression are shown to be higher among irregular attendees compared with regular attendees [43]. The vast majority (83%) amongst our ASD group had a regular dental contact and, notably, there were no differences regarding the anxiety between those with ASD who had a regular contact and those who did not.

5. Conclusion and Clinical Implication

In conclusion, people with ASD reported more painful dental experiences and more often felt they were forced to dental treatment they were not prepared for, they have more dental anxiety and emphasize different aspects of dental anxiety compared to typically developing people. Dental treatment and methods for supporting the communication with patients with ASD need to be developed, in order to reduce the negative dental experiences and dental anxiety in people with ASD.

Acknowledgments

The authors express their gratitude to all the participants of this study for their time and effort. The authors also thank Sara Ekman who helped with the statistical analysis and Stephany Plenty for proofreading. This study was partly funded through the regional agreement for support for research between Stockholm County Council (ALF) and Karolinska Institutet, Stockholm, Sweden, and The Swedish Medical Research Council (Grant no. 523-2011-3646).

References

[1] U. Wide Boman, V. Carlsson, M. Westin, and M. Hakeberg, "Psychological treatment of dental anxiety among adults: a systematic review," *European Journal of Oral Sciences*, vol. 121, no. 3, part 2, pp. 225–234, 2013.

[2] P. Milgrom, P. Weinstein, and T. Getz, *Treating Fearful Dental Patients: A Patient Management Handbook*, Continuing Dental Education, University of Washington, Seattle, Wash, USA, 2nd edition, 1995.

[3] G. Klingberg, U. Berggren, S. G. Carlsson, and J. G. Noren, "Child dental fear: cause-related factors and clinical effects," *European Journal of Oral Sciences*, vol. 103, no. 6, pp. 405–412, 1995.

[4] E. Skaret, M. Raadal, E. Berg, and G. Kvale, "Dental anxiety and dental avoidance among 12 to 18 year olds in Norway," *European Journal of Oral Sciences*, vol. 107, no. 6, pp. 422–428, 1999.

[5] G. Humphris and K. King, "The prevalence of dental anxiety across previous distressing experiences," *Journal of Anxiety Disorders*, vol. 25, no. 2, pp. 232–236, 2011.

[6] E. Skaret, M. Raadal, E. Berg, and G. Kvale, "Dental anxiety among 18-yr-olds in Norway: prevalence and related factors," *European Journal of Oral Sciences*, vol. 106, no. 4, pp. 835–843, 1998.

[7] G. Klingberg and A. G. Broberg, "Dental fear/anxiety and dental behaviour management problems in children and adolescents: a review of prevalence and concomitant psychological factors," *International Journal of Paediatric Dentistry*, vol. 17, no. 6, pp. 391–406, 2007.

[8] L. Krekmanova, M. Bergius, A. Robertson et al., "Everyday-and dental-pain experiences in healthy Swedish 8–19 year olds: an epidemiological study," *International Journal of Paediatric Dentistry*, vol. 19, no. 6, pp. 438–447, 2009.

[9] P. Wogelius, S. Poulsen, and H. T. Sørensen, "Asthma, ear problems, and dental anxiety among 6- to 8-yr-olds in Denmark: a population-based cross-sectional study," *European Journal of Oral Sciences*, vol. 111, no. 6, pp. 472–476, 2003.

[10] J. M. Armfield, "Cognitive vulnerability: a model of the etiology of fear," *Clinical Psychology Review*, vol. 26, no. 6, pp. 746–768, 2006.

[11] J. M. Armfield, G. D. Slade, and A. J. Spencer, "Cognitive vulnerability and dental fear," *BMC Oral Health*, vol. 8, no. 1, article 2, 2008.

[12] American Psychiatric Association, *Diagnostic and Statistical Manual of Mental Disorders*, American Psychiatric Association, Washington, DC, USA, 5th edition, 2013.

[13] American Psychiatric Association, *Diagnostic and Statistical Manual of Mental Disorders*, American Psychiatric Association, Washington, DC, USA, 4th edition, 2000.

[14] L. Klintwall, A. Holm, M. Eriksson et al., "Sensory abnormalities in autism: a brief report," *Research in Developmental Disabilities*, vol. 32, no. 2, pp. 795–800, 2011.

[15] L. I. Stein, J. C. Polido, Z. Mailloux, G. G. Coleman, and S. A. Cermak, "Oral care and sensory sensitivities in children with autism spectrum disorders," *Special Care in Dentistry*, vol. 31, no. 3, pp. 102–110, 2011.

[16] M. Gomot and B. Wicker, "A challenging, unpredictable world for people with Autism Spectrum Disorder," *International Journal of Psychophysiology*, vol. 83, no. 2, pp. 240–247, 2012.

[17] H. Anckarsäter, O. Stahlberg, T. Larson et al., "The impact of ADHD and autism spectrum disorders on temperament, character, and personality development," *The American Journal of Psychiatry*, vol. 163, no. 7, pp. 1239–1244, 2006.

[18] S. Baron-Cohen, S. Wheelwright, R. Skinner, J. Martin, and E. Clubley, "The autism-spectrum quotient (AQ): evidence from Asperger syndrome/high-functioning autism, males and females, scientists and mathematicians," *Journal of Autism and Developmental Disorders*, vol. 31, no. 1, pp. 5–17, 2001.

[19] S. L. Bishop and M. M. Seltzer, "Self-reported autism symptoms in adults with autism spectrum disorders," *Journal of Autism and Developmental Disorders*, vol. 42, no. 11, pp. 2354–2363, 2012.

[20] N. L. Corah, "Development of a dental anxiety scale," *Journal of Dental Research*, vol. 48, no. 4, article 596, 1969.

[21] N. L. Corah, E. N. Gale, and S. J. Illig, "Assessment of a dental anxiety scale," *The Journal of the American Dental Association*, vol. 97, no. 5, pp. 816–819, 1978.

[22] U. Berggren and S. G. Carlsson, "Usefulness of two psychometric scales in Swedish patients with severe dental fear," *Community Dentistry and Oral Epidemiology*, vol. 13, no. 2, pp. 70–74, 1985.

[23] R. Moore, U. Berggren, and S. G. Carlsson, "Reliability and clinical usefulness of psychometric measures in a self-referred population of odontophobics," *Community Dentistry and Oral Epidemiolog*, vol. 19, no. 6, pp. 347–351, 1991.

[24] K. H. Abrahamsson, M. Hakeberg, J. Stenman, and K. Öhrn, "Dental beliefs: evaluation of the Swedish version of the revised Dental Beliefs Survey in different patient groups and in a non-clinical student sample," *European Journal of Oral Sciences*, vol. 114, no. 3, pp. 209–215, 2006.

[25] Y. Asahi, K. Kubota, and S. Omichi, "Dose requirements for propofol anaesthesia for dental treatment for autistic patients compared with intellectually impaired patients," *Anaesthesia and Intensive Care*, vol. 37, no. 1, pp. 70–73, 2009.

[26] A. Lucas, G. Holtmann, G. Gerken et al., "Visceral pain and public speaking stress: neuroendocrine and immune cell responses in healthy subjects," *Brain, Behavior, and Immunity*, vol. 20, no. 1, pp. 49–56, 2006.

[27] U. Klages, Ö. Ulusoy, S. Kianifard, and H. Wehrbein, "Dental trait anxiety and pain sensitivity as predictors of expected and experienced pain in stressful dental procedures," *European Journal of Oral Sciences*, vol. 112, no. 6, pp. 477–483, 2004.

[28] S. A. Green and A. Ben-Sasson, "Anxiety disorders and sensory over-responsivity in children with autism spectrum disorders: is there a causal relationship?" *Journal of Autism and Developmental Disorders*, vol. 40, no. 12, pp. 1495–1504, 2010.

[29] U. Berggren, C. J. Pierce, and I. Eli, "Characteristics of adult dentally fearful individuals. A cross-cultural study," *European Journal of Oral Sciences*, vol. 108, no. 4, pp. 268–274, 2000.

[30] S. Saalasti, T. Lepistö, E. Toppila et al., "Language abilities of children with Asperger syndrome," *Journal of Autism and Developmental Disorders*, vol. 38, no. 8, pp. 1574–1580, 2008.

[31] A. Antonovsky, *Unrevealing the Mystery of Health: How People Manage Stress and Stay Well*, Jossey-Bass, London, UK, 1987.

[32] S. Jaakkola, P. Rautava, M. Saarinen et al., "Dental fear and sense of coherence among 18-yr-old adolescents in Finland," *European Journal of Oral Sciences*, vol. 121, no. 3, part 2, pp. 247–251, 2013.

[33] E. Hesselmark, S. Plenty, and S. Bejerot, "Comparing group cognitive behavioural therapy and group recreational activity for adults with disorders: a preliminary randomised controlled open trial," *Autism*, vol. 18, no. 6, pp. 672–683, 2013.

[34] K. H. Abrahamsson, U. Berggren, M. Hakeberg, and S. G. Carlsson, "The importance of dental beliefs for the outcome of dental-fear treatment," *European Journal of Oral Sciences*, vol. 111, no. 2, pp. 99–105, 2003.

[35] C.-O. Brahm, J. Lundgren, S. G. Carlsson, P. Nilsson, J. Hultqvist, and C. Hägglin, "Dentists' skills with fearful patients: education and treatment," *European Journal of Oral Sciences*, vol. 121, no. 3, pp. 283–291, 2013.

[36] A. De Jongh, P. Adair, and M. Meijerink-Anderson, "Clinical management of dental anxiety: what works for whom?" *International Dental Journal*, vol. 55, no. 2, pp. 73–80, 2005.

[37] G. Righi, A. L. Tierney, H. Tager-Flusberg, and C. A. Nelson, "Functional connectivity in the first year of life in infants at risk for autism spectrum disorder: an EEG study," *PLoS ONE*, vol. 9, no. 8, Article ID e105176, 2014.

[38] B. Bäckman and O. C. Pilebro, "Visual pedagogy in dentistry for children with autism," *ASDC Journal of Dentistry for Children*, vol. 66, no. 5, pp. 325–331, 1999.

[39] L. M. Orellana, S. Martínez-Sanchis, and F. J. Silvestre, "Training adults and children with an autism spectrum disorder to be compliant with a clinical dental assessment using a TEACCH-based approach," *Journal of Autism and Developmental Disorders*, vol. 44, no. 4, pp. 776–785, 2014.

[40] P. E. Langdon, G. H. Murphy, E. Wilson et al., "Asperger syndrome and anxiety disorders (PAsSA) treatment trial: a study protocol of a pilot, multicentre, single-blind, randomised crossover trial of group cognitive behavioural therapy," *BMJ Open*, vol. 3, no. 7, Article ID e003449, 2013.

[41] A. de Jongh, M. Schutjes, and I. H. A. Aartman, "A test of Berggren's model of dental fear and anxiety," *European Journal of Oral Sciences*, vol. 119, no. 5, pp. 361–365, 2011.

[42] V. Pohjola, S. Lahti, M. M. Vehkalahti, M. Tolvanen, and H. Hausen, "Association between dental fear and dental attendance among adults in Finland," *Acta Odontologica Scandinavica*, vol. 65, no. 4, pp. 224–230, 2007.

[43] J. M. Bernson, M. L. Elfström, and M. Hakeberg, "Dental coping strategies, general anxiety, and depression among adult patients with dental anxiety but with different dental-attendance patterns," *European Journal of Oral Sciences*, vol. 121, no. 3, pp. 270–276, 2013.

Permissions

All chapters in this book were first published in Journal of Allergy, by Hindawi Publishing Corporation; All chapters in this book were first published in AR&T, by Hindawi Publishing Corporation; hereby published with permission under the Creative Commons Attribution License or equivalent. Every chapter published in this book has been scrutinized by our experts. Their significance has been extensively debated. The topics covered herein carry significant findings which will fuel the growth of the discipline. They may even be implemented as practical applications or may be referred to as a beginning point for another development.

The contributors of this book come from diverse backgrounds, making this book a truly international effort. This book will bring forth new frontiers with its revolutionizing research information and detailed analysis of the nascent developments around the world.

We would like to thank all the contributing authors for lending their expertise to make the book truly unique. They have played a crucial role in the development of this book. Without their invaluable contributions this book wouldn't have been possible. They have made vital efforts to compile up to date information on the varied aspects of this subject to make this book a valuable addition to the collection of many professionals and students.

This book was conceptualized with the vision of imparting up-to-date information and advanced data in this field. To ensure the same, a matchless editorial board was set up. Every individual on the board went through rigorous rounds of assessment to prove their worth. After which they invested a large part of their time researching and compiling the most relevant data for our readers.

The editorial board has been involved in producing this book since its inception. They have spent rigorous hours researching and exploring the diverse topics which have resulted in the successful publishing of this book. They have passed on their knowledge of decades through this book. To expedite this challenging task, the publisher supported the team at every step. A small team of assistant editors was also appointed to further simplify the editing procedure and attain best results for the readers.

Apart from the editorial board, the designing team has also invested a significant amount of their time in understanding the subject and creating the most relevant covers. They scrutinized every image to scout for the most suitable representation of the subject and create an appropriate cover for the book.

The publishing team has been an ardent support to the editorial, designing and production team. Their endless efforts to recruit the best for this project, has resulted in the accomplishment of this book. They are a veteran in the field of academics and their pool of knowledge is as vast as their experience in printing. Their expertise and guidance has proved useful at every step. Their uncompromising quality standards have made this book an exceptional effort. Their encouragement from time to time has been an inspiration for everyone.

The publisher and the editorial board hope that this book will prove to be a valuable piece of knowledge for researchers, students, practitioners and scholars across the globe.

List of Contributors

Brandy E. Strahan
University of West Florida, 11000 University Parkway, Building 37, Pensacola, FL 32514, USA

Jennifer H. Elder
University of Florida, College of Nursing, Gainesville, FL 32610-0187, USA

Nahit Motavalli Mukaddes and Mustafa Deniz Tutkunkardas,
Child Psychiatry Department, Istanbul School of Medicine, Istanbul University, 34080 Istanbul, Turkey

Nahit Motavalli Mukaddes
Istanbul Institute of Child and Adolescent Psychiatry, 34365 Istanbul, Turkey

Oktay Sari and Aydan Aydin
Department of Special Education, Marmara University, 34730 Istanbul, Turkey

Pinar Kozanoglu
Private Education Center, 34140 Istanbul, Turkey

Johanna K. Lake Andrea Perry and Yona Lunsky
Dual Diagnosis Service, Centre for Addiction and Mental Health, 501 Queen StreetWest, Toronto, ON, Canada M5V 2B4

Johanna K. Lake and Yona Lunsky
Department of Psychiatry, University of Toronto, 250 College Street, 8th Floor, Toronto, ON, Canada M5T 1R8

Joanna C. Hamlin and Tina A. Crook
Department of Dietetics and Nutrition, University of Arkansas for Medical Sciences, Little Rock, AR 72202, USA

Margaret Pauly, Stepan Melnyk, Oleksandra Pavliv, William Starrett and S. Jill James
Department of Pediatrics, University of Arkansas for Medical Sciences, Little Rock, AR 72202, USA

S. Jill James
Department of Pediatrics, University of Arkansas for Medical Sciences, Arkansas Children's Hospital Research Institute, 13 Children'sWay Slot 512-41B, Little Rock, AR 72202, USA

Richard E. Frye Stepan Melnyk George Fuchs Tyra Reid Stefanie Jernigan Oleksandra Pavliv Amanda Hubanks, Laura Walters and S. Jill James
Department of Pediatrics, Arkansas Children's Hospital Research Institute, University of Arkansas for Medical Sciences, Little Rock, AR 72202, USA

David W. Gaylor
Department of Biostatistics, Arkansas Children's Hospital Research Institute, University of Arkansas for Medical Sciences, Little Rock, AR 72202, USA

Soichiro Matsuda, Yasuyo Minagawa and Junichi Yamamoto
Department of Psychology, Keio University, 2-15-45 Mita, Minato-ku, Tokyo 108-0073, Japan

Soichiro Matsuda
Japan Society for the Promotion of Science, 5-3-1 Kojimachi, Chiyoda-ku, Tokyo 102-0083, Japan

Yasuyo Minagawa and Junichi Yamamoto
CREST, Japan Science and Technology Agency, 4-1-8 Honcho, Kawaguchi-shi, Saitama 332-0012, Japan

M. Ghaziuddin
Department of Psychiatry, University of Michigan Medical Center, Plymouth Road, Ann Arbor, MI 48109-0277, USA

K. Welch
Center for Statistical Consultation and Research (CSCAR), University of Michigan Medical Center, Plymouth Road, Ann Arbor, MI 48109-0277, USA

Dan Ehninger
German Center for Neurodegenerative Diseases (DZNE), Ludwig-Erhard-Allee 2, 53175 Bonn, Germany

SudhaM. Srinivasan, Maninderjit Kaur and Anjana N. Bhat
Department of Physical Therapy, Biomechanics and Movement Sciences, University of Delaware,Newark, DE 19713, USA

Isabel K. Park and Anjana N. Bhat
Physical Therapy Program, Department of Kinesiology, University of Connecticut, Storrs, CT 06269, USA

Timothy D. Gifford, Kerry L. Marsh, and Anjana N. Bhat
Center for Health, Intervention, and Prevention, Department of Psychology, University of Connecticut, Storrs, CT 06269, USA

Anjana N. Bhat
Behavioral Neuroscience Program, Department of Psychology, University of Delaware, Newark, DE 19713, USA

Tafari Mbadiwe and Richard M. Millis
Department of Physiology and Biophysics, The Howard University College of Medicine,Washington, DC 20059, USA

Marie Guimard-Brunault, Catherine Barthélémy, and Frédérique Bonnet-Brilhault
CHRU de Tours, Centre Universitaire de Pédopsychiatrie, 2 Boulevard Tonnellé, 37044 Tours Cedex 9, France

Marie Guimard-Brunault, Catherine Barthélémy, Joëlle Martineau and Frédérique Bonnet-Brilhault
Université François Rabelais de Tours, 60 rue du Plat D'Etain, 37020 Tours Cedex 1, France

Marie Guimard-Brunault, Nadia Hernandez, Laetitia Roché, Sylvie Roux, Catherine Barthélémy, Joëlle Martineau and Frédérique Bonnet-Brilhault
UMR Inserm U 930, Équipe 1: Imagerie et Cerveau, Université François Rabelais de Tours, Tours, France

Marie Guimard-Brunault
UMR Inserm U 930, Équipe 1: Imagerie et Cerveau, CHRU de Tours-Hôpital Bretonneau, 2 boulevard Tonnellé, Bât B1A, 1er Etage, 37044 Tours Cedex 9, France

Audrée Jeanne Beaudoin, Guillaume Sébire, and Mélanie Couture
Université de Sherbrooke, Sherbrooke, QC, Canada J1H 5N4

Louisa M. T. Silva, Mark Schalock, Kristen R. Gabrielsen and Martha Buenrostro
Teaching Research Institute, Western Oregon University, 345 N. Monmouth Avenue, Monmouth, OR 97361, USA

Sarojini S. Budden
Providence Neurodevelopmental Center for Children, St. Vincent's Hospital, Portland, OR, USA

Gretchen Horton
Sikhara Group, 3434 NWSavier Street, Portland, OR 97210, USA

Jordan Hashemi and Mariano Tepper
Department of Electrical and Computer Engineering, Duke University, Durham, NC 27708, USA

Thiago Vallin Spina
Institute of Computing, University of Campinas, 13083 Campinas, SP, Brazil

Amy Esler
Department of Pediatrics, University of Minnesota, Minneapolis, MN 55455, USA

Vassilios Morellas and Nikolaos Papanikolopoulos
Department of Computer Science and Engineering, University of Minnesota, Minneapolis, MN 55455, USA

Helen Egger
Department of Psychiatry and Behavioral Sciences, Duke University, Durham, NC 22708, USA

Geraldine Dawson
Department of Psychiatry and Behavioral Sciences and School of Medicine, Duke University, Durham, NC 27708, USA

Guillermo Sapiro
Department of Electrical and Computer Engineering, Department of Computer Science, and Department of Biomedical Engineering, Duke University, Durham, NC 27708, USA

Esther I. de Bruin
Research Institute of Child Development and Education (RICDE), University of Amsterdam, 1018WS Amsterdam, The Netherlands
Research Priority Area Yield, University of Amsterdam, 1018 WS Amsterdam,The Netherlands

John H. Graham
Department of Biology, Berry College, Mount Berry, GA 30149, USA

Anneke Louwerse
Department of Child and Adolescent Psychiatry/ Psychology, Erasmus MC-Sophia, 3015 CN Rotterdam,The Netherlands

Anja C. Huizink
Department of Developmental Psychology, Faculty of Psychology and Education, VU University Amsterdam, 1081 BT Amsterdam,The Netherlands

Lucia Perez Repetto, Emmanuelle Jasmin, and Mélanie Couture
Ecole de Réadaptation, Faculté de M´edecine et des Sciences de la Santé, Université de Sherbrooke, Sherbrooke, QC, Canada J1H 5N4
Axe Mére-Enfant, Centre de Recherche du Centre Hospitalier Universitaire de Sherbrooke (CRCHUS),Sherbrooke, QC, Canada J1H 5N4

Emmanuelle Jasmin and Mélanie Couture
Axe le Développement de l'Enfant dans sa Famille et sa Communauté, Institut de Premiére Ligne en Santé et Services Sociaux, CIUSSS de l'Estrie-CHUS, Sherbrooke, QC, Canada J1H 4C4

Eric Fombonne
Department of Psychiatry and Institute for Development and Disability, Oregon Health and Science University, Portland, OR 97239, USA

Erika Gisel
Center for Interdisciplinary Research in Rehabilitation, Montreal, QC, Canada H2H 2N8
School of Physical and OccupationalTherapy, Faculty of Medicine, McGill University, Montreal, QC, Canada H3G 1Y5

Patricia O. Towle and Patricia A. Patrick
Westchester Institute for Human Development, Valhalla, NY, USA
School of Health Sciences and Practice, New York Medical College, Valhalla, NY, USA

Patricia A. Patrick
Department of Pediatrics, New York Medical College, Valhalla, NY, USA

Costanza Colombi and Mohammad Ghaziuddin
University of Michigan, Ann Arbor, MI, USA

Shawn E. Christ, Kimberly Bodner and Amanda J. Moffitt
Department of Psychological Sciences, University of Missouri, Columbia, MO, USA

Shawn E. Christ and Janine P. Stichter
Thompson Center for Autism and Neurodevelopmental Disorders, University of Missouri, Columbia, MO, USA

Janine P. Stichter, Karen V. O'Connor and Melissa J. Herzog
Department of Special Education, University of Missouri, Columbia, MO, USA

Lei Xu, Alice R. Richman and Kaitlyn Clawson
Department of Health Education and Promotion, College of Health and Human Performance, Greenville, East Carolina University, Greenville, NC 27858, USA

Linda CraneMitchell
Department of Child Development and Family Relations, College of Health and Human Performance, East Carolina University, Greenville, NC 27858, USA

Martin A. Volker and Gloria K. Lee
Department of Counseling, Educational Psychology, and Special Education, College of Education, Michigan State University, East Lansing, MI 48824-1034, USA

Elissa H. Dua and Joshua R. Popkin
Department of Counseling, School and Educational Psychology, Graduate School of Education, University at Buffalo, The State University ofNew York, Buffalo, NY 14260-1000, USA

Christopher Lopata, Marcus L. Thomeer and Jonathan D. Rodgers
Institute for Autism Research, Canisius College, 2001 Main Street, Buffalo, NY 14208, USA

Jennifer A. Toomey and Andrew T. Nelson
Summit Educational Resources, 150 Stahl Road, Getzville, NY 14068, USA

Audrey M. Smerbeck
Psychology Department, College of Liberal Arts, Rochester Institute of Technology, Rochester, NY 14230, USA

Malinda L. Pennington
Special Education, Department of Curriculum, Instruction, and Counselor Education, NC State University, Poe Hall 602, Campus Box 7801, Raleigh, NC 27695-7801,USA

Douglas Cullinan and Louise B. Southern
North Carolina State University, Raleigh, NC 27607, USA

Anne M. Roux, Paul T. Shattuck, Jessica E. Rast, Julianna A. Rava and Amy D. Edwards
A.J. Drexel Autism Institute, Drexel University, 3020 Market Street, Suite 560, Philadelphia, PA 19104-3734, USA

Xin Wei, Mary McCracken and Jennifer W. Yu
SRI International, 333 Ravenswood Avenue, BS 162, Menlo Park, CA 94025-3493, USA

Kathleen Dickinson and Maurice Place
School of Health and Life Sciences, Northumbria University, Coach Lane Campus, Newcastle Upon Tyne NE7 7XA, UK

Kyleen Luhrs
University of Washington School of Medicine, Seattle,WA 91895, USA

Tracey Ward
School of Psychology, Family, and Community, Seattle Pacific University, Seattle,WA 98119, USA

Caitlin M. Hudac, Jennifer Gerdts and Raphael A. Bernier
Department of Psychiatry and Behavioral Sciences, University of Washington, Seattle,WA 91895, USA

Holly A. F. Stessman and Evan E. Eichler
Department of Genome Sciences, University of Washington, Seattle, WA 91895, USA

Holly A. F. Stessman
Department of Pharmacology, Creighton University Medical School, Omaha, NE 68178, USA

Evan E. Eichler
Howard Hughes Medical Institute, Seattle, WA 91895, USA

Sheri R. Kiami
Department of PhysicalTherapy, Movement and Rehabilitation Sciences, Northeastern University, 301 Robinson Hall, 360 Huntington Avenue, Boston, MA 02115, USA

Shelley Goodgold
Simmons College, Boston, MA, USA

My Blomqvist and Göran Dahllöf
Division of Paediatric Dentistry, Department of Dental Medicine, Karolinska Institutet, 141 04 Huddinge, Sweden

Susanne Bejerot
Department of Clinical Neuroscience, Karolinska Institutet and Northern Stockholm Psychiatry, St. Göran Hospital, 112 81 Stockholm, Sweden

Index

A

Accessing Services, 17, 19, 21

Adaptive Behavior, 33-37, 65, 78, 114, 126, 168, 212, 223, 225

Asperger Disorder, 23, 50, 53, 266-267

Autism Diagnosis, 3, 7, 103, 111, 113, 124, 204, 231

Autism Spectrum Disorder, 1, 17, 22, 24-25, 29, 33, 40, 48, 50, 62, 89, 96, 111, 126-127, 138, 145, 151-153, 155, 159, 162, 185, 187, 209, 235, 248, 256, 268, 273-274

B

Betaine, 26-30, 32

Body Mass Index, 2, 239, 241-244

C

Childhood Autism Rating Scale, 7-9, 15, 35, 42-43, 91-93, 114, 126

Choline, 26-32

Chromosomal Microarray, 200, 207-208

Cognitive Behaviour Therapy, 20, 23

Cognitive Flexibility, 187-190, 195, 198

Computer Vision Tools, 127-128,135-136

Coping Strategies, 256-260, 262-264

D

Dental Anxiety, 266-270, 272-274

Dental Anxiety Scale, 268-270, 273

Dermatoglyphics, 139, 143-144

Developmental Disabilities, 1, 6, 14-15, 19, 22, 24-25, 31, 40-41, 87, 98, 107, 125, 138, 151-154, 162-163, 177, 197, 207, 209, 211-213, 227, 235, 245-246, 264-265

Developmental Disorders, 1, 6, 9, 14-16, 18, 22-25, 43, 48, 54, 60-61, 75-77, 79, 94-96, 125-128, 137-138, 151-152, 177-180, 197-199, 211, 227, 237, 246, 255, 273-274

Dietary Intake, 26-29, 32

E

Early Intensive Behavioral Intervention, 7-9

Educational Interventions, 13, 205, 219

Educational Programs, 7, 9

Epigenetics, 80, 84-87

Executive Function, 183, 187-190, 194-196, 198-199, 258

Eye-tracking, 42-43, 47-48, 89-91, 94, 138, 155

F

Facial Expressions, 42-45, 47-48, 64, 187-188, 190

Facial Features, 127, 129-130, 132-133, 136-137, 190

Fetal Brain, 55-61

Folinic Acid Treatment, 31, 33, 38, 40

G

Gaze Behavior, 42-45, 47-48

Gene Expression, 27, 30, 80, 82, 86-88

Genetic Etiology, 248-249, 252

Gestational Immune Activation, 55-56, 60-61

Gilliam Autism Rating Scale, 209-210, 212, 219-220

Glutathione Metabolism, 33, 39

Glutathione Redox Status, 31, 33-38, 40

H

Haploinsufficiency, 55-57, 60-61

High-functioning Autism, 6-8, 17, 22-25, 48, 50-52, 54, 76, 185-186, 197-198, 246, 273

I

Inhibitory Control, 187-196, 198

Intensive Behavioral Intervention, 7-9, 96

Internal Consistency, 114-116, 147, 209-213, 216, 218

Interpersonal Synchrony, 62-64, 66-68, 72-74

M

Maternal Stress, 256-257, 259-260, 262-264

Mental Disorders, 14, 17, 22-24, 34, 48, 53, 61, 75, 125, 137, 139, 143-144, 151, 181, 186, 197, 208, 219-221, 225-228, 249, 264, 273

Mental Health, 17-23, 25, 226, 235-236, 238, 246, 249, 254-255

Mental Health Services, 17-18, 20-23, 25

Metabolic Abnormalities, 26-27, 33

Methylation, 26-27, 30-31, 33-34, 37-40, 80-88

Methylation Metabolism, 33-34

Methylcobalamin, 33-39

Motor Performance, 62-65, 68, 72-75, 78

N

Naturalistic Behavioral Program, 7

Neurocognitive Processes, 155, 187, 195

Neurodevelopmental Disorder, 33, 187

Neuropsychiatric Disorders, 9, 55, 255

Nutritional Treatment, 33, 38-39

O
Obese Adolescent, 1
Obesity, 1-3, 5-6, 239, 244-246

P
Parent Training Interventions, 96-98, 103, 106-107, 152
Pervasive Developmental Disorder, 9, 24, 31, 97, 165, 185, 199, 222, 224, 228, 266
Polymorphisms, 27, 31, 84-85, 87
Psychiatric Disorders, 18, 22, 50-52, 88, 139-141, 237, 248-255, 266

Q
Quality of Life, 18, 23, 126, 150, 182, 234, 257

R
Robotic Interventions, 62-64, 72, 74

S
Screening Instrument, 115, 126, 154-157, 159, 161, 163, 209, 212
Sensory Abnormalities, 111-113, 118, 124, 267
Sensory Features, 145-151
Social Challenges, 19, 188, 237
Social Communication, 24, 42, 54, 62, 64-65, 70, 74, 78, 96, 103, 109, 124, 154-155, 165, 170, 179, 182, 187-189, 192, 194, 197-198, 202
Social Competence Intervention, 24, 187-189, 197, 199
Social Development, 80, 178, 257
Social Interaction, 7, 9, 13, 17, 20, 24, 26, 33, 51-52, 64, 80, 89, 92, 96, 102, 108, 111, 120, 145, 155, 187, 189, 194, 196-197, 210, 212, 214-216, 221-222, 224, 239, 244
Social Skills, 3, 9, 19-21, 23-24, 33-34, 36-38, 154, 174, 187-188, 195-197, 221, 229-230
Social Skills Intervention, 187
Support Services, 229-230, 235, 256-257, 262-263

T
Tactile Abnormalities, 111-112, 119, 124
Task Switching, 168, 187, 191-194, 197
Typically Developing, 1-2, 6, 8, 34-35, 38-39, 42-44, 47, 63, 89, 103, 115, 117, 119, 139-140, 149, 154, 160, 162, 165, 190, 230, 239-240, 244, 246, 257, 266-267, 272-273

V
Visual Attention, 47-48, 89-91, 93-95, 104, 127-129, 131, 135-136, 138, 151, 164, 183

W
Working Memory, 182-191, 193-199